Primer on the Autonomic Nervous System

Primer on the Autonomic Nervous System

Editor in Chief
David Robertson
Vanderbilt University

Editors
Italo Biaggioni
Vanderbilt University

Geoffrey Burnstock
Royal Free & University College London

Phillip A. Low
The Mayo Clinic

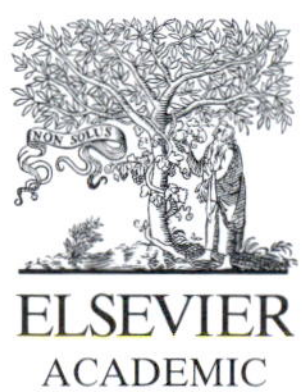

ELSEVIER
ACADEMIC
PRESS

AMSTERDAM • BOSTON • HEIDELBERG • LONDON
NEW YORK • OXFORD • PARIS • SAN DIEGO
SAN FRANCISCO • SINGAPORE • SYDNEY • TOKYO

Elsevier Academic Press
525 B Street, Suite 1900, San Diego, California 92101-4495, USA
84 Theobald's Road, London WC1X 8RR, UK

This book is printed on acid-free paper. ♾

Library of Congress Cataloging-in-Publication Data

Primer on the autonomic nervous system / editor in chief, David Robertson; editors, Italo Biaggioni, Geoffrey Burnstock, Phillip A. Low.—2nd ed.
p. ; cm.
Includes bibliographical references and index.
ISBN 0-12-589762-6
1. Autonomic nervous system—Diseases. 2. Autonomic nervous system—Physiology. I. Robertson, David, 1947–
[DNLM: 1. Autonomic Nervous System Diseases—physiopathology. 2. Autonomic Nervous System—physiology. WL 600 P953 2004]
RC407.P75 2004
616.8′56—dc22 2003070923

British Library Cataloguing in Publication Data
A catalogue record for this book is available from the British Library

ISBN: 0-12-589762-6

For all information on all Academic Press publications
visit our Web site at www.academicpress.com

Printed in the United States of America
04 05 06 07 08 09 9 8 7 6 5 4 3 2 1

Contents

5. Peripheral Autonomic Nervous System

ROBERT W. HAMILL AND ROBERT E. SHAPIRO

6. The Autonomic Neuroeffector Junction

GEOFFREY BURNSTOCK

7. Autonomic Neuromuscular Transmission

MAX R. BENNETT

8. Dopaminergic Neurotransmission

CHRISTOPHER BELL

9. Dopamine Receptors

AKI LAAKSO AND MARC G. CARON

10. Noradrenergic Neurotransmission

DAVID S. GOLDSTEIN

11. α_1-Adrenergic Receptors

ROBERT M. GRAHAM

12. α_2-Adrenergic Receptors

LEE E. LIMBIRD

13. β-Adrenergic Receptors

STEPHEN B. LIGGETT

14. Purinergic Neurotransmission

GEOFFREY BURNSTOCK

15. Adenosine Receptors and Autonomic Regulation

ITALO BIAGGIONI

16. Acetylcholine and Muscarinic Receptors

B. V. RAMA SASTRY AND DAVID ROBERTSON

17. Nicotinic Acetylcholine Receptors: Structure and Functional Properties

PALMER TAYLOR

18. Acetylcholinesterase and Its Inhibitors

ALBERT ENZ

19. Amino Acid Neurotransmission

WILLIAM TALMAN

20. Peptidergic Neurotransmission

GRAHAM J. DOCKRAY

21. Leptin Signaling in the Central Nervous System

KAMAL RAHMOUNI, WILLIAM G. HAYNES, AND ALLYN L. MARK

22. Nitrergic Neurotransmission

JILL LINCOLN

23. Serotonin Receptors and Neurotransmission

ELAINE SANDERS-BUSH AND CHARLES D. NICHOLS

24. Antidepressant-Sensitive Norepinephrine Transporters: Structure and Regulation

RANDY D. BLAKELY

PART III PHYSIOLOGY

25. Cardiac and Other Visceral Afferents

JOHN C. LONGHURST

26. Skeletal Muscle Afferents

MARC P. KAUFMAN

27. Entrainment of Sympathetic Rhythms

MICHAEL P. GILBEY

28. Sexual Function

JOHN D. STEWART

29. Gastrointestinal Function

MICHAEL CAMILLERI

30. Regulation of Metabolism

ROBERT HOELDTKE

31. The Sweat Gland

PHILLIP A. LOW

32. Temperature Regulation

MIKIHIRO KIHARA, JUNICHI SUGENOYA, AND PHILLIP A. LOW

33. Autonomic Control of Airways

PETER J. BARNES

44. Autonomic Effects of Anesthesia

THOMAS J. EBERT

45. Peripheral Dopamine Systems

GRAEME EISENHOFER AND DAVID S. GOLDSTEIN

46. Dopamine Mechanisms in the Kidney

ROBERT M. CAREY

PART

IV

STRESS

47. Exercise and the Autonomic Nervous System

VERNON S. BISHOP

48. Effects of High Altitude

LUCIANO BERNARDI

49. Hypothermia

BRUCE C. PATON

50. Psychological Stress and the Autonomic Nervous System

MICHAEL G. ZIEGLER

51. Aging and the Autonomic Nervous System

VERA NOVAK AND LEWIS A. LIPSITZ

52. Mind-Body Interactions

DANIEL TRANEL

PART V

NEUROPATHOLOGY

53. Oxidative Processes

JING ZHANG AND THOMAS J. MONTINE

54. α-Synuclein and Neurodegeneration

MICHEL GOEDERT

55. Experimental Autoimmune Autonomic Neuropathy

STEVEN VERNINO

PART VI

EVALUATION OF AUTONOMIC FAILURE

56. Clinical Assessment of Autonomic Failure

DAVID ROBERTSON

57. Evaluation of the Patient with Syncope

HORACIO KAUFMANN

58. Evaluation of the Patient with Orthostatic Intolerance

RONALD SCHONDORF

59. Sympathetic Microneurography

B. GUNNAR WALLIN

PART

XII

OTHER CLINICAL CONDITIONS

95. Disorders of Sweating

ROBERT D. FEALEY

96. Male Erectile Dysfunction

DOUGLAS F. MILAM

97. Sleep-Disordered Breathing and Autonomic Failure

SUDHANSU CHOKROVERTY

98. Hypoadrenocorticism

DAVID H. P. STREETEN

99. Mastocytosis

L. JACKSON ROBERTS, II

100. Cocaine Overdose

WANPEN VONGPATANASIN AND RONALD G. VICTOR

101. Sympathetic Nervous System and Pain

WILFRID JÄNIG

102. Baroreflex Functioning in Monogenic Hypertension

FRIEDRICH C. LUFT

113. Dihydroxyphenylserine

ROY FREEMAN

114. Adrenergic Agonists and Antagonists in Autonomic Failure

ROY FREEMAN

115. Erythropoietin in Autonomic Failure

ITALO BIAGGIONI

116. Bionic Baroreflex

TAKAYUKI SATO, ANDRÉ DIEDRICH, AND KENJI SUNAGAWA

117. Acupuncture

JOHN C. LONGHURST

PART XIV

EXPERIMENTAL AUTONOMIC NEUROSCIENCE

118. Autonomic Disorders in Animals

MATTHEW J. PICKLO, SR.

119. Transgenic Strategies in Autonomic Research

KAZUTO KOBAYASHI AND TOSHIHARU NAGATSU

120. Mouse Homologous Recombination Models

NANCY R. KELLER

Contributors

Valentina Accurso
Department of Medicine
Mayo Clinic
200 First Street SW
Rochester, MN 55905

Marlies Alvarenga
Baker Medical Research Institute
P.O. Box 6492
St. Kilda Road Central
Melbourne Victoria 8008
Australia

Lauren A. Arnold
Department of Neurochemistry
Kimberly H. Courtwright and Joseph W. Summers Institute of Metabolic Diseases
Baylor University Medical Center
2812 Elm Street
Dallas, TX 75226

David B. Averill
Hypertension and Vascular Disease Center
Bowman Gray Campus
Medical Center Blvd.
Winston-Salem, NC 27156-1032

Felicia B. Axelrod
Director, Dysautonomia Treatment and Evaluation Center
New York University School of Medicine
530 First Avenue, Suite 9Q
New York, NY 10016

Peter J. Barnes
Department of Thoracic Medicine
National Heart and Lung Institute
Dovehouse St.
London SW3 6LY
United Kingdom

Christopher Bell
Department of Physiology
Trinity College Dublin
Dublin 2
Ireland

Eduardo E. Benarroch
Department of Neurology
Mayo Clinic
200 First Street SW
Rochester MN 55905

Max R. Bennett
Neurobiology Laboratory
Department of Physiology
Institute for Biomedical Research
University of Sydney
Sydney, NSW 2006
Australia

Neal L. Benowitz
Clinical Pharmacology Unit
Bldg 30, 5th Floor
University of California, San Francisco
San Francisco, CA 94110

Luciano Bernardi
Clinica Medica 2—Dipartimento Medicina Interna
IRCCS S. Matteo
Universita di Pavia
27100 Pavia
Italy

Italo Biaggioni
Vanderbilt University
1500 21st Avenue South, Suite 3500
Nashville, TN 37232

Vernon S. Bishop
Department of Pharmacology
University of Texas Health Sciences Center
7703 Floyd Curl Drive
San Antonio, TX 78284-7764

Randy D. Blakely
Center for Molecular Neuroscience
Vanderbilt University
7140A Medical Research Building III
Nashville, TN 37232-8548

Frans Boomsma
Department of Internal Medicine
Erasmus Medical Center
Rotterdam, The Netherlands

Alba Larre Borges
University of Uruguay
Montevideo, Uruguay

Daniel Bulla
University of Uruguay
Montevideo, Uruguay

Geoffery Burnstock
Autonomic Neuroscience Institute
Rowland Hill Street
London NW3 2PF
United Kingdom

David A. Calhoun
Vascular Biology and Hypertension Program
520 ZRB
University of Alabama Birmingham
703 South 19th Street
Birmingham AL 35294-0007

Michael Camilleri
Mayo Clinic
Charlton 7154
200 First Street, SW
Rochester, MN 55905

Robert M. Carey
Division of Endocrinology
Box 801414
University of Virginia Health Systems
Charlottesville, VA 22908-1414

Marc G. Caron
Howard Hughes Medical Institute Laboratories
Department of Cell Biology
Box 3287
Duke University Medical Center
Durham, NC 27710

P. David Charles
Director, Movement Disorders Clinic
Medical Center South
Vanderbilt University
2100 Pierce Avenue
Nashville, TN 37232-3375

Sudhansu Chokroverty
St. Vincent's Catholic Medical Center
170 West 12th Street
Cronin 466
New York, NY 10011

Victor A. Convertino
U.S. Army Institute of Surgical Research
Fort Sam Houston, Texas

Allen W. Cowley, Jr.
Department of Physiology
Medical College of Wisconsin
8701 Watertown Plank Road
Milwaukee, WI 53226

Stephen N. Davis
Division of Diabetes, Metabolism and Endocrinology
715 Preston Research Building
Vanderbilt University
Nashville, TN 37232-6303

Thomas L. Davis
Department of Neurology
352 Medical Center South
Vanderbilt University
Nashville TN 37232-3375

Jaap Deinum
Department of Internal Medicine
Erasmus Medical Center
Rotterdam, The Netherlands

André Diedrich
Divison of Clincial Pharmacology
AA3228 Medical Center North
Vanderbilt University
Nashville, TN 37232-2195

Debra I. Diz
Hypertension and Vascular Disease Center
Bowman Gray Campus
Medical Center Boulevard
Winston-Salem, NC 27157-1032

Graham J. Dockray
Physiological Laboratory
University of Liverpool
Crown Street
P.O. Box 147
Liverpool L69 3BX
United Kingdom

Thomas J. Ebert
Department of Anesthesiology
Medical College of Wisconsin
8701 Watertown Plank Road
Milwaukee, WI 53226

Dwain L. Eckberg
Cardiovascular Physiology
Hunter Holmes McGuire Department of Veterans Affairs Medical Center
1201 Broad Rock Boulevard
Richmond, VA 23249

Graeme Eisenhofer
Clinical Neurocardiology Section
National Institutes of Neurological Disorders and Stroke
National Institutes of Health
Bethesda, MD 28016

Albert Enz
Novartis Pharma AG
Nervous System Research
Bldg. WSJ-386.762
Lichtstrasse 35
CH-4002 Basel
Switzerland

Andrew C. Ertl
Division of Diabetes, Metabolism and Endocrinology
715 Preston Research Building
Vanderbilt University
Nashville, TN 37232-6303

Murray Esler
Baker Medical Research Institute
P.O. Box 6492
St. Kilda Road Central
Melbourne Victoria 8008
Australia

Robert D. Fealey
Department of Neurology
Mayo Clinic
200 First Street SW
Rochester, MN 55905

Stanley F. Fernandez
Department of Pharmacology and Toxicology
SUNY-Buffalo
120 Shoshone Street
Buffalo, NY 14214

F. Fouad-Tarazi
Cardiovascular Medicine
Cleveland Clinic Foundation
9500 Euclid Avenue
Cleveland, OH 55195

Kleber G. Franchini
Department of Internal Medicine
State University of Campinas
Campinas, Brazil

Roy Freeman
Center for Autonomic and Peripheral Nerve Disorders
Beth Israel Deaconess Medical Center
1 Deaconess Road
Boston, MA 02215-5321

Raffaello Furlan
Medicina Interna II
Ospedale L. Sacco
University of Milan
Via G.B. Grassi 74
20157 Milan
Italy

Emily M. Garland
Division of Clinical Pharmacology
AA3228 Medical Center North
Vanderbilt University
Nashville, TN 37232-2195

Ray W. Gifford, Jr.
Emeritus
Cleveland Clinic Foundation
9500 Euclid Avenue
Cleveland, OH 44195

Michael P. Gilbey
Department of Physiology
University College London
Royal Free Campus
Rowland Hill Street
London NW3 2PF
United Kingdom

Janice L. Gilden
Division of Diabetes and Endocrinology
University of Health Sciences/The Chicago Medical School
3333 Greenbay Road (#111E)
North Chicago, IL 60064

Peter J. Goadsby
Headache Group
Institute of Neurology
The National Hospital for Neurology and Neurosurgery
Queen Square
London, WCIN 3BG
United Kingdom

Michel Goedert
MRC Laboratory of Molecular Biology
Hills Road
Cambridge CB2 2QH
England

David S. Goldstein
National Institutes of Health
Building 10, Room 6N252
10 Center Drive MSC-1620
Bethesda MD 20892-1620

Robert M. Graham
Victor Chang Cardiac Research Institute
384 Victoria Street
Darlinghurst, NSW 2010
Australia

Maureen K. Hahn
Center for Molecular Neuroscience and Department of Pharmacology
7141 Medical research Building III
Vanderbilt University Medical Center
Nashville, TN 373237-6420

Robert W. Hamill
Department of Neurology
University of Vermont College of Medicine
89 Beaumont Drive, Given C225
Burlington, VT 05405

Kenneth R. Hande
Division of Medical Oncology
777 Preston Research Building
Nashville, TN 37232-6420

Yadollah Harati
Department of Neurology
Baylor College of Medicine
6550 Fannin Street #1800
Houston, TX 77030-2717

Jacqui Hastings
Baker Medical Research Institute
P.O. Box 6492
St. Kilda Road Central
Melbourne Victoria 8008
Australia

William G. Haynes
University of Iowa
Cardiovascular Center
524 MRC
Iowa City, IA 52242

Caryl E. Hill
Division of Neuroscience
John Curtin School of Medical Research
Australian National University
GPO 334
Canberra, ACT 2601
Australia

Max J. Hilz
Director of Clinical Neurophysiology
University Erlangen-Nuremberg, Germany
New York University School of Medicine
550 First Avenue, NB 7W11
New York, NY 10016

Robert Hoeldtke
Director, Division of Endocrinology
West Virginia University
Morgantown, WV 26505

Keith Hyland
Department of Neurochemistry
Kimberly H. Courtwright and Joseph W. Summers Institute of Metabolic Diseases
Baylor University Medical Center
2812 Elm Street
Dallas, TX 75226

Joseph L. Izzo, Jr.
Clinical Professor of Medicine
601 Elmwood Avenue
Rochester, NY 14642

Edwin K. Jackson
Center for Clinical Pharmacology
623 Scaife Hall
3550 Terrace Street
Pittsburgh, PA 15261

Wilfrid Jänig
Physiologisches Institut
Christian-Albrechts-Universität zu Kiel
Olshausenstr. 40
24098 Kiel, Germany

Karen M. Joos
Department of Ophthalmology
Vanderbilt Eye Center
8000 Medical Center East
Nashville, TN 37232-8808

Jens Jordan
Franz-Vohard-Klinik
Haus 129
Humboldt University
Wiltberstr. 50
13125 Berlin, Germany

Stephen G. Kaler
National Institute for Child Health and Human Development
National Institutes of Health
Building 10, Room 9S259
Bethesda, MD 28092

Marc P. Kaufman
Division of Cardiovascular Medicine
Departments of Internal Medicine and Human Physiology TB-1712
University of California at Davis
Davis, CA 95616

Horacio Kaufmann
Autonomic Nervous System Laboratory
Department of Neurology
Mount Sinai School of Medicine
New York, NY 10029-6574

David Kaye
Baker Medical Research Institute
P.O. Box 6492
St. Kilda Road Central
Melbourne Victoria 8008
Australia

Nancy R. Keller
Autonomic Dysfunction Center
Vanderbilt University
Nashville, TN 37232-2195

Terry Ketch
Autonomic Dysfunction Center
AA3228 MCN
Vanderbilt University
Nashville, TN 37232-2195

Mazhar H. Khan
Pennsylvania State University College of Medicine
Milton S. Hershey Medical Center
500 University Drive
Hershey, PA 17033

Ramesh K. Khurana
FAAN
Chief, Division of Neurology
Union Memorial Hospital
201 East University Parkway
Baltimore, MD 21218

Mikihiro Kihara
Kinki University School of Medicine
Department of Neurology
377-2 Ohno-Higashi/Osaka-Sayam
Osaka 589 Japan

Kwang-Soo Kim
Molecular Neurobiology Laboratory
MRC216
McLean Hospital
Harvard Medical School
Belmont, MA 02478

Kazuto Kobayashi
Department of Molecular Genetics
Institute of Biomedical Sciences
Fukushima Medical University
Hikarigaoka, Fukushima 960-1295
Japan

Aki Laakso
Howard Hughes Medical Institute Laboratories
Department of Cell Biology
Box 3287
Duke University Medical Center
Durham, NC 27710

Gavin Lambert
Baker Medical Research Institute
P.O. Box 6492
St. Kilda Road Central
Melbourne Victoria 8008
Australia

Jacques W. M. Lenders
Department of Internal Medicine
St. Radboud University Medical Center
Nijmegen, The Netherlands

Vanda A. Lennon
Departments of Immunology and Laboratory
Medicine and Pathology
Mayo Clinic
Guggenheim 811
200 First Street SW
Rochester, MN 55905

Stephen B. Liggett
University of Cincinnati College of Medicine 2
Albert Sabin Way, Room G062
Cincinnati, OH 45267-0564

Lee E. Limbird
Associate Vice Chancellor for Research
Vanderbilt University
D-3300 Medical Center North
1161 21st Avenue South
Nashville, TN 37232-2104

Jill Lincoln
Autonomic Neurosciences Institute
Department of Anatomy and Developmental Biology
University College London
Royal Free Campus
Rowland Hill Street
London NW3 2PF
United Kingdom

Lewis A. Lipsitz
Division of Gerontology
Beth Israel Deaconess Medical Center
Harvard Medical School
1200 Centre Street
Boston, MA 02131

John C. Longhurst
Department of Medicine
C40 Medical Sciences 1
University of California, Irvine
Irvine, CA 92697-4075

Phillip A. Low
Department of Neurology
Mayo Clinic
Guggenheim 811
200 first Street SW
Rochester, MN 55905

Friedrich C. Luft
Franz Volhard Klinik
HELIOS Klinikum-Berlin
Germany

Hazem Machkhas
Department of Neurology
Baylor College of Medicine
6550 Fannin Street
Houston, TX 77030-2717

James G. McLeod
Department of Neurophysiology
University of New South Wales
Liverpool, NSW 2170
Australia

Alberto Malliani
Medicina Interna II
Ospedale L. Sacco
University of Milan
Via G.B. Grassi 74
20157 Milan
Italy

William M. Manger
New York University Medical Center
National Hypertension Association
324 East 30th Street
New York, NY 10016

Allyn L. Mark
University of Iowa
Cardiovascular Center
218 CMAB
Iowa City, Iowa 52242-1101

Christopher J. Mathias
Neurovascular Medicine Unit
Imperial College London at St. Mary's Hospital
& Autonomic Unit
National Hospital for Neurology & Neurosurgery
& Institute of Neurology, University College London
United Kingdom

Mario Medici
Institute of Neurology
University of Uruguay
Montevideo, Uruguay

Douglas F. Milam
Department of Urologic Surgery
Vanderbilt University
Nashville, TN 37232-2765

Thomas J. Montine
Department of Pathology
University of Washington
Harborview Medical Center
Box 359791
Seattle, WA 98104

Margaret Morris
Baker Medical Research Institute
P.O. Box 6492
St. Kilda Road Central
Melbourne Victoria 8008
Australia

Toshiharu Nagatsu
Institute of Comprehensive Medical Science
Fujita Health University
Toyake 470-1192
Japan

Opas Nawasiripong
Department of Neurology
Baylor College of Medicine
6550 Fannin Street
Houston, TX 77030-2717

James L. Netterville
Division of Otolaryngology
S-2100 Medical Center North
Vanderbilt University
Nashville, TN 37232

Charles D. Nichols
Department of Pharmacology
Vanderbilt University
8148A Medical Research Building III
Nashville, TN 37232-8548

Vera Novak
Division of Gerontology
Beth Israel Deaconess Medical Center
Harvard Medical School
1200 Center Street
Boston, MA 02131

Suzanne Oparil
Vascular Biology and Hypertension Program
520 ZRB
University of Alabama Birmingham
703 South 19th Street
Birmingham, AL 35294-0007

Bruce C. Paton
University of Colorado HSC
4200 E. Ninth Avenue
Denver, CO 80262

Michael Pfeifer
Division of Endocrinology
East Carolina University
600 Moye Avenue
Greenville, NC 27834

Matthew J. Picklo, Sr.
Department of Pharmacology, Physiology and Therapeutics
University of North Dakota School of Medicine and Health Sciences
Grand Forks, ND 58203

Raquel Ponce de Leon
University of Uruguay
Montevideo, Uruguay

Niall Quinn
Sobell Department of Motor Neuroscience and Movement Disorders
Institute of Neurology
Queen Square
London WC1 N 3BG United Kingdom

Alejandro A. Rabinstein
Department of Neurology
Mayo Clinic
200 First Street SW
Rochester, MN 55905

Kamal Rahmouni
University of Iowa
Cardiovascular Center
524 MRC
Iowa City, IA 52242

Satish R. Raj
Autonomic Dysfunction Unit
Division of Clincal Pharmacology
Vanderbilt University
Nashville, TN 37232-2195

Jeff Richards
Baker Medical Research Institute
P.O. Box 6492
St. Kilda Road Central
Melbourne Victoria 8008
Australia

L. Jackson Roberts, II
Division of Clinical Pharmacology
522 Robinson Research Building
Vanderbilt University
Nashville, TN 37232-2195

David Robertson
Vanderbilt University Medical Center
Clinical Research Center
AA-3228 MCN
Nashville, TN 37232-2195

Rose Marie Robertson
Division of Cardiology
351 Preston Research Building
Vanderbilt University
Nashville, TN 37232

Dan M. Roden
Director, Division of Clincal Pharmacology
532 Robinson Research Building
Vanderbilt University
Nashville, TN 37232

Elaine Sanders-Bush
Department of Pharmacology
Vanderbilt University
8140 Medical Research Building III
Nashville, TN 37232-8548

B.V. Rama Sastry
Department of Pharmacology
504 Oxford House
Vanderbilt University
Nashville, TN 37232-4125

Takayuki Sato
Department of Cardiovascular Control
Kochi Medical School
Nankoku, Kochi 783-8505
Japan

Irwin J. Schatz
John A. Burns School of Medicine
University of Hawaii at Manoa
Department of Medicine
1356 Lusitana Street 7th Floor
Honolulu, Hawaii 96813

Ronald Schondorf
Department of Neurology
Sir Mortimer B. Davis Jewish General Hospital
3755 Chemin del la Côte St. Catherine
Montreal, Quebec
Canada H3T 1E2

Rosemary Schwarz
Baker Medical Research Institute
P.O. Box 6492
St. Kilda Road Central
Melbourne Victoria 8008
Australia

Robert E. Shapiro
Department of Neurology
University of Vermont College of Medicine
89 Beaumont Drive, Given C225
Burlington, VT 05405

Lawrence I. Sinoway
Pennsylvania State University College of Medicine
Milton S. Hershey Medical Center
500 University Drive
Hershey, PA 17033

Virend K. Somers
Department of Medicine
Mayo Clinic
200 First Street SW
Rochester, MN 55905

Michaela Stampfer
Movement Disorders Section
Department of Neurology
University Hospital
Anichstreasse 35
6020 Innsbruck
Austria

John D. Stewart
Montreal Neurological Hospital
3801 University Street, Room 365
Montreal, QC
Canada H3A 2B4

David H.P. Streeten

Junichi Sugenoya
Aichi Medical University
Department of Physiology
Nagakute, Aichi, 480-1195, Japan

Kenji Sunagawa
Department of Cardiovascular Dynamics
National Cardiovascular Center Research Institute
5-7-1 Fujishirodai, Suita, Osaka 565-8565
Japan

William Talman
Department of Neurology
University of Iowa and Veterans Affairs Medical Center
200 Hawkins Drive, #2RCP
Iowa City, Iowa 52242-1009

Palmer Taylor
Department of Pharmacology
School of Medicine
School of Pharmacy and Pharmaceutical Sciences
University of California, San Diego
9500 Gilman Drive
La Jolla, CA 92093-0636

Jane Thompson
Baker Medical Research Institute
P.O. Box 6492
St. Kilda Road Central
Melbourne Victoria 8008
Australia

H. Stanley Thompson
Department of Ophthalmology
University of Iowa
Iowa City, Iowa 52242

Daniel Tranel
Department of Neurology
University of Iowa College of Medicine
200 Hawkins Drive #2007 RCP
Iowa City, Iowa 52242-1053

Anton H. van den Meiracker
Department of Internal Medicine
Erasmus Medical Center
Rotterdam, The Netherlands

Steven Vernino
Department of Neurology
Mayo Clinic
200 First Street SW
Rochester, MN 55905

Ronald G. Victor
Division of Hypertension
University of Texas Southwestern Medical Center
5323 Harry Hines Blvd., J4. 134
Dallas, TX 75390-8586

Simi Vincent
Division of Clinical Pharmacology
AA3228 Medical Center North
Vanderbilt University
Nashville, TN 37232-2195

Wanpen Vongpatanasin
Division of Hypertension
University of Texas Southwestern Medical Center
5323 Harry Hines Blvd., J4.134
Dallas, TX 75390-8586

B. Gunnar Wallin
The Sahlgren Academy at Göteborg University
Institute of Clinical Neuroscience
Sahlgren University Hospital
S413 45 Göteborg, Sweden

Gregor K. Wenning
Movement Disorders Section
Department of Neurology
University Hospital
Anichstreasse 35
6020 Innsbruck
Austria

Wouter Wieling
Department of Medicine
Amsterdam Medical Center
Meibergdreef 9
P.O. Box 22660
1100 DD Amsterdam
The Netherlands

Eelco F. M. Wijdicks
Department of Neurology, W8B
Mayo Clinic
200 First Street SW
Rochester, MN 55905

Jing Zhang
Department of Pathology
Vanderbilt University
U4220A Medical Center North
1161 21st Avenue South
Nashville, TN 37232-2562

Michael G. Ziegler
UCSD Medical Center
200 West Arbor Drive
San Diego, CA 92103-8341

Preface

The *Primer on the Autonomic Nervous System* aims to provide a concise and accessible overview of autonomic neuroscience for students, scientists, and clinicians. In spite of its compact size, its 119 chapters draw on the expertise of 200 scientists and clinicians.

We thank the American Autonomic Society for its continued interest and moral support of this project. We especially express our appreciation to our contributors, who, along with the editors, prepared their chapters without compensation in order to keep the cost of the *Primer* within the reach of students.

We are delighted with the enthusiastic reception of the first edition of the *Primer on the Autonomic Nervous System*, which sold more copies than any previous text on autonomic neuroscience. With this edition we welcome two new editors, Geoffrey Burnstock and Italo Biaggioni, and express our gratitude to retiring editor Ronald J. Polinsky, who was pivotal in the planning and execution of the first edition.

The new *Primer* would have been impossible without Mrs. Dorothea Boemer, whose efficiency and wisdom, combined with her mastery of lucid English prose, facilitated the preparation of this substantially enlarged edition. We also thank Dr. Noelle Gracy at Academic Press, who kept all of us on track and on schedule.

In the first edition, readers were encouraged to email their criticisms and advice for improving the text in the second edition. We thank the many of you who took time to do just that. Several new sections and a number of clarifications are included in response to these suggestions. If you have comments or advice for further improvement, please send them to david.robertson@vanderbilt.edu.

David Robertson
Italo Biaggioni
Geoffrey Burnstock
Phillip A. Low

PART I

ANATOMY

1 Development of the Autonomic Nervous System

Caryl E. Hill
Division of Neuroscience
John Curtin School of Medical Research
Australian National University
Canberra, Australia

The sympathetic, parasympathetic, and enteric neurons and adrenal chromaffin cells of the autonomic nervous system develop from the specific axial migration of neural crest cells. Growth factors released by structures along the migratory route contribute to the specification of the cells to particular lineages. After ganglion formation, the neuroblasts extend neurites toward their target organs in a stereotyped manner independent of the presence of their putative targets. This growth and the expansion of the neural plexus within the target tissue again depends on specific growth factors that regulate the further differentiation and survival of the innervating neurons. These processes contribute to the specificity of synaptic integration found within the autonomic nervous system.

The autonomic nervous system is composed of neurons and nonneuronal cells of the sympathetic, parasympathetic, and enteric ganglia and the chromaffin cells of the adrenal medulla. All of these cells are derived from neural crest cells, which migrate early during embryonic development from the dorsolateral margin of the neural folds following fusion to form the neural tube. After migration, the presumptive neurons aggregate into ganglia and grow axons to their targets, to provide homeostatic control for organ systems such as the cardiovascular, urinogenital, respiratory, and gastrointestinal systems. The neurons of the autonomic nervous system, in turn, are under the control of the central nervous system through preganglionic neurons, which are located in the spinal cord and receive inputs from different brain regions. Many studies have shown that the development of both ganglionic and peripheral innervation proceeds in a rostrocaudal manner with a correspondence between the rostrocaudal position of preganglionic and postganglionic elements [1, 2]. Different targets located at the same axial level are also innervated in a stereotyped and specific manner, suggesting the existence of particular subpopulations of neurons governing different functions [1, 2]. Such a degree of specificity invites a question concerning its origin during development.

PATHWAYS AND FATE OF NEURAL CREST CELLS

Migration of the neural crest cells proceeds in two main streams: dorsolateral to the somites and ventromedially through the rostral portion of the somites (Fig. 1.1). It is the latter stream that produces the neurons and nonneuronal cells of the autonomic nervous system, while the former stream produces pigment cells or melanocytes. The fate of the neural crest cells is, however, different at different axial levels [3]. Thus, the sympathetic ganglia and adrenal medulla arise from truncal neural crest, whereas parasympathetic ganglia arise from cranial and sacral levels (Fig. 1.2). The enteric nervous system, in contrast, is derived from crest cells migrating predominantly from the vagal regions and colonizing the gut in a unidirectional manner from anterior to posterior, although a small contribution to the hindgut is made by the sacral neural crest [4].

Because the neural crest gives rise to a number of divergent cell types, including autonomic neurons and glia, it has been of considerable interest to determine whether these cells are committed to a particular phenotype from the onset of migration or whether they are truly pluripotent—that is, their final fate is dependent on interactions with molecules along their migration pathways and at their final destination. Whereas some of the neural crest derivatives, such as the melanocytes, appear to be already committed before migration, recent data suggest that sympathetic neuroblasts, chromaffin cells, and enteric neurons may arise from pluripotent cells that develop a restriction in their fate as migration proceeds [3].

FACTORS OPERATING DURING NEURAL CREST MIGRATION

The majority of sympathetic neurons, adrenal chromaffin cells, and a subpopulation of enteric neurons are capable of synthesizing and releasing catecholamines such as

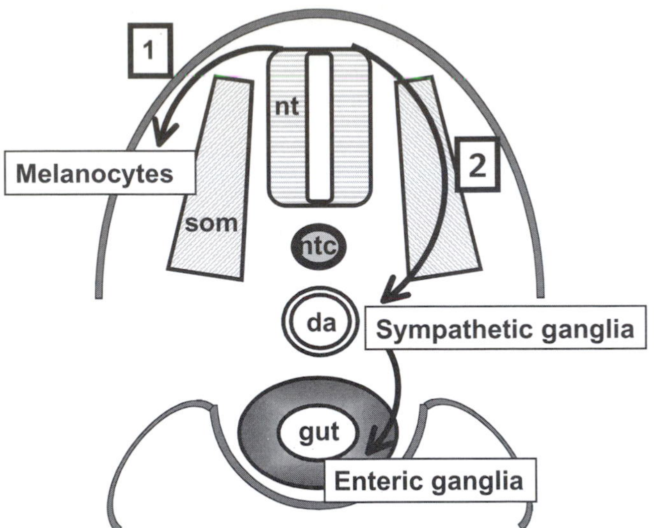

FIGURE 1.1 Migration pathways for the neural crest. The dorsolateral stream (*1*) gives rise solely to melanocytes, whereas the ventromedial stream (*2*) gives rise to four cell lineages of the autonomic nervous system—for example, sympathetic ganglia and enteric neurons—depending on the axial level. da, dorsal aorta; gut, gastrointestinal tract; nt, neural tube; ntc, notochord; som, somite.

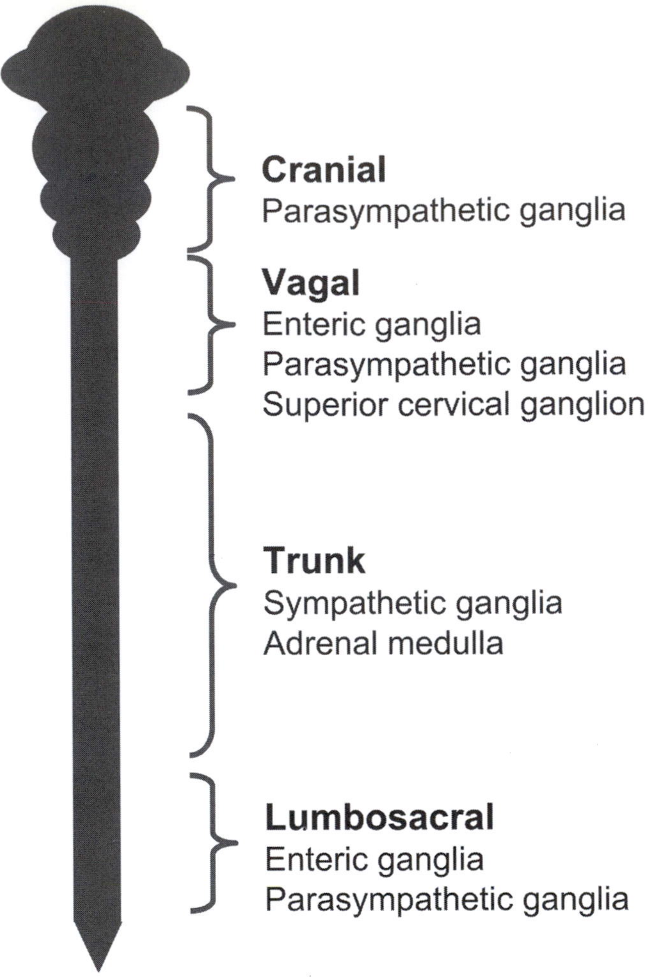

FIGURE 1.2 Fate of neural crest cells. The migration of neural crest cells at different axial levels gives rise to the four components of the autonomic nervous system. The superior cervical ganglion is the most anterior of the paravertebral sympathetic chain ganglia.

noradrenaline, although the enteric neurons only express this trait transiently. This characteristic develops during migration of the neural crest because of proximity with several structures. Of particular importance are the notochord and the dorsal aorta, the latter having been shown to release bone morphogenetic proteins, which can induce expression of several transcription factors important for the differentiation of adrenergic neurons [3, 5].

In the case of the enteric neurons and chromaffin cells, migration away from these inductive structures permits the influence of other environmental factors. For adrenal chromaffin cells, glucocorticoid hormones produced by the adrenal cortex have been suggested to play an important role in their subsequent neuroendocrine development, although recent studies with glucocorticoid receptor–deficient mice indicate the involvement of additional factors [6]. Studies of mice deficient in growth factors, their receptors, and particular transcription factors that regulate developmental fates have provided evidence for the existence of different subpopulations of enteric neurons [4]. In these mice, large regions of the gut were devoid of enteric neurons. Because these regions corresponded to the sites at which neural crest cells from different rostrocaudal levels colonized the gut, these data provide evidence that different neural crest populations have different growth factor requirements during early development.

Although the majority of sympathetic neurons use noradrenaline as their principal neurotransmitter, many of these neurons also express during development properties associated with the neurotransmitter acetylcholine [7]. These cholinergic properties develop in many sympathetic neurons long before contact with their target, often even before they have extended their axons. The fate and purpose of these early cholinergic neurons and the growth factors that affect them are currently unknown.

NEURITE OUTGROWTH AND TARGET CONTACT

The rudimentary sympathetic chain forms as a uniform column of cells alongside the dorsal aorta and subsequently elongates into individual ganglia [1]. Similarly, in the gut, the enteric ganglia form secondarily to the initial colonization of a particular gut region [4]. As the presumptive neurons leave the cell cycle they begin to extend axons. The progress of both the preganglionic axons to their targets in the autonomic ganglia and of the postganglionic axons to their targets in the periphery occurs at a similar time and in a stereotyped way, guided by factors elaborated in the intervening environment [1, 2]. Thus, in both systems the target is not required to direct this nerve growth, because axons take the correct path to the periphery despite target ablation. Within the target organ, the axons branch and form a network. Swellings or varicosities along the axons, containing the neurotransmitter vesicles, come into close contact with the target cells to form the functional autonomic synapses [8].

FACTORS INVOLVED IN NEURITE OUTGROWTH AND NEURONAL SURVIVAL

For both the preganglionic and postganglionic autonomic neurons, the removal of the target tissue leads to significant neuronal death [5, 9]. These observations have led to the proposal that particular factors are synthesized and released by target organs and taken up by nerve fibers to ensure the survival of the innervating neurons. Nerve growth factor (NGF) is the archetypal neurotrophic factor, and recent experiments with mutant mice lacking either NGF or its receptor have confirmed its essential role in the survival and differentiation of sympathetic neurons [5]. A related molecule, neurotrophin-4 (NT-4), has been shown to serve a similar role for preganglionic neurons because significant neuronal losses occur in mice deficient in NT-4 [9]. The equivalent factors for parasympathetic and enteric neurones are unknown.

In addition to NGF, sympathetic neurons are also dependent on the related molecule, neurotrophin-3 (NT-3). NT-3 is produced by target tissues and blood vessels, which frequently form the scaffolding for neurite growth. It is therefore possible that NT-3 operates to stimulate nerve growth and maintain neurons during the process of neurite growth to peripheral target organs. Within the target, NGF is available to stimulate axonal branching and enable continued neuronal survival [5].

SYNAPSE FORMATION AND NEURONAL DIFFERENTIATION

Functional responses can be elicited after neural stimulation early in development, soon after preganglionic and postganglionic axons are detected within target organs [8]. For the majority of catecholaminergic neurons, there is little evidence that significant changes in the expression of neurotransmitter receptors and development of the target organ occur as a result of the presence of innervating axons. Conversely, studies of cholinergic sympathetic neurons, which form a small subpopulation of neurons in sympathetic ganglia, do show significant reciprocal interactions with their targets. For this population, which does not correspond with the one that expresses cholinergic properties early during development, cholinergic differentiation is a late event, completely dependent on target contact [2, 5, 7]. Indeed, neurotransmitter release from these neurons promotes the release of a cytokine, which, in turn, induces a change in the innervating neurons from a catecholaminergic to a cholinergic phenotype. The close association between the neurotransmitter release sites on the varicosities and the target membranes is likely to facilitate these short-range inductive events [8].

CONCLUSIONS

Development of the autonomic nervous system proceeds in a stereotyped manner from the migration of the neural crest cells from particular rostrocaudal levels of the spinal cord through to the growth of axons to their peripheral targets. This specificity arises through the response of the cells to growth factors released into the environment through which the neural crest cells migrate or the axons grow. The final differentiation and survival of the autonomic neurons relies on the acquisition of additional growth factors from their presumptive targets. The release of these factors may be reciprocal, in response to release of transmitters from the growing axons. Complex responses to multiple factors may assist in the development of specifically coupled neurons and effectors.

References

1. Hill, C. E., and M. Vidovic. 1992. Connectivity in the sympathetic nervous system and its establishment during development. In *Development, regeneration, and plasticity of the autonomic nervous system*, ed. I. A. Hendry and C. E. Hill, 179–229. Chur, Switzerland: Harwood Academic Publishers.
2. Ernsberger, U. 2001. The development of postganglionic sympathetic neurons: Coordinating neuronal differentiation and diversification. *Auton. Neurosci.* 94:1–13.
3. Sieber-Blum, M. 2000. Factors controlling lineage specification in the neural crest. *Int. Rev. Cytol.* 197:1–33.
4. Young, H. M., and D. Newgreen. 2001. Enteric neural crest-derived cells: Origin, identification, migration, and differentiation. *Anat. Rec.* 262:1–15.
5. Francis, N. J., and S. C. Landis. 1999. Cellular and molecular determinants of sympathetic neuron development. *Annu. Rev. Neurosci.* 22:541–566.
6. Schober, A., K. Krieglstein, and K. Unsicker. 2000. Molecular cues for the development of adrenal chromaffin cells and their preganglionic innervation. *Eur. J. Clin. Invest.* 30(Suppl. 3):87–90.
7. Ernsberger, U., and H. Rohrer. 1999. Development of the cholinergic neurotransmitter phenotype in postganglionic sympathetic neurons. *Cell Tissue Res.* 297:339–361.
8. Hill, C. E., J. K. Phillips, and S. L. Sandow. 1999. Development of peripheral autonomic synapses: Neurotransmitter receptors, neuroeffector associations and neural influences. *Clin. Exp. Pharmacol. Physiol.* 26:581–590.
9. Schober, A., and K. Unsicker. 2001. Growth and neurotrophic factors regulating development and maintenance of sympathetic preganglionic neurons. *Int. Rev. Cytol.* 205:37–76.

2 Mechanisms of Differentiation of Autonomic Neurons

Kwang-Soo Kim
Molecular Neurobiology Laboratory
McLean Hospital
Harvard Medical School
Belmont, Massachusetts

During the last decade, impressive progress has been achieved in identifying the extracellular signaling molecules and key transcription factors that critically govern the development and fate determination of the autonomic nervous system (ANS). In particular, molecular and cellular mechanisms underlying the specification of the neurotransmitter phenotype have been elucidated. Several key fate-determining transcription factors such as Mash1, Phox2a, and Phox2b have been identified to be responsible for development of the ANS. One important emerging feature is that those key transcription factors regulate not only development, but also final properties of differentiated neurons such as neurotransmitter identity. In line with this concept, those factors directly or indirectly regulate the expression of both cell type–specific markers and panneuronal markers. Second, these transcription factors function in an intricate regulatory cascade, starting from key signaling molecules such as bone morphogenic proteins (BMPs). Finally, as evidenced by the study of *dopamine β-hydroxylase* (*DBH*) gene regulation, multitudes of cell type–specific factors (e.g., Phox2a and Phox2b), and general transcription factors (e.g., CREB and Sp1) cooperatively regulate the expression of cell type–specific marker genes. This new molecular information will facilitate our understanding of the function of the ANS in the normal and the diseased brain.

The ANS (also called the autonomic division or the autonomic motor system) is one of two major divisions of the peripheral nervous system. The ANS has three major subdivisions that are spatially segregated: the sympathetic, the parasympathetic, and the enteric nervous systems. Whereas the sympathetic system controls the *fight-or-flight* reactions during emergencies by increasing the sympathetic outflow to the heart and other viscera, the parasympathetic system is responsible for the basal autonomic functions such as heart rate and respiration in normal conditions. The enteric system regulates peristalsis of the gut wall and modulates the activity of the secretory glands. During the last decade, impressive progress has been made in regard to the molecular mechanisms underlying the development of the ANS. Among many different aspects, this chapter focuses primarily on the transcriptional regulatory code that underlies the development and neurotransmitter identity determination of the ANS.

THE AUTONOMIC NERVOUS SYSTEM IS DERIVED FROM NEURAL CREST CELLS

During the early developmental period of vertebrate embryo, the neural tube and notochord are formed from the ectodermal and mesodermal layers, respectively. At this time, neural crest cells originate from the dorsolateral edge of the neural plate and are generated at the junction of the neural tube and the ectoderm (Fig. 2.1). Interactions between the nonneural ectodermal layer and neural plate critically influence the formation of neural crest cells at their interface [1]. On formation, neural crest cells migrate along specific routes to diverse destinations and differentiate into a variety of cell types that include all neurons and glial cells of the peripheral nervous system and the neurons of the gastric mucosal plexus. In addition, some other cell types such as smooth muscle cells, pigment cells, and chromatophores are known to arise from neural crest cells. Much progress has been achieved in the identification of signaling molecules and downstream transcription factors that control lineage determination and differentiation of neural crest cells [2, 3].

SIGNALING MOLECULES REGULATE THE DEVELOPMENTAL PROCESSES OF THE AUTONOMIC NERVOUS SYSTEM

Studies have demonstrated that various signaling molecules—for example, members of the BMP family, Wnt, sonic hedgehog, and fibroblast growth factor—play critical roles in the early formation of neural crest cells and for final determination of neuronal identity [1, 4, 5]. These signals

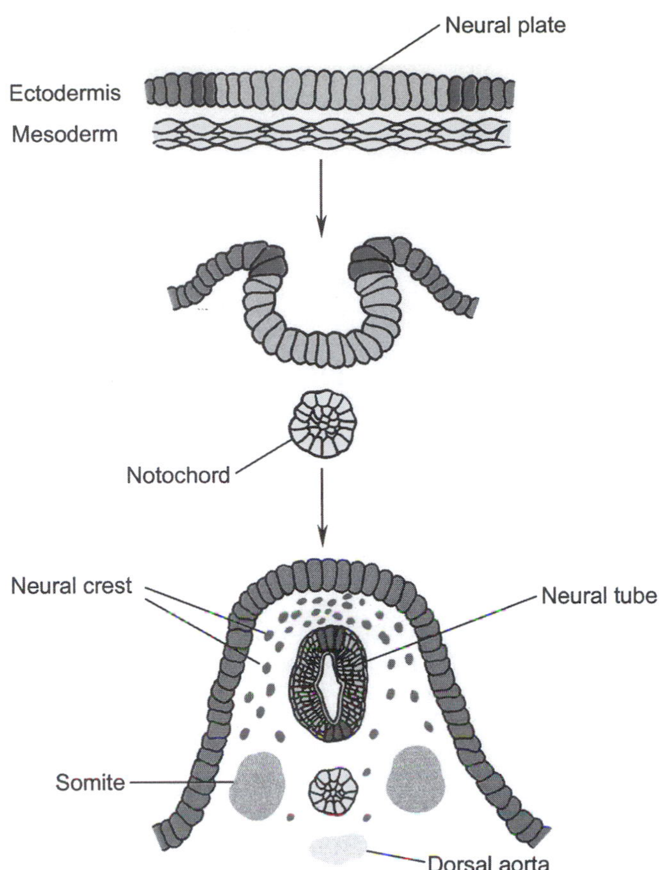

FIGURE 2.1 All cell types of the autonomic nervous system (ANS) are derived from neural crest cells. Neural crest cells are formed at the dorsal neural tube and migrate along diverse routes. Depending on their specific routes and interactions with the target tissues, they differentiate into a variety of cell types including pigment cells, different types of neurons and glia of the ANS, and parts of the adrenal gland. (See Color Insert)

are often provided from the neighboring tissues during migration of neural crest cells. For instance, grafting and ablation experiments in chick embryos demonstrate that the notochord is necessary but not sufficient to induce adrenergic phenotypes of neural crest–derived sympathetic ganglia [6, 7]. A possible candidate for notochord-derived molecule(s) is sonic hedgehog [7]. In addition, a series of elegant experiments has established that BMP family members, expressed from the dorsal aorta, play a crucial role in the differentiation and fate determination of the sympathetic nervous system [see Reference 8, and references therein]. Notably, these extracellular signaling molecules seem to work in concert with intracellular signals such as cyclic adenosine monophosphate (cAMP). Consistent with this, using neural crest cell culture, induction of differentiation and neurotransmitter phenotypes by BMP is enhanced by cAMP-increasing agents [9, 10]. Interestingly, it appears that cAMP signaling acts as a bimodal regulator of sympathoadrenal (SA) cell development in neural crest cultures because its moderate activation promotes SA cell development, whereas its robust activation opposes, even in the presence of BMP-2, SA cell development and the expression of the SA lineage–determining genes [10]. Finally, during the last decade, numerous studies demonstrate that different neurotrophic factors such as nerve growth factor, glial-derived neurotrophic factor, neurotrophin-3, and/or their receptor signals critically regulate the survival and development of all three divisions of ANS [2, 11].

TRANSCRIPTIONAL CODE UNDERLYING THE DEVELOPMENT AND PHENOTYPIC SPECIFICATION OF THE AUTONOMIC NERVOUS SYSTEM

Various signaling molecules and factors are thought to trigger a regulatory cascade by inducing the expression of downstream transcription factors, which eventually activate or repress the final target genes [4, 12]. Some transcription factors in these cascades may be cell type–specific and responsible for determination of neuronal phenotypes including neurotransmitter identity. Several key transcription factors that play critical roles in the development of the ANS have been identified as detailed in the following sections.

Mash1

Mash1 (also called CASH1), a basic helix-loop-helix protein, is the first transcription factor shown to be essential for development of the ANS. In Mash1$^{-/-}$ mice, virtually all noradrenaline (NA) neurons of the nervous system were affected, suggesting that Mash1 is a critical factor for determining the NA fate. Mash1 appears to relay the signals of BMP molecules for sympathetic development. Consistent with this idea, Mash1 expression was induced by BMPs in neural crest cultures and was largely diminished in sympathetic ganglia after the inhibition of BMP function [13]. In the Mash1-inactivated mouse embryos, neural crest cells migrated to the vicinity of the dorsal aorta, but they did not develop into mature sympathetic neurons, as evidenced by the lack of the expression of *tyrosine hydroxylase* (*TH*), *DBH*, and panneuronal markers [14]. In addition, Mash1 directly or indirectly affects the expression of another key transcription factor, Phox2a (see below); however, neither the immediate downstream targets nor the mechanisms of how BMP signals control Mash1 expression are defined in detail.

Phox2 Genes

Phox2a and Phox2b are two closely related homeodomain transcription factors that are expressed in virtually all neurons that transiently or permanently express the NA neurotransmitter phenotype [15]. Gene inactivation studies have demonstrated that Phox2a or Phox2b, or both, are essential for proper development of all three divisions of ANS and some NA-containing structures of the central nervous system (CNS). For instance, in both Phox2a$^{-/-}$ and Phox2b$^{-/-}$ mouse brain, the major NA population in the locus ceruleus does not form, strongly suggesting that both genes are required for its development [16, 17]. In contrast, only Phox2b seems to be required for the development of sympathetic neurons. In Phox2a$^{-/-}$ mice, sympathetic neuron development was largely normal. Interestingly, however, both genes are able to induce sympathetic neuronlike phenotype when ectopically expressed in chick embryos [18]. During sympathetic development, Phox2b expression is induced by BMP molecules independently of Mash1, whereas Phox2a expression is regulated by both Mash1 and Phox2b (Fig. 2.2). Recent promoter studies showed that Phox2a and Phox2b are able to directly activate the *DBH* promoter by interacting with multiple sequence motifs residing in the 5′ flanking region (see later). Collectively, Phox2a and Phox2b appear to regulate both development and neurotransmitter identity of sympathetic neurons and other NA neurons.

GATA3

Transcription factors belonging to the GATA family contain the C_4 zinc finger DNA-binding motif and bind to nucleotide sequences with the consensus motif, GATA. Among the six known GATA family members, GATA3 emerges to be a candidate factor that may regulate development of ANS and neurotransmitter identity. First, GATA3 is expressed in the CNS, peripheral nervous system, adrenal glands, and other tissues during development. Second, in Gata3$^{-/-}$ mutant mouse, sympathetic ganglia are formed but fail to express NA-synthesizing enzymes and die because of the lack of NA [19]. Finally, our recent data show that GATA3 is able to directly activate the promoter function of the *TH* and *DBH* genes (Hong and Kim, unpublished data). Taken together, it is likely that GATA3 plays a critical role for specification of NA neurotransmitter phenotype in ANS development.

Activator Protein 2

Activator protein 2 (AP2) is a retinoic acid–inducible and developmentally regulated transcription factor. Because AP2 has a deleterious effect on early development of the embryo, its precise role on ANS development has not been established. However, AP2 can robustly transactivate the promoter activities of both the *TH* and *DBH* genes, and specific *cis*-regulatory elements that mediate transactivation by AP2 are identified in the upstream promoters. Therefore, it is likely that AP2 may play a direct role in specification of NA phenotype in sympathetic development. In support of this, AP2 is abundantly expressed in neural crest cell lineages and neuroectodermal cells.

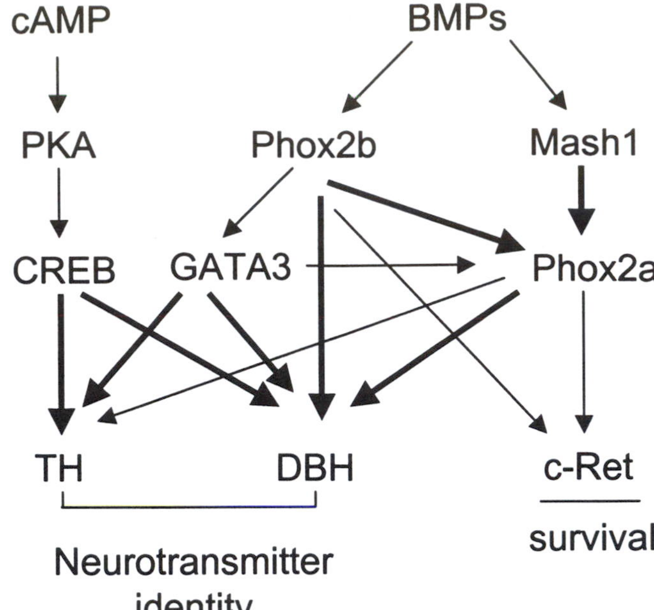

FIGURE 2.2 Diagram depicting the regulatory network of the noradrenaline (NA) phenotype determination and maintenance. Diagram shows the possible regulatory interactions in the cascade of development and NA phenotype expression of autonomic nervous system (ANS) neurons. *Thick arrows* indicate likely direct regulation and *thin arrows* indicate direct or indirect regulation. Bone morphogenic proteins (BMPs) are secreted from the dorsal aorta and activate the expression of MASH1/CASH1 and Phox2b. Phox2b then activates the expression of Phox2a. Phox2a or Phox2b, or both, in turn activate neurotransmitter-specifying genes *tyrosine hydroxylase* (*TH*) and *dopamine β-hydroxylase* (*DBH*). Direct action of Phox2a/2b on *DBH* transcription has been demonstrated. The transcription factor CREB has been shown to interact with the 5′ promoter and directly activates transcription of the *TH* and *DBH* genes. The cyclic adenosine monophosphate (cAMP) signaling pathway appears to regulate NA phenotype determination in concert with Phox2a/2b. A zinc finger factor GATA3, presumably downstream of Phox2b, also appears to be required for expression of NA-specific genes. Phox2a and 2b also regulate the expression of panneuronal genes including the glial-derived neurotrophic factor (GDNF) receptor c-Ret, which may relate to their role in formation or survival, or both, of ANS neurons.

Other Transcriptional Factors

Although the above transcription factors are the most promising candidates, additional factors are emerging to be important for ANS development and phenotype specification. For example, dHand is another basic helix-loop-helix transcription factor whose expression is induced by BMPs and is dependent on Mash1. On the basis of its specific expression in sympathetic neurons, dHand may directly contribute to ANS development. However, analysis of dHand function was hampered because the knockout mice died before sympathetic neuron development. Notably, transcriptional regulation of ANS and phenotype identity may require the combinatorial action of cell type–specific factors (e.g., Phox2a and Phox2b) and general transcription factors. Such examples may include cAMP response element binding protein and Sp1, which are required for transcriptional activity of both the *TH* and *DBH* gene (see later).

NEUROTRANSMITTER PHENOTYPES OF THE AUTONOMIC NERVOUS SYSTEM

Among the various phenotypes of a particular neuron, neurotransmitter identity is an essential feature because it determines the nature of the chemical neurotransmission a given neuron will mediate and influences the specific connectivity with target cells. For specification of the neurotransmitter identity, the given neurons should express relevant genes encoding the biosynthetic enzymes and cofactors, as well as the specific reuptake protein. In addition, expression of these genes needs to be matched with the appropriate receptors of the target tissues. Therefore, expression of the particular neurotransmitter phenotypes should be coordinated with the differentiation and phenotype specification of the target tissues. Molecular mechanisms underlying the specification of neurotransmitters in the nervous system have been investigated extensively, and key signaling molecules and transcriptional factors have been identified. Among these, specification of the NA phenotype of sympathetic nervous system and CNS is well characterized. Therefore, the discussion in this chapter focuses on molecular characterization of NA phenotype determination and its phenotypic switch to cholinergic phenotype.

Noradrenaline Phenotype

NA is a major neurotransmitter of the ANS, especially in sympathetic neurons, and fundamentally mediates the function of the ANS. Consistent with this, a rare human disease called the *DBH*-deficient disease, in which NA was undetectable, was identified to have a severe autonomic function failure ([20]; also see Chapter 80). NA is one of the catecholamine neurotransmitters that are synthesized from tyrosine by three consecutive enzymatic steps. Whereas *TH* is responsible for the first step of catecholamine biosynthesis, converting tyrosine to L-dopa, and is expressed in all catecholamine neurons, *DBH* is responsible for conversion of dopamine to NA and is specifically expressed in NA neurons. Thus, *DBH* is a hallmark protein of NA neurons and the control mechanism of its expression is an essential feature in the development of NA neurons.

Control Mechanism of *DBH* Gene Expression Is Closely Related to Autonomic Nervous System Development

DBH gene regulation has been studied by numerous investigators using both *in vivo* transgenic mouse approaches and *in vitro* cell culture systems. As schematically summarized in Figure 2.3, the 1.1 kb region of the 5′ upstream *DBH* gene promoter has three functional domains that can drive reporter gene expression in an NA cell type–specific manner. More detailed deletional and site-directed mutational analyses indicate that as little as 486 base pair (bp) of the upstream sequence of the human *DBH* gene can direct expression of a reporter gene in a cell-specific manner [21]. Whereas the distal region spanning −486 to −263 bp appears to have a cell-specific silencer function, the proximal part spanning −262 to +1 bp is essential for high-level and cell-specific *DBH* promoter activity. In this 262-bp proximal area, four protein-binding regions (domains I to IV), initially identified by DNase I footprinting analysis, were found to encompass functionally important, multiple *cis*-regulatory elements [21], including the cAMP response element (CRE), YY1, AP2, Sp1, and core motifs of homeodomain binding sites. Site-directed mutagenesis of each sequence motif has revealed that these multiple *cis*-acting elements synergistically or cooperatively, or both, regulate the transcriptional activity of the *DBH* gene [22]. Among these, two ATTA-containing motifs in domain IV and another motif in domain II were identified to be NA-specific, *cis*-acting motifs in that their mutation diminished the *DBH* promoter function only in NA cell lines. Another NA-specific *cis*-regulatory element was identified between domain II and III (Fig. 2.3). Interestingly, analysis of DNA–protein interactions on the *DBH* promoter demonstrated that all of these four NA-specific, *cis*-regulatory elements are Phox2-binding sites [23]. Taken together, this experimental evidence establishes that the *DBH* gene is an immediate downstream target of Phox2 proteins.

Cholinergic Phenotype and the Switch of Neurotransmitter Phenotypes by the Target Cell Interactions

Another major neurotransmitter in the ANS is acetylcholine, and those neurons that generate this neurotransmitter are designated cholinergic. The number of cholinergic neurons is much less than NA neurons among sympathetic neurons. Although differentiation and cholinergic specification are extensively investigated in central motor neurons [4], development of cholinergic ANS neurons is not well characterized. Therefore, it is of great interest to understand if key transcription factors, such as HB9 and MNR2, like-

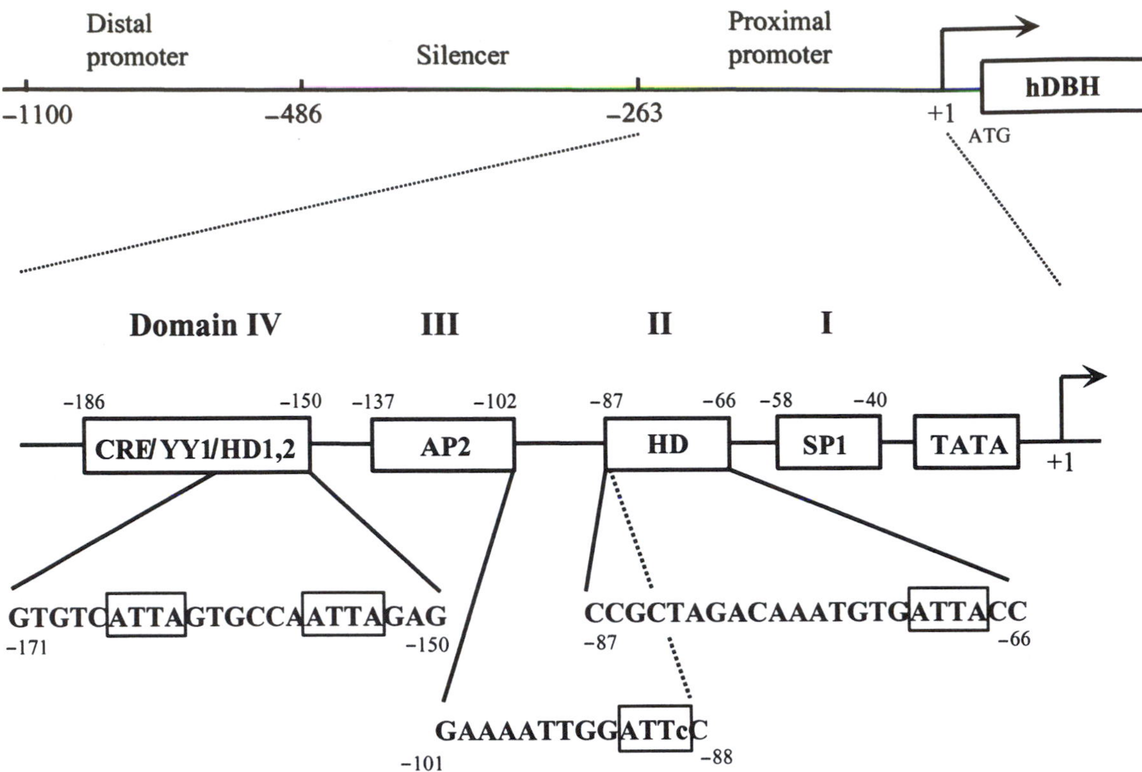

FIGURE 2.3 Schematic diagram depicting the structure of the human *dopamine β-hydroxylase* (*DBH*) gene promoter. **Top**, Three functional promoter domains that are characterized by either *in vivo* transgenic mice or *in vitro* cell culture studies are shown. **Bottom**, Four footprinted domains (I–IV) and specific *cis*-acting elements characterized within the proximal promoter (−263 to +1) are shown. *In vitro* analysis of *DBH* promoter function showed that multiple transcription factors including cell type–specific (e.g., Phox2a and 2b), cell-preferred (e.g., AP2), and general factors (e.g., CREB and Sp1) cooperatively regulate the NA cell type–specific and stage-specific expression of the *DBH* gene [22]. Four nucleotide sequence motifs containing homeodomain core motif (ATTA; *open boxes*) are identified to be binding sites for Phox2 proteins [23]. A nucleotide deviated from the consensus motif is shown in lower case.

wise play key roles in determining cholinergic phenotype during ANS development. Interestingly, it is well described that the NA phenotype of sympathetic axons is switched into the cholinergic phenotype, on contact with the developing sweat glands [2]. The presumable cholinergic-inducing factor secreted from the sweat gland remains to be defined, although leukemia inhibitory factor and ciliary neurotrophic factor are candidates. Consistent with the observation that expression of *TH* and *DBH* remain even after neurotransmitter switch from NA to cholinergic phenotype, a recent study reported that *TH* cofactor tetrahydrobiopterin (BH4) levels decreased significantly during the neurotransmitter switch [24]. Immunoreactivity for the BH4-synthesizing guanosine triphosphate cyclohydrolase became undetectable in the sweat gland neurons during this phenotypic switch, suggesting that suppression of cofactor expression underlies the neurotransmitter switch during development.

Acknowledgments

This work was supported by grants MH48866, DAMD-17-01-1-0763, and NARSAD Independent Award.

References

1. Liem, K. F., Jr., G. Tremml, H. Roelink, and T. M. Jessell. 1995. Dorsal differentiation of neural plate cells induced by BMP-mediated signals from epidermal ectoderm. *Cell* 82:969–979.
2. Francis, N. J., and S. C. Landis. 1999. Cellular and molecular determinants of sympathetic neuron development. *Annu. Rev. Neurosci.* 22:541–566.
3. Christiansen, J. H., E. G. Coles, and D. G. Wilkinson. 2000. Molecular control of neural crest formation, migration and differentiation. *Curr. Opin. Cell Biol.* 12:719–724.
4. Edlund, T., and T. M. Jessell. 1999. Progression from extrinsic to intrinsic signaling in cell fate specification: A view from the nervous system. *Cell* 96:211–224.
5. Wilson, S. I., A. Rydstrom, T. Trimborn, K. Willert, R. Nusse, T. M. Jessell, and T. Edlund. 2001. The status of Wnt signalling regulates neural and epidermal fates in the chick embryo. *Nature* 411:325–330.
6. Stern, C. D., K. B. Artinger, and M. Bronner-Fraser. 1991. Tissue interactions affecting the migration and differentiation of neural crest cells in the chick embryo. *Development* 113:207–216.
7. Ernsberger, U., and H. Rohrer. 1996. The development of the noradrenergic transmitter phenotype in postganglionic sympathetic neurons. *Neurochem. Res.* 21:823–829.
8. Schneider, C., H. Wicht, J. Enderich, M. Wegner, and H. Rohrer. 1999. Bone morphogenetic proteins are required in vivo for the generation of sympathetic neurons. *Neuron* 24:861–870.

9. Lo, L., X. Morin, J. F. Brunet, and D. J. Anderson. 1999. Specification of neurotransmitter identity by Phox2 proteins in neural crest stem cells. *Neuron* 22:693–705.
10. Bilodeau, M. L., T. Boulineau, R. L. Hullinger, and O. M. Andrisani. 2000. Cyclic AMP signaling functions as a bimodal switch in sympathoadrenal cell development in cultured primary neural crest cells. *Mol. Cell. Biol.* 20:3004–3014.
11. Taraviras, S., and V. Pachnis. 1999. Development of the mammalian enteric nervous system. *Curr. Opin. Genet. Dev.* 9:321–327.
12. Goridis, C., and J. F. Brunet. 1999. Transcriptional control of neurotransmitter phenotype. *Curr. Opin. Neurobiol.* 9:47–53.
13. Goridis, C., and H. Rohrer. 2002. Specification of catecholaminergic and serotonergic neurons. *Nat. Rev. Neurosci.* 3:531–541.
14. Guillemot, F., L. C. Lo, J. E. Johnson, A. Auerbach, D. J. Anderson, and A. L. Joyner. 1993. Mammalian achaete-scute homolog 1 is required for the early development of olfactory and autonomic neurons. *Cell* 75:463–476.
15. Brunet, J. F., and A. Pattyn. 2002. Phox2 genes—from patterning to connectivity. *Curr. Opin. Genet. Dev.* 12:435–440.
16. Morin, X., H. Cremer, M. R. Hirsch, R. P. Kapur, C. Goridis, and J. F. Brunet. 1997. Defects in sensory and autonomic ganglia and absence of locus coeruleus in mice deficient for the homeobox gene Phox2a. *Neuron* 18:411–423.
17. Pattyn, A., C. Goridis, and J. F. Brunet. 2000. Specification of the central noradrenergic phenotype by the homeobox gene Phox2b. *Mol. Cell. Neurosci.* 15:235–243.
18. Stanke, M., D. Junghans, M. Geissen, C. Goridis, U. Ernsberger, and H. Rohrer. 1999. The Phox2 homeodomain proteins are sufficient to promote the development of sympathetic neurons. *Development* 126:4087–4094.
19. Lim, K. C., G. Lakshmanan, S. E. Crawford, Y. Gu, F. Grosveld, and J. D. Engel. 2000. Gata3 loss leads to embryonic lethality due to noradrenaline deficiency of the sympathetic nervous system. *Nat. Genet.* 25:209–212.
20. Robertson, D., M. R. Goldberg, J. Onrot, A. S. Hollister, R. Wiley, J. G. Thompson, Jr., and R. M. Robertson. 1986. Isolated failure of autonomic noradrenergic neurotransmission: Evidence for impaired beta-hydroxylation of dopamine. *N. Engl. J. Med.* 314:1494–1497.
21. Seo, H., C. Yang, H. S. Kim, and K. S. Kim. 1996. Multiple protein factors interact with the *cis*-regulatory elements of the proximal promoter in a cell-specific manner and regulate transcription of the *dopamine beta-hydroxylase* gene. *J Neurosci.* 16:4102–4112.
22. Kim, H. S., H. Seo, C. Yang, J. F. Brunet, and K. S. Kim. 1998. Noradrenergic-specific transcription of the *dopamine beta-hydroxylase* gene requires synergy of multiple *cis*-acting elements including at least two Phox2a-binding sites. *J. Neurosci.* 18:8247–8260.
23. Seo, H., S. J. Hong, S. Guo, H. S. Kim, C. H. Kim, D. Y. Hwang, O. Isacson, A. Rosenthal, and K. S. Kim. 2002. A direct role of the homeodomain proteins Phox2a/2b in noradrenaline neurotransmitter identity determination. *J. Neurochem.* 80:905–916.
24. Habecker, B. A., M. G. Klein, N. C. Sundgren, W. Li, W. R. Woodward. 2002. Developmental regulation of neurotransmitter phenotype through tetrahydrobiopterin. *J. Neurosci.* 22:9445–9452.

3 Milestones in Autonomic Research

Max R. Bennett
Neurobiology Laboratory
Department of Physiology
Institute for Biomedical Research
University of Sydney
Sydney, Australia

RECEPTORS

Classical Transmitters: The Discovery of Noradrenaline, Acetylcholine, and Their Receptors

Langley [1] first showed that suprarenal extract (adrenaline) contracts and relaxes different smooth muscles, as does stimulation of their sympathetic nerve supply. Then, his student, Elliott, determined that adrenaline most likely acts at the junction between nerves and smooth muscle cells, not on nerve terminals, and made the audacious suggestion that "adrenaline might then be the chemical stimulant liberated on each occasion when the impulse arrives at the periphery" [4]. Langley [2] subsequently developed the concept that a "receptive substance" exists for alkaloids such as nicotine and curare at the junction between motor–nerve and muscle. Thus was developed the concept of transmitter release, the idea of receptors and identification of the first transmitter substance. Dale [5] showed that acetylcholine, which at that time was not known to be a natural constituent of the body, had similar actions on smooth muscles and cardiac muscle, as did stimulating parasympathetic nerves, such as the vagus, which Loewi [6] subsequently showed released a "Vagusstoff" possessing the properties of acetylcholine. Dale [7] concluded this classical research period with a comment that was to erect a paradigm that is still taught to this day, namely that "We can then say that postganglionic parasympathetic fibers are predominantly, and perhaps entirely 'cholinergic' and that postganglionic sympathetic fibers are predominantly, though not entirely, 'adrenergic', while some, and probably all of the preganglionic fibers of the whole autonomic system are 'cholinergic'."

This chapter, which summarizes the milestones in autonomic research, begins with Langley's great papers (1901–1906) [1, 2] on peripheral transmission establishing the concept of the synapse and concludes at the time of Bennett's monograph [3] on "Autonomic Neuromuscular Transmission" in 1972.

The Discovery of New Transmitters, Including Nucleotides, Peptides, and Nitric Oxide

A search for new transmitters, other than acetylcholine and noradrenaline, was prompted by the discovery in the early 1960s that the paradigm established by Dale [7] more than 30 years earlier was not correct. Nerves that relax some smooth muscles were found that did not involve the release of noradrenaline or acetylcholine [8]. A variety of non-adrenergic, noncholinergic transmitters were subsequently identified, including adenosine triphosphate, vasoactive intestinal polypeptide, nitric oxide, and neuropeptide Y.

VARICOSITIES

Varicosities Shown to be the Source of Transmitters

Hillarp [9] described the autonomic neuromuscular junction as consisting of smooth muscle innervated by a "very dense plexus, consisting of coarse non-varicose nerve fibers and of finer nerves which as a rule are set with an abundance of fairly gross varicosities." The "extremely fine nerve fibers" are "generally finely-varicose." Bennett and Merrillees [10] argued that each varicosity possesses the potential to release transmitter, not just the terminating varicosity, commenting that "transmitter is released from the varicosities which occur about every 1–3 μm along an axon."

Varicosities Have the Capacity to Take Up Transmitters After Their Release

Hertting and his colleagues [11] discovered that the principal method of removal of catecholamines after their release from varicosities is not by enzymatic breakdown but rather by reuptake into the varicosities by an active process [11].

Varicosities Possess Receptors That on Activation Modulate Further Transmitter Release

Starke [12] showed an inhibition through alpha-adrenoceptors of noradrenaline overflow from the isolated, sympathetically stimulated and perfused rabbit heart, which does not possess postsynaptic alpha-adrenoceptors, indicating an inhibition of noradrenaline release caused by its action on the nerve terminal varicosities.

Generation of Currents and Second Messengers on Receptor Activation After Transmitter Release from Varicosities

Synaptic Potential May Occur in Smooth Muscle and Cardiac Muscle on Transmitter Release from Varicosities

del Castillo and Katz [13] obtained the first intracellular recording of transmission at an autonomic neuroeffector junction, observing hyperpolarizing inhibitory junction potentials (IJPs) in the frog's heart on stimulating the vagus nerve. This provided the electrical signs of the effects of the "Vagusstoff" of Loewi [6], first described some 34 years earlier. Subsequently, Burnstock and Holman [14] made the first intracellular recordings of excitatory junction potentials (EJPs) in the vas deferens on stimulating its sympathetic nerves.

Currents Generated by the Release of Transmitter from a Varicosity Flow in an Electrical Syncytium

Bozler [15] showed that action potentials initiated at a point in a smooth muscle could propagate away from the muscle-stimulating electrode for distances much longer than that of a single smooth muscle cell, indicating that the smooth muscle cells must be electrically coupled together in some kind of electrical syncytium. Bennett [16] subsequently showed that the currents initiated in smooth muscle cells by released transmitter flowed in this electrical syncytium and were not constrained to the cell in which they were initiated, commenting that "It is therefore possible that some cells are very little affected by chemical transmitter and the EJP in these cells being predominantly due to electrical coupling between the cells during transmission." This provided an explanation for how currents initiated at the adventitial surface of a blood vessel could affect cells at the intimal surface of the vessel.

Second Messengers May Be Generated by the Release of Transmitter from a Varicosity and Subsequently Flow in a Syncytium: The Distinction Between Metabotropic and Ionotropic Receptors

The concept that second messengers could result in control of the generation of potentials, such as IJPs, was established by experiments that showed that introduction of cyclic adenosine monophosphate (cAMP) into a cardiac cell increases calcium currents during the plateau phase of the action potential in the cell, thus mimicking the effects of beta-adrenoceptor activation with noradrenaline [17]. Such receptors were subsequently referred to as metabotropic to distinguish them from those receptors that are ligand-gated ion channels, referred to as ionotropic. Second messengers were subsequently shown to diffuse through the syncytial couplings of the muscle cells.

Action Potentials, Initiated by the Generation of Junction Potentials, Are Caused by the Influx of Calcium Ions

The pathways for raising the intracellular calcium in smooth and cardiac muscle cells were identified in the 1960s. The action potential in smooth muscle is solely caused by the influx of calcium ions through potential dependent calcium channels [18].

The action of noradrenaline on beta-adrenoceptors in the heart is to greatly increase the inward calcium current associated with the plateau phase of the action potential [19], which with the discovery of second messengers, is now known to be consequent on the phosphorylation of the calcium channel through cAMP. Activation of second messenger pathways may also release calcium from intracellular stores as a consequence of activation of inositol 1,4,5-triphosphate receptors and ryanodine receptors located on the membranes of these stores.

Control of the Influx of Calcium Ions Is a Principal Means of Decreasing Blood Pressure

Identification of pathways for raising the calcium in vascular smooth and cardiac muscle cells has led to the development of some of the main blood pressure decreasing agents, including calcium channel blockers and beta-adrenoceptor blockers.

References

1. Langley, J. N. 1901. Observations on the physiological action of extracts of suprarenal bodies. *J. Physiol.* (*Cambridge*) 27:237–256.
2. Langley, J. N. 1906. Croonian Lecture of the Royal Society: On nerve endings and on special excitable substances in cells. *Proc. R. Soc. Lond. B* LXXVIII:170–194.
3. Bennett, M. R. 1972. Autonomic neuromuscular transmission. In *Monographs of the Physiological Society No. 30*. Cambridge, UK: Cambridge University Press.
4. Elliott, T. R. 1904. On the action of adrenalin. *J. Physiol.* (*Cambridge*) 34:xx–xxi.
5. Dale, H. H. 1914. The action of certain esters and ethers of choline and their relation to muscarine. *J. Pharmacol. Exp. Ther.* 6:147–190.

6. Loewi, O. 1921. Über humorale Übertragbarkeit der Herznervenwirkung. I. Mitteilung. *Pflügers Arch. Gesamte. Physiol. Menschen. Tiere.* 1989:239–242.
7. Dale, H. H. 1934. Nomenclature of fibres in the autonomic system and their effects. *J. Physiol.* (*Cambridge*) 80:10P.
8. Bennett, M. R., G. Burnstock, M. E. Holman. 1966. Transmission from intramural inhibitory nerves to the smooth muscle of the guinea-pig taenia coli. *J. Physiol.* (*Cambridge*) 182:541–558.
9. Hillarp, N. A. 1946. Structure of the synapse and the peripheral innervation apparatus of the autonomic nervoius system. *Acta. Anat. Suppl.* IV:1–153.
10. Bennett, M. R., and N. C. R. Merrillees. 1966. An analysis of the transmission of excitation from autonomic nerves to smooth muscle. *J. Physiol.* (*Cambridge*) 185:520–535.
11. Hertting, G., J. Axelrod, I. J. Kopin, and L. G. Whitby. 1961. Lack of uptake of catecholamines after chronic denervation of sympathetic nerves. *Nature* (*London*) 189:66.
12. Starke, K. 1971. Influence of alpha receptor stimulants on noradrenaline release. *Naturwissenschaften* 58:420.
13. del Castillo, J., and B. Katz. 1957. Modifications del la membrane produites par des influx nerveux dans la region du pacemaker du coeur. Microphysiolgie comparée des elements excitables. *Colloq. Int. CNRS* (*Paris*) 67:271–279.
14. Burnstock, G., and M. E. Holman. 1961. The transmission of excitation from autonomic nerve to smooth muscle. *J. Physiol.* (*Cambridge*) 155:115–133.
15. Bozler, E. 1941. Action potentials and conduction of excitation in muscle. *J. Cell. Comp. Physiol.* 18:385–391.
16. Bennett, M. R. 1967. The effect of intracellular current pulses in smooth muscle cells of the guinea pig vas deferens at rest and during transmission. *J. Gen. Physiol.* 50:2459–2475.
17. Tsien, R. W., W. Giles, and P. Greengard. 1972. Cyclic AMP mediates the effects of adrenaline on cardiac Purkinje fibres. *Nat. New Biol.* 240:181–183.
18. Bennett, M. R. 1967. The effect of cations on the electrical properties of the smooth muscle cells of the guinea pig vas deferens. *J. Physiol.* (*Cambridge*) 190:465–479.
19. Reuter, H. 1967. The dependence of slow inward current in Purkinje fibres on the extracellular calcium concentration. *J. Physiol.* (*Cambridge*) 192:479–492.

P A R T II

PHARMACOLOGY

4 Central Autonomic Control

Eduardo E. Benarroch
Department of Neurology
Mayo Clinic
Rochester, Minnesota

The central autonomic control areas are distributed throughout the neuroaxis. They include the insular cortex, anterior cingulate gyrus, amygdala, and bed nucleus of the stria terminalis; hypothalamus; periaqueductal gray (PAG) matter of the midbrain, parabrachial nucleus (PBN); nucleus tractus solitarii (NTS); ventrolateral medulla (VLM) and caudal raphe nuclei. These areas are reciprocally interconnected, receive converging visceral and nociceptive information, contain neurons that are affected by visceral inputs, and generate patterns of autonomic responses through direct or indirect inputs to preganglionic sympathetic and parasympathetic neurons [1–3].

ANATOMY OF CENTRAL AUTONOMIC AREAS

Forebrain

The insular cortex is the primary visceral sensory cortex. It contains an organotropic visceral sensory map; the anterior insula is the primary area for taste, whereas the posterior insula is the general visceral afferent area [3, 4]. The insular cortex has reciprocal, topographically, and functionally specific interconnections with the NTS and PBN, which relay viscerosensory information carried by the vagus and other cranial afferents to the insular cortex, through projections to the parvicellular subdivisions of the ventral posterior medial nucleus of the thalamus. The posterior dorsal insula is also the primary cortical area receiving pain, temperature, and spinal visceroceptive information from lamina I of the spinal cord, through a spinothalamic connection with the posterior portion of the ventromedial nucleus of the thalamus, which projects to the insular cortex [3, 5].

The anterior cingulate cortex is critically involved in initiation, motivation, and execution of emotional and goal-directed behaviors. Through its widespread interconnections with central autonomic regions, it participates in high-level regulation of autonomic and endocrine function. The ventromedial prefrontal cortex also has extensive reciprocal connections with the amygdala, and these interactions modulate emotional responses. Bilateral lesions of the ventromedial prefrontal cortex selectively impair autonomic "preparatory" reactions in response to emotionally significant stimuli [4].

The amygdala plays a critical role in emotional responses, including conditioned fear. It has reciprocal interactions with the cerebral cortex, basal forebrain, and limbic striatum. The central nucleus of the amygdala (CeNA) projects to the hypothalamus PAG and autonomic areas of the brainstem and integrates autonomic, endocrine, and motor responses associated with emotion [6].

The preoptic–hypothalamic unit is subdivided into three functionally distinct longitudinal zones: periventricular, medial, and lateral. The periventricular zone includes the suprachiasmatic nucleus, involved in circadian rhythms and nuclei-controlling endocrine function. The median preoptic nucleus, the paraventricular nucleus (PVN), and arcuate nucleus produce regulatory hormones that control anterior pituitary function. Magnocellular neurons in the supraoptic nucleus and PVN produce vasopressin (AVP) and oxytocin. The medial preoptic nucleus contains thermosensitive and osmosensitive neurons, and the arcuate and ventromedial nuclei are involved in regulation of appetite and reproductive function. The lateral hypothalamus controls food intake, sleep wake cycle and motivated behavior. Neurons of the posterior lateral hypothalamus secrete hypocretin/orexin and regulate the switch between wakefulness and sleep through projections to monoaminergic and cholinergic brainstem nuclei. The PVN, dorsomedial nucleus, and lateral hypothalamic innervate separate subsets of preganglionic sympathetic and parasympathetic neurons. The PVN gives rise to the most widespread autonomic output of the hypothalamus. The lateral hypothalamic area relays influences of the insula and amygdala on autonomic nuclei [7].

Brainstem

The PAG integrates autonomic, motor, and antinociceptive responses to stress. It receives multiple input from the amygdala, preoptic area, and dorsal horn of the spinal cord. It is subdivided into longitudinal columns, with specific inputs and outputs and specific functions. The lateral PAG initiates opioid-independent analgesia and sympathoexcitatory responses through projection to the VLM. The ventrolateral PAG initiates opioid-dependent analgesia and sympathoinhibitory responses through its projection to the medullary raphe nuclei [8].

The PBN includes several subnuclei that receive visceral inputs through the NTS and inputs from nociceptors, thermoreceptors, and muscle receptors through the spinoparabrachial tract originating in lamina I of the dorsal horn. The PBN projects to the hypothalamus, amygdala, and the thalamus and is involved in taste, salivation, gastrointestinal activity, cardiovascular activity, respiration, osmoregulation, and thermoregulation. This region includes the Kölliker-Fuse nucleus (pontine respiratory group), which regulates activity of respiratory and cardiovascular neurons of the medulla. The dorsal pons also contains the Barrington nucleus, corresponding to the "pontine micturition center." It innervates sacral preganglionic neurons innervating the bladder, bowel, and sexual organs, as well as the Onuf nucleus motor neurons innervating the pelvic floor and external sphincters. It is critical for coordinated contraction of the bladder detrusor and relaxation of the external sphincter during micturition [2, 3].

The NTS is the first relay station for general visceral and taste afferents [2, 3]. It is critically involved in medullary reflexes and relays viscerosensory information to all central autonomic regions. The NTS consists of several subnuclei with specific inputs and outputs and has a viscerotropic organization. Taste afferents relay in its rostral, gastrointestinal afferents in its intermediate portion, and cardiovascular and respiratory afferents in the caudal half of the NTS. The NTS sends descending projections to spinal respiratory and preganglionic parasympathetic and sympathetic neurons; propriobulbar projections to neuronal cell groups of the medullary reticular–mediating baroreceptor, chemoreceptor, cardiopulmonary, and gastrointestinal reflexes; and ascending projections to all other rostral components of the central autonomic network, including the PBN, PAG, amygdala, medial preoptic, paraventricular, dorsomedial, and lateral hypothalamic nuclei, subfornical organ, and medial orbitofrontal cortex. The area postrema is a chemosensitive region with abundant connections with other central autonomic areas. It has long been considered the "chemoreceptor trigger zone" for vomiting and contains receptors for circulating angiotensin II, AVP, natriuretic peptides, and other humoral signals involved in cardiovascular regulation.

The VLM contains the premotor neurons controlling vasomotor tone, cardiac function, and respiration. Neurons of the rostral VLM provide a major excitatory input to sympathetic preganglionic vasomotor neurons of the intermediolateral cell column (IML) [9]. Neurons of the caudal VLM are an integral component of several medullary reflexes. The VLM contains catecholaminergic neurons corresponding to the rostral C1 (adrenergic) and caudal A1 (noradrenergic) groups. C1 neurons project to the IML and A1 neurons to the hypothalamus. The VLM contains the ventral respiratory group (VRG), including the pre-Bötzinger complex, which has a critical role in generation of the respiratory rhythm. Inspiratory neurons of the rostral VRG and expiratory neurons of the caudal VRG project to phrenic, intercostal, and abdominal spinal motor neurons [2]. The central chemosensitive region, located in the ventral surface of the medulla, contains neurons that respond to increased P_{CO_2} and decreased pH in the cerebrospinal fluid. Neurons of the rostral ventromedial medulla, including the caudal raphe nuclei, also provide direct inputs to the sympathetic preganglionic neurons and may contribute to control of arterial pressure. The function of the raphe–spinal pathway is complex and includes both sympathoexcitatory and sympathoinhibitory influences. These neurons may be involved in sympathetic control to endocrine organs and to skin effectors for thermoregulation.

LEVELS OF INTEGRATION OF CENTRAL AUTONOMIC CONTROL

Bulbospinal Level

Baroreceptor, cardiac receptor, chemoreceptor, and pulmonary mechanoreceptor afferents preferentially activate neurons located on separate NTS subnuclei. These neurons generate several medullary reflexes by projecting to sympathoinhibitory neurons of the caudal VLM, sympathoexcitatory neurons of the rostral VLM, vagal cardiomotor neurons of the nucleus ambiguus and the dorsal vagal nucleus, respiratory neurons of the VRG and dorsal respiratory group, and AVP-producing magnocellular hypothalamic neurons [2].

Pontomesencephalic Level

The PBN is a site of viscerosomatic convergence and serves as a substrate for integration of noxious, thermoreceptive, metaboreceptive, and viscerosensitive inputs with motivational, emotional, and homeostatic responses [3]. The lateral PAG initiates integrated sympathoexcitatory "fight or flight" responses, whereas the ventrolateral PAG elicits hyporeactive immobility and sympathoinhibition (the "playing death" response) [8].

Forebrain Level

The cortical autonomic areas, the amygdala, hypothalamus, and PAG form a functional unit involved both in the assessment of emotional content of stimuli and initiation and regulation of emotional autonomic, endocrine, and motor responses. The PVN plays a central role in the integrated response to stress, because it secretes corticotrophin releasing factor (CRF) and AVP and projects to the rostral

VLM and to the preganglionic sympathetic and sympathoadrenal neurons. It is activated by hypoglycemia, hypovolemia, cytokines, or other internal stressors. The CRF neurons of the PVN are involved in reciprocal excitatory interactions with the noradrenergic neurons of the locus ceruleus, which selectively respond to novel, potentially threatening external stimuli. The CeNA, lateral hypothalamus, and PAG are involved in the cardiovascular, visceromotor, somatomotor, and antinociceptive components of the defense response [8].

References

1. Benarroch, E. E. 1997. *Central autonomic network: Functional organization and clinical correlations.* Armonk, NY: Futura.
2. Blessing, W. W. 1997. *The lower brainstem and bodily homeostasis.* New York: Oxford University Press.
3. Saper, C. B. 2002. The central autonomic nervous system: conscious visceral perception and autonomic pattern generation. *Annu. Rev. Neurosci.* 25:433–469.
4. Verberne, A. J., and N. C. Owens. 1998. Cortical modulation of the cardiovascular system. *Prog. Neurobiol.* 54:149–168.
5. Craig, A. D. 1996. An ascending general homeostatic afferent pathway originating in lamina I. In *Progress in brain research*, Vol. 107. ed. G. Holstege, R. Bandler, and C. B. Saper, 225–242. Amsterdam: Elsevier.
6. Amaral, D. G., J. I. Price, A. Pitkanen, and S. T. Charmichael. 1992. Anatomical organization of the primate amygdaoid complex. In *The amygdala: Neurobiological aspects of emotion*, ed. J. P. Aggleton, 1–66. New York: Wiley-Lyss.
7. Swanson, L. W. 1991. Biochemical switching in hypothalamic circuits mediating responses to stress [Review]. *Prog. Brain Res.* 87:181–200.
8. Bandler, R., and M. T. Shipley. 1994. Columnar organization in the midbrain periaqueductal gray: Modules for emotional expression? *Trends Neurosci.* 17:379–389.
9. Guyenet, P. G. 1990. Role of the ventral medulla oblongata in blood pressure regulation. In *Central regulation of autonomic functions*, ed. A. D. Loewy and K. M. Spyer, 145–167. New York: Oxford University Press.

5 Peripheral Autonomic Nervous System

Robert W. Hamill
Department of Neurology
University of Vermont
College of Medicine
Burlington, Vermont

Robert E. Shapiro
Department of Neurology
University of Vermont
College of Medicine
Burlington, Vermont

The autonomic nervous system (ANS) is structurally and functionally positioned to interface between the internal and external milieu, coordinating bodily functions to ensure homeostasis (cardiovascular and respiratory control, thermal regulation, gastrointestinal motility, urinary and bowel excretory functions, reproduction, and metabolic and endocrine physiology), and adaptive responses to stress (flight or fight response). Thus, the ANS has the daunting task of ensuring the survival and the procreation of the species. These complex roles require complex responses and depend on the integration of behavioral and physiologic responses that are coordinated centrally and peripherally. In 1898, Langley, a Cambridge University physiologist, coined the term "autonomic nervous system" and identified three separate components: sympathetic, parasympathetic, and enteric. The following section focuses on the first two aspects of the peripheral ANS: the sympathetic nervous system (SNS), including the adrenal medulla, and the parasympathetic nervous system (PNS). The following précis addresses the neuroanatomy of the SNS, adrenal medulla, and PNS, and then presents a more detailed, albeit brief, review of the functional neuroanatomy, physiology, and pharmacology of the peripheral ANS. Importantly, the role of the ANS at multiple interfaces in normal and abnormal physiology is emerging as a key mediator of pathophysiology in a range of complex disorders (anxiety and panic, chronic fatigue syndrome, regional pain syndromes, autonomic failure) and as a critical substrate underpinning the field of neurocardiology. The following information serves as a framework from which to view the complexity of the ANS as revealed in the more detailed descriptions that follow.

SYMPATHETIC NERVOUS SYSTEM

The SNS (Fig. 5.1) is organized at a spinal and peripheral level such that cell bodies within the thoracolumbar sections of the spinal cord provide preganglionic efferent innervation to sympathetic neurons that reside in ganglia dispersed in three arrangements: paravertebral, prevertebral, and previsceral or terminal ganglia. Paravertebral ganglia are paired structures that are located bilaterally along the vertebral column. They extend from the superior cervical ganglia (SCG), located rostrally at the bifurcation of the internal carotid arteries, to ganglia located in the sacral region. There are 3 cervical ganglia (the SCG, middle cervical ganglion, and inferior cervical ganglion, which is usually termed the cervicothoracic or stellate ganglion because it is a fused structure combining the inferior cervical and first thoracic paravertebral ganglia), 11 thoracic ganglia, 4 lumbar ganglia, and 4 to 5 sacral ganglia. More caudally, two paravertebral ganglia join to become the ganglion impar. Prevertebral ganglia are midline structures located anterior to the aorta and vertebral column and are represented by the celiac ganglia, aorticorenal ganglia, and the superior and inferior mesenteric ganglia. Previsceral, or terminal ganglia, are small collections of sympathetic ganglia located close to target structures; they are also referred to as short noradrenergic neurons because their axons cover limited distances. Generally, the preganglionic fibers are relatively short and the postganglionic fibers are quite long in the SNS. The axons of these postsynaptic neurons are generally unmyelinated and of small diameter ($<5\,\mu m$). The target organs of sympathetic neurons include smooth muscle and cardiac muscle, glandular structures, and parenchymal organs (e.g., liver, kidney, bladder, reproductive organs, muscles, and others [see Fig. 5.1]), as well as other cutaneous structures.

The spinal cells of origin for the presynaptic input to sympathetic peripheral ganglia are located from the first thoracic to the second lumbar level of the cord, although minor variations exist. The principal neurons generally have been viewed as located in the lateral horn of the spinal gray matter (intermediolateral cell column), but four major groups of autonomic neurons exist: intermediolateralis pars principalis (ILP), intermediolateralis pars funicularis, nucleus intercalatus spinalis, and the central autonomic nucleus or dorsal commissural nucleus (anatomic nomenclature is nucleus intercalatus pars paraependymalis). For paravertebral ganglia, more than 85 to 90% of the presynaptic fibers originate from cell bodies in ILP or intermediolateralis pars

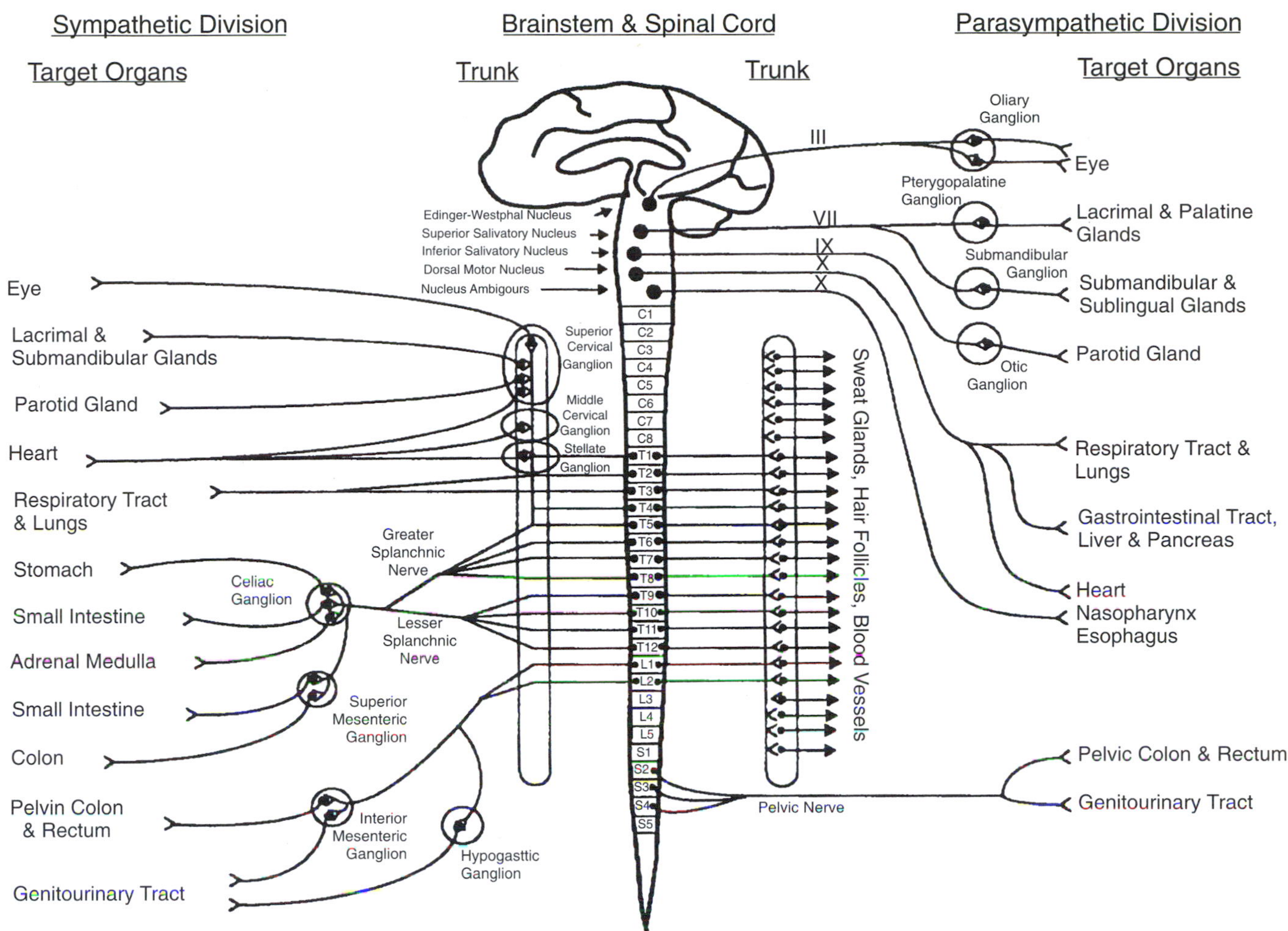

FIGURE 5.1 Schematic diagram of the sympathetic and parasympathetic divisions of the peripheral autonomic nervous system. The paravertebral chain of the sympathetic division is illustrated on both sides of the spinal outflow to demonstrate the full range of target structures innervated. Although the innervation pattern is diagrammatically illustrated to be direct connections between preganglionic outflow and postganglionic neurons, there is overlap of innervation such that more than one spinal segment provides innervation to neurons within the ganglia.

funicularis. Prevertebral ganglia and terminal ganglia receive a larger proportion of preganglionic terminals from the central autonomic nucleus/dorsal commissural nucleus. The nucleus intercalatus also contributes preganglionic fibers, but the exact extent of these is not fully understood and is probably limited. These spinal autonomic nuclei receive substantial supraspinal input from multiple transmitter systems located at multiple levels of the neuraxis, diencephalon (hypothalamus), and brainstem (raphe, locus coeruleus, reticular formation, and ventral lateral medulla) provide the largest input, and the pattern of innervation viewed in horizontal sections reveals a ladderlike arrangement of the distribution of nerve terminals [1]. Without detailing the source or course of specific systems, it is important to point out that the following different neurotransmitter (NT) systems impinge on preganglionic neurons within this ladderlike structure: monoamines—epinephrine, norepinephrine (NE), and serotonin; neuropeptides—substance P, thyrotropin-releasing hormone, metenkephalin, vasopressin, oxytocin, and neuropeptide Y (NPY); amino acids—glutamate, gamma-aminobutyric acid, and glycine. Undoubtedly, others exist and more will be found. It is apparent that dysfunction of these supraspinal systems or alterations of these NTs by disease or pharmacologic agents will alter the spinal control of peripheral ganglia and result in clinical dysfunction.

The outflow from the spinal cord to peripheral ganglia is segmentally organized with some overlap. Retrograde tracing studies indicate that there is a rostral–caudal gradient: SCG receives innervation from spinal segments T1–3; stellate ganglia T1–6; adrenal gland T5–11; celiac and superior mesenteric ganglia T5–12; and inferior mesenteric and hypogastric ganglion from L1–2. These presynaptic fibers, which are small in diameter (2–5 µm) and thinly myelinated, exit the ventral roots through the white rami communicantes to join the paravertebral chain either directly innervating their respective ganglion at the same level or traveling along the chain to innervate a target ganglion many levels away (Fig. 5.2). The distribution of postsynaptic fibers also follow a regional pattern with the head, face, and neck receiving innervation from the cervical ganglia (spinal segments T1–4), the upper limb and thorax from the stellate and upper thoracic ganglia (spinal segments T1–8), the lower trunk and abdomen from lower thoracic ganglia (spinal segments T4–12), and the pelvic region and lower limbs from lumbar and sacral ganglia (spinal segments T10-L2). More recently, with the introduction of transneuronal tracing techniques, using such molecules as the pseudorabies virus, it has been possible to inject ganglia in the periphery and examine the transneuronal passage of tracer. Thus, supraspinal neurons projecting to the specific sets of preganglionic neurons that innervate the peripheral ganglia injected may be examined. Interestingly, a surprisingly common set of central pathways influencing the thoracolumbar sympathetic outflow were labeled. For example, after injections in either the SCG, stellate or celiac ganglia, or the adrenal gland, the following five brain areas are labeled: ventromedial and rostral ventrolateral medulla, caudal raphe nuclei, A5 noradrenergic cell group, and the paraventricular nucleus of the hypothalamus [2]. Apparently, these central loci must share regulatory functions that are coordinated through similar pathways of thoracolumbar outflow. These same studies indicate that other brain areas are only labeled from specific ganglia; thus, site-specific central control also exists. Of additional interest, numerous small interneurons in Rexed laminae VII and X of the spinal cord were labeled, providing structural support for the observation that spinal intersegmental and intrasegmental autonomic interactions (including autonomic reflexes) exist.

It is apparent that the structural organizational of the SNS permits the integration and dissemination of responses depending on demand. Multiple supraspinal descending pathways provide a dense innervation of all four major autonomic cell groups in the spinal cord, but clearly specific topographic responses also exist. In turn, each preganglionic neuron innervates anywhere from 4 to 20 postganglionic sites (estimates), and each spinal outflow level may reach multiple peripheral ganglia, which, in turn, supply multiple targets, permitting additional dispersion of sympathetic responses when indicated. At each thoracic level there are

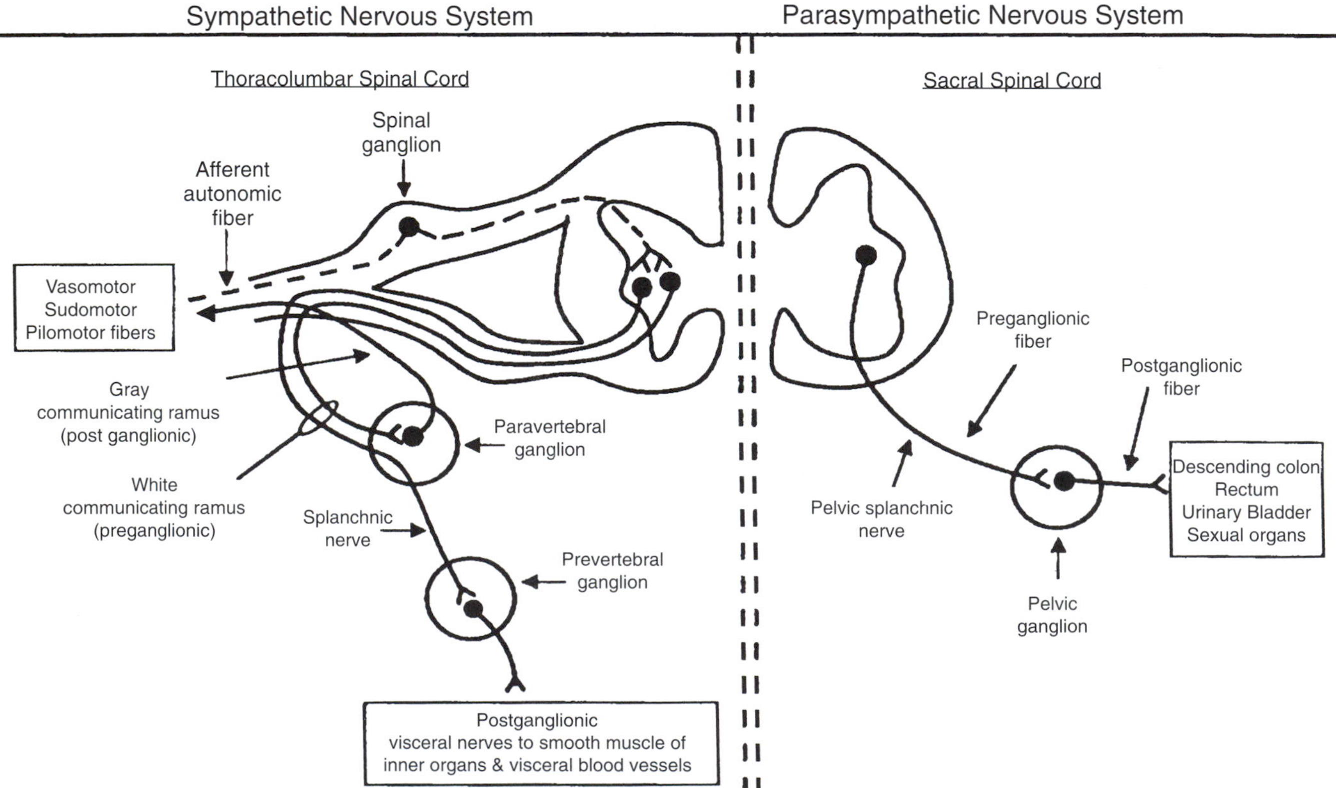

FIGURE 5.2 Schematic illustration of the segmental spinal arrangement of the sympathetic and parasympathetic nervous system. Although segmental interactions exist, they are polysynaptic, operating through interneurons; the primary input to spinal preganglionic neurons is supraspinal originating from brainstem structures (not shown).

an estimated 5000 preganglionic neurons (these counts have generally been limited to the cells located in the ILP). Because preganglionic output to prevertebral ganglia originates from more medially placed cell bodies, it is conceivable that a greater number of neurons at certain segmental levels contribute to the output. Thus, a given spinal segment has a powerful base to influence greater than 100,000 postganglionic neurons. Although previous thinking suggested that responses were "all or none and widespread," anatomic studies continue to reveal subtleties of structural arrangements that indicate that the system is not only poised for generalized activation of the peripheral SNS, but is also able to exert control of relatively specific sites and functions.

The postganglionic fibers in the SNS travel quite lengthy paths to arrive at target organs. For instance, fibers from the SCG traverse the extracranial and intracranial vasculature to reach such targets as the lacrimal glands, parotid glands, pineal gland, and pupils. Fibers from the stellate ganglia course through the branchial plexus to reach vascular and cutaneous targets in the upper limb and hand. Within the abdomen, axons originating from the paravertebral ganglia supply the viscera and the mesenteric vasculature. Lumbar and sacral paravertebral ganglia course distally along peripheral nerves and blood vessels to reach the distal vasculature and cutaneous structures in the feet. In humans, the innervation to the leg requires a sympathetic axon to be 50 cm in length, and with an estimated overall diameter of 1.2 μm the axonal volume is approximately 565,000 μm^3. This axonal cytoskeleton and its metabolic requirements are supported by a perikaryon of about 30 μm with a somal volume of 14,000 μm^3. With this structural architecture to maintain, these neurons are vulnerable to various metabolic and structural insults. Although most preganglionic fibers have a relatively short course to their ganglion targets, the upper thoracic preganglionic fibers travel relatively longer distances to reach the stellate and SCG, and preganglionic fibers to the adrenal medulla and prevertebral ganglia course through the paravertebral chain, reaching these visceral targets as the splanchnic nerves. Along the course, fiber systems may be interrupted, resulting in local autonomic dysfunction. For example, the Horner syndrome results from lesion of either preganglionic fibers to the SCG or the postganglionic axons, which leave the SCG to innervate Müller's muscle of the upper eyelid, pupillodilator muscles, facial vasculature, and sudomotor structures of the face (see Fig. 5.1).

The autonomic neuroeffector junction is generally a poorly defined synaptic structure lacking the prejunctional and postjunctional specializations that are observed in the central nervous system or skeletal muscle motor endplates. The unmyelinated highly branched postganglionic fibers become beaded with varicosities as they approach their targets. The varicosities are not static; they move along as structures with a diameter of 0.5 to 2 μm and a length of approximately 1.0 μm. The number of varicosities varies from 10,000/mm^3 to more than 2,000,000/mm^3 depending on the target being innervated. The varicosities are packed with mitochondria and vesicles containing various transmitters and are at varying distances from their target organs. For instance, for smooth muscle targets, this distance varies from 20 nm in the vas deferens to 1–2 μm in large arteries. In a sense the release of transmitter is accomplished *en passage* as the impulse travels along an autonomic axon. The lack of a restrictive synaptic arrangement permits the released NTs to diffuse various distances along a target organ and activate multiple receptors, again expanding the overall effect of sympathetic activation. Between 100 and 1000 vesicles exist in each varicosity in noradrenergic fibers. Traditional teaching suggests that vesicle characteristics indicate the transmitter system: small granular vesicles are noradrenergic; small agranular vesicles are cholinergic; and large granular vesicles are peptidergic. However, exceptions to these correlations exist.

The principal neuronal phenotype in peripheral sympathetic ganglia is the noradrenergic neuron, which is generally multipolar in character with synapses mainly located more on dendrites than somata. Depending on which ganglia are examined, studies indicate that from 80 to 95% of ganglion cells will stain positively for tyrosine hydroxylase, the rate-limiting enzyme in catecholamine biosynthesis, or will have positive catecholamine fluorescence. The remaining cells have a mixture of transmitters, or are postganglionic cholinergic cells (the sudomotor and periosteal components of sympathetic function). Within sympathetic ganglia there is a small group of small, intensely fluorescent neurons. The transmitters identified in small, intensely fluorescent cells include dopamine, epinephrine, or serotonin. As described later in this chapter, the original concept that preganglionic neurons in the SNS are cholinergic and postganglionic neurons are noradrenergic has given way to new information that a whole array of molecules (cholinergic, catecholaminergic, monoaminergic, peptidergic, "noncholinergic, nonadrenergic," and gaseous) appear to be involved in neurotransmission either as agents themselves or as neuromodulators (*vide infra*).

SYMPATHOADRENAL AXIS AND THE ADRENAL GLAND

Interactions between the adrenal cortex and adrenal medulla constitute a critical link between the autonomic and endocrine systems. The adrenal cortex is largely regulated by the hypothalamic-pituitary-adrenocortical axis, whereas the adrenal medulla is primarily under neural control. Both adrenal cortex and medulla respond to stress and metabolic aberrations. The coordinated response of increased plasma cortisol and catecholamines during stress indicate that central limbic and hypothalamic centers exert combined influences to ensure the needed neurohumoral adaptations. The interdependence of these two components of the adrenal gland arises early in development: migrating sympathoblasts destined for the adrenal medulla require the presence of the cortical tissue to change their developmental fate from neurons to that of chromaffin cells. These cells, named because they exhibit brown color when treated with "chrome salts," do not develop neural processes but instead serve an endocrine function by releasing their neurohumors (epinephrine, NE, and neuropeptides) into the bloodstream. During adulthood the presence of the cortex is critical for maintaining the levels of epinephrine, because the induction of the enzyme phenylethanolamine-*N*-methyltransferase is dependent on local levels of cortisol. Although traditional teaching emphasizes the preganglionic cholinergic splanchnic innervation of the adrenal medulla, there is also evidence that postganglionic sympathetic fibers, vagal afferents, and other sensory afferents are present.

Tracing studies indicate that dye placed within the adrenal medulla is transported retrogradely within spinal preganglionic sympathetic neurons in a somewhat bell-shaped distribution from approximately T2-L1, with the predominant innervation originating from T7–T10. Neuronal cell bodies are primarily within the nucleus ILP, with the pars funicularis and pars intercalatus providing a relatively small portion of the innervation. The exiting nerve roots pass through the sympathetic chain, join to form the greater splanchnic nerve, and distribute themselves beneath the adrenal capsule and within the medulla. A small number of nerve cells are labeled in ganglia within the sympathetic chain, suggesting that postganglionic sympathetic fibers innervate the gland. Whether these terminals are labeled as they pass along blood vessels within the gland or they innervate medullary or cortical cells is not fully resolved. Also, at least in the guinea pig, tracing studies indicate that the PNS may contribute a small efferent innervation to the gland, because neurons in the dorsal motor nucleus of the vagus are labeled after injections in the medulla. Also, cell bodies within the dorsal root ganglia and vagal sensory ganglia (nodose) are also labeled after tracer studies of the adrenal medulla, indicating an afferent innervation as well. Lastly, although not a prominent innervation pattern, there appears to be an intrinsic innervation that arises from ganglion cells sparsely populating the subcapsular, cortical, and medullary regions of the gland. The innervation pattern of the adrenal medulla is thus more complex than the traditionally listed thoracolumbar preganglionic cholinergic outflow, although the major adaptive responses depend on the preganglionic cholinergic innervation because surgical section of these nerves or pharmacologic blockade with cholinergic antagonists preclude the induction of tyrosine hydroxylase and appropriate release of catecholamines after various stress paradigms.

Morphologic studies of the adrenal medulla have revealed the presence of two basic types of granules in chromaffin cells. A diffuse spherical granule contains the predominant monoamine secreted by medullary cells, epinephrine, whereas eccentrically located dense core granules contain NE. As indicated earlier for ganglion neurons, chromaffin cells of the adrenal medulla also co-contain other molecules. For example, the opioid molecules are well represented: enkephalin is co-contained in vesicles with the monoamines. The signaling cascade responsible for enhancing the synthesis and release of these neurohormonal agents is complicated and includes preganglionic innervation, steroid hormones (glucocorticoids), and growth factors (nerve growth factor).

PARASYMPATHETIC NERVOUS SYSTEM

The craniosacral outflow is the source of central neuronal pathways providing the efferent innervation of peripheral ganglia of the PNS (see Fig. 5.1). The cranial nerves involved include cranial nerves III, VII, IX, and X, and the sacral outflow is largely restricted to sacral cord levels 2, 3, and 4. As indicated for the SNS, the preganglionic innervation is largely cholinergic with these terminals releasing acetylcholine (ACh) at the ganglion synapses. In contrast to the SNS, the major transmitter postsynaptically is also ACh. These cholinergic neurons also co-contain other transmitter substances: preganglionic neurons contain enkephalins, and ganglionic cholinergic neurons frequently contain vasoactive intestinal peptide (VIP) or NPY, or both. The parasympathetic fibers in cranial nerve III originate in the Edinger-Westphal nuclei of the midbrain and travel in the periphery of the nerve (where they are subject to dysfunction secondary to nerve compression), exiting along with the nerve to the inferior oblique to supply the ciliary ganglion. Second-order postganglionic fibers exit in the ciliary nerves and supply the pupilloconstrictor fibers of the iris and the ciliary muscle where their combined action permits the near response, including accommodation. The salivatory nuclei, located near the pontomedullary junction, provide the preganglionic parasympathetic innervation for cranial nerves VII and IX. The superior salivatory nucleus sends preganglionic fibers, which leave the facial nerve at the level of the geniculate ganglion (nonparasympathetic sensory ganglion) to form the greater superficial petrosal nerve to the pterygopalatine (sphenopalatine) ganglia that provides postganglionic secretomotor and vasodilator fibers to the lacrimal glands through the maxillary nerve. Other preganglionic fibers in the facial nerve continue and subsequently leave through the chorda tympani to join the lingual nerve, eventually synapsing in the submandibular ganglion. Postsynaptic cholinergic fibers supply the sublingual and submandibular glands. Postganglionic fibers from the pterygopalatine and submandibular ganglia also supply glands and vasculature in the mucosa of the sinuses, palate, and nasopharynx. The inferior salivatory nucleus sends preganglionic fibers through the glossopharyngeal nerve (cranial nerve IX) to the otic ganglion, which, in turn, relays postganglionic fibers to the parotid gland through the auriculotemporal nerve. The preganglionic fibers in cranial nerve IX branch from the nerve at the jugular foramen and contribute to the tympanic plexus and form the lesser superficial petrosal nerve. This nerve exits the intracranial compartment through the foramen ovale along the third division of the trigeminal nerve to reach the otic ganglion.

The most caudal cranial nerve participating in the preganglionic parasympathetic system is the vagus nerve (cranial nerve X). The dorsal motor nucleus of the vagus is located in the medulla and sends preganglionic fibers to innervate essentially all organ systems within the chest and abdomen, including the gastrointestinal tract as far as the left colonic flexure (splenic flexure). Also, the nucleus ambiguus supplies preganglionic fibers to the vagus and these fibers are believed to be involved mostly with regulating visceral smooth muscle, whereas the dorsal motor vagus neurons may be secretomotor in nature. The glossopharyngeal and vagus nerves also contain a substantial number of afferent fibers (in the vagus, afferent fibers may exceed the efferent fiber system by a ratio of 9 : 1) so that a sensory component related to autonomic control exists within cranial nerves IX and X. These afferents provide a critical component of the baroreceptor reflex arc, relaying information regarding the systemic blood pressure to central cardiovascular areas in the nucleus tractus solitarii and other medullary centers involved in blood pressure and heart rate control.

The parasympathetic cell bodies in the spinal cord are located in the intermediolateral cell column of second, third, and fourth sacral segments (see Fig. 5.2). These neurons send preganglionic nerve fibers through the pelvic nerve to ganglia located close to or within the pelvic viscera. Postganglionic fibers are relatively short, in contradistinction to their length in the SNS, and supply cholinergic terminals to structures involved in excretory (bladder and bowel) and reproductive (fallopian tubes and uterus, prostate, seminal vesicles, vas deferens, and erectile tissue) functions. Of interest, the pelvic ganglia involved in some of these functions appear to be mixed ganglia (especially in rodents) in which sympathetic and parasympathetic neurons are components of the same pelvic ganglion. They appear to receive their traditional preganglionic input, but may have local interconnections that are not fully revealed by current studies. As indicated later, there is clear evidence that the cholinergic postganglionic neurons in the pelvic ganglion in the rodent co-contain VIP and nitric oxide (NO) as two other transmitter molecules. These neurons are believed to be integrally involved in sexual functions in the male, permitting the development and maintenance of potency. The exact regulatory factors controlling the synthesis and release of these transmitter molecules and the specific receptor systems involved remain to be fully explored.

THE CONCEPT OF PLURICHEMICAL TRANSMISSION AND CHEMICAL CODING

The notion of the presence of multiple transmitters and a chemical coding system of autonomic neurons is now firmly established. Originally it was posited that principal neurons were only noradrenergic (contained NE), but during the last two decades it has become clear that within a single neuron multiple transmitter systems may exist, and that within a given ganglion the variety and pattern of NTs may be quite extensive (Table 5.1). Also, the composition of NTs may change depending on the location of the ganglia: paravertebral ganglia tend to have fewer transmitters, whereas prevertebral and terminal ganglia may have various NTs, although as noted for the guinea pig SGC (Fig. 5.3), some paravertebral ganglia have a broad array of transmitters. The

TABLE 5.1 Neurotransmitter Phenotypes in Autonomic Neurons

Autonomic neurons	Transmitter characteristics (not all inclusive)
Sympathetic neurons	
Paravertebral ganglia	NE, CCK, somatostatin,
Prevertebral ganglia	SP, Enk, ACh
Terminal ganglia (previsceral ganglia)	VIP, 5-HT, NPY, DYN1-8, DYN1-17
Parasympathetic neurons	
Major parasympathetic ganglia	
Ciliary	
Sphenopalatine	ACh, VIP, SP, CAs-SIF, NPY, NO
Otic	
Submandibular/sublingual	
Pelvic ganglia	
Terminal parasympathetic ganglia (previsceral ganglia)	
Enteric neurons	
Myenteric plexus (Auerbach's)	GABA, ACh, VIP, 5-HT
Submucosal plexus (Meisner's)	SP, Enk, SRIF, motilinlike peptide, bombesinlike peptide
Enteric ganglia	
Chromaffin cells of adrenal medulla	E, NE, Enk, NPY, APUD
Paraganglia-chromaffin	
SIF cells, ganglia	

5-HT, 5-hydroxyltryptamine; ACh, acetylcholine; APUD, amine precursor uptake and decarboxylation; CAs-SIF, catecholamines-small intensely fluorescent; CCK, cholecystokinin; DA, dopamine; DYN, dynorphin A (DYN 1-8, or DYN 1-17; neurons with dynorphin A also contain dynorphin B and "-neo-endorphine"); E, epinephrine; Enk, enkephalin; GABA, gamma-aminobutyric acid; NE, norepinephrine; NO, nitric oxide; NPY, neuropeptide Y; SP, substance P; SRIF, somatostatin; VIP, vasoactive intestinal polypeptide.

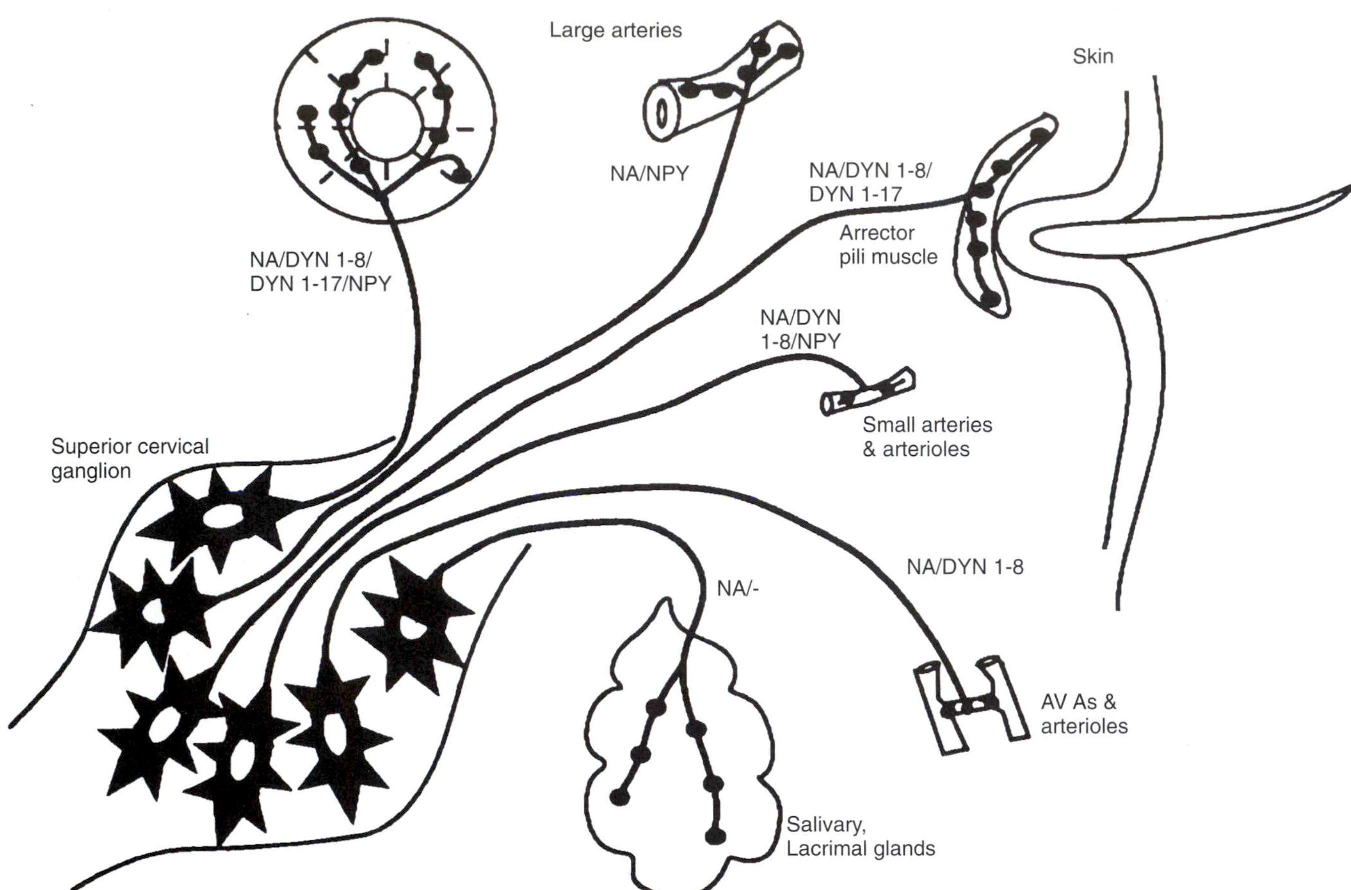

FIGURE 5.3 Chemical coding and target organization. Chemical coding of sympathetic neurons projecting from the superior cervical ganglion to various targets in the head of guinea pigs. Each population of neurons has a specific combination of neuropeptides. Note that all neurons containing a form of dynorphin A (DYN 1–8 or DYN 1–17) also contain dynorphin B and "-neo-endorphin. No neuropeptides have been found in neurons projecting to secretory tissue in the salivary or lacrimal glands. Neurons with similar peptide combinations also occur in other paravertebral ganglia of guinea pigs, except that the salivary secretomotor neurons are absent. Conversely, the paravertebral ganglia have many nonnoradrenergic vasodilatory neurons containing prodynorphin-derived peptides VIP and NPY. AVAs, arteriovenous anastomoses; NA, noradrenaline; NPY, neuropeptide Y. (See Reference 7.)

exact colocation and functions of these multiple transmitters are not fully understood, but some general principles exist. NPY is probably the most prominent peptide in sympathetic ganglia and is highly colocalized with NE. The sudomotor component of ganglia is dependent on a population of cells, which are cholinergic in character (i.e., contain ACh as NT), and the most frequent peptide colocalized with ACh is VIP. The distribution of these cholinergic cells varies: in paravertebral ganglia they may represent 10 to 15% of the neuronal population, whereas they represent less than 1% of the neurons in prevertebral ganglia. NE + NPY and ACh + VIP are believed to be released together, but some degree of activity-chemical coding exists; that is, at lower levels of activation NE is preferentially released, whereas greater levels of stimulation result in NPY being released. Both agents have vasoconstrictor properties and are integral in cardiovascular control, especially in the maintenance of blood pressure. Of course, the eventual action and effect of a transmitter rests with the receptor system that is activated (*vide infra*).

Purinergic neurotransmission expands the cotransmission motif. Presynaptic and postsynaptic mechanisms exist: the purine nucleotide adenosine triphosphate is in high concentration in sympathetic synaptic vesicles, and after release adenosine triphosphate is catabolized to adenosine moieties. There are at least eight receptors (four purinergic and four adenosinergic) that serve to translate purinergic and adenosinergic effects (vasoconstriction and vasodilation) to vascular beds through endothelium-dependent and endothelium-independent mechanisms.

Chemical coding also reveals that ganglion neurons with specific transmitter molecules innervate specific targets or receive specific afferent inputs. Apparently, anterograde and retrograde transsynaptic information appears to determine the transmitter phenotype of the neuron. Thus, studies of neuronal circuitry indicate that pathway-specific combinations determine the presence and combinations of specific peptides within autonomic neurons. This is particularly true in the prevertebral ganglia, but studies in the guinea pig SCG demonstrate that the transmitter molecules vary depending on the target organ supplied (see Fig. 5.3). Although all principal cells portrayed are noradrenergic in character (as indicated by NA), the neuropeptides co-contained in neurons vary depending on whether the targets are secretory (salivary and lacrimal glands), vascular (small vs large arteries, arterioles vs arteriovenous anastomoses), pupil, or skin. Detailed pictures of these chemically coded circuits are beginning to emerge from studies of paravertebral (SCG), prevertebral (superior mesenteric), and previsceral (pelvic) ganglia. This phenomenon pertains to both the SNS and PNS.

Preganglionic sympathetic neurons in the spinal cord have traditionally been viewed as cholinergic neurons. More recently, it has been recognized that neuronal cell bodies in the cat ILP may contain a variety of transmitters including enkephalin, neurotensin, somatostatin, and substance P. In rodents, VIP and calcitonin gene–related peptide–containing neurons also have been localized to the ILP by immunocytochemistry. Also, preganglionic fibers in the sacral parasympathetic outflow co-contain enkephalin. It is apparent that neurotransmission is plurichemical in both preganglionic and postganglionic fiber systems.

FUNCTIONAL NEUROANATOMY AND BIOCHEMICAL PHARMACOLOGY

The peripheral ANS is well structured to provide the physiologic responses critical for homeostasis and acute adaptations to stressful, perhaps life-threatening, circumstances. As outlined in Figure 5.1 and Table 5.2, multiple organ systems respond to NTs released from autonomic endings and circulating catecholamines released from the adrenal medulla. Traditional teaching is that the effects of activation of the SNS and PNS are generally antagonistic; this is still largely the case. However, viewed more specifically, the relationships between these two major components of the ANS are far from simple. For instance, not all organs receive an equal number of both sets of fibers, and, in some situations, both SNS and PNS effects are similar. It is important to remember that receptor systems, including the signal transduction components, on the target organs are the critical molecular proteins that determine the actual effects of ligand receptor interactions on the cell membrane. Thus, when the SNS is stimulated with its capability to produce a widespread response, a host of receptor systems are activated to affect the necessary and desired change. An example of these responses includes the following aspects of SNS activation: dilatation of the pupil, slight increase in glandular secretions, bronchodilation, increased heart rate and force of contraction, decreased gastrointestinal tract motility, decreased function of the reproductive organs, and mobilization of energy substrates to meet demands. The receptor systems mediating these responses include α_{1A}, α_{1B}, α_{1D}, α_{2A}, α_{2B}, α_{2C}, β_1, β_2, and β_3 receptors. α_1 Receptors have subtype-selective distributions, second messenger systems, and functions. Activation of these receptors occurs after interaction with NE and variously results in contraction of smooth muscle in the vasculature and iris and relaxation of smooth muscle in the gut. α_1 Receptors exert a limited positive inotropic effect on the heart and mediate salivary gland secretion and contraction of the prostate gland. α_2 Receptors also have discrete subtype-specific localizations and functions in brain, peripheral nerve, and target tissues. α_2 Receptors serve as autoreceptors on sympathetic nerve terminals and inhibit the release of NE as part of a negative feedback loop. They also can act as constrictors of both arterial and venous vascular smooth muscle. Furthermore, these receptors play important roles in nociception and also mediate metabolic and endocrine changes such as inhibition of lipolysis in adipose tissue and reduction of insulin release from the pancreas. Beta receptors (β_1) provide positive inotropic and chronotropic effects on the heart and stimulate renin release from the kidney. β_2 Receptors relax smooth muscle of the bronchi and pelvic organs, as well as the vascular

TABLE 5.2 Autonomic Nervous System Functions

Organ	Sympathetic nervous system	Parasympathetic nervous system
Eye		
Pupil	Dilatation	Constriction
Ciliary muscle	Relax (far vision)	Constrict (near vision)
Lacrimal gland	Slight secretion	Secretion
Parotid gland	Slight secretion	Secretion
Submandibular gland	Slight secretion	Secretion
Heart	Increased rate	Slowed rate
	Positive inotropism	Negative inotropism
Lungs	Bronchodilation	Bronchodilation
Gastrointestinal tract	Decreased motility	Increased motility
Kidney	Decreased output	None
Bladder	Relax detrusor	Contract detrusor
	Contract sphincter	Relax sphincter
Penis	Ejaculation	Erection
Sweat glands	Secretion	Palmar sweating
Piloerection muscles	Contraction	None
Blood vessels		
Arterioles	Constriction	None
Muscle		
Arterioles	Constriction or dilatation	None
Metabolism	Glycogenolysis	None

structures of the gut and skeletal muscle. β_2 Receptors located in liver and skeletal muscle elicit activation of glycogenolysis and gluconeogenesis. This receptor system is particularly activated by epinephrine rather than NE.

The PNS is poised for more focal responses, but some effects may be quite broad, particularly with the wide-ranging innervation of the vagus nerve. Activation of parasympathetic pathways leads to pupillary constriction, substantial secretion from lacrimal and salivary glands, slowed cardiac rate and negative inotropism, bronchoconstriction, enhanced gastrointestinal motility, and contraction of the detrusor muscle of the bladder. In contrast to the SNS, the PNS does not appear to influence metabolic or endocrine processes in any major way. However, recent evidence indicates that preganglionic vagal fibers originating in the dorsal motor nucleus innervate postganglionic parasympathetic ganglia in the pancreas and appear to influence exocrine and endocrine function. Thus, as new data emerge, the integrated roles of the SNS and PNS will continue to expand.

An understanding of the receptor systems mediating the responses to PNS activation is incomplete. Preganglionic cholinergic receptors, which exist in the SNS and PNS, are nicotinic in character, whereas postganglionic cholinergic receptors are muscarinic. Molecular cloning studies have revealed multiple subtypes of both sets of receptors. The subtypes of muscarinic receptors, which are termed M1, M2, M3, M4, M5, are more fully understood (at least for the first three subtypes): M1 receptors are excitatory to neurons in ganglia and lead to noradrenaline release in sympathetic neurons; M2 receptors mediate the bradycardia and decrease contractility of the heart after vagal activation; M3 stimulation leads to contraction of smooth muscle and enhanced secretion from glandular tissues. The discovery that multiple subtypes of nicotinic receptors also exist will lead to new understanding of how these cholinergic receptor systems function with both the presynaptic and postsynaptic components of the peripheral ANS.

The complexity of autonomic control and the range of mechanisms available to peripheral sympathetic and parasympathetic neurons and their targets are expanded by presynaptic gaseous molecules (NO) and postsynaptic endothelium released peptides. Also, central nervous system centers involved in autonomic control contain NO synthase, and evidence suggests that NO may mediate sympathoinhibition or sympathoexcitation depending on the nuclear groups involved. Peripherally, NO exerts tonic vasodilation and mediates ACh-induced vasodilation, as well as mediating catecholamine release and action. Endothelins, released abluminally by endothelial cells, bind to endothelial and adrenoceptors on vascular smooth muscle and endothelial cells and appear also to regulate sympathetic terminals.

The discoveries that a number of neurotrophic factors (neurotrophins) and their receptors are part and parcel of the development and integrity of the SNS and PNS expand the horizons regarding how anatomic pathways are established and maintained and adapt to intrinsic and extrinsic demands. Because of its relatively simple anatomic architecture, the peripheral ANS continues to serve as a model system to understand neuronal development, structural and functional linkages among neurons and their targets, and the integrative role(s) these "little brains" (6000–30,000 neurons) serve. As the structure–function relationships and molecular pharmacology of the peripheral ANS are clarified, new approaches to understanding its functions and treatments of its maladies will undoubtedly emerge. The following sections in this Primer will expand on these issues.

References

1. Romagnano, M. A., and R. W. Hamill. 1984. Spinal sympathetic pathway: An enkephalin ladder. *Science* 225:737–739.
2. Strack, A. M., W. B. Sawyer, J. H. Hughes, K. B. Platt, A. D. Loewy. 1989. A general pattern of CNS innervation of the sympathetic outflow demonstrated by transneuronal pseudorabies viral infections. *Brain Res.* 491:156–162.
3. Baloh, R. H., H. Enomoto, E. M. Johnson, Jr., and J. Milbrandt. 2000. The GDNF family ligands and receptors-implications for neural development [Review]. *Curr. Opin. Neurobiol.* 10:103–110.
4. Burnstock, G., and P. Milner. 1999. Structural and chemical organization of the autonomic nervous system with special reference to non-adrenergic, non-cholinergic transmission. In *Autonomic failure,* ed 4. R. Banister, and C. J. Mathias, Eds, 66. New York: Oxford University Press.
5. Chowdhary, S., and J. N. Townend. 1999. Role of nitric oxide in the regulation of cardiovascular autonomic control. *Clin. Sci. (Lond).* 97:5–17.
6. Dinner, D. S. 1993. The autonomic nervous system [Review]. *J. Clin. Neurophysiol.* 10:1–82.
7. Elfvin, L.-G., B. Lindh, and T. I. Hokfelt. 1993. The chemical neuroanatomy of sympathetic ganglia. *Ann. Rev. Neurosci.* 16:471–507.
8. Gibbins, I. 1995. Chemical neuroanatomy of sympathetic ganglia. In *Autonomic ganglia.* E. M. McLachlan, Ed, 73–121. Luxembourg: Harwood Academic Publishers.
9. Goldstein, D. S. 2001. *The autonomic nervous system in health and disease.* 23–135. New York: Marcel Dekker.
10. Janig, W., and H. J. Habler. 2000. Specificity in the organization of the autonomic nervous system: A basis for precise neural regulation of homeostatic and protective body functions. *Prog. Brain Res.* 122: 351–367.
11. Schober, A., and K. Unsicker. 2001. Growth and neurotrophic factors regulating development and maintenance of sympathetic preganglionic neurons. *Int. Rev. Cytol.* 205:37–76.
12. Zansinger, J. 1999. Role of nitric oxide in the neural control of cardiovascular function. *Cardiovasc. Res.* 43:639–649.

6 The Autonomic Neuroeffector Junction

Geoffrey Burnstock
Autonomic Neuroscience Institute
London, United Kingdom

The autonomic neuromuscular junction differs in several important respects from the better known skeletal neuromuscular junction; it is not a synapse with the well-defined prejunctional and postjunctional specializations established for the skeletal neuromuscular synapse or ganglionic synapses. A model of the autonomic neuroeffector junction has been proposed on the basis of combined electrophysiologic, histochemical, and electron-microscopical studies. The essential features of this model are that the terminal portions of autonomic nerve fibers are varicose, transmitter being released *en passage* from varicosities during conduction of an impulse, although excitatory and inhibitory junction potentials are probably elicited only at close junctions. Furthermore, the effectors are muscle bundles rather than single smooth muscle cells, which are connected by low-resistance pathways (gap junctions) that allow electrotonic spread of activity within the effector bundle. In blood vessels, the nerves are confined to the adventitial side of the media muscle coat, and this geometry appears to facilitate dual control of vascular smooth muscle by perivascular nerves and by endothelial relaxing and contracting factors. Neuroeffector junctions do not have a permanent geometry with postjunctional specializations, but rather the varicosities are continuously moving and their special relation with muscle cell membranes changes with time, including dispersal and reformation of receptor clusters. For example, varicosity movement is likely to occur in cerebral blood arteries, where there is a continuously increasing density of sympathetic innervation during development and aging and in hypertensive vessels or those that have been stimulated chronically *in vivo*, where there can be an increase in innervation density of up to threefold.

STRUCTURE OF THE AUTONOMIC NEUROMUSCULAR JUNCTION

Varicose Terminal Axons

In the vicinity of the effector tissue, axons become varicose, varicosities occurring at 5–10 µm intervals (Fig. 6.1A), and branches intermingle with other axons to form the autonomic ground plexus, first described by Hillarp in 1946. The extent of the branching and the area of effector tissue affected by individual neurons varies with the tissue. Autonomic axons combined in bundles are enveloped by Schwann cells. Within the effector tissue they partially lose their Schwann cell envelope, usually leaving the last few varicosities naked.

The density of innervation, in terms of the number of axon profiles per 100 muscle cells in cross section, also varies considerably in different organs. For example, it is very high in the vas deferens (Fig. 6.2A), iris, nictitating membrane, and sphincteric parts of the gastrointestinal tract, but low in the ureter, uterus, and longitudinal muscle coat of the gastrointestinal tract. In most blood vessels, the varicose nerve plexus is placed at the adventitial border and fibers rarely penetrate into the medial muscle coat (Fig. 6.2B).

Junctional Cleft

The width of the junctional cleft varies considerably in different organs. In the vas deferens, nictitating membrane, sphincter pupillae, rat parotid gland, and atrioventricular and sinoatrial nodes in the heart, the smallest neuromuscular distances range from 10 to 30 nm [1, 2]. The minimum neuromuscular distance varies considerably in different blood vessels [3]. Generally, the greater the vessel diameter, the greater the separation of nerve and muscle. Thus, minimal neuromuscular distances in arterioles and in small arteries and veins are about 50 to 100 nm, in medium to large arteries the separation is 200 to 500 nm, whereas in large elastic arteries where the innervation is sparser, the minimum neuromuscular distances are as wide as 1000 to 2000 nm. Serial sectioning has shown that at close junctions in both visceral and vascular organs there is fusion of prejunctional and postjunctional basal lamina (see Fig. 6.1B). In the longitudinal muscle coat of the gastrointestinal tract, autonomic nerves and smooth muscle are rarely separated by less than 100 nm. However, in the circular muscle coat, close (20 nm) junctions are common, sometimes several axon profiles being closely apposed with single muscle cells.

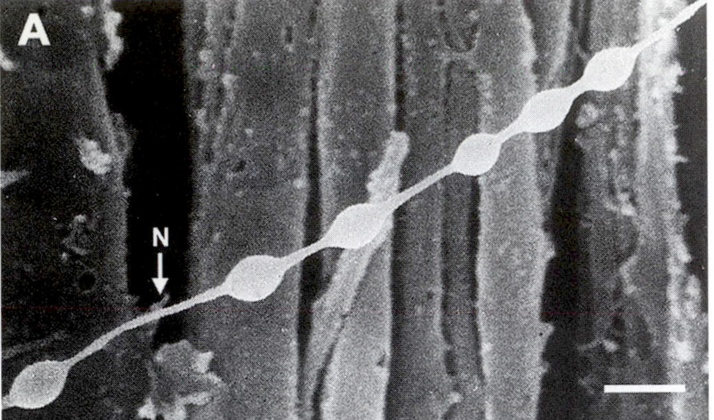

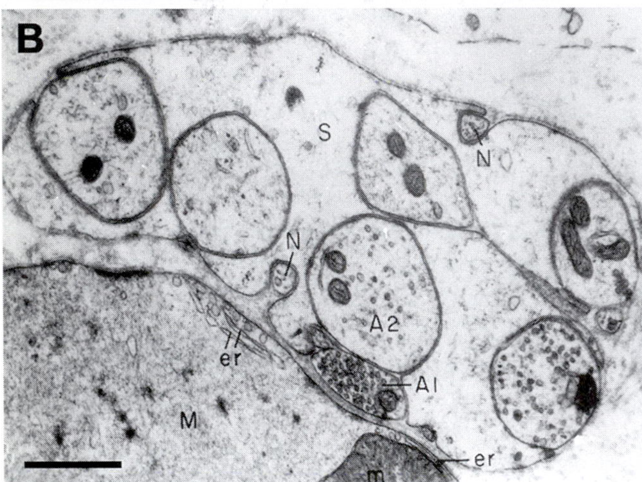

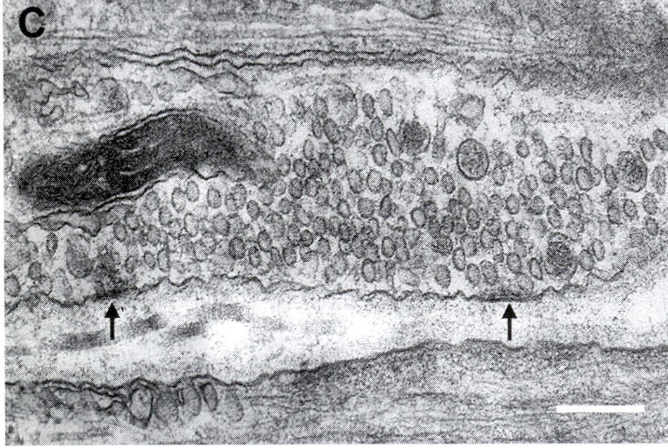

FIGURE 6.1 **A**, Scanning electron micrograph of a single terminal varicose nerve fiber lying over smooth muscle of small intestine of rat. Intestine was pretreated to remove connective tissue components by digestion with trypsin and hydrolysis with HCl. Scale bar = 3 µm. (Reproduced with permission from Burnstock, G. 1988. Autonomic neural control mechanisms. With special reference to the airways. In *The airways. Neural control in health and disease.* M. A. Kaliner, and P. J. Barnes, Eds, 1–22. New York: Marcel Dekker.) **B**, A medium-sized intramuscular bundle of axons within a single Schwann cell (S). There is no perineurial sheath. Some axons, free of Schwann cell processes, contain "synaptic" vesicles (e.g., *A1* and *A*). For nerve profile A1, there is close proximity (about 80 nm) to smooth muscle (*M*; *m*, mitochondria; *er*, endoplasmic reticulum) with fusion of nerve and muscle basement membranes. Most of the axons in bundles of this size have few vesicles in the plane of section, but they resemble the vesicle-containing axons of the larger trunks in that they have few large neurofilaments. The small profiles (*N*), less than 0.25 µm in diameter, are probably intervaricosity regions of terminal axons. Scale bar = 1 µm. (Reproduced with permission from Merrillees, N. C. R., G. Burnstock, and M. E. Holman. 1963. Correlation of fine structure and physiology of the innervation of smooth muscle in the guinea pig vas deferens. *J. Cell Biol.* 19:529–550.) **C**, Autonomic varicosities with dense prejunctional thickenings and bunching of vesicles, probably representing transmitter release sites (*arrows*), but there is no postjunctional specialization. Scale bar = 0.25 µm. (Courtesy of Phillip R. Gordon-Weeks.)

Prejunctional and Postjunctional Specialization

Although there are many examples of prejunctional thickenings of nerve membranes in varicosities associated with accumulations of small synaptic vesicles, representing sites of transmitter release (see Fig. 6.1C), there are no convincing demonstrations of postjunctional specializations, such as membrane thickening or folding or indeed absence of micropinocytic vesicles; this is in keeping with the view that even close junctions might be temporary liaisons.

Muscle Effector Bundles and Gap Junctions

The smooth muscle effector is a muscle bundle rather than a single muscle cell—that is, individual muscle cells being connected by low-resistance pathways that allow electrotonic spread of activity within the effector bundle. Sites of electrotonic coupling are represented morphologically by areas of close apposition between the plasma membranes of adjacent muscle cells. High-resolution electron micrographs have shown that the membranes at these sites consist of "gap junctions" (see Fig. 6.2C). Gap junctions (or nexuses) vary in size between punctate junctions, which are not easily recognized except in freeze-fracture preparations, and junctional areas more than 1 µm in diameter. The number and arrangement of gap junctions in muscle effector bundles of different sizes in different organs and their relation to density of autonomic innervation have not been fully analyzed. It is interesting that partial denervation has been shown to result in an increase in gap junctions.

AUTONOMIC NEUROTRANSMISSION

Electrophysiology

Excitatory and inhibitory junction potentials can be recorded in smooth muscle cells in response to stimulation of the autonomic nerves in both visceral (Fig. 6.3A and B) and vascular organs, which represent the responses to

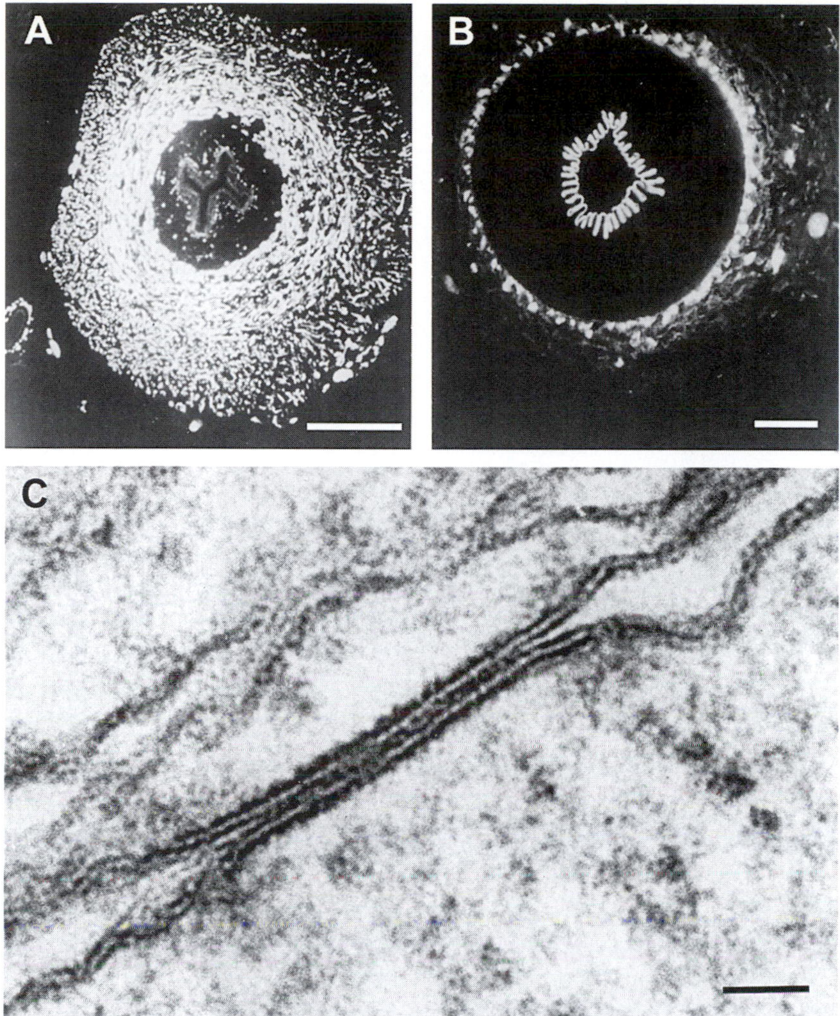

FIGURE 6.2 Comparison between the adrenergic innervation of the densely innervated vas deferens of the guinea pig (**A**) and the rabbit ear artery (**B**) in which the adrenergic fibers are confined to the adventitial–medial border. The inner elastic membrane shows a nonspecific fluorescence (autofluorescence). (**A** and **B**, Reproduced with permission from Burnstock, G., and M. Costa. 1975. *Adrenergic neurones: Their organisation, function and development in the peripheral nervous system*. London: Wiley & Sons Ltd.) **C**, A gap junction between two smooth muscle cells grown in tissue culture. (Reproduced with permission from Campbell, G. R., Y. Uehara, G. Mark, and G. Burnstock. 1971. Fine structure of smooth muscle cells grown in tissue culture. *J. Cell Biol.* 49:21–34.) Scale bar = 500 μm (**A**), 50 μm (**B**), and 50 nm (**C**).

adenosine triphosphate, released as a cotransmitter with noradrenaline from sympathetic nerves, as a cotransmitter with acetylcholine from parasympathetic nerves in the bladder, and as a cotransmitter with nitric oxide from nonadrenergic, noncholinergic inhibitory enteric nerves. Detailed analysis of these responses revealed that transmitter released from varicosities close (10–100 nm) to smooth muscle cells would produce junction potentials, although transmitter released from varicosities up to 500 to 1000 nm away (especially in large blood vessels) was likely to produce some muscle response; and that only about 1 to 3% of the varicosities release transmitter with a single impulse, although the probability for release increased to about 25% with repetitive nerve stimulation [4, 5, 6].

Receptor Localization on Smooth Muscle Cells

The distribution of P2X purinoceptors on smooth muscle cells in relation to autonomic nerve varicosities in urinary bladder, vas deferens, and blood vessels has been examined recently by using immunofluorescence and confocal microscopy. Antibodies against the $P2X_1$ receptor, the dominant receptor subtypes found in smooth muscle, and an antibody against the synaptic vesicle proteoglycan SV2

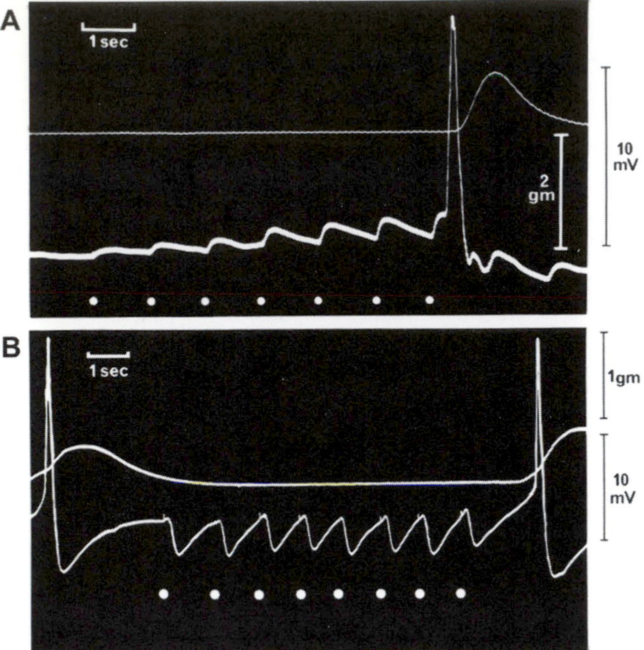

FIGURE 6.3 Electrophysiology of transmission at autonomic neuromuscular junctions. **Top trace**, Mechanical record. **Bottom trace**, Changes in membrane potential recorded with a sucrose-gap method (Burnstock & Straub, 1958). The junction potentials recorded with this method are qualitatively similar to those recorded with intracellular microelectrodes. **A**, Excitatory junction potentials (EJPs) recorded in smooth muscle of the guinea pig vas deferens in response to repetitive stimulation of postganglionic sympathetic nerves (*white dots*). Note both summation and facilitation of successive EJPs. At a critical depolarization threshold, an action potential is initiated that results in contraction. **B**, Inhibitory junction potentials (IJPs) recorded in smooth muscle of the atropinized guinea pig taenia-coli in response to transmural stimulation (*white dots*) of the intramural nerves remaining after degeneration of the adrenergic nerves by treatment of the animal with 6-hydroxydopamine (250 mg/kg intraperitoneally for 2 successive days) 7 days previously. Note that the IJPs in response to repetitive stimulation results in inhibition of spontaneous spike activity and relaxation. (Reproduced with permission from Burnstock, G. 1973. The autonomic neuroeffector system. *Proc. Aust. Physiol. Pharmacol. Soc.* 4:6–22.)

showed clusters of receptors (about $0.9 \times 0.2\,\mu m$ in size) located beneath varicosities [7, 8]. Many more small clusters (about $0.4 \times 0.04\,\mu m$) were present on the whole surface of smooth muscle cells unrelated to varicosities; they may represent pools of receptors that can migrate toward varicosities to form large clusters. In blood vessels, small clusters of P2X receptors are present on cells throughout the medial muscle coat, whereas large clusters are restricted to the muscle cells at the adventitial surface. Alpha-adrenoceptors appear to be located only in extrajunctional regions, so that the possibility that noradrenaline is released from more distant varicosities has been raised. There are hints from studies of receptor-coupled green fluorescent protein chimeras that the receptor clusters are labile, dispersing when a varicosity moves to a new site where clusters reform, perhaps within a 20- to 30-minute time scale.

MODEL OF AUTONOMIC NEUROEFFECTOR JUNCTION

A model of the autonomic neuromuscular junction has been proposed on the basis of combined electrophysiologic, histochemical, and electron-microscopical studies described earlier (Fig. 6.4A and B) [1, 9, 10]. The essential features of this model are that the terminal portions of autonomic nerve fibers are varicose, transmitter being released *en passage* from varicosities during conduction of an impulse, although excitatory junction potentials and inhibitory junction potentials are probably elicited only at close junctions. Furthermore, the effectors are muscle bundles rather than single smooth muscle cells, which are connected by low-resistance pathways (gap junctions) that allow electrotonic spread of activity within the effector bundle. In blood vessels, the nerves are confined to the adventitial side of the media muscle coat, and this geometry appears to facilitate dual control of vascular smooth muscle by endothelial relaxing and contracting factors and perivascular nerves.

Neuroeffector junctions do not have a permanent geometry with postjunctional specializations, but rather the varicosities are continuously moving and their special relation with muscle cell membranes changes with time. For example, it is likely to occur in cerebral blood arteries, where there is a continuously increasing density of sympathetic innervation during development until old age, and in vessels that have been stimulated chronically *in vivo*, where there can be an increase in innervation density of up to threefold, including an increase in the number of varicosities per unit length of nerve from 10 to 20 per $100\,\mu m$ to 30 per $100\,\mu m$.

Autonomic effector junctions appear to be suitable not only for neurotransmission, but also for neuromodulation. A neuromodulator is defined as any substance that modifies the process of neurotransmission. It may achieve this either by prejunctional action that increases or decreases transmitter release or by postjunctional action that alters the time course or extent of action of the transmitter, or both (Fig. 6.4B).

Finally, it should be emphasized that if this model of the autonomic effector junction is true, then the earlier emphasis on looking for images of specialized nerve–cell close apposition may not be appropriate; even if a varicosity has a passing close relation with a cell, releasing transmitter for which receptors are expressed on that cell (e.g., mast cells, epithelial cells, or even immune cells) then, in effect, that cell is innervated.

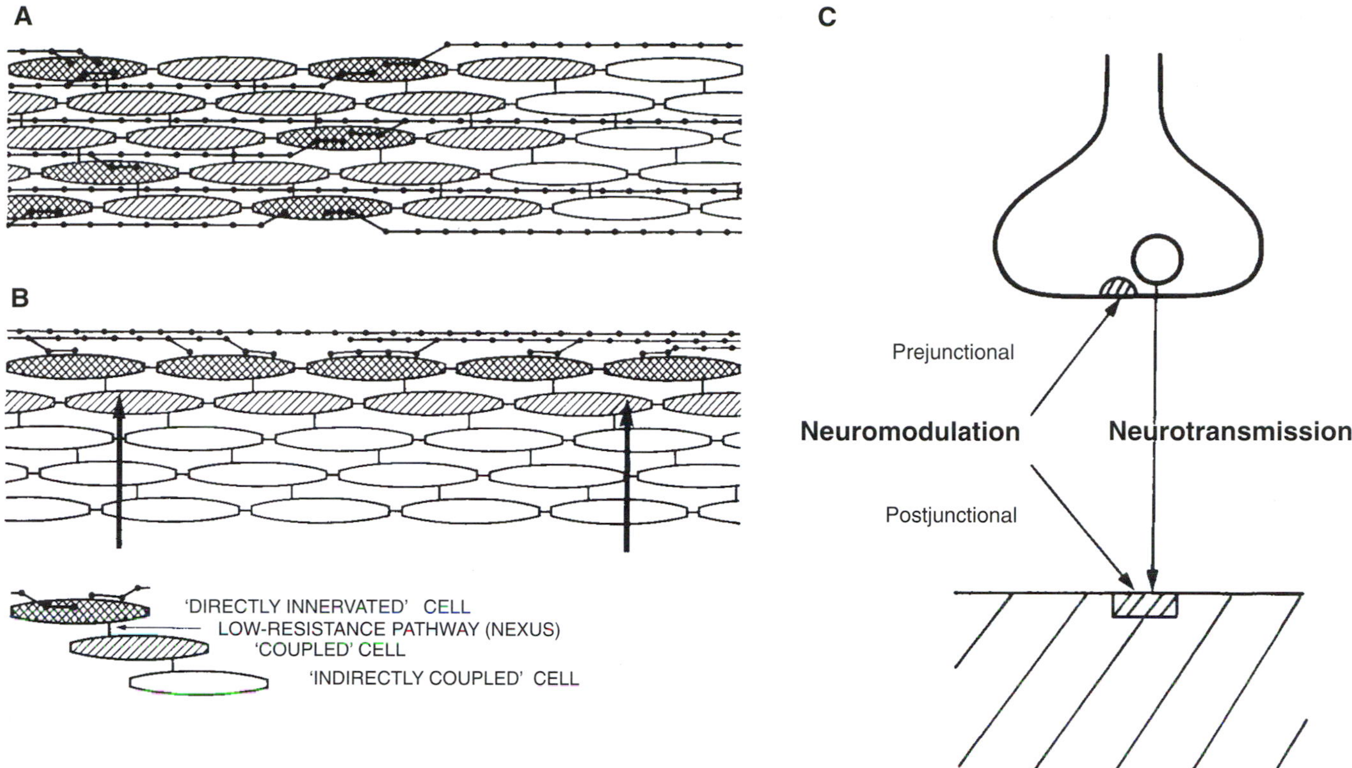

FIGURE 6.4 **A**, Schematic representation of control of visceral smooth muscle. "Directly innervated" cells (*cross-hatched*) are those that are directly activated by neurotransmitter; "coupled cells" (*hatched*) are those where junction potentials spread from "directly innervated" cells, when a sufficient area of the muscle effector bundle is depolarized, a propagated action potential will activate the "indirectly coupled" cells (*white*). **B**, Schematic representation of control of vascular smooth muscle by nerves (-●●-) and endothelial factors (*arrows*). (**A** and **B**, Reproduced with permission from Burnstock, G. 1975. Control of smooth muscle activity in vessels by adrenergic nerves and circulating catecholamines. In *Smooth muscle pharmacology and physiology. Les colloques de l'INSERM, Vol. 50*, 251–264. Paris: INSERM.) **C**, Schematic representation of prejunctional and postjunctional neuromodulation. (Reproduced with permission from Burnstock, G. 1982. Neuromuscular transmitters and trophic factors. In *Advanced medicine 18*, M. Sarner, Ed, 143–148. London: Pitman Medical.)

References

1. Burnstock, G., and T. Iwayama. 1971. Fine structural identification of autonomic nerves and their relation to smooth muscle. In *Progress in Brain Research, 34, Histochemistry of Nervous Transmission*. O. Eränkö, Ed, 389–404. Amsterdam: Elsevier.
2. Sandow, S. L., D. Whitehouse, and C. E. Hill. 1998. Specialised sympathetic neuroeffector associations in rat iris arterioles. *J. Anat.* 192(Pt 1):45–57.
3. Luff, S. E. 1996. Ultrastructure of sympathetic axons and their structural relationship with vascular smooth muscle. *Anat. Embryol. (Berl)* 193:515–531.
4. Bennett, M. R., and W. G. Gibson. 1995. On the contribution of quantal secretion from close-contact and loose-contact varicosities to the synaptic potentials in the vas deferens. *Philos. Trans. R. Soc. Lond B Biol. Sci* 347:187–204.
5. Brain, K. L., V. M. Jackson, S. J. Trout, and T. C. Cunnane. 2002. Intermittent ATP release from nerve terminals elicits focal smooth muscle Ca2+ transients in mouse vas deferens. *J. Physiol.* 541:849–862.
6. Stjärne, L. 1989. Basic mechanisms and local modulation of nerve impulse-induced secretion of neurotransmitters from individual sympathetic nerve varicosities. *Rev. Physiol Biochem. Pharmacol.* 112:1–137.
7. Dutton, J. L., P. Poronnik, G. H. Li, C. A. Holding, R. A. Worthington, R. J. Vandenberg, D. I. Cook, J. A. Barden, and M. R. Bennett. 2000. $P2X_1$ receptor membrane redistribution and down-regulation visualized by using receptor-coupled green fluorescent protein chimeras. *Neuropharmacology* 39:2054–2066.
8. Hansen, M. A., V. J. Balcar, J. A. Barden, and M. R. Bennett. 1998. The distribution of single P_{2X1}-receptor clusters on smooth muscle cells in relation to nerve varicosities in the rat urinary bladder. *J. Neurocytol.* 27:529–539.
9. Burnstock, G. 1979. Autonomic innervation and transmission. *Br. Med. Bull.* 35:255–262.
10. Burnstock, G. 1986. Autonomic neuromuscular junctions: Current developments and future directions. The Third Anatomical Society Review Lecture. *J. Anat.* 146:1–30.
11. Burnstock, G., and R. W. Straub. 1958. A method for studying the effects of ions and drugs on the resting and action potentials in smooth muscle with external electrodes. *J. Physiol.* 140:156–167.

7 Autonomic Neuromuscular Transmission

Max R. Bennett
Neurobiology Laboratory
Department of Physiology
Institute for Biomedical Research
University of Sydney
Sydney, Australia

NEW TRANSMITTERS AND THE CONCEPT OF COTRANSMITTERS

The greatest surprise in the study of autonomic neuroeffector transmission, after the discovery that transmitters other than noradrenaline and acetylcholine exist (see Chapter 3), followed from the observation of Furchgott and Zawadzki [2] on the obligatory role of endothelial cells in the relaxation of arterial smooth muscle by acetylcholine. This pointed to the existence of a substance that, when released from endothelial cells, acts on vascular smooth muscle cells to relax them. The subsequent identification of this substance as nitric oxide (see, e.g., Reference 3) led to the discovery that nitric oxide is a principal transmitter at some autonomic neuromuscular junctions. The identity of new transmitters other than the classical noradrenaline and acetylcholine (see Chapter 3) raises the question as to the relation between the new and the classical transmitters in the control of the viscera and the vasculature. Burnstock [4] proposed that nerve terminals may release more than one transmitter, in many cases the release of a classical transmitter from a terminal being accompanied with that of a new transmitter, which he referred to as a cotransmitter. This concept, which seemed radical at the time, is now well established [5].

VARICOSITIES, VESICLE-ASSOCIATED PROTEINS, AND CALCIUM FLUXES

By 1972, it was known that varicosities are the source of transmitter release at autonomic nerve endings, that once a transmitter is released it may act back on the varicosities to modify their capacity to secrete further, and that in the case of catecholamines, the varicosities also remove the transmitter by an active uptake process (see Chapter 3). More recently, it has been established that synaptic vesicles in these varicosities possess proteins required for exocytosis, namely synaptobrevin and SNAP25, and that these are accumulated at a site that is defined by a high concentration of syntaxin on the varicosity membrane necessary for vesicle docking [6]. Furthermore, introduction of methods that allow identification of the calcium influx into nerve terminals necessary to trigger transmitter release show that all varicosities receive a calcium influx on propagation of the terminal action potential [7]. Each varicosity along the length of a sympathetic terminal collateral branch then has the capacity to secrete transmitter on arrival of the nerve impulse.

IONOTROPIC RECEPTORS ARE LOCALIZED TO THE MUSCLE MEMBRANE AT VARICOSITIES

Although there are many different receptor types on the muscular effectors of the autonomic nervous system (see Chapter 3), only the spatial distribution of the purinergic subtype P2X1 ionotropic receptor has been described in detail at reasonably high resolution. Two size classes of P2X1 receptor patches, one about 1 μm in diameter and the other about 0.4 μm in diameter, occur in smooth muscles, with a large size uniquely associated with varicosities (see, e.g., Reference 6). It has generally been taken for granted that metabotropic receptors will not be located in any special way with respect to varicosities, but this is yet to be tested with adequate techniques.

METABOTROPIC AND IONOTROPIC RECEPTORS ARE INTERNALIZED AND RECYCLED AFTER BINDING TRANSMITTER

The question arises as to the stability of receptors located in the membranes of muscle cells—that is, whether they are of the metabotropic or ionotropic type (see Chapter 3).

This chapter begins at the time of publication of Bennett's (1972) monograph [1], "Autonomic Neuromuscular Transmission" and ends in 2000. See Chapter 3, "Milestones in Autonomic Research," for further comments on the autonomic neuroeffector junction.

Chuang and colleagues showed more than 20 years ago that desensitization of the beta-adrenergic receptor on binding transmitter is associated with receptor internalization [8] into lysosomes [9]. Subsequently, Lefkowitz and colleagues showed that such internalized receptors could recycle to the membrane [10] and that desensitization of the beta-adrenergic receptor after activation involved its phosphorylation before internalization [11]. This work on the beta-adrenergic receptor formed the basis for studies of desensitization and internalization of all the other metabotropic receptors on autonomic effectors. It has been taken for granted that because no evidence has accrued for internalization and recycling of the nicotinic receptor at the somatic neuromuscular junction on binding ligand, the other ionotropic receptors would likewise fail to undergo such recycling. Therefore, it came as a surprise when the P2X1 ionotropic receptor on smooth muscle was subsequently shown to internalize on bindings to its transmitter [12].

SOURCES OF INTRACELLULAR CALCIUM IN SMOOTH MUSCLE FOR INITIATING CONTRACTION

An increase in intracellular calcium ion concentration is required for the initiation of contraction in muscle effectors [13]. After identification of calcium as the ion responsible for the action potential in smooth muscle (see Chapter 3), second messenger pathways were identified that also trigger the release of calcium from intracellular stores [14] (see Chapter 3). A further source of calcium is provided by the action of certain transmitters on their receptors, which increases the intracellular calcium concentration as a consequence of the relatively high calcium permeability of the channel opened by the receptor. Such is the case for adenosine triphosphate acting on P2X1 purinoceptors in smooth muscle [15]. The increases in calcium concentration in smooth muscle from these different sources have been directly observed by Fay and colleagues on the introduction of techniques for observing calcium in single smooth muscle cells using appropriate calcium indicators [16].

MODULATION OF CALCIUM INFLUX AND THE CONTROL OF HYPERTENSION

There is considerable evidence for altered calcium channel function in vascular smooth muscle during hypertension, suggesting that deficiencies in the action of the calcium channel per se contributes in a major way to the etiology of this condition [17]. Identification of the pathways for increasing calcium in vascular smooth muscle cells and cardiac muscle cells has led to the development of some of the main blood pressure lowering agents, including calcium channel blockers and beta-adrenoceptor blockers [18].

References

1. Bennet, M. R. 1972. Autonomic neuromuscular transmission. *Monographs of the Physiological Society, No. 30.* Cambridge, UK: Cambridge University Press.
2. Furchgott, R. F., and J. V. Zawadzki. 1980. The obligatory role of endothelial cells in the relaxation of arterial smooth muscle by acetylcholine. *Nature (London)* 288:373–376.
3. Ignarro, L. J., G. M. Buga, K. S. Wood, R. E. Byrns, and G. Chaudhuri. 1987. Endothelium derived relaxing factor produced and released from artery and vein is nitric oxide. *Proc. Natl. Acad. Sci. USA* 84:9265–9269.
4. Burnstock, G. 1976. Do some nerve cells release more than one transmitter? *Neuroscience (Oxford)* 1:239–248.
5. Hokfelt, T., K. Fuxe, and B. Pernow B, Eds. 1986. Coexistence of neuronal messengers: A new principle in chemical transmission. *Prog. Brain. Res.* 68:3–405. Amsterdam: Elsevier.
6. Barden, J. A., L. J. Cottee, and M. R. Bennett. 1999. Vesicle associated proteins and P2X receptor clusters at single sympathetic varicosities in mouse vas deferens. *J. Neurocytol.* 28:469–480.
7. Brain, K. L., and M. R. Bennett. 1997. Calcium in sympathetic varicosities of mouse vas deferens during facilitation, augmentation and autoinhibition. *J. Physiol. (Cambridge)* 502:521–536.
8. Chuang, D. M., L. Farber, W. J. Kinnier, and E. Costa. 1980. Beta-adrenergic receptors from frog erythrocytes: Receptor internalization as a mechanism for receptor desensitization. *Adv. Biochem. Psychopharmacol.* 21:143–150.
9. Chuang, D. M. 1982. Internalization of beta-adrenergic receptor binding sites: Involvements of lysosomal enzymes. *Biochem. Biophys. Res. Commun.* 105:1466–1472.
10. Stadel, J. M., P. Nambi, R. G. Shorr, D. F. Sawyer, M. G. Caron, and R. J. Lefkowitz. 1983. Catecholamine-induced desensitization of turkey erythrocyte adenylate cyclase is associated with phosphorylation of the beta-adrenergic receptor. *Proc. Natl. Acad. Sci. USA* 80:3173–3177.
11. Strulovici, B., and R. J. Lefkowitz. 1984. Activation, desensitization, and recycling of frog erythrocyte beta-adrenergic receptors: Differential perturbation by in situ trypsinizaton. *J. Biol. Chem.* 259:4389–4395.
12. Dutton, J. L., P. Poronnik, G. H. Li, C. A. Holding, R. A. Worthington, R. J. Vandenberg, D. I. Cook, J. A. Barden, and M. R. Bennett. 2000. P2X1 receptor membrane redistribution and down regulation visualized by using receptor coupled green fluorescent protein chimeras. *Neuropharmacology* 39:2054–2066.
13. Somlyo, A. P., and A. V. Somlyo. 1994. Signal transduction and regulation in smooth muscle. *Nature (London)* 372:231–236.
14. Ehrlich, B. E., and J. Watras. 1988. Inositol 1,4,5-triphosphate activates a channel from smooth muscle sarcoplasmic reticulum. *Nature (London)* 336:583–586.
15. Benham, C. D., and R. W. Tsien. 1987. A novel receptor-operated calcium permeable channel activated by ATP in smooth muscle. *Nature (London)* 328:275–278.
16. Fay, F. S., H. H. Shlevin, W. C. Granger, Jr., and S. R. Taylor. 1979. Aequorin luminescence during activation of single isolated smooth muscle cells. *Nature (London)* 280:506–508.
17. Hermsmeyer, K. 1993. Calcium channel function in hypertension. *J. Hum. Hypertens.* 7:173–176.
18. Parving, H. H. 2001. Hypertension and diabetes: The scope of the problem. *Blood Press. Suppl.* (Suppl 2):25–31.

8 Dopaminergic Neurotransmission

Christopher Bell
Department of Physiology
Trinity College Dublin
Dublin, Ireland

The catecholamines share a common synthetic pathway, with dopamine (DA) being the immediate precursor of noradrenaline (NA) (Fig. 8.1), so it is not surprising that dopaminergic and noradrenergic neurons have many similarities. The existence of a large dopaminergic pool of neurons in the striatum has allowed the chemical, functional, and pharmacologic characteristics of this phenotype to be explored in detail. In the sympathetic nervous system, there is evidence for dopaminergic neural influences on a variety of visceral functions, particularly renal function, digestive tract motility, and vascular resistance. However, these dopaminergic neurons are admixed with larger populations of noradrenergic cells. It is therefore necessary to be able to accurately define the differences between the two types. Classification of the receptors on which neurogenic DA acts, and some of its functional correlates, may be found in later chapters of this book. This chapter is concerned solely with the neurochemical features that can be exploited to distinguish dopaminergic from noradrenergic phenotypes. The reading list does not attempt to be comprehensive, but provides sources with useful summaries of specific aspects of the field.

TRANSMITTER NEUROCHEMISTRY

Transmitter Synthesis

Both dopaminergic and noradrenergic neurons synthesize their transmitters primarily from plasma tyrosine; thus, both contain tyrosine hydroxylase (TH), and the levels and presence of this enzyme throughout the neuron are similar for both types. Because only noradrenergic cells convert DA to NA, only these cells require dopamine β-hydroxylase (DBH). In these cells, DBH also is present throughout the length of the neuron at similar levels. However, antigenically active DBH is absent from dopaminergic cells [1, 2].

The intermediate enzyme, dopa decarboxylase (DDC), is present in low concentrations within proximal parts of noradrenergic cells, but is absent, at least in immunologically demonstrable amounts, from the terminal regions [1, 2]. It has been suggested that the absence of DDC from noradrenergic terminals is a consequence of down-regulation by high local levels of end product. However, experimental depletion of NA stores for up to seven days does not result in demonstrable levels of DDC, suggesting that at least in the short term, the absence is a phenotypic characteristic [3]. By contrast, the terminal regions of dopaminergic axons contain levels of DDC equivalent to those in cell bodies and proximal axons, probably reflecting partial reliance of transmitter synthesis on uptake of plasma dopa and on intraneuronal hydroxylation of tyrosine. This is consistent with the fact that after total catecholamine depletion with reserpine, transmitter stores in dopaminergic neurons, but not in noradrenergic neurons, can be partially repleted by systemic administration of L-dopa. The membrane uptake process is not restricted to terminal axons because repletion also can be demonstrated in cell bodies. Repletion occurs only in the presence of monoamine oxidase inhibition, confirming that conversion of dopa to DA is cytoplasmic in location, as it is in noradrenergic neurons [1, 2].

Transmitter Storage and Release

Ultrastructural and ultracentrifugation studies indicate that storage of transmitter in dopaminergic and noradrenergic axons occurs in the same type of small vesicle, the storage matrices of which can be visualized by creation of electron-dense chromate complexes. These vesicular stores are depleted equally effectively from both dopaminergic and noradrenergic nerves by the alkaloid reserpine, which enters the neuron by passive diffusion and displaces catecholamine molecules from their protein-binding sites.

At noradrenergic synapses, presynaptic adrenoceptors exist, whose activation reduces further NA release. Studies suggest that a comparable feedback process exists at dopaminergic synapses, with autoinhibition of release by activation of presynaptic D_2 receptors [4].

Transmitter Recycling

After activation-induced release, both NA and DA are taken back into the axon terminals through specific trans-

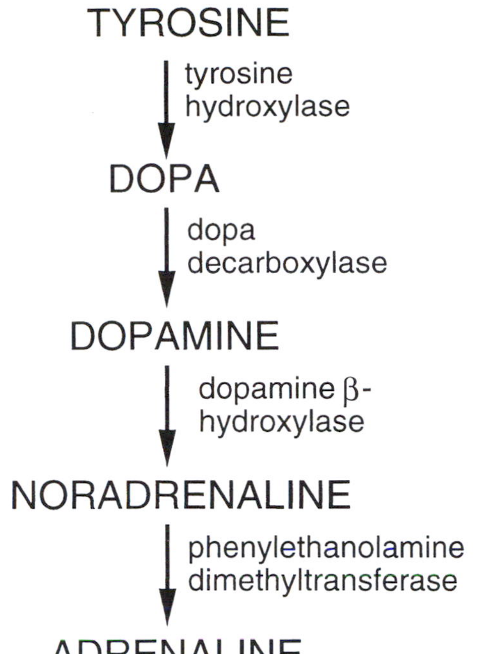

FIGURE 8.1 The neuronal synthetic pathway for catecholamines.

porters [5, 6]. The transporter on the noradrenergic plasma membrane is denoted as $Uptake_1$ and can be selectively inhibited by tricyclic antidepressants such as imipramine. The dopaminergic membrane transporter is not sensitive to $Uptake_1$ inhibitors, but is selectively inhibited by a series of aryl dialkylpiperazine molecules typified by GBR12909. Some antiparkinsonian drugs such as benztropine also inhibit DA transport, but they exert a degree of inhibition on $Uptake_1$ at the same concentrations.

The presence of these selective transporters allows differential entry to dopaminergic and noradrenergic axons of some pharmacologic agents that affect vesicular catecholamine binding. Thus, guanethidine, which preferentially uses the NA transporter ($Uptake_1$), depletes transmitter stores from noradrenergic axons at doses that do not affect dopaminergic terminals [7]. The synthetic DA analog 6-hydroxydopamine is taken up equally avidly by both transporters, but it can be restricted to dopaminergic and noradrenergic axons in the presence of an appropriately selective transport inhibitor.

The characteristics of noradrenergic and dopaminergic neurons are summarized in Table 8.1, and Table 8.2 outlines the procedures that can be applied experimentally to distinguish the dopaminergic phenotype. Notably, the criteria to be applied are not restricted to the autonomic nervous system, and there is no reason to believe that they are applicable only to mammalian species.

TABLE 8.1 Summary of Major Neurochemical Features Characterizing Noradrenergic and Dopaminergic Neurons

Feature	Noradrenergic	Dopaminergic
Synthesis	Tyrosine hydroxylation throughout neuron	Tyrosine hydroxylation throughout neuron
	Dopa decarboxylation only in proximal neuron	Dopa decarboxylation throughout neuron
	Transmitter synthesis solely from plasma tyrosine	Transmitter synthesis from both plasma tyrosine and plasma dopa
	Final step in transmitter synthesis intravesicular	Final step in transmitter synthesis cytoplasmic
Storage	Some vesicular storage of precursor dopamine with noradrenaline in ratio c. 1:20–1:100	Not known if any dopa costored in vesicles with DA
Release	Inhibitory feedback on release through presynaptic α-adrenoreceptors	Inhibitory feedback on release by presynaptic D_2 receptors
Inactivation	Inactivation by reuptake through NA transporter ($Uptake_1$)	Inactivation by reuptake through DA transporter

DA, dopamine; NA, noradrenaline.

FUTURE QUESTIONS

A major uncertainty is the extent to which the distinction between noradrenergic and dopaminergic neurons is immutable. The demonstration that cholinergic and catecholaminergic sympathetic neurons originate from a single neural crest precursor [8] indicates that dopaminergic and noradrenergic cells share a common ancestry and that the phenotypic distinction is because of environmental influences. However, the fact that dopaminergic and noradrenergic sympathetic axons innervate the same effector cells argues against this environmental influence being a simple retrograde neurotrophic one. Studies of developing mesencephalic cells have indicated that the trophic cocktail necessary for expression of TH is considerably less complex than that needed for coexpression of other characteristics of the dopaminergic phenotype, such as DDC and the DA transporter [9]. It is therefore possible that chronic alterations in availability of various factors in adulthood could affect changes in noradrenergic and dopaminergic phenotype or the reverse.

A further possibility is that chronic alteration of transmitter function could influence expression of the phenotypic markers. For example, sympathetic noradrenergic axons in patients with DBH deficiency store substantial amounts of DA and this is released in response to reflex sympathetic stimulation [10]. The plasma membranes of these axons must therefore be exposed chronically to far greater levels of DA than normal, and this could alter expression of the DA transporter. Such questions are of considerable biological and some clinical significance and warrant further research.

TABLE 8.2 Checklist of Useful Experimental Approaches to Identification of Dopaminergic Autonomic Neurons

Criterion	Comments	Methodologies
Synthesis		
Intraneuronal level of TH typical of catecholaminergic cell	Use noradrenergic neuron as positive control.	Immunohistochemistry
Absence of dopamine β-hydroxylase	Use noradrenergic neuron as positive control.	Immunohistochemistry
Dopa decarboxylase in terminal axon	Use noradrenergic neuron as negative control; use colocalization of TH to exclude "amine-handling" neurons.	Immunohistochemistry
Storage		
High intraneuronal concentration of endogenous DA, stored in chromaffin-reactive vesicles	For immunohistochemical studies, use noradrenergic neuron as negative control. For biochemical studies, pharmacologic manipulations may be needed to show independence from noradrenergic neurons (see below).	Immunohistochemistry, biochemistry, electron microscopy
Axon carries DA transporter	Use noradrenergic neuron as negative control. Some pharmacologic approaches also target the transporter (see below).	Immunohistochemistry
DA stores resistant to guanethidine depletion	Use noradrenergic neuron as positive control.	Immunohistochemistry, biochemistry, electron microscopy
DA stores depleted by reserpine	Exclude nonneuronal cellular origin in SIF, SNIF, or enterochromaffin cells. Similar effect on noradrenergic storage of NA and DA.	Immunohistochemistry, biochemistry
After reserpine, DA stores repleted by exogenous L-dopa	Monoamine oxidase inhibition may be necessary. Use noradrenergic neuron as negative control.	Immunohistochemistry, biochemistry, electron microscopy
DA depletion by 6-hydroxydopamine prevented by DA transporter inhibition, not by $Uptake_1$ inhibition	Check that in noradrenergic neuron depletion of both NA and DA prevented by $Uptake_1$ inhibition, not by DA transporter inhibition.	Immunohistochemistry, biochemistry, electron microscopy
Action potential-dependent release of DA independent of NA	Remember that some DA is released from noradrenergic neurons.	Biochemistry
Postsynaptic effect abolished by inactivation of DA receptors, not affected by adrenoreceptor antagonists	Beware nonspecificity of some antagonists.	Function
DA release, postsynaptic effects enhanced by inhibition of DA transporter, not by $Uptake_1$ inhibition	Check that comparable parameters at noradrenergic synapses enhanced by $Uptake_1$ blockade, not by DA transporter inhibition.	Biochemistry, function

Note the importance of using known noradrenergic neurons (same species, same preparative procedures, preferably same individual) as controls. DA, dopamine; NA, noradrenaline; TH, tyrosine hydroxylase.

References

1. Bell, C. 1991. Peripheral dopaminergic nerves. In *Novel peripheral neurotransmitters*, ed. C. Bell, 135–160. Oxford: Pergamon Press.
2. Ferguson, M., and C. Bell. 1993. Autonomic innervation of the kidney and ureter. In *Nervous control of the urogenital system*, ed. C. A. Maggi, 1–31. London: Harwood Academic Publishers.
3. Mann, R., and C. Bell. 1991. Neuronal metabolism and DOPA decarboxylase immunoreactivity in terminal noradrenergic sympathetic axons of rat. *J. Histochem. Cytochem.* 39:663–668.
4. Benoit-Marand, M., E. Borelli, and F. Gonon. 2001. Inhibition of dopamine release via presynaptic D2 receptors: Time course and function characteristics in vivo. *J. Neuorsci.* 21:9134–9141.
5. Eisenhofer, G. 2001. The role of neuronal and extraneuronal plasma membrane transporters in the inactivation of peripheral catecholamines. *Pharmacol. Ther.* 91:35–62.
6. Holzschuh, J., S. Ryu, F. Aberger, and W. Driever, W. 2001. Dopamine transporter expression distinguishes dopaminergic neurons from other catecholaminergic neurons in the developing zebrafish embryo. *Mech. Dev.* 101:237–243.
7. Villanueva, I., M. Pinon, L. Quevedo-Corona, R. Martinez-Olivares, and R. Racotta. 2003. Epinephrine and dopamine colocalization with norepinephrine in various peripheral tissues: guanethidine effects. *Life Sci.* 73:1645–1653.
8. Yamamori, T. 1996. Leukemia inhibitory factor and phenotypic specialization. In *Chemical factors in neural growth, degeneration and repair*, ed. C. Bell, 265–292. Amsterdam: Elsevier Science.
9. Ling, Z. D., E. D. Potter, L. W. Lipton, and P. M. Carvey. 1998. Differentiation of mesencephalic progenitor cells in dopaminergic neurons by cytokines. *Exp. Neurol.* 149:411–423.
10. Thompson, J. M., C. J. O'Callaghan, B. A. Kingwell, G. W. Lambert, G. L. Jennings, and M. D. Esler. 1995. Total norepinephrine spillover, muscle sympathetic nerve activity and heart-rate spectral analysis in a patient with dopamine β-hydroxylase deficiency. *J. Auton. Nerv. Syst.* 55:198–206.

9 Dopamine Receptors

Aki Laakso
Howard Hughes Medical Institute Laboratories
Department of Cell Biology
Duke University Medical Center
Durham, North Carolina

Marc G. Caron
Howard Hughes Medical Institute Laboratories
Department of Cell Biology
Duke University Medical Center
Durham, North Carolina

Dopamine is a catecholamine that has a crucial physiologic role in the regulation of movement, affect, cognition, reward, and hormone release. Its involvement in several neuropsychiatric disorders has become increasingly evident since 1958, when it was discovered to act as a neurotransmitter by Nobel laureate Arvid Carlsson. Parkinson's disease, for example, is caused by a specific degeneration of dopaminergic neurons in the brain, leading to dopamine deficiency and a neurologic syndrome characterized by muscle rigidity, tremor, and difficulty in initiating movements. Conversely, practically all addictive drugs of abuse—as well as naturally reinforcing behaviors such as eating and having sex—cause pleasure by increasing synaptic dopamine concentrations in the brain reward areas, such as nucleus accumbens (also called ventral striatum in humans and other primates). Furthermore, the brain dopaminergic system seems to be overactive in schizophrenic psychosis, and dopamine receptor antagonists have formed the mainstay of antipsychotic pharmacotherapy for more than 40 years.

Dopamine released from presynaptic nerve terminals elicits its effect through a family of G protein–coupled dopamine receptors. In the 1970s it became evident that at least two classes of dopamine receptors (D1 and D2) were required to explain all the physiologic effects of dopamine and the pharmacologic profile of drugs blocking its actions. This traditional classification was mainly based on the ability of D1 receptors to stimulate the signal transduction enzyme adenylate cyclase, whereas D2 receptors either did not have an effect or inhibited it. Development of molecular cloning techniques subsequently led to the identification of all five dopamine receptors, but physiologic classification to D1-like (D1 and D5) and D2-like (D2, D3, and D4) receptors still seems practical today, because many properties in structure, signaling, and pharmacology are shared within subfamilies.

STRUCTURAL AND FUNCTIONAL CHARACTERISTICS OF DOPAMINE RECEPTORS

Gene Structure

The genomic organization of dopamine receptor genes supports the idea that dopamine receptors have evolved from two distinct gene families, giving rise to D1-like and D2-like subfamilies [1–5]. Like many genes for G protein–coupled receptors, the coding regions of D1 and D5 receptor genes lack introns (Table 9.1). Interestingly, the human genome contains two D5 receptor pseudogenes, D5ψ1 and D5ψ2, that are almost identical (95%) with the D5 gene, but have premature termination codons. Although they are expressed with distribution similar to the D5 receptor, the mRNA appear not to be translated. D2-like receptor genes, in contrast, have several introns in their coding regions (see Table 9.1). Two isoforms of the D2 receptor, D2-short (D2S) and D2-long (D2L), are formed by alternative splicing of an 87-base pair (bp) exon between introns 4 and 5. Although they are expressed in the same regions, D2L is more ubiquitous. The functional significance of the two D2 isoforms is discussed later. Several splice variants of the D3 receptor mRNA also exist, although these seem to be species-specific and many of them are not translated to functional proteins. The human D4 receptor gene shows considerable allelic variation. The number and sequence of 48-bp repeat insertions in the coding region for third intracellular loop are variable, with a four repeat allele being the most frequent in studied populations. The functional consequences of this polymorphism still remain obscure.

Receptor Structure

All dopamine receptors belong to a superfamily of G protein–coupled receptors with seven transmembrane regions (Fig. 9.1) [1–5]. D1-like receptors have a relatively

TABLE 9.1 Molecular Biology, Structure, and Pharmacology of Human Dopamine Receptors

	D1-like		D2-like		
	D1	**D5**	**D2**	**D3**	**D4**
Chromosomal localization	5q35.1	4p15.1–16.1	11q22–23	3q13.3	11p15.5
Introns	No	No	6	5	3
mRNA size	3.8 kb	3.0 kb	2.5 kb	8.3 kb	5.3 kb
Amino acids	446	477	414 (D2S) 443 (D2L)	400	387–515[a]
Agonists	Fenoldopam SKF 38393 SKF 81297 Apomorphine Dopamine	Fenoldopam SKF 38393 SKF 81297 Apomorphine Dopamine	Lisuride R(−)-NPA Bromocriptine Pergolide Dopamine Apomorphine Quinpirole	R(−)-NPA Lisuride Pergolide PD 128,907 7-OH-DPAT Quinpirole Bromocriptine Dopamine Apomorphine	Lisuride PD 168,077 Dopamine Pergolide Quinpirole
Antagonists	SCH 23390 SKF 83566 (+)-Butaclamol *cis*-Flupentixol	SCH 23390 SKF 83566 (+)-Butaclamol *cis*-Flupentixol	Spiperone Eticlopride Haloperidol (+)-Butaclamol Raclopride Chlorpromazine Sulpiride	Eticlopride Spiperone Raclopride (+)-Butaclamol Chlorpromazine Haloperidol Sulpiride	Spiperone L-745,870 Haloperidol Chlorpromazine Clozapine

[a] Depending on the number of 16 amino acid tandem repeats in the third cytoplasmic loop.

short third cytoplasmic loop and long C-terminal tail, whereas D2-like receptors have a considerably longer third cytoplasmic loop and short C-terminal tail. These structural properties are common in many G protein–coupled receptors that stimulate and inhibit adenylate cyclase, respectively. D1 and D5 receptors have two potential asparagine-linked glycosylation sites, one in the N-terminal region and the other in the second extracellular loop, whereas the D2 receptor has three glycosylation sites in the N-terminal region and one in the second extracellular loop, D3 has three, and D4 only one. All dopamine receptors have cysteine residues in the first and second extracellular loops, which form a disulfide bond and stabilize the receptor structure. The long C-terminal tail of D1-like receptors is anchored to the membrane with a palmitoylated cysteine residue near the last transmembrane region, whereas the short tail of D2-like receptors ends with a palmitoylated cysteine (see Fig. 9.1). Hydrophobic membrane-spanning regions seem to determine the ligand recognition, and thus the pharmacologic profile of these receptors. Accordingly, the sequence homology between receptor subtypes is greatest in these regions, being 78% between D1 and D5 receptors, 75% between D2 and D3, but only 53% between D2 and D4. Finally, the 29 amino acid insertion in the third cytoplasmic loop of the D2 receptor that differentiates between the short and long variants of the D2 receptor affects the coupling of the receptor to different G proteins. Therefore, it is not surprising that D2S and D2L seem to have differing physiologic functions in different neuronal cell types [6, 7].

SIGNAL TRANSDUCTION

D1-like Receptors

Since the early 1970s dopamine has been known to stimulate adenylate cyclase activity in the brain, leading to accumulation of the second messenger cyclic adenosine monophosphate [1–5]. This effect is mediated primarily through D1 receptors, although D5 receptors also are able to stimulate adenylate cyclase and may even display constitutive agonist-independent activity on this effector. Whereas D1 receptors can mediate this effect by coupling to $G_s\alpha$ subunits of G proteins, the most likely counterpart in the brain is $G_{olf}\alpha$, which is much more ubiquitous in brain regions where the D1 receptor is mostly expressed, such as the striatum. D1 receptors also can modulate the actitivity of Na^+/K^+-adenosine triphosphatase, affecting the neuronal depolarization state of neurons, as well as fluid absorption in the kidney. In kidney cells, D1 stimulation also inhibits the activity of the Na^+/H^+ ion pump. D1 receptors are also able to increase intracellular calcium levels through a variety of mechanisms, including the activation of phosphatidyli-

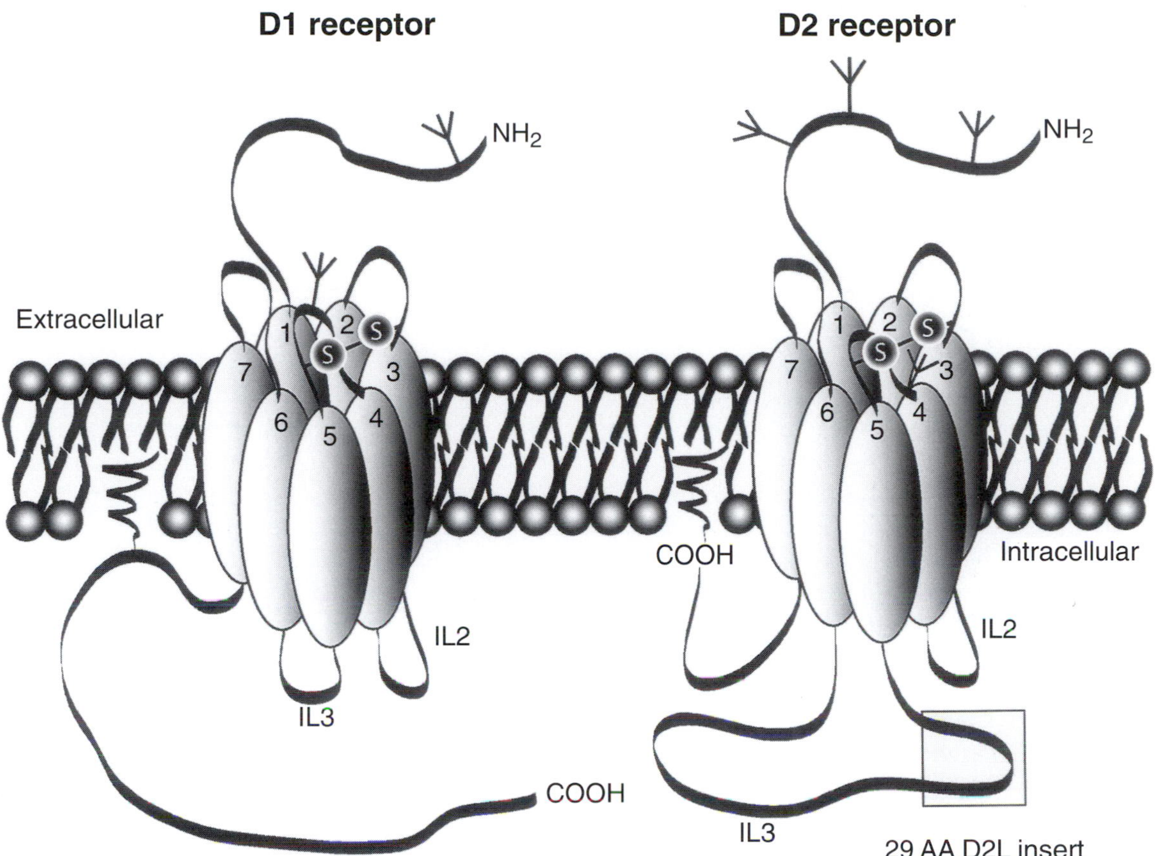

FIGURE 9.1 The structure of D1 and D2 dopamine receptors. Both are G protein–coupled receptors with seven transmembrane domains (numbered 1–7). The D1 receptor has a short third intracellular loop and a long C-terminal tail, which is palmitoylated and anchored to the membrane near the seventh transmembrane domain. The D2 receptor has a long third intracellular loop (containing the 29 amino acid insert in the D2L splice variant) and a short C-terminal tail, which ends with a palmitoylated cysteine. A disulfide bond connects the first and second extracellular loops of all dopamine receptors. The D1 receptor has two asparagine-linked glycosylation sites, whereas the D2 receptor has four. IL2, intracellular loop 2; IL3, intracellular loop 3.

nositol hydrolysis and modulation of calcium channels by protein kinase A activation.

D2-like Receptors

The ability of D2 receptors to inhibit adenylate cyclase was first observed in the anterior pituitary, where this signaling pathway is crucial for the regulation of prolactin release. Later, D3 and D4 receptors also were shown to inhibit adenylate cyclase. At least in the brain, this effect is most likely mediated by coupling of D2 receptors to the $G_o\alpha$ subunit, instead of various $G_i\alpha$ proteins [8]. In addition, D2-like receptors also can decrease intracellular calcium levels and induce cell hyperpolarization by increasing outward potassium currents. Physiologically, these effects are important for D2 receptor–mediated inhibition of prolactin release from lactotrophic cells in the anterior pituitary and for its function as an autoreceptor controlling dopamine release.

Oligomerization

Only recently, G protein–coupled receptor signaling, including that of dopamine receptors, was recognized to be regulated by the formation of receptor oligomers [9]. Oligomers or dimers may consist of the same receptors (homodimers) or even receptors for different neurotransmitters (heterodimers). D1 receptors have been found to dimerize at least with adenosine A1 receptors, D2 receptors with somatostatin SSTR5 receptors, and D5 with γ_2 subunits of $GABA_A$ receptor, which actually is a multimeric ion channel receptor. Oligomers usually have slightly different pharmacologic properties and may have surprisingly different signaling properties, when compared with interacting receptors expressed or activated alone. In the near future, this field of research may greatly increase our understanding of neurotransmitter interactions in the brain and periphery.

PHARMACOLOGY

The number of clinically used or scientifically interesting compounds acting as agonists or antagonists at dopamine receptors is enormous and cannot be thoroughly listed in this chapter. Rather, we will try to give a useful overview and name some drugs as typical examples (see Table 9.1) [1, 3–5]. Although several ligands display selectivity for D1-like dopamine receptors over D2-like receptors or vice versa, the development of truly subtype-specific ligands has proven difficult. Dopamine itself has a 10- to 100-fold greater affinity for D2 than D1 receptors, a 10-fold greater affinity for D5 than D1, and a 10- to 20-fold greater affinity for D3 and D4 than D2 receptors. D2 and D4 receptors also exist in high and low agonist affinity states, where the low affinity state probably represents spare receptors unable to couple to G proteins, perhaps because of subcellular localization. Clinically, dopamine receptor agonists, such as bromocriptine, are used as adjuvant therapy in Parkinson's disease and in the treatment of hyperprolactinaemia caused by benign pituitary adenomas, whereas antagonists of D2-like receptors, like haloperidol, are widely used as neuroleptic drugs in the treatment of schizophrenia and other psychoses. Some D2-like receptor antagonists, such as metoclopramide, also are effective as antiemetic drugs. Typical side effects of drugs blocking dopamine receptors include extrapyramidal neurologic symptoms resembling Parkinson's disease, and hyperprolactinemia. Radiolabeled receptor ligands have been used to study the distribution and density of dopamine receptors in brain slices and other organs such as the kidney, and also in humans using *in vivo* brain imaging. Examples for this include [^{3}H]/[^{11}C]SCH-23390 for D1-like receptors and [^{3}H]/[^{11}C]raclopride and [^{3}H]spiperone for D2 and D3 receptors.

DISTRIBUTION

The most striking feature of dopamine receptor distribution, especially in the brain, is that D1 and D2 receptors are expressed at the levels that are an order of magnitude or two greater compared with the other subtypes [3–5]. Moreover, the brain distribution of D1 and D2 receptors closely follows that of dopaminergic innervation, whereas D3, D4, and D5 receptors are expressed in more specialized patterns. However, it has been difficult to determine the actual distribution of these less common subtypes in the absence of truly specific radioligands. The most specific means of assessing the distribution is by *in situ* hybridization, but in the case of presynaptic receptors, the hybridization signal may be located far from the final localization of mature receptor proteins, which are subject to axonal transport.

DISTRIBUTION IN THE BRAIN

D1 Receptors

The D1 receptor is a postsynaptic dopamine receptor, and its highest levels are found in GABAergic medium spiny neurons in brain regions receiving dense dopaminergic innervation, including caudate and putamen, nucleus accumbens, and olfactory tubercle. In these regions, its density is approximately three times greater than the density of D2 receptors. Lower levels are found in cerebral cortex, amygdala, thalamus, hypothalamus, and hippocampus. In entopeduncular nucleus, globus pallidus, and substantia nigra pars reticulata, it is probably expressed in axon terminals of GABAergic neurons projecting from caudate and putamen.

D2 Receptors

D2 receptors are present both as postsynaptic receptors and presynaptic autoreceptors in dopaminergic neurons regulating neurotransmitter release. Recent evidence from genetically engineered animals suggests that D2L is more important in mediating postsynaptic responses (seen behaviorally, for example, as haloperidol-induced catalepsy in experimental animals), whereas D2S might be predominant, or at least sufficient, as an autoreceptor [6, 7]. Greatest densities are found in caudate and putamen, nucleus accumbens, and olfactory tubercle, where D2 is expressed as a postsynaptic receptor in medium spiny neurons and cholinergic interneurons, and as a presynaptic receptor in dopaminergic nerve terminals. D1 and D2 have opposite effects on adenylate cyclase, and their expression is actually mostly segregated to distinct populations of medium spiny neurons in these brain regions. Lower levels are expressed in substantia nigra pars compacta and ventral tegmental area, where most of the dopaminergic cell bodies are located, followed by prefrontal, cingulate, temporal and entorhinal cortices, septum, amygdala, and hippocampus.

D3 receptors

Like D2 receptors, D3 receptors also are expressed both as presynaptic and postsynaptic dopamine receptors. Their expression in the brain is limited to more limbic regions, including shell of the nucleus accumbens, islands of Calleja, and olfactory tubercle. Very low levels are found in substantia nigra, ventral tegmental area, hippocampus, cerebral cortex, and Purkinje cells of cerebellum.

D4 Receptors

The greatest levels of D4 receptor are found in frontal cortex, amygdala, olfactory tubercle, and hypothalamus, whereas only very low levels are seen in caudate, putamen, and nucleus accumbens.

D5 Receptors

The D5 receptor displays a restricted distribution, and at least mRNA is expressed in hippocampus, lateral mamillary nucleus, and parafascicular nucleus of the thalamus. Sensitive polymerase chain reaction methods also have revealed expression in few cells in caudate and putamen.

DOPAMINE RECEPTORS IN THE PERIPHERY

Outside the central nervous system, the most prominent function of dopamine receptors is probably the inhibition of prolactin release from anterior pituitary by D2 and possibly D4 receptors [5]. All dopamine receptor subtypes are also expressed in the kidney, where they participate in the regulation of fluid and sodium reabsorption and renin release. D1- and D2-like receptors are also found in both cortex and medulla of the adrenal gland, where they regulate aldosterone and catecholamine release, respectively. D2-like receptors in sympathetic ganglia and nerve terminals inhibit norepinephrine release, and both D1- and D2-like receptors are present in blood vessels controlling vasodilation. Moderately high levels (10 times greater than in the brain) of D4 receptors are found in the heart, but its function there is still unknown.

REGULATION

Dopamine receptors are under constant regulation [2, 3]. Chronic treatment with antipsychotic drugs that block dopamine receptors leads to increased expression and upregulation of D2 receptors in the brain. In contrast, in mice that lack the dopamine transporter, and thus have increased extracellular levels of dopamine, the expression of both D1 and D2 receptors is decreased by 50%. These long-term changes take place at the level of gene expression, but dopamine receptors also can undergo much more rapid regulation when stimulated by an agonist [10]. This agonist-dependent desensitization leads to phosphorylation of serine and threonine residues of the receptor, uncoupling from the effectors, and finally the internalization of the receptor, where it can be dephosphorylated and recycled back to the membrane.

References

1. Gingrich, J. A., and M. G. Caron. 1993. Recent advances in the molecular biology of dopamine receptors. *Annu. Rev. Neurosci.* 16:299–321.
2. Civelli, O., J. R. Bunzow, and D. K. Grandy. 1993. Molecular diversity of the dopamine receptors. *Annu. Rev. Pharmacol. Toxicol.* 32:281–307.
3. Jaber, M., S. W. Robinson, C. Missale, and M. G. Caron. 1996. Dopamine receptors and brain function. *Neuropharmacology* 35: 1503–1519.
4. Lachowicz, J. E., and D. R. Sibley. 1997. Molecular characteristics of mammalian dopamine receptors. *Pharmacol. Toxicol.* 81:105–113.
5. Missale, C., S. R. Nash, S. W. Robinson, M. Jaber, and M. G. Caron. 1998. Dopamine receptors: From structure to function. *Physiol. Rev.* 78:189–225.
6. Wang, Y., R. Xu, T. Sasaoka, S. Tonegawa, M. P. Kung, and E. B. Sankoorikal. 2000. Dopamine D2 long receptor-deficient mice display alterations in striatum-dependent functions. *J. Neurosci.* 20:8305–8314.
7. Usiello, A., J. H. Baik, F. Rougé-Pont, R. Picetti, A. Dierich, M. LeMeur, P. V. Piazza, and E. Borrelli. 2000. Distinct functions of the two isoforms of dopamine D2 receptors. *Nature* 408:199–203.
8. Jiang, M., K. Spicher, G. Boulay, Y. Wang, and L. Birnbaumer. 2001 Most central nervous system D2 dopamine receptors are coupled to their effectors by Go. *Proc. Natl. Acad. Sci. USA* 98:3577–3582.
9. Bouvier, M. 2001. Oligomerization of G protein–coupled transmitter receptors. *Nat. Rev. Neurosci.* 2:274–286.
10. Tiberi, M., S. R. Nash, L. Bertrand, R. J. Lefkowitz, and M. G. Caron. 1996. Differential regulation of dopamine D1A receptor responsiveness by various G protein–coupled receptor kinases. *J. Biol. Chem.* 271:3771–3778.

10 Noradrenergic Neurotransmission

David S. Goldstein
National Institutes of Health
Bethesda, Maryland

The chemical transmitter at sympathetic nerve endings is norepinephrine (NE). Sympathetic stimulation releases NE, and noradrenergic binding to adrenoceptors on cardiovascular smooth muscle cells causes the cells to contract. Sympathoneural NE therefore satisfies the main criteria defining a neurotransmitter: a chemical released from nerve terminals by electrical action potentials that interacts with specific receptors on nearby structures to produce specific physiologic responses.

Different stressors can elicit different patterns of sympathoneural outflows, and therefore differential NE release, in the various vascular beds. This redistributes blood flows. Local sympathoneural release of NE also markedly affects cardiac function and glandular activity. The adjustments usually are not sensed, and the organism usually does not feel distressed. Examples of situations associated with prominent changes in sympathoneural outflows include orthostasis, mild exercise, postprandial hemodynamic changes, mild changes in environmental temperature, and performance of nondistressing locomotor tasks.

In contrast, in response to perceived global threats, whether from external physical or internal psychologic or metabolic stimuli—especially when the organism senses an inability to cope with those stimuli—increased neural outflow to the adrenal medulla elicits catecholamine secretion into the adrenal venous drainage. In humans, the predominant catecholamine in the adrenal venous drainage is epinephrine (EPI). EPI rapidly reaches all cells of the body (with the exception of most of the brain), producing a wide variety of hormonal effects at low blood concentrations. One can comprehend all of the many effects of EPI in terms of countering acute threats to survival that mammals have faced perennially, such as sudden lack of metabolic fuels, trauma with hemorrhage, and antagonistic confrontations. Thus, even mild hypoglycemia elicits marked increases in plasma levels of EPI, in contrast with small increases in plasma levels of NE. Distress accompanies all these situations, the experience undoubtedly fostering the long-term survival of the individual and the species by motivating avoidance learning and producing signs universally understood among other members of the species.

Increases in adrenomedullary activity, as indicated by plasma EPI levels, often correlate more closely with increases in pituitary-adrenocortical activity, as indicated by plasma levels of corticotropin (ACTH), than with increases in sympathoneural activity, as indicated by plasma NE levels. For example, insulin-induced hypoglycemia produces drastic increases in plasma EPI and ACTH levels, with rather mild NE responses.

NORADRENERGIC INNERVATION OF THE CARDIOVASCULAR SYSTEM

Sympathetic nerves to the ventricular myocardium travel through the ansae subclaviae, branches of the left and right stellate ganglia. The fibers in the ansae subclaviae pass along the dorsal surface of the pulmonary artery into the plexus that supplies the left main coronary artery. In primates, cardiac sympathetic nerves originate about equally from the superior, middle, and inferior cervical (stellate) ganglia. Individual cardiac nerves supply relatively localized regions of myocardium, with the right sympathetic chain generally projecting to the anterior left ventricle and the left sympathetic chain to the posterior left ventricle. Sympathetic innervation of the sinus and atrioventricular nodes also has a degree of sidedness, the right sympathetics projecting more to the sinus node and the left to the atrioventricular node. Thus, left stellate stimulation produces relatively little sinus tachycardia.

Epicardial sympathetic nerves provide the main source of noradrenergic terminals in the myocardium. Sympathetic nerves travel with the coronary arteries in the epicardium before penetrating into the myocardium, whereas vagal nerves penetrate the myocardium after crossing the atrioventricular groove and then continue in the subendocardium. Postganglionic noradrenergic fibers reach all parts of the heart. The sinus and atrioventricular nodes and the atria receive the densest innervation, the ventricles less dense innervation, and the Purkinje fibers the least. Sympathetic and vagal afferents follow similar intracardiac routes to those of the efferents.

The heart contains high concentrations of NE compared with concentrations in other body organs. Atrial myocardium possesses the greatest concentrations. In humans, ventricular myocardial NE levels range from 3.5

to 14 nmol/g. Myocardial cells do not store NE; instead, myocardial NE is localized to vesicles in sympathetic nerves.

Although the coronary arteries possess sympathetic noradrenergic innervation, assessing the regulation and physiologic role of this innervation has proven to be difficult, because several interacting factors complicate neural control of the coronary vasculature. Alterations in myocardial metabolism and systemic hemodynamics change coronary blood flow, coronary vasomotion in response to sympathetic stimulation depends on the functional integrity of the endothelium, and coronary arteries appear to receive less dense innervation than do other arteries.

The body's myriad arterioles largely determine total resistance to blood flow and therefore contribute importantly to blood pressure. Sympathetic nerves enmesh blood vessels in lattice-like networks in the adventitial surface that extend inward to the adventitial–medial border, with the concentration of sympathetic nerves increasing as arterial caliber decreases, so that small arteries and arterioles, the smallest nutrient vessels possessing smooth muscle cells, possess the most intense innervation. The unique architectural association between sympathetic nerves and the vessels that determine peripheral resistance has enticed cardiovascular researchers, particularly in the area of autonomic regulation, for many years. Sympathetic vascular innervation varies widely among vascular beds, with dense innervation of resistance vessels in the gut, kidneys, skeletal muscle, and skin. Sympathetic stimulation in these beds produces profound vasoconstriction, whereas stimulation in the coronary, cerebral, and bronchial beds elicits weaker constrictor responses, consistent teleologically with the "goal" of preserving blood flow to vital organs.

NE released from sympathetic nerve terminals acts mainly locally, with only a small proportion of released NE reaching the bloodstream. One must therefore keep in mind the indirect and distant relation between plasma NE levels and sympathetic nerve activity in interpreting plasma NE levels in response to stressors, pathophysiologic situations, and drugs.

NOREPINEPHRINE: THE SYMPATHETIC NEUROTRANSMITTER

Norepinephrine Synthesis

Enzymatic steps in NE synthesis have been characterized in more detail than those for any other neurotransmitter. Catecholamine biosynthesis begins with uptake of the amino acid tyrosine (TYR) into the cytoplasm of sympathetic neurons, adrenomedullary cells, possibly paraaortic enterochromaffin cells, and specific centers in the brain. Tyrosine hydroxylase (TH) catalyzes the conversion of TYR to dihydroxyphenylalanine (dopa). This is the enzymatic rate-limiting step in catecholamine synthesis. The enzyme is almost saturated under normal conditions. Thus, although alterations in dietary TYR intake normally should not affect the rate of catecholamine biosynthesis under baseline conditions, after prolonged rapid turnover of catecholamines, TYR availability may become a limiting factor. The enzyme is stereospecific. Concentrations of tetrahydrobiopterin, Fe^{2+}, and molecular oxygen regulate TH activity. Dihydropteridine reductase (DHPR) catalyzes the reduction of dihydropterin produced during the hydroxylation of TYR. Because the reduced pteridine, tetrahydrobiopterin, is a key cofactor for TH, DHPR deficiency decreases the amount of TYR hydroxylation for a given amount of TH enzyme. Both phenylalanine hydroxylase and TH require tetrahydrobiopterin as a cofactor. Therefore, DHPR deficiency also inhibits phenylalanine metabolism and presents clinically as an atypical form of phenylketonuria.

Catecholamines and dopa feedback-inhibit TH, and α-methyl-*para*-TYR inhibits the enzyme competitively. Conversely, stressors that increase sympathetic neuronal and adrenomedullary hormonal outflows augment the synthesis and concentration of TH in sympathetic ganglia, sympathetically innervated organs, the adrenal gland, and the locus ceruleus of the pons. Multiple and complex mechanisms contribute to TH activation. Short-term mechanisms include feedback inhibition and phosphorylation of the enzyme, the latter depending on membrane depolarization, contractile elements, and receptors. Long-term mechanisms include changes in TH synthesis. During stress-induced sympathetic stimulation, acceleration of catecholamine synthesis in sympathetic nerves helps to maintain tissue stores of NE. Even with diminished stores after prolonged sympathoneural activation, increased nerve traffic can maintain extracellular fluid levels of the transmitter.

L-Aromatic amino acid decarboxylase (L-AAADC, also called dopa decarboxylase [DDC]) catalyzes the rapid conversion of dopa to dopamine (DA). Many types of tissues contain this enzyme—especially the kidneys, gut, liver, and brain. Activity of the enzyme depends on pyridoxal phosphate. Although DDC metabolizes most of the dopa formed in catecholamine-synthesizing tissues, some of the dopa enters the circulation unchanged. This provides the basis for using plasma dopa levels to examine catecholamine synthesis. α-Methyl-dopa, an effective drug in the treatment of high blood pressure, inhibits DDC and therefore NE synthesis. This inhibition does not explain the antihypertensive action of the drug; rather, α-methyl-NE, formed from α-methyl-dopa in catecholamine-synthesizing tissues, stimulates α-adrenoceptors in the brain, thereby inhibiting sympathetic outflows. Other DDC inhibitors include carbidopa and benserazide. These catechols do not readily penetrate the blood–brain barrier, and by inhibiting conversion of dopa to DA in the periphery, they enhance the efficacy of

L-dopa treatment of Parkinson's disease. DDC blockade increases dopa levels and decreases levels of dihydroxyphenylacetic acid (DOPAC), a DA metabolite. The rates of increase in extracellular fluid dopa levels and of decrease in DOPAC levels after acute DDC inhibition provide *in vivo* indexes of TH activity.

Dopamine β-hydroxylase (DBH) catalyzes the conversion of DA to NE. DBH is localized to tissues that synthesize catecholamines, such as noradrenergic neurons and chromaffin cells. DBH is confined to the vesicles. Thus, treatment with reserpine, which blocks the translocation of amines from the axonal cytoplasm into vesicles, prevents the conversion of DA to NE in sympathetic nerves. DBH contains, and its activity depends on, copper. Because of this dependence, children with Menkes disease, a rare, X-linked recessive inherited disorder of copper metabolism, have neurochemical evidence of concurrently increased catecholamine biosynthesis and decreased conversion of DA to NE, with high plasma and cerebrospinal fluid ratios of dopa:dihydroxyphenylglycol (DHPG, the neuronal NE metabolite). Patients with congenital absence of DBH have virtually undetectable levels of NE and DHPG and high levels of DA and DOPAC. DBH activity also requires ascorbic acid, which provides electrons for the hydroxylation. Phenylethanolamine-*N*-methyltransferase catalyzes the conversion of NE to EPI in the cytoplasm of chromaffin cells.

STORAGE

Varicosities in sympathetic nerves contain two types of cytoplasmic vesicles: small dense core (diameter 40–60 nm) and large dense core (diameter 80–120 nm). Vesicles generated near the Golgi apparatus of the cell bodies travel by axonal transport in the axons to the nerve terminals. Noradrenergic vesicles may also form by endocytosis within the axons. Because reserpine eliminates the electron-dense cores of the small but not the large vesicles, the cores of the small vesicles may represent NE, whereas the electron-dense cores of the large vesicles may represent additional components.

Cores of both types of vesicle contain adenosine triphosphate (ATP). The vesicles also contain at least three types of polypeptides: chromogranin A, an acidic glycoprotein; enkephalins; and neuropeptide Y (NPY). Extracellular fluid levels of each of these compounds have been considered as indexes of exocytosis. Vesicles in sympathetic nerves actively remove and trap axoplasmic amines. Vesicular uptake favors L- over D-NE, Mg^{2+} and ATP accelerate the uptake, and reserpine effectively and irreversibly blocks it. The vesicular uptake carrier protein resembles the neuronal uptake carriers. In the brain, mRNA for the vesicular transporter is expressed in monoamine-containing cells of the locus ceruleus, substantia nigra, and raphe nucleus, corresponding to noradrenergic, dopaminergic, and serotonergic centers. Neurotransmitter specificity appears to depend on different transporters in the cell membrane, rather than on different vesicular transporters.

Tissue NE stores are maintained by a balance of synthesis and turnover. Under resting conditions, the main determinant of NE turnover—that is, irreversible loss of NE from the tissue—is net leakage of NE from the vesicles into the axoplasm, with subsequent enzymatic breakdown of the axoplasmic NE.

Sympathetic neuroimaging using radio-iodinated meta-iodobenzylguanidine, positron-emitting analogs of sympathomimetic amines, and 6-[^{18}F]fluorodopamine depends on uptake of the imaging agents via the cell membrane NE transporter and then translocation into vesicles via the vesicular monoamine transporter. Visualization of sympathetic innervation in organs such as the heart therefore results from radiolabeling of the vesicles in sympathetic nerves.

RELEASE

Adrenomedullary chromaffin cells, much easier to study than sympathetic nerves, have provided the most commonly used model for studying mechanisms of catecholamine release. Agonist occupation of nicotinic acetylcholine receptors releases catecholamines from the cells. Because nicotinic receptors mediate ganglionic neurotransmission, researchers have presumed that the results obtained in adrenomedullary cells probably apply to postganglionic sympathoneural cells.

According to the exocytotic theory of NE release, acetylcholine depolarizes terminal membranes by increasing membrane permeability to sodium. The increased intracellular sodium levels directly or indirectly enhance transmembrane influx of calcium, through voltage-gated calcium channels. The increased cytoplasmic calcium concentration evokes a cascade of as yet incompletely defined biomechanical events resulting in fusion of the vesicular and axoplasmic membranes. The interior of the vesicle exchanges briefly with the extracellular compartment, and the soluble contents of the vesicles diffuse into the extracellular space. As predicted from this model, manipulations other than application of acetylcholine that depolarize the cell, such as electrical stimulation or increased K^+ concentrations in the extracellular fluid, also activate the voltage-gated calcium channels and trigger exocytosis. During cellular activation, simultaneous, stoichiometric release of soluble vesicular contents—ATP, enkephalins, chromogranins, and DBH—without similar release of cytoplasmic macromolecules, has provided biochemical support for the exocytosis theory. Electron micrographs occasionally have shown an "omega sign," with an apparent gap in the cell membrane at the site of fusion of vesicle with the axoplasmic membrane.

At least two storage pools of NE appear to exist in sympathetic nerve terminals—a small, readily releasable pool of newly synthesized NE and a large reserve pool in long-term storage. The relation between the two pools of NE and the two forms of vesicles, large and small dense core, has not been established.

Sympathetic nerve endings also can release NE by calcium-independent, nonexocytotic mechanisms. One such mechanism probably is reverse transport through the neuronal uptake carrier. The indirectly acting sympathomimetic amine, tyramine, releases NE nonexocytotically, because tyramine releases NE independently of calcium and does not release DBH. Myocardial ischemic hypoxia also evokes calcium-independent release of NE.

The hydrophilic nature of catecholamines and their ionization at physiologic pH probably prevent NE efflux by simple diffusion. As noted earlier, sympathetic stimulation releases other compounds besides NE. Some of these compounds may function as neurotransmitters. ATP, adenosine, NPY, acetylcholine, and EPI have received the most attention.

Pharmacologic stimulation of a large variety of receptors on noradrenergic terminals affects the amount of NE released during cellular activation. Compounds inhibiting NE release include acetylcholine, gamma-aminobutyric acid (GABA), prostaglandins of the E series, opioids, adenosine, and NE itself. Compounds enhancing NE release include angiotensin II, acetylcholine (at nicotinic receptors), ACTH, GABA (at $GABA_A$ receptors), and EPI (through stimulation of presynaptic β_2-adrenoceptors). In general, whether at physiologic concentrations these compounds exert modulatory effects on endogenous NE release remains unproven, especially in humans. An exception, however, is inhibitory presynaptic modulation by NE itself, through autoreceptors on sympathetic nerves. This modulatory action appears to vary with the vascular bed under study, being prominent in skeletal muscle beds such as the forearm, relatively weak in the kidneys, and virtually absent in the adrenals.

In addition to local feedback control of NE release, reflexive "long-distance" feedback pathways, through high- and low-pressure baroreceptors, elicit reflexive changes in sympathoneural impulse activity. Alterations in receptor numbers or of intracellular biomechanical events after receptor activation also affect responses to agonists. Therefore, these factors may regulate NE release by transsynaptic local and reflexive long-distance mechanisms.

DISPOSITION

Unlike acetylcholine, which is inactivated mainly by extracellular enzymes, NE is inactivated mainly by uptake into cells, with subsequent intracellular metabolism or storage (Fig. 10.1). Reuptake into nerve terminals—

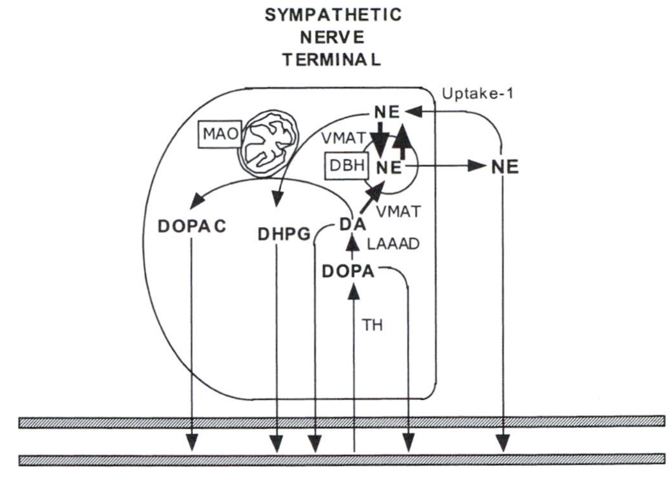

FIGURE 10.1 Sources of catechols in sympathetic nerve terminals and the circulation. DA, dopamine; DBH, dopamine β-hydroxylase; DHPG, dihydroxyphenylglycol; DOPAC, dihydroxyphenylacetic acid; LAAAD, L-aromatic amino acid decarboxylase; MAO, monoamine oxidase; NE, norepinephrine; TH, tyrosine hydroxylase; VMAT, vesicular monoamine transporter.

$Uptake_1$—through the cell membrane NE transporter is the predominant means of terminating the actions of released NE. $Uptake_1$ is energy requiring and can transport catecholamines against large concentration gradients. The only common structural feature of all known substrates for $Uptake_1$ is an aromatic amine, with the ionizable nitrogen moiety not incorporated in the aromatic system. $Uptake_1$ does not require a catechol nucleus. Alkylation of the primary amino group decreases the effectiveness of the transport, explaining why sympathetic nerves take up NE more efficiently than they do EPI and why they do not take up isoproterenol, an extensively alkylated catecholamine, at all. Methylation of the phenolic hydroxyl groups also markedly decreases susceptibility to $Uptake_1$; therefore, sympathetic nerves do not take up O-methylated catecholamine metabolites such as normetanephrine.

Neuronal uptake by dopaminergic neurons differs from that by noradrenergic neurons, because the former take up DA more avidly than they take up NE, whereas the latter take up both catecholamines about equally well. Desipramine and other tricyclic antidepressants block uptake by noradrenergic neurons more effectively than they block uptake by dopaminergic neurons. These pharmacologic differences fit with the existence of distinct transporters for NE and DA. The human NE transporter protein includes 12 to 13 hydrophobic and therefore membrane-spanning domains. This structure differs substantially from that of adrenoceptors and other receptors coupled with G proteins, but is very similar to that of the DA, GABA, serotonin, and vesicular transporters, all members of a family of neurotransmitter transporter proteins.

Neuronal uptake absolutely requires intracellular K^+ and extracellular Na^+ and functions most efficiently when Cl^- accompanies Na^+. Transport does not directly require ATP; however, maintaining ionic gradients across cell membranes depends on ATP, and the carrier uses the energy expended in maintaining the transmembrane Na^+ gradient to cotransport amines with Na^+. Many drugs or *in vitro* conditions inhibit $Uptake_1$, including cocaine, tricyclic antidepressants, low extracellular Na^+ concentrations, and Li^+.

NE taken up into the axoplasm by the $Uptake_1$ transporter is subject to two fates: translocation into storage vesicles and deamination by monoamine oxidase (MAO). The combination of enzymatic breakdown and vesicular uptake constitute an intraneuronal "sink," keeping cytoplasmic concentrations of NE very low. Reserpine, which effectively blocks the vesicular transport, not only shuts down conversion of DA to NE but also prevents the conservative recycling of NE. Reserpine therefore rapidly depletes NE stores. After reserpine injection, plasma DHPG levels increase first, reflecting marked net leakage of NE from vesicular stores, and then decline to very low levels, reflecting the abolition of vesicular uptake and β-hydroxylation of DA.

Neural and nonneural tissues contain MAO, which catalyzes the oxidative deamination of DA to form DOPAC and NE to form DHPG (Fig. 10.2). Because of the efficient uptake and reuptake of catecholamines into the axoplasm of catecholamine neurons, and because of the rapid exchange of amines between the vesicles and axoplasm, the neuronal pool of MAO, located in the outer mitochondrial membrane, figures prominently in the overall functioning of catecholamine systems. Two isozymes of MAO, MAO-A and MAO-B, have been described. Clorgyline blocks MAO-A, and deprenyl and pargyline block MAO-B. MAO-A predominates in neural tissue, whereas both subtypes exist in nonneuronal tissue. Inhibitors of MAO-A potentiate pressor effects of tyramine, whereas inhibitors of MAO-B do not. NE and EPI are substrates for MAO-A, and DA is a substrate for both MAO-A and MAO-B. The deaminated products are short-lived aldehydes. For DA, the aldehyde intermediate is converted rapidly to DOPAC by aldehyde dehydrogenase; for NE, the aldehyde intermediate is converted mainly to DHPG by an aldehyde reductase. The formation of the aldehydes reduces a flavine component of the enzyme. The reduced enzyme reacts with molecular oxygen, regenerating the enzyme but also producing hydrogen peroxide, which may be toxic to cells, because the peroxidation releases free radicals. The aldehydes themselves are also neurotoxic.

Because catechol-O-methyltransferase (COMT) in nonneuronal cells catalyzes the O-methylation of DHPG to form methoxyhydroxyphenylglycol (MHPG) and of DOPAC to form homovanillic acid, plasma levels of DHPG and DOPAC probably mainly reflect neuronal metabolism of NE and DA.

MAO inhibitors are effective antidepressants. A phenomenon known as the "cheese effect" limits their clinical use. In patients taking MAO inhibitors, administration of sympathomimetic amines such as in many nonprescription

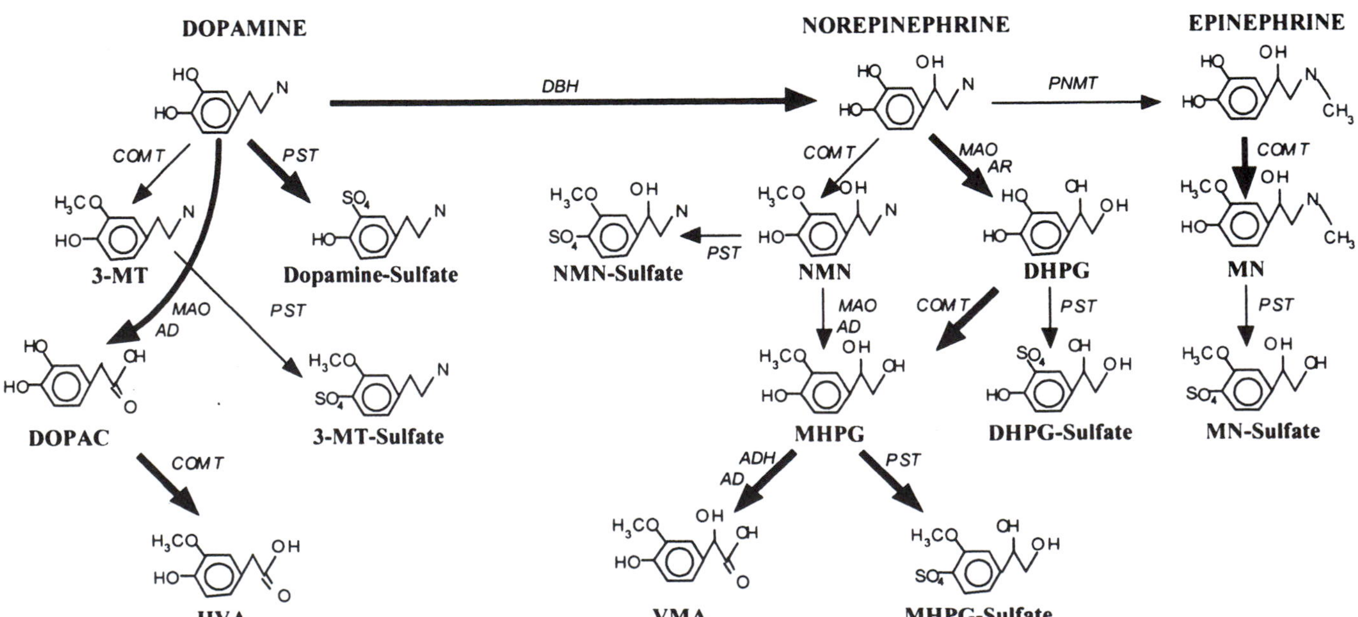

FIGURE 10.2 Main enzymatic steps in catecholamine metabolism. AR, aldehyde reductase; COMT, catechol-O-methyltransferase; HVA, homovanillic acid; MHPG, methoxyhydroxyphenylglycol; 3-MT, 3-methoxytyramine; MN, metanephrine; NMN, normetanephrine; VMA, vanillylmandelic acid.

decongestants, or ingestion of foods such as aged cheese, wine, or meat, which contain tyramine, can produce paroxysmal hypertension. Because tyramine and other sympathomimetic amines displace NE from sympathetic vesicles into the axoplasm, blockade of MAO in this setting causes axoplasmic NE to accumulate, and outward transport of the NE stimulates cardiovascular smooth muscle cells, producing intense vasoconstriction and hypertension.

Nonneuronal cells remove NE actively by a process called Uptake_2, characterized by the ability to transport isoproterenol; susceptibility to blockade by O-methylated catecholamines, corticosteroids, and ß-haloalkylamines; and an absence of susceptibility to blockade by the Uptake_1 blockers cocaine and desipramine. In contrast with Uptake_1, Uptake_2 functions independently of extracellular Na^+. The Uptake_2 carrier has little if any stereoselectivity and has low affinity and specificity for catecholamines. For example, extraneuronal cells remove imidazolines such as clonidine by Uptake_2. Whereas reverse transport through the Uptake_1 carrier requires special experimental conditions, one can readily demonstrate reverse transport through the Uptake_2 carrier. Thus, during infusion of a catecholamine at a high rate, the catecholamine can accumulate in extraneuronal cells, with reentry of the catecholamine into the extracellular fluid through the Uptake_2 carrier after the infusion ends.

COMT catalyzes the conversion of NE to normetanephrine and EPI to metanephrine. Uptake_2 and COMT probably act in series to remove and degrade circulating catecholamines. The methyl group donor for the reaction is *S*-adenosyl methionine. COMT not only is expressed in nonneuronal cells but also by adrenomedullary chromaffin cells. Ongoing production of normetanephrine and metanephrine in such cells explains the high sensitivity of plasma levels of free (unconjugated) metanephrines in the diagnosis of pheochromocytomas, which are chromaffin cell tumors. Vanillylmandelic acid and MHPG, the products of the combined O-methylation and deamination of NE, are the two main end products of NE metabolism, with vanillylmandelic acid formed mainly in the liver.

References

1. Goldstein, D. S. 1995. *Stress, catecholamines, and cardiovascular disease.* New York: Oxford University Press.
2. Goldstein, D. S. 2001. *The autonomic nervous system in health and disease.* New York: Marcel Dekker.

11

α_1-Adrenergic Receptors

Robert M. Graham
Victor Chang Cardiac Research Institute
Darlinghurst, New South Wales, Australia

SUBTYPES

α_1-Adrenergic receptors are integral membrane glycoproteins and members of the biogenic amine or class A family (which also includes α_2- and β-ARs, as well as the light-activated photoreceptor, rhodopsin) of G protein–coupled receptors (GPCRs) [1]. Like other members of the GPCR superfamily, the largest family of membrane receptors and possibly the largest gene family in the human genome, α_1-ARs are long, single-chain polypeptides. Three subtypes have been identified by molecular cloning in several species including humans. They are classified as the α_{1A}- (previously the $\alpha_{1A/c}$), the α_{1B}-, and the α_{1D}-ARs (previously the α_{1a} or $\alpha_{1a/d}$) (for a detailed consideration of α_1-AR subtype-classification, see References 1–3). For the α_{1A}-AR, four splice variants ($\alpha_{1A\text{-}1}$, $\alpha_{1A\text{-}2}$, $\alpha_{1A\text{-}3}$, $\alpha_{1A\text{-}4}$) have been identified, and they are expressed at different levels in various tissues, including the liver, heart, and prostate [4]. However, the functional significance of these splice variants is unclear, because they all display similar ligand-binding and functional activity when expressed in heterologous cell systems. The characteristics of the various α_1-AR subtypes are shown in Table 11.1. In addition to these subtypes, a putative fourth subtype, the α_{1L}-AR, which displays low affinity for prazosin and other α_1-antagonists, has been identified by functional but not by molecular studies [4]. This subtype is postulated to mediate contraction of prostate smooth muscle, but it remains unclear if it is a distinct subtype or a merely a functional variant of one of the cloned α_1 subtypes, such as the α_{1A} splice variants, because the latter all display some of the characteristics of an α_{1L} subtype when expressed in heterologous cell systems.

Another molecular variant of the α_{1A}-AR is a coding region polymorphism that involves an arginine to cysteine ($Arg^{492}Cys$) substitution in an arginine-rich region of the C-terminal tail [5]. This polymorphic receptor is found with greater frequency in black individuals, but it is not associated with the essential hypertension. In addition, it is unclear if it alters receptor regulation or produces any other functional effects.

STRUCTURE AND SIGNALING

Like rhodopsin, the only GPCR for which a high-resolution structure is available, α_1-ARs contain seven transmembrane (TM)-spanning α-helical domains linked by three intracellular and three extracellular loops [1]. In addition, the juxtamembranous portion of the C-terminal tail likely forms an eighth α-helix that lies parallel to the plain of the membrane and is significantly involved in receptor signaling. The N-terminus of α_1-AR subtypes is located extracellularly, and their C-terminus is located intracellularly (Fig. 11.1). The ligand-binding pocket is formed by the clustering of the seven α-helical domains to form a water-accessible region for agonist to bind, and it is located in the outer (extracellular) one third of the membrane-spanning domain (Fig. 11.2). Residues of the intracellular (cytoplasmic) domains, particularly the third intracellular loop, mediate specific interactions with the cognate G proteins, and thus are involved in receptor engagement with its signaling and regulatory pathways. All three subtypes couple to phospholipase C, and thus to Ca^{2+}-activation through members of the $G\alpha_{q/11}$ G protein family [1]. The α_{1B} and α_{1D}, but not the α_{1A} subtype may also couple to phospholipase δ_1 activation through G_h. In addition, α_1-ARs may increase intracellular Ca^{2+} levels by enhancing Ca^{2+} influx, both through voltage-dependent and -independent Ca^{2+} channels, and may augment arachidonic acid release, as well as phospholipase D, mitogen-activated protein kinase, and rho kinase activation.

LIGAND BINDING AND ACTIVATION

Binding of catecholamines to α_1-AR involves an ionic interaction between the basic aliphatic nitrogen atom common to all sympathomimetic amines and an aspartate (Asp^{125} in the hamster α_{1B}-AR) in the third transmembrane-spanning segment (TMIII) [1]. In the ground state, this TMIII aspartate forms a salt bridge with a lysine residue (Lys^{331} in the α_{1B}-adrenergic receptor) in TMVII. Activation

TABLE 11.1 Characteristics of the Cloned α_1ARs

Characteristics	Receptor Subtype		
	α_{1A}	α_{1B}	α_{1D}
M_r*	68	80	≈65
Amino acids§	431–501	515–520	561–572
Glycosylation sites (N-terminus)	3	4	2
Phosphorylation sites	PKA	PKA	—
Genomic organization			
Introns	1	1	2
Exons	2	2	
Chromosomal localization†	8	5	20 p13
Pharmacologic selectivity			
Subtype-selective agents	5-Methylurapidil, (+)niguldipine, oxymetazoline, A-61603, SNAP-5089, KMD-3213, RS17053	AH11110A, L-765,314	(+) Norepinephrine, BMY 7378, SKF105854
Nonselective agents‡	—	Prazosin, phentolamine, benoxathian, abanoquil, terazosin, doxazosin, tamulosin, phenylephrine, methoxamine, cirazoline	—
Prototypic tissues	Rat kidney and submaxillary gland, rabbit liver, human heart and liver	Rat spleen, liver, and heart	Rat aorta, lung, and cerebral cortex
Receptor-coupled signaling‡	—	Ca^{2+} mobilization, PLC, PLA_2, PLD	—
G protein coupling	$G_{q/11/4}$	$G_{q/11/4/16}$, G_h	G_{q11}, G_h

*Apparent molecular weights (M_r) determined by sodium dodecyl sulfate–polyacrylamide gel electrophoresis are shown.
PKA, protein kinase A; PLA_2, phospholipase A_2; PLC, phospholipase C; PLD, phospholipase D.
†Refers to the human genome.
‡These characteristics are the same for all subtypes.
§Differences because of species variability or splice variants, or both.
Adapted from Graham, R., D. Perez, J. Hwa, and M. Piascik. 1996. Alpha$_1$-adrenergic receptor subtypes: Molecular structure, function, and signalling. *Circ. Res.* 78:737–749.

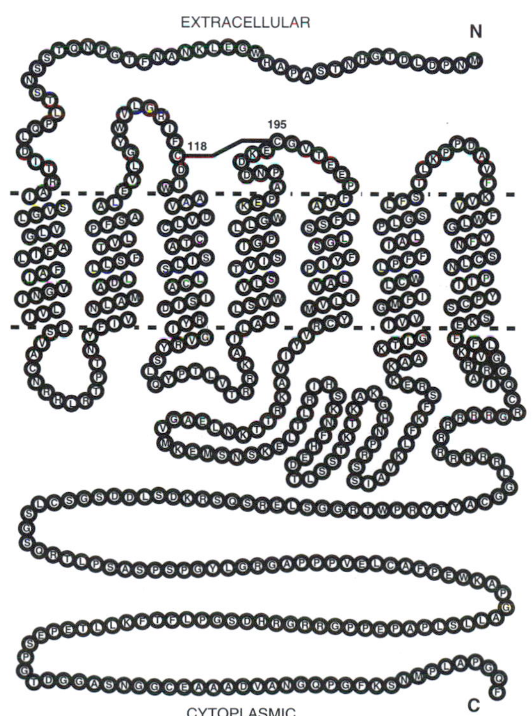

FIGURE 11.1 Secondary structure model of the hamster α_{1B}-AR. *Dotted lines* indicate the approximate boundaries of the plasma membrane. A putative solvent-inaccessible disulfide bond between Cys^{118} and Cys^{195} [1], which likely stabilizes the receptor's tertiary structure by linking the first two extracellular loops, is shown.

of α_1-ARs likely involves disruption of this ionic interaction. This is because of competition between the protonated amine of catecholamines and the TMVII lysine, which is just favored by the slightly more basic pK_a of the protonated amine (pK_a 11.0) versus the lysine (pK_a 10.5). Agonist binding to α_1-ARs also involves an H-bond interaction between the *meta* hydroxyl group of catecholamines and a serine residue (Ser^{188}, α_{1A}-receptor numbering) in TMV, whereas an interaction between the *para* hydroxyl and another TMV serine (Ser^{192}) contributes only minimally to receptor activation.

A further important interaction, for both binding and activation, involves aromatic–aromatic bonding between the catecholamine ring and that of a phenylalanine (Phe^{310} for the α_{1B}-adrenergic receptor) in TMVI [6]. This interaction also is important in receptor activation, which in addition to the TMIII-TMVII salt bridge disruption mentioned earlier, involves movement of TMVI that is likely required to allow interaction between the intracellular third loop and the receptor's cognate G protein. Aromatic–aromatic interactions between two phenylalanines (Phe^{163} and Phe^{187}) in TMIV and TMV, respectively, and the catecholamine ring, also have been suggested to be important for agonist binding [7], but not for activation, although that with Phe^{163} may be

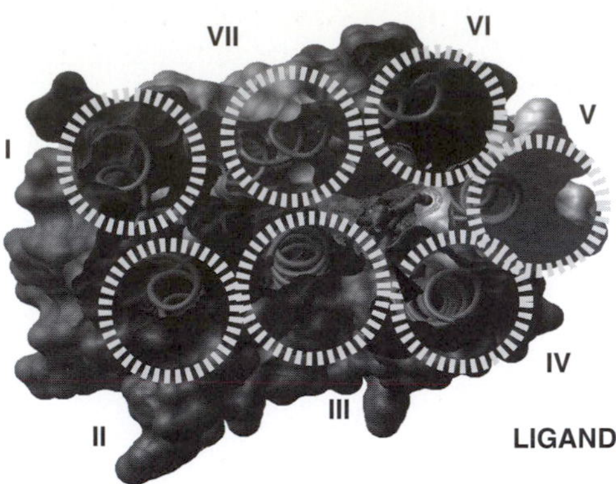

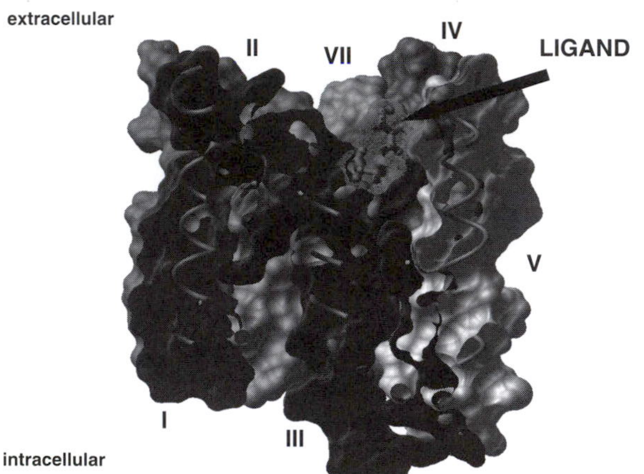

FIGURE 11.2 Cutaway three-dimensional model of the hamster α_{1B}-AR, showing the seven α-helical transmembrane domains indicated by *Roman numerals* and by *dashed circles* and backbone ribbons (*yellow corkscrews*), with the catecholamine agonist, epinephrine (*magenta ball and stick model with surrounding dot surface*), modeled in its binding pocket. **Top**, Top view (looking down onto the plane of the membrane). **Bottom**, Side view. This model was kindly provided by Dr. J. Novotny. (See Color Insert)

indirect, because this residue is replaced by a leucine in the α_{1B}- and α_{1D}-adrenergic receptors.

Residues critical for subtype-selective agonist recognition have been evaluated and, importantly, just 2 of the approximately 172 residues in the transmembrane domains (Ala^{204} in TMV and Leu^{314} in TMVI, and Val^{185} in TMV and Met^{293} in TMVI of the α_{1B}- and α_{1A}-receptors, respectively) have been shown to account entirely for the selective agonist-binding profiles of the α_{1A} and α_{1B} subtypes [1].

Interactions between antagonists and α_1-ARs are less well defined, although the selectivity of two α_{1A}-antagonists, phentolamine and WB4101, involves interactions with three consecutive residues (Gly^{196}, Val^{197}, and Thr^{198}) in the second extracellular loop [7].

REGULATION

α_1-Adrenergic receptors are subject to agonist-induced regulation that results in both short- and long-term desensitization of signaling. These regulatory responses are mediated by agonist-induced conformational changes that lead to C-terminal tail receptor phosphorylation, both by receptor-linked protein kinase C and G protein–coupled receptor kinases, followed by the binding of arrestins and internalization by the clathrin pathway. These responses have been studied in most detail for the α_{1A} and α_{1B} receptors, whereas less information is available for the α_{1D} subtype [8].

VASCULAR SUBTYPES

Despite the critical role of α-ARs in mediating arteriolar vasoconstriction, the particular subtype(s) responsible remains unclear. Consistent with findings in rodents, clinical trials of α_{1A}-selective blockers have implicated this subtype as a major regulator of blood pressure. In contrast, studies of a patient with sympathotonic orthostatic hypotension indicate that the α_{1B}-AR may be a major regulator of vascular resistance in humans [9]. Moreover, expression of this subtype increases in the elderly at a time when hypertension is commonly manifested. Thus, there is evidence for both the α_{1A}- and α_{1B}-adrenergic receptors being involved in blood pressure control in humans. Studies in the rat and in mouse knockout models indicate that the α_{1D} subtype also can play a role in blood pressure regulation. Indeed, such studies of genetically engineered animal models [reviewed in References 7 and 10] indicate that sympathetic regulation of vascular tone by the various α_1 subtypes is complex and may involve cross-regulation of their contractile effects or of their expression, or both. For example, inactivation of the α_{1A}-adrenergic receptor results in a small but significant decrease in basal blood pressure and in pressor responses to the α_1-agonist, phenylephrine [11]. Inactivation of the α_{1D}-adrenergic receptor, however, also partially impairs vasoconstrictor responses, but without a change in basal blood pressure. Given that overexpression of the α_{1B}-adrenergic receptor in transgenic mice does not increase systemic arterial blood pressure, and that inactivation of this subtype results in only a small attenuation of phenylephrine pressor responses with no change in basal blood pressure, it could reasonably be suggested that the α_{1A}- and α_{1D}-, but not the α_{1B}-ARs, are the mediators of vasoconstriction. However, mice lacking both the α_{1A} and α_{1B} receptors, or both the α_{1B} and α_{1D} receptors show profound attenuation of phenylephrine pressor responses. Thus, under appropriate circumstances, the α_{1B}-subtype may contribute significantly to sympathetic regulation of arteriolar tone. Further studies are required to fully elucidate the mechanisms involved in this apparent latent contribution of the α_{1B}-AR to peripheral resistance and to determine if these findings in animal models are also germane to the regulation of vascular resistance and blood pressure in humans.

References

1. Graham, R., D. Perez, J. Hwa, and M. Piascik. 1996. Alpha$_1$-adrenergic receptor subtypes: Molecular structure, function, and signalling. *Circ. Res.* 78:737–749.
2. Graham, R., D. M. Perez, M. Piascik, R. Riek, and J. Haw. 1995. Characterisation of alpha$_1$-adrenergic receptor subtypes. *Pharmacol. Commun.* 6:15–22.
3. Hieble, J., D. Bylund, D. Clarke, D. Eikenburg, S. Langer, R. Lefkowitz, K. Mineman, and B. Ruffolo. 1995. International Union of Pharmacology. X. Recommendation for nomenclature of alpha$_1$-adrenoceptors: Consensus update. *Pharmacol. Rev.* 47:267–270.
4. Chang, D., T. K. Chang, S. Yamanishi, F. R. Salazar, A. Kosaka, R. Khare, S. Bhakta, J. Jasper, I. S. Shieh, J. Lesnick, A. Ford, D. Daniels, R. Eglen, D. Clarke, C. Bach, and H. Chan. 1998. Molecular cloning, genomic characterization and expression of novel human alpha$_{1A}$-adrenoceptor isoforms. *FEBS Lett.* 422:279–283.
5. Xie, H., R. Kim, C. Stein, J. Gainer, N. Brown, and A. Wood. 1999. Alpha1A-adrenergic receptor polymorphism: Association with ethnicity but not essential hypertension. *Pharmacogenetics* 9:651.
6. Chen, S., M. Xu, F. Lin, D. Lee, R. Riek, and R. Graham. 1999. Phe^{310} in transmembrane Vl of the alpha$_{1B}$-adrenergic receptor is a Key Switch Residue involved in activation and catecholamine ring aromatic bonding. *J. Biol. Chem.* 274:16,320–16,330.
7. Piascik, M., and D. Perez. 2001. α_1-Adrenergic receptors: New insights and directions. *J. Pharmacol. Exp. Ther.* 298:403–410.
8. Garcia-Sainz, J., F. Vazquez-Cuevas, and M. Romero-Avila. 2001. Phosphorylation and desensitization of alpha$_{1D}$-adrenergic receptors. *Biochem. J.* 353:603–610.
9. Shapiro, R., B. Winters, M. Hales, T. Barnett, D. Schwinn, N. Flavahan, and D. Berkowitz. 2000. Endogenous circulating sympatholytic factor in orthostatic intolerance. *Hypertension* 36:553.
10. Koshimizu, T. A., J. Yamauchi, A. Hirasawa, A. Tanoue, and G. Tsujimoto. 2002. Recent progress in α_1-adrenoceptor pharmacology. *Biol. Pharm. Bull.* 24(4):401–408.
11. Rokosh, D., and P. Simpson. 2002. Knockout of the $\alpha_{1A/C}$-adrenergic receptor subtype: The $\alpha_{1A/C}$ is expressed in resistance arteries and is required to maintain arterial blood pressure. *Proc. Natl. Acad. Sci. USA* 99:9474–9479.

12

α_2-Adrenergic Receptors

Lee E. Limbird
Associate Vice Chancellor for Research
Vanderbilt University
Nashville, Tennessee

α_2-Adrenergic receptors (α_2-ARs) bind to their endogenous ligands, epinephrine and norepinephrine, and are blocked by the antagonist yohimbine. There are three subtypes of α_2-AR, encoded by three independent, intronless genes. These subtypes are denoted as α_{2A} (human chromosome 10), α_{2B} (human chromosome 2), and α_{2C} (human chromosome 4).

Ligand selectivity for pharmacologic agents does exist for the various α_2-AR subtypes, although this selectivity has been observed principally *in vitro*, because not all of these ligands have been evaluated for their pharmacokinetic properties *in vivo* (Table 12.1).

The lack of truly specific ligands for each of the α_2-AR subtypes, particularly antagonists, has prevented the unequivocal assignment of the differing α_2-AR subtypes to various physiologic responses. However, tools to genetically manipulate the mouse genome to create mutant (e.g., D79N α_{2A}-AR) or null alleles of each of these subtypes now provide an understanding of many of the roles of the different α_2-AR subtypes, as outlined in Table 12.2. For example, the α_{2A}-AR appears to be critical for agonist-mediated decreasing of blood pressure, suppression of pain perception, anesthetic sparing, and working memory. The α_{2A}-AR also appears to respond to endogenous catecholamines to suppress epileptogenesis (kindling) and depressive symptoms, the latter measured in mouse behavioral studies. The α_{2C}-AR elicits depressive behaviors, behaving functionally the opposite of the α_{2A}-AR subtype. The α_{2B}-AR, in contrast to the α_{2A}-AR, is involved in the vascular hypertensive effect of α_2-AR agonists. Both the α_{2A}- and α_{2C}-AR are involved in suppression of catecholamine release from central and peripheral neurons. The α_{2C}-AR is critical for suppression of epinephrine release from the adrenal cortex. Taken together, these findings suggest that subtype-selective agonists may be useful in manipulating one versus another adrenergic response *in vivo*.

An even more refined therapeutic selectivity might be achieved using *partial* agonists of α_2-ARs. We have observed that agonist-mediated decreasing of blood pressure can occur in mice heterozygous for the α_{2A}-AR, whereas agonist-evoked sedation cannot. These data suggest that partial agonists with less than 50% intrinsic activity (efficacy) might be useful in a number of therapeutic settings, such as treatment of attention deficit hyperactivity disorder and improvement of cognition in the elderly, where sedation as a side effect would undermine the therapeutic value of these agents.

Interestingly, imidazoline compounds, for which there is evidence of a role in the central nervous system in regulating blood pressure, nonetheless appear to decrease blood pressure through α_2-ARs when administered *peripherally*. Thus, moxonidine and rilmenidine, developed as imidazoline I_1-selective agents, are unable to decrease blood pressure in D79N α_{2A}-AR or α_{2A}-AR knockout mice. Also of interest is the finding that these agents are *partial* agonists at the α_{2A}-AR, which may explain their ability to decrease blood pressure without evoking sedative side effects.

All three subtypes of the α_2-AR share the same signaling pathways in native cells: decrease in adenylyl cyclase activity, suppression of voltage-gated Ca^{2+} currents, and activation of receptor-operated K^+ currents. In some target cells, α_2-ARs also regulate mitogen-activated protein kinase activity. In heterologous cells, the α_{2A}-AR has been shown to activate phospholipases A_2 and D, although these responses have yet to be observed in native target cells.

Despite the similarity of the signaling pathways of the α_2-AR subtypes, there are interesting differences in the trafficking itineraries of these receptors (Table 12.3). In polarized epithelial cells (using MDCKII cells as a model system), the α_{2A}-AR and α_{2C}-AR are delivered directly to the basolateral surface, whereas the α_{2B}-AR is randomly delivered. The steady-state localization of all three α_2-AR subtypes is at the basolateral surface; however, the α_{2B}-AR rapidly turns over at the apical surface (minutes), in contrast to its $t_{1/2}$ of 10 to 12 hours on the basolateral surface. (The half-life of the α_{2A}- and α_{2C}-AR subtypes is similarly 10 to 12 hours on the basolateral surface.) Whereas the α_{2A}- and α_{2B}-AR subtypes are enriched on the surface in MDCKII cells, the α_{2C}-AR distributes between the surface and intracellular compartments in MDCK and other heterologous cells (see Table 12.3).

Agonist-evoked receptor redistribution also varies among the α_2-AR subtypes (see Table 12.3). Agonist occupancy of the α_{2B}-AR evokes rapid sequestration, endocytosis, and

TABLE 12.1 Relative Selectivity for Ligands at the Three α_2-Adrenergic Receptor Subtypes

Agonists	**Shared:** norepinephrine, epinephrine, aproclinodine **Selective:** oxymetazoline (A > C ≫ B), clonidine, guanabenz (A,C), UK 14303 (A > C), dexmedetomidine (A,B)
Antagonists	**Shared:** yohimbine, rauwolscine, phentolamine, idazoxan, RX 44408 **Selective:** ARC 239 (B > C ≫ A), prazosin (B,C > A), BRL 44408 (A ≫ C), mianserin (A,B)

Modified from Saunders, C., and L. E. Limbird. 1999. Localization and trafficking of alpha2-adrenergic receptor subtypes in cells and tissues. *Pharmacol. Ther.* 84:193–205.

recycling of the receptor. In contrast, agonists do not accelerate α_{2A}-AR turnover at the cell surface. The functional relevance of these different trafficking itineraries for the arrival of nascent receptors at polarized surfaces or for agonist-redirected trafficking of the receptors is yet to be established.

A number of individual human polymorphisms have been identified for each of the α_2-AR subtypes. Some of these have resulted in alterations in G protein coupling, desensitization, or G protein receptor kinase–mediated phosphorylation, at least when assessed in heterologous cells expressing each of the α_2-AR polymorphisms. What will be of particular interest is to ascertain the *in vivo* consequences of these polymorphisms and their impact as genetic risk factors for pathophysiology linked to α_2-AR function or response to α_2-AR–directed therapeutic agents.

TABLE 12.2 Physiologic Effects of Altering α_2-Adrenergic Receptor Gene Expression in Mice

	Genetic alterations			
Physiologic or behavioral effect	**D 79Nα_{2A}-AR**	**KO α_{2A}-AR**	**KO α_{2B}-AR**	**KO α_{2C}-AR**
Hypotensive effects of α_2-AR agonist	X	X	'''	—
Bradycardic effects of α_2-AR agonist	↓	↓	—	—
Hypertensive effects of α_2-AR agonist	↓*	—	X	—
Hypotensive effects of centrally administered imidazolines	↓	—		
Hypotensive effects of peripherally administered	X	X		
Resting heart rate	—	↑	—	—
Resting blood pressure	—	—	—	—
Salt-induced hypertension			X†	—
Sedative effects of dexmedetomidine	X	X	—	—
Antinociceptive effects of α_2-AR agonist	X/↓‡		—	—
Antinociceptive effects of moxonidine	↓			
Adrenergic-opioid synergy in spinal antinociception	X			
Anesthetic-sparing effects of dexmedetomidine	X	X		
Hypothermic effects of dexmedetomidine	X		—	—/↓
Antiepileptogenic effects of endogenous catecholamines	X			
Presynaptic inhibition of norepinephrine release	—	↓	—	↓§
Inhibition of epinephrine release from adrenal cortex				X
Startle reflex				↑
Prepulse inhibition of startle reflex				↓
Latency to attack after isolation				↓
General aggression				—
Locomotor stimulation of D-amphetamine				↑
L-5-hydroxytryptophan-induced serotonin syndrome				↓
L-5-hydroxytryptophan-induced head twitches				—
Performance in T-maze	—	—	—	↓
Working memory enhancement of α_2-AR agonist		X		—
Forced swim stress and behavioral despair test		↑		↓
Anxiety in open field test		↑¶		—
Stimulus-response learning in passive avoidance test				—

Data summarized previously in Kable, J. W., L. C. Murrin, and D. B. Bylund. 2000. *In vivo* gene modification elucidates subtype-specific functions of alpha(2)-adrenergic receptors. *J. Pharmacol. Exp. Ther.* 293:1–7; and Rohrer, D. K., and B. K. Kobilka. 1998. G protein-coupled receptors: Functional and mechanistic insights through altered gene expression. *Physiol. Rev.* 78:35–52.

*Dependent on site of agonist administration.

†Mice were heterozygous (+/–) for α_{2B}-null mutation.

‡Extent of attenuation depended on test used.

§In α_{2AC}-double KO mice.

¶Only after injection (e.g., saline) as a stressor.

X, abolished; —, no effect; ↓, attenuated; α_2-AR, α_2-adrenergic receptor; KO, knockout; blank spaces denote effects unstudied.

TABLE 12.3 Differing Trafficking Itineraries of α_2-Adrenergic Receptor Subtypes

Subtype	Polarization in renal epithelial cells (MDCKII cultures)	Response to agonist pretreatment (heterologous systems)
α_{2A}-AR	**Steady state:** basolateral **Targeting:** direct to basolateral surface	**Desensitization:** minor, delayed **Down-regulation:** minor delayed
α_{2B}-AR	**Steady state:** basolateral **Targeting:** random delivery; rapid turnover on apical surface (<60 min); $t_{1/2}$ = 10–12 hours on basolateral surface	**Desensitization:** extensive, rapid **Down-regulation:** extensive
α_{2C}-AR	**Steady state:** basolateral and intracellular **Targeting:** direct to basolateral surface	**Desensitization:** minor, delayed **Down-regulation:** minor, delayed

From von Zastrow, M., R. Link, D. Daunt, G. Barsh, and B. Kobilka. 1993. Subtype-specific differences in the intracellular sorting of G protein-coupled receptors. *J. Biol. Chem.* 268:763–766; Wozniak, M., and L. E. Limbird. 1996. The three alpha 2-adrenergic receptor subtypes achieve basolateral localization in Madin-Darby canine kidney II cells via different targeting mechanisms. *J. Biol. Chem.* 271:5017–5024; Schramm, N. L., and L. E. Limbird. 1999. Stimulation of mitogen-activated protein kinase by G protein-coupled alpha(2)-adrenergic receptors does not require agonist-elicited endocytosis. *J. Biol. Chem.* 274:24,935–24,940; Kurose, H. and R. J. Lefkowitz. 1994. Differential desensitization and phosphorylation of three cloned and transfected alpha 2-adrenergic receptor subtypes. *J. Biol. Chem.* 269:10,093–10,099; Jewell-Motz, E. A., and S. B. Liggett. 1996. G protein-coupled receptor kinase specificity for phosphorylation and desensitization of alpha2-adrenergic receptor subtypes. *J. Biol. Chem.* 271:18,082–18,087; and reviewed in Heck, D. A., and D. B. Bylund. 1998. Differential down-regulation of alpha 2-adrenergic receptor subtypes. *Life Sci.* 62:1467–1472.

Given the new understanding of the α_2-AR subtypes in manipulating different physiologic effects and the refinement of this understanding with regard to partial agonists at the receptor, it would seem that pathway-selective agents might soon be developed for therapeutic intervention in settings that currently are not adequately addressed.

References

1. Kable, J. W., L. C. Murrin, and D. B. Bylund. 2000. In vivo gene modification elucidates subtype-specific functions of alpha(2)-adrenergic receptors. *J. Pharmacol. Exp. Ther.* 293:1–7.
2. Limbird, L. E. 1988. Receptors linked to inhibition of adenylate cyclase: Additional signaling mechanisms. *FASEB J.* 2:2686–2695.
3. Rohrer, D. K., and B. K. Kobilka. 1998. G protein-coupled receptors: Functional and mechanistic insights through altered gene expression. *Physiol. Rev.* 78:35–52.
4. Rohrer, D. K., and B. K. Kobilka. 1998. Insights from in vivo modification of adrenergic receptor gene expression. *Annu. Rev. Pharmacol. Toxicol.* 38:351–373.
5. Saunders, C., and L. E. Limbird. 1999. Localization and trafficking of alpha2-adrenergic receptor subtypes in cells and tissues. *Pharmacol. Ther.* 84:193–205.
6. Small, K. M., and S. B. Liggett. 2001. Identification and functional characterization of alpha(2)-adrenoceptor polymorphisms. *Trends Pharmacol. Sci.* 22:471–477.
7. Tan, C. M., M. H. Wilson, L. B. MacMillan, B. K. Kobilka, and L. E. Limbird. 2002. Heterozygous alpha 2A-adrenergic receptor mice unveil unique therapeutic benefits of partial agonists. *Proc. Natl. Acad. Sci. USA* 99:12,471–12,476.
8. von Zastrow, M., R. Link, D. Daunt, G. Barsh, and B. Kobilka. 1993. Subtype-specific differences in the intracellular sorting of G protein-coupled receptors. *J. Biol. Chem.* 268:763–766.
9. Wozniak, M., and L. E. Limbird. 1996. The three alpha 2-adrenergic receptor subtypes achieve basolateral localization in Madin-Darby canine kidney II cells via different targeting mechanisms. *J. Biol. Chem.* 271:5017–5024.

13

β-Adrenergic Receptors

Stephen B. Liggett
University of Cincinnati
College of Medicine 2
Cincinnati, Ohio

Of the nine adrenergic receptors, three are classified by traditional pharmacologic and molecular criteria as β-adrenergic receptors: β_1-AR, β_2-AR, and β_3-AR (Fig. 13.1; Table 13.1). Of the three subtypes, the β_2-AR is by far the most extensively expressed in the body [1]. Indeed, virtually every cell/tissue expresses some level of β_2-AR expression, although in some cases expression is very low and no physiologic role is known. Despite this essentially ubiquitous expression, their function is robust in many tissues, and therefore one can predict the effects of dysfunctional β_2-AR and administration of β_2-AR agonists and antagonists. Endogenous activation is primarily through epinephrine, because norepinephrine has a significantly lower affinity for β_2-AR. The β_1-AR has a more restricted expression, most notably in the heart, adipose tissue, and the kidney. Epinephrine and norepinephrine both display high affinity for the β_1-AR. The β_3-AR is expressed primarily in brown and white adipose tissue, with a greater affinity for norepinephrine. These ligand-binding properties are consistent with the lack of postsynaptic localization of β_2-ARs, whereas β_1AR (and likely β_3ARs) is primarily in neurotransmitter pathways.

SIGNALING OF β-AR SUBTYPES

All β-ARs serve to activate adenylyl cyclase through interaction with the stimulatory guanine nucleotide binding protein termed G_s. Like other G proteins, G_s is heterotrimeric, consisting of α, β, and γ subunits. Classically, signal transduction has been considered to be carried out by the disassociated $G_{s\alpha}$ subunit, but it is also clear that the βγ subunits can activate additional signaling and that β-AR signal in the absence of agonist, by spontaneously "toggling" to the active conformation [2]. Binding of agonists stabilize the active conformation, whereas neutral antagonists have no effect on this equilibrium, and inverse agonists favor stabilization of the inactive conformation (Fig. 13.2). In regards to the latter two agents, the physiologic response to a neutral antagonist may be negligible if there are minimal preexisting levels of agonists. In contrast, the physiologic response to an inverse agonist should theoretically be observed regardless of whether agonist is present. Taken together, β-AR responsiveness at the cellular level is highly dependent on multiple factors including expression levels of receptors, G proteins and effectors, the specifics of various G protein coupling, and conditions that favor spontaneous activation.

REGULATION OF β-AR FUNCTION

With continuous agonist exposure, many G protein–coupled receptors undergo a waning of function, which is termed desensitization [3]. Desensitization is an adaptive response, necessary for the cell to integrate multiple signaling events, and is critical for maintenance of homeostasis, whereas in some pathologic states, desensitization may be maladaptive. This loss of effectiveness with repetitive agonist exposure is observed clinically as tachyphylaxis. The β_2-AR is prototypic of receptors that undergo such regulation. Rapid desensitization, which occurs over seconds to minutes after agonist exposure, is caused by phosphorylation of the β_2-AR by the β-AR kinase and by the cyclic adenosine monophosphate (cAMP)–dependent protein kinase A. Only those receptors that are activated (in essence, those bound by agonist) are phosphorylated by the β-AR kinase. The phosphorylated receptor is subsequently bound by β-arrestin [4], which acts to partially uncouple the receptor from G_s. Protein kinase A–mediated desensitization does not require the activated state (i.e., receptor occupancy) and is one mechanism of heterologous desensitization, because the activation of any receptor that increases cAMP in the cell will result in kinase activation, β_2-AR phosphorylation, and partial uncoupling. The β_1-AR also undergoes agonist-promoted functional desensitization, which appears to be mediated by the β-AR kinase and protein kinase A. Short-term, agonist-promoted desensitization of the β_3-AR is highly dependent on cell type, but appears to be less than the other two subtypes.

With longer exposure to agonists, many G protein–coupled receptors also undergo a more extensive functional desensitization, which is caused by a loss of cellular expression of the receptor. This appears to be true for all three β-

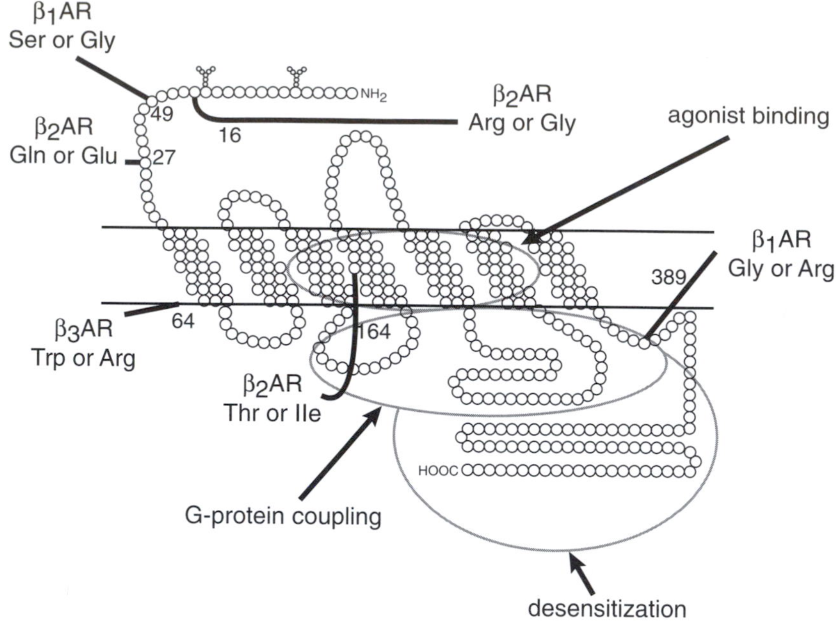

FIGURE 13.1 Structural and genetic features of β-adrenergic receptors.

TABLE 13.1 β-Adrenergic Receptor Subtypes

Receptor	Localization	Function
β_1-AR	Heart	Inotropy, chronotropy
	White adipocytes	Lipolysis
	Kidney	Renin release
	Vasculature	Dilatation
β_2-AR	Airway, uterus	Smooth muscle relaxation
	Eye	Ciliary muscle relaxation
	Bladder	Relaxation
	Vasculature	Relaxation
	White adipocytes	Lipolysis
	Skeletal muscle	Glycogenolysis, contraction
	Liver	Glycogenolysis, gluconeogenesis
	Pancreatic islet cells	Insulin secretion
β_3-AR	Brown adipocytes	Nonshivering thermogenesis, lipolysis
	White adipocytes	Lipolysis
	Skeletal muscle	

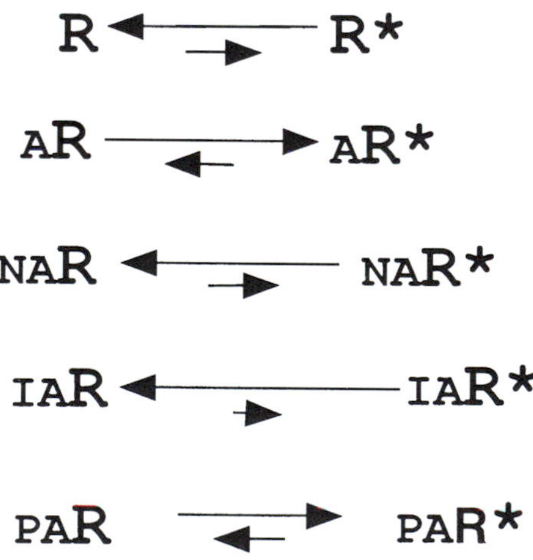

FIGURE 13.2 Spontaneous activation of G protein–coupled receptors. A, agonist; IA, inverse agonist; NA, neutral antagonist; PA, partial agonist; R, receptor.

AR subtypes, although again there appears to be a high degree of cell type specificity. The mechanisms of down-regulation include decreases in receptor transcription, enhanced degradation of mRNA, and an enhanced degradation of receptor protein. When testing for a functional receptor *in vivo*, it is important to consider whether there has been recent exposure to pathologically elevated catecholamines or exogenous agonists, or antagonists. If this is not considered, then the basis of a perceived defect may be obscured.

POLYMORPHISMS OF β-AR

With virtually any abnormality of the autonomic nervous system that involves catecholamines, it is clear that there is interindividual variation in expression of the phenotype. In addition, in many diseases, the clinical response to agonists and antagonists also displays this variability from one person to another, which cannot be explained by the extent of the underlying pathophysiology [5, 6]. These observations suggest that genetic variability of the receptors may be

TABLE 13.2 β-Adrenergic Receptor Polymorphisms

Position			Alleles		Minor Allele Frequency (%)		
Receptor	**Nucleotide**	**Amino Acid**	**Major**	**Minor**	**White Individuals**	**Black Individuals**	***In Vitro* Phenotype**
β_1-AR	145	49	Ser	Gly	15	13	Down-regulation: Gly49 > Ser49
	1165	389	Arg	Gly	27	42	G_s coupling: Arg389 > Gly389
β_2-AR	46	16	Gly	Arg	39	50	Down-regulation: Gly16 > Arg16
	79	27	Gln	Glu	43	27	Down-regulation: Gln27 > Glu27
	491	164	Thr	Ile	2–5	2–5	G_s coupling: Ile164 < Thr164
β_3-AR	190	64	Trp	Arg	10	12	G_s coupling: Arg64 < Trp64

playing a role in risk, disease modification, or response to therapy. These common variations, which occur with frequencies greater than 1%, are termed polymorphisms and should be distinguished from rare mutations. Each of the β-AR subtypes has been found to have single nucleotide polymorphisms (SNPs) in their coding regions that alter the encoded amino acid (nonsynonymous SNPs). Their location, allele frequencies, and functional effects *in vitro* are shown in Figure 13.1 and Table 13.2. Because of the relatively high frequency of these β-AR SNPs, it has been considered to be unlikely that SNPs in one receptor can be a major cause of disease. In part, this may be because of the redundancy of signaling pathways, spare receptors, and other means by which the body can counter-regulate aberrant receptor function at the physiologic level. However, combinations of SNPs from several adrenergic receptors may represent a significant risk, as has been suggested with an α_{2C}AR and β_1-AR polymorphism combination and heart failure [7]. Disease modification, such as severity, progression, or association with clinical subsets, has been shown for a number of diseases and β-AR SNPs [8]. β_2AR SNPs have been associated with the bronchodilatory response to the agonist albuterol in asthma [9, 10]. Other studies are likely to show that β-AR polymorphisms are pharmacogenetic loci for the treatment of other diseases where the receptors are targets for agonists and antagonists.

References

1. Krief, S., F. Lonnqvist, S. Raimbault, B. Baude, A. Van Spronsen, P. Arner, A. D. Strosberg, D. Ricquier, and L. J. Emorine. 1993. Tissue distribution of beta 3-adrenergic receptor mRNA in man. *J. Clin. Invest.* 91:344–349.
2. Pierce, K. L., R. T. Premont, and R. J. Lefkowitz. 2002. Seven-transmembrane receptors. *Nat. Rev. Mol. Cell. Biol.* 3:639–650.
3. Lohse, M. J., S. Engelhardt, S. Danner, and M. Bohm. 1996. Mechanisms of beta-adrenergic receptor desensitization: From molecular biology to heart failure. *Basic Res. Cardiol.* 91:29–34.
4. Luttrell, L. M., and R. J. Lefkowitz. 2002. The role of beta-arrestins in the termination and transduction of G-protein-coupled receptor signals. *J. Cell Sci.* 115:455–465.
5. Drazen, J. M., E. K. Silverman, and T. H. Lee. 2000. Heterogeneity of therapeutic responses in asthma. *Br. Med. Bull.* 56:1054–1070.
6. van Campen, L. C., F. C. Visser, and C. A. Visser. 1998. Ejection fraction improvement by beta-blocker treatment in patients with heart failure: An analysis of studies published in the literature. *J. Cardiovasc. Pharmacol.* 32(Suppl. 1):S31–S35.
7. Small, K. M., L. E. Wagoner, A. M. Levin, S. L. R. Kardia, and S. B. Liggett. 2002. Synergistic polymorphisms of β_1- and α_{2C}-adrenergic receptors and the risk of congestive heart failure. *N. Engl. J. Med.* 347:1135–1142.
8. Small, K. M., D. W. McGraw, and S. B. Liggett. 2003. Pharmacology and physiology of human adrenergic receptor polymorphisms. *Annu. Rev. Pharmacol. Toxicol.* 43:381–411.
9. Israel, E., J. M. Drazen, S. B. Liggett, H. A. Boushey, R. M. Cherniack, V. M. Chinchilli, D. M. Cooper, J. V. Fahy, J. E. Fish, J. G. Ford, M. Kraft, S. Kunselman, S. C. Lazarus, R. F. Lemanske, R. J. Martin, D. E. McLean, S. P. Peters, E. K. Silverman, C. A. Sorkness, S. J. Szefler, S. T. Weiss, and C. N. Yandava. 2000. The effect of polymorphisms of the β_2-adrenergic receptor on the response to regular use of albuterol in asthma. *Am. J. Respir. Crit. Care Med.* 162:75–80.
10. Drysdale, C. M., D. W. McGraw, C. B. Stack, J. C. Stephens, R. S. Judson, K. Nandabalan, K. Arnold, G. Ruano, and S. B. Liggett. 2000. Complex promoter and coding region β_2-adrenergic receptor haplotypes alter receptor expression and predict *in vivo* responsiveness. *Proc. Natl. Acad. Sci. USA* 97:10,483–10,488.
11. Mialet-Perez, J., D. A. Rathz, N. N. Petrashevskaya, H. S. Hahn, L. E. Wagoner, A. Schwartz, G. W. Dorn, and S. B. Liggett. 2003. Beta 1-adrenergic receptor polymorphisms confer differential function and predisposition to heart failure. *Nat. Med.* 9:1300–1305.

14 Purinergic Neurotransmission

Geoffrey Burnstock
Autonomic Neuroscience Institute
London, United Kingdom

Adenosine triphosphate (ATP) is a primitive extracellular signaling molecule and is now established as a cotransmitter in most nerve types in the peripheral and central nervous systems (CNS). There is purinergic cotransmission from sympathetic nerves (together with noradrenaline [NA] and neuropeptide Y), parasympathetic nerves (together with acetylcholine [ACh]), sensory-motor nerves (together with calcitonin gene–related peptide and substance P), enteric nerves (together with nitric oxide [NO] and vasoactive intestinal polypeptide [VIP]) and in subpopulations of central neurons with glutamate, dopamine, NA, γ-aminobutyric acid, and 5-hydroxytryptamine. Postjunctional purinergic P2X ionotropic receptors are involved in neurotransmission both at neuroeffector junctions in the periphery and synapses in ganglia and in the CNS, whereas prejunctional modulation of neurotransmission is mediated largely by P1 (A1 subtypes) and P2Y G protein–coupled receptors.

An increase in the role of ATP as a cotransmitter has been demonstrated in pathologic conditions including interstitial cystitis and hypertension. In addition to rapid signaling during neurotransmission, ATP appears to act as a long-term (trophic) signaling molecule during development and regeneration, sometimes synergistically with growth factors. Purinergic mechanosensory transduction has been proposed where ATP released from epithelial cells closely associated with sensory nerve terminals labeled with $P2X_3$ receptors leads to activation of sensory nerve activity related to physiologic events such as bladder voiding, or to nociception, or both. The therapeutic potential of purinoceptor agonists and antagonists, ATP transport inhibitors and promoters, and adenosine triphosphatase (ATPase) inhibitors is being explored.

It is now more than 30 years since purinergic neurotransmission was proposed by Burnstock in 1972, but it is only in the past few years that ATP has become widely accepted as a neurotransmitter [1]. The early evidence that nonadrenergic, noncholinergic (NANC) nerves used ATP as a transmitter when supplying the smooth muscle of the intestine and bladder was based on the criteria generally regarded as necessary for establishing a substance as a neurotransmitter. The criteria was summarized by Eccles in 1964 as the following: synthesis and storage of transmitter in nerve terminals; release of transmitter during nerve stimulation; postjunctional responses to exogenous transmitters that mimic responses to nerve stimulation; enzymes that inactivate the transmitter and/or an uptake system for the transmitter or its breakdown products; and drugs that produce parallel blocking of potentiating effects on the responses of both exogenous transmitter and nerve stimulation. There is evidence for neuronal synthesis, storage, and release of ATP and for inactivation of released ATP by ectoATPases. The model proposed for purinergic neurotransmission in 1972 is shown in Figure 14.1.

Receptors for ATP are implicit in the process of purinergic neurotransmission, and the early proposal by Burnstock in 1978 to distinguish receptors for adenosine (P1-purinoceptors) from those for ATP (P2-purinoceptors) was the start of many subsequent studies of both P1- and P2-purinoceptor subtypes. In 1994, on the basis of molecular cloning, transduction mechanisms, and selective agonist potencies, Abbracchio and Burnstock made the proposal, which has been widely adopted, that P2-purinoceptors should be considered in terms of two major families: a P2X receptor family, which are ligand-gated ion channel receptors, and a P2Y receptor family, which are G protein–coupled receptors. This subdivision into ionotropic and metabotropic families brings receptors for ATP in line with most of the other major neurotransmitters (Table 14.1). Four subtypes of the P1 receptor, seven subtypes of the P2X receptor family, and seven subtypes of the P2Y receptor family are currently recognized and have been characterized (Table 14.2) [2, 3].

Following the proposal by Burnstock in 1976 that nerves might store and release more than one transmitter, there is now considerable experimental support for ATP as a cotransmitter with classical transmitters and neuropeptides in most major nerve types (Fig. 14.2) [4, 5, 6]. ATP released from nerves may also act as a prejunctional modulator of cotransmitter release (often through adenosine) or as a postjunctional modulator of cotransmitter actions.

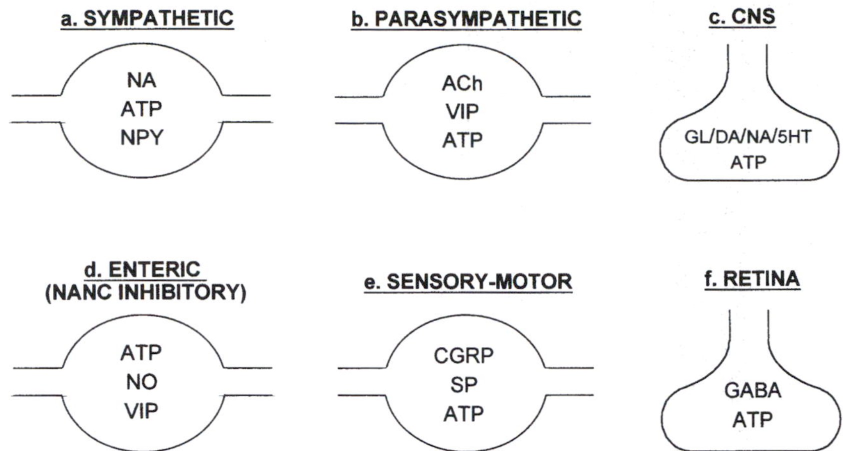

FIGURE 14.1 Schematic representation of purinergic neuromuscular transmission depicting the synthesis, storage, release and inactivation of adenosine triphosphate, and autoregulation through prejunctional adenosine (P1) receptors. (Modified with permission from Burnstock, G. 1999. Purinergic cotransmission. *Brain Res. Bull.* 50:355–357.)

TABLE 14.1 Comparison of Fast Ionotropic and Slow Metabotropic Receptors for Acetylcholine, γ-Aminobutyric Acid, Glutamate, and 5-Hydroxytryptamine with Those for Purines and Pyrimidines

	Receptors	
Messenger	**Fast ionotropic**	**Slow metabotropic**
ACh	Nicotinic Muscle type Neuronal type	Muscarinic M_1–M_5
GABA	$GABA_A$	$GABA_B$
Glutamate	AMPA Kainate NMDA	$mGlu_1$–$mGlu_7$
5-HT	$5\text{-}HT_3$	$5\text{-}HT_{1A\text{-}F}$ $5\text{-}HT_{2A\text{-}C}$ $5\text{-}HT_4$ $5\text{-}HT_{5A\text{-}B}$ $5\text{-}HT_6$ $5\text{-}HT_7$
ATP	$P2X_{1\text{-}7}$	$P2Y_{1,2,4,6,11,12,13}$

Modified from Abbracchio, M. P., and G. Burnstock. 1998. Purinergic signalling: Pathophysiological roles. *Jpn. J. Pharmacol.* 78:113–145.

5-HT, 5-hydroxytryptamine; ACh, acetylcholine; AMPA, 2-(aminomethyl)phenylacetic acid; ATP, adenosine triphosphate; GABA, γ-aminobutyric acid; NMDA, *N*-methyl-D-aspartate.

SYMPATHETIC NERVES

The first hint about sympathetic purinergic cotransmission was in an article published by Burnstock and Holman in 1962, in which they recorded excitatory junction potentials (EJPs) in smooth muscle cells of the vas deferens through stimulation of the hypogastric nerves. Although these junction potentials were blocked by guanethidine, which prevents the release of sympathetic neurotransmitters, at the time it was surprising that adrenoceptor antagonists were ineffective. It was more than 20 years before selective desensitization of the ATP receptor by α,β-methylene ATP was shown to block the EJPs, when it became clear that we were looking at the responses to ATP as a cotransmitter in sympathetic nerves [7]. Release of ATP was shown to be abolished by tetrodotoxin, guanethidine, and, after destruction of sympathetic nerves, by 6-hydroxydopamine, but not by reserpine, which blocked the second slow noradrenergic phase of the response but not the initial fast phase. Spritzing ATP onto single smooth muscle cells of the vas deferens mimicked the EJP, whereas spritzed NA did not.

Sympathetic purinergic cotransmission also has been demonstrated in a variety of blood vessels. The proportion of NA to ATP is extremely variable in the sympathetic nerves supplying the different blood vessels. The purinergic component is relatively minor in rabbit ear and rat tail arteries, is more pronounced in the rabbit saphenous artery, and has been claimed to be the sole transmitter in sympathetic nerves supplying arterioles in the mesentery and the submucosal plexus of the intestine, whereas NA released from these nerves acts as a modulator of ATP release.

PARASYMPATHETIC NERVES

Parasympathetic nerves supplying the urinary bladder use ACh and ATP as cotransmitters, in variable proportions in different species; and by analogy with sympathetic nerves, ATP again acts through P2X ionotropic receptors, whereas the slow component of the response is mediated by a metabotropic receptor, in this case muscarinic. There is

TABLE 14.2 Characteristics of Purine-Mediated Receptors

Receptor	Main distribution	Agonists	Antagonists	Transduction mechanisms
P1 (adenosine)				
A_1	Brain, spinal cord, testis, heart, autonomic nerve terminals	CCPA, CPA	DPCPX, CPX, XAC	G_i (1–3); ↓cAMP
A_{2A}	Brain, heart, lungs, spleen	CGS 21680	KF17837, SCH58261	G_S; ↑cAMP
A_{2B}	Large intestine, bladder	NECA	Enprofylline	G_S; ↑cAMP
A_3	Lung, liver, brain, testis, heart	DB-MECA, DBX RM	MRS1222, L-268,605	G_i (2,3), $G_{q/11}$; ↓cAMP ↑IP_3
P2X				
$P2X_1$	Smooth muscle, platelets, cerebellum, dorsal horn spinal neurones	αβmeATP = ATP = 2meSATP (rapid desensitization)	TNP-ATP, IP_5I, NF023	Intrinsic cation channel (Ca^{2+} and Na^+)
$P2X_2$	Smooth muscle, CNS, retina, chromaffin cells, autonomic and sensory ganglia	ATP ≥ ATPγS ≥ 2mSATP ≫ αβme ATP (pH + Zn^{2+} sensitive)	Suramin, PPADS	Intrinsic ion channel (particularly Ca^{2+})
$P2X_3$	Sensory neurones, NTS, some sympathetic neurones	2mSATP ≥ ATP ≥ αβmeATP (rapid desensitization)	TNP-ATP, suramin, PPADS	Intrinsic cation channel
$P2X_4$	CNS, testis, colon	ATP ≫ αβmeATP	—	Intrinsic ion channel (especially Ca^{2+})
$P2X_5$	Proliferating cells in skin, gut, bladder, thymus, spinal cord	ATP ≫ αβmeATP	Suramin, PPADS	Intrinsic ion channel
$P2X_6$	CNS, motor neurones in spinal cord	(does not function as homomultimer)	—	Intrinsic ion channel
$P2X_7$	Apoptotic cells in immune system, pancreas, skin, etc.	BzATP > ATP ≥ 2meSATP ≫ αβme ATP	KN62, KN04 Coomassie brilliant blue	Intrinsic cation channel and a large pore with prolonged activation
P2Y				
$P2Y_1$	Epithelial and endothelial cells, platelets, immune cells, osteoclasts	2meSADP > 2meSATP = ADP > ATP	MRS2279, MRS2179	G_q/G_{11}; PLCβ activation
$P2Y_2$	Immune cells, epithelial and endothelial cells, kidney tubules, osteoblasts	UTP = ATP	Suramin	G_q/G_{11} and possibly G_i; PLCβ activation
$P2Y_4$	Endothelial cells	UTP ≥ ATP	Reactive blue 2, PPADS	G_q/G_{11} and possibly G_i; PLCβ activation
$P2Y_6$	Some epithelial cells, placenta, T cells, thymus	UDP > UTP ≫ ATP	Reactive blue 2, PPADS, suramin	G_q/G_{11}; PLCβ activation
$P2Y_{11}$	Spleen, intestine, granulocytes	ARC67085MX > BzATP ≥ ATPγS > ATP	Suramin, reactive blue 2	G_q/G_{11} and G_S; PLCβ activation
$P2Y_{12}$	Platelets, glial cells	ADP = 2meSADP	ARC67085MX, ARC69931MX	G_i (2); inhibition of adenylate cyclase
$P2Y_{13}$	Spleen, brain, lymph nodes, bone marrow	ADP = 2meSADP ≫ ATP and 2meSATP		G_i

Modified from Burnstock, G. 2001. Purine-mediated signalling in pain and visceral perception. *Trends Pharmacol. Sci.* 22:182–188.

α,βme-ATP, α,β-methylene ATP; 2meSATP, 2-methylthioATP; ATP, adenosine triphosphate; BzATP, 2′3′-*O*-(4-benzoyl-benzoyl) ATP; cAMP, cyclic adenosine monophosphate; CCPA, 2-chloro-N^6-cyclopentyladenosine; CPA, N^6-cyclopentyladenosine; CPX, 8-cyclopentyl-1,3-dipropylxanthine; DBX RM, 1–3-dibutylxanthine-1-riboside-5′-*N*-methylcarboxamide; DPCPX, 8-cyclopentyl-1,3-dipropylxanthine; Ins (1,4,5)P_3, inositol (1,4,5)-triphosphate; IB-MECA, N^6-(3-iodobenzyl)-5′-*N*-methylcarboxamidoadenosine; IP_5I, di-inosine pentaphosphate; NECA, *N*-ethylcarboxamidoadenosine; NTS, nucleus of the solitary tract; PLC-β, phospholipase C-β; PPADS, pyridoxalphosphate-6-azophenyl-2′,4′-disulfonic acid; RB2, Reactive blue 2; TNP-ATP, 2′3′-*O*-(2,4,6-trinitrophenyl)adenosine 5′-triphosphate; XAC, xanthine amine congener.

some evidence to suggest parasympathetic, purinergic cotransmission to resistance vessels in the heart and airways.

SENSORY-MOTOR NERVES

It has been well established since the seminal studies of Lewis in 1927 that transmitters released after the passage of antidromic impulses down sensory nerve collaterals during "axon reflex" activity produces vasodilation of skin vessels. It is now known that axon reflex activity is widespread in autonomic effector systems and forms an important physiologic component of autonomic control. Calcitonin gene–related peptide and substance P are well established to coexist in sensory-motor nerves and, in some subpopulations, as first proposed by Holton in the 1950s, ATP is a cotransmitter.

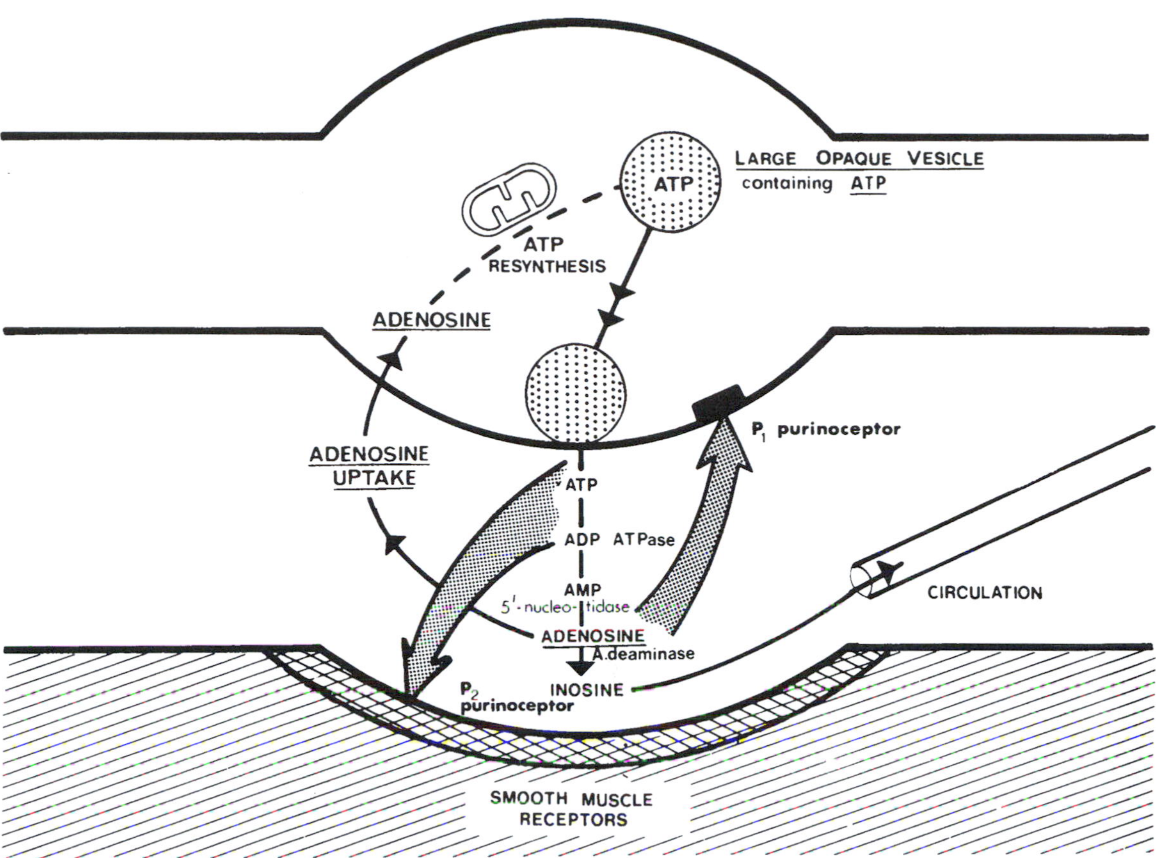

FIGURE 14.2 Schematic showing the chemical coding of cotransmitters in autonomic and sensory-motor nerves and in neurons in the central nervous system and retina. (Modified with permission from Burnstock, G. 1972. Purinergic nerves. *Pharmacol. Rev.* 24:509–581.)

INTRAMURAL (INTRINSIC) NERVES

Intrinsic neurons exist in most of the major organs of the body. Many of these are part of the parasympathetic release system; but certainly in the gut and perhaps also in the heart, some of these intrinsic neurons are derived from neural crest tissue that differs from that which forms the sympathetic and parasympathetic systems and appear to represent an independent control system. In the heart, subpopulations of intrinsic nerves in the atrial and intraatrial septum have been shown to contain and/or release ATP, NO, neuropeptide Y, ACh, and 5-hydroxytryptamine. Many of these nerves project to the microvasculature and produce potent vasomotor actions.

The enteric nervous system contains several hundred million neurons located in the myenteric plexuses between muscle coats and the submucous plexus. The chemical coding of these nerves has been examined in detail. A subpopulation of these intramural enteric nerves provides NANC inhibitory innervation of the gastrointestinal smooth muscle. It seems likely that three major cotransmitters are released from these nerves: ATP produces fast inhibitory junction potentials, NO also produces inhibitory potentials but with a slower time course, whereas VIP produces slow tonic relaxations. The proportions of these three transmitters vary considerably in different regions of the gut and in different species; for example, in some sphincters, the NANC inhibitory nerves largely use VIP and others largely use NO, whereas in nonsphincteric regions of the intestine, ATP is more prominent.

SKELETAL NEUROMUSCULAR JUNCTIONS

ATP coexists and is released with ACh in motor nerves supplying skeletal muscle and, indeed, in developing myotubes ATP, acting through P2X receptors, is equally effective with ACh, acting through nicotinic receptors. However, in adults, the cotransmitter role of ATP is lacking, but the ATP released acts both as a postjunctional potentiator of the nicotinic actions of ACh and as a prejunctional modulator of ACh release after its breakdown to adenosine and action on prejunctional P1 receptors.

SYNAPTIC PURINERGIC TRANSMISSION IN GANGLIA AND BRAIN

Two articles published in *Nature* in 1992 made a strong impression on the neuroscience community, both showing that excitatory postsynaptic potentials were mimicked by ATP and blocked by the P2 receptor antagonist, suramin. One concerned the guinea pig celiac ganglion, and the other concerned the rat medial habenula. Since that time, purinergic synaptic transmission has been demonstrated in other ganglia and other regions of the brain. Although the distribution and modulatory roles of P1 receptors in the CNS have been recognized for many years, the role of P2 receptors has been neglected. However, there is growing evidence for multiple roles for ATP receptors in ganglia and in the CNS. Wide distribution of immunoreactivity to the antibodies for $P2X_2$, $P2X_4$, and $P2X_6$ receptors including $P2X_{2/6}$ and $P2X_{4/6}$ heteromultimers and, to a lesser extent, $P2X_1$ and $P2X_3$ receptors, as well as $P2Y_1$ receptors, have been described in many different regions of the brain and spinal cord and have been correlated with electrophysiologic studies. Synaptic purinergic transmission also has been demonstrated in the myenteric plexus. Some elegant studies have shown a complex distribution of different P2 receptor subtypes in different cells in the inner ear and in the retina.

GLIAL CELLS

P2 receptor subtypes have been identified on cell types closely associated with neurons, including astrocytes, oligodendrocytes, Schwann cells, and enteric glial cells. Glial cells have been shown to release ATP.

PLASTICITY OF EXPRESSION OF PURINERGIC COTRANSMITTERS

The expression of cotransmitters and receptors in the autonomic nervous system shows marked plasticity during development and aging in the nerves that remain after trauma or surgery, under the influence of hormones, and in various disease situations [8]. There are examples where the role of ATP is significantly enhanced in disease—for example, in interstitial cystitis and obstructed bladder, the purinergic component of parasympathetic cotransmission is increased by up to 40%. There is a significantly greater role for ATP compared with NA in various blood vessels of spontaneously hypertensive rats.

LONG-TERM (TROPHIC) SIGNALING

In addition to the examples of short-term signaling described earlier, there are now many examples of purinergic signaling concerned with long-term events in development and regeneration, including cell proliferation, differentiation, migration, and death. For example, α,β-meATP produces proliferation of glial cells, whereas adenosine inhibits proliferation. A P2Y receptor was cloned from the frog embryo, which appears to be involved in the development of the neural plate. An example of synergism between purines and trophic factors comes from studies of the transplantation of the myenteric plexus into the brain where the myenteric plexus was shown to cause a marked proliferation of nerve fibers in the corpus striatum.

$P2X_3$ RECEPTORS AND NOCICEPTION

There have been various reports over the years concerning ATP on sensory nerves [9, 10]. In 1995, the $P2X_3$ receptor was cloned and shown to be expressed predominantly on nociceptive neurons in sensory ganglia. Sensory nerve terminals in the tongue are strongly immunopositive for the $P2X_3$ receptor, and a tongue sensory nerve preparation has been developed to examine the properties of purinergic sensory signaling. ATP and α,β-meATP applied to the tongue were shown to preferentially activate sensory afferent fibers in the lingual nerve, but not the taste fibers in the chorda tympani.

A new hypothesis for purinergic mechanosensory transduction in visceral organs involved in initiation of pain was proposed by Burnstock in 1999, in which it was suggested that distension of tubes, such as the ureter, salivary ducts, and gut, and sacs, such as urinary and gallbladders, leads to the release of ATP from the lining epithelial cells, which diffuses to the subepithelial sensory nerve plexus to stimulate $P2X_3$ or $P2X_{2/3}$ receptors, or both, which mediate messages to pain centers in the CNS. ATP has been shown to be released from the epithelial cells in the distended bladder, gut, and ureter, and $P2X_3$ receptors have been identified in subepithelial nerves in these organs. Recording in a $P2X_3$ knockout mouse, it has been shown that the micturition reflex is impaired and that responses of sensory fibers to $P2X_3$ receptor agonists are gone, suggesting that $P2X_3$ receptors on sensory nerves in the bladder have a physiologic and a nociceptive role. Similarly, $P2X_3$ receptors on projections of neurons from the nodose ganglia supplying neuroepithelial bodies in the lining of the lung may also mediate pathophysiologic events, perhaps involved in protective responses to hyperventilation or to noxious gases.

FUTURE DEVELOPMENTS

Future developments are likely to include purinergic signaling in the brain, focusing on physiologic and behavioral roles and long-term trophic roles of purines and pyrimidines in the nervous system, particularly in embryonic development and in regeneration.

There is likely to be substantial interest in the therapeutic development of purinergic agents for a variety of diseases of the nervous system. The therapeutic strategies are likely to extend beyond the development of selective agonists and antagonists for different P2 receptor subtypes, to the development of agents that control the expression of P2 receptors, to the development of inhibitors of extracellular ATP breakdown, and to the development of ATP transport enhancers and inhibitors. The interactions of purinergic signaling with other established signaling systems in the nervous system also will be an important way forward.

References

1. Burnstock, G. 1972. Purinergic nerves. *Pharmacol. Rev.* 24:509–581.
2. Burnstock, G. 1997. The past, present and future of purine nucleotides as signalling molecules. *Neuropharmacology* 36:1127–1139.
3. Ralevic, V., and G. Burnstock. 1998. Receptors for purines and pyrimidines. *Pharmacol. Rev.* 50:413–492.
4. Burnstock, G. 1976. Do some nerve cells release more than one transmitter? *Neuroscience* 1:239–248.
5. Burnstock, G. (Guest Ed.). 1996. Purinergic neurotransmission. *Semin. Neurosci.* 8:171–257.
6. Burnstock, G. 1999. Purinergic cotransmission. *Brain Res. Bull.* 50:355–357.
7. Burnstock, G. 1995. Noradrenaline and ATP: Cotransmitters and neuromodulators. *J. Physiol. Pharmacol.* 46:365–384.
8. Abbracchio, M. P., and G. Burnstock. 1998. Purinergic signalling: Pathophysiological roles. *Jpn. J. Pharmacol.* 78:113–145.
9. Burnstock, G. 2000. P2X receptors in sensory neurones. *Br. J. Anaesth.* 84:476–488.
10. Dunn, P. M., Y. Zhong, and G. Burnstock. 2001. P2X receptors in peripheral neurones. *Prog. Neurobiol.* 65:107–134.
11. Burnstock, G. 1999. Current status of purinergic signalling in the nervous system. *Prog. Brain Res.* 120:3–10.

15 Adenosine Receptors and Autonomic Regulation

Italo Biaggioni
Vanderbilt University
Nashville, Tennessee

Adenosine is an endogenous nucleoside formed by the degradation of adenosine triphosphate (ATP) during energy-consuming processes. Extracellular concentrations of adenosine are increased when energy demands exceed oxygen supply—that is, during ischemia. Adenosine modulates many physiologic processes through activation of four subtypes of G protein–coupled membrane receptors: A_1, A_{2A}, A_{2B}, and A_3. Its physiologic importance depends on the affinity of these receptors and the extracellular concentrations reached. In general, adenosine is considered a "retaliatory" metabolite, whose actions are apparent only during ischemic conditions. However, adenosine may have tonic actions even during physiologic conditions, mostly through activation of high-affinity A_{2A}, and perhaps A_1 receptors.

Adenosine has perhaps the shortest half-life of all autocoids, particularly in humans. It is rapidly and extensively metabolized to inactive inosine by adenosine deaminase. It also is quickly transported back into cells by an energy-dependent uptake mechanism, which is part of a purine salvage pathway designed to maintain intracellular levels of ATP. The effectiveness of this adenosine transport system is species dependent. It is particularly active in humans, and it is mainly responsible for the extremely short half-life of adenosine in human blood, which is probably less than 1 second. Adenosine mechanisms are the target of commonly used drugs. Dipyridamole (Persantine, Aggrenox) acts by blockade of adenosine reuptake, thus potentiating its actions. Conversely, caffeine and theophylline are antagonists of adenosine receptors.

Adenosine receptors are ubiquitous and, depending on their localization, may mediate opposite effects. This phenomenon is particularly evident in the interaction of adenosine and the autonomic nervous system; adenosine can produce either inhibition or excitation of autonomic neurons [1]. This chapter first outlines the effects of adenosine in the efferent, central, and afferent autonomic pathways, emphasizing those with clinical relevance. Then an integrated view is proposed that may explain how these seemingly contradictory effects may work together.

POSTSYNAPTIC ANTIADRENERGIC EFFECTS OF ADENOSINE

Adenosine A_1 receptors are found in target organs innervated by the sympathetic nervous system. A_1 receptors are coupled to inhibition of adenylate cyclase, and their effects are opposite those of β-adrenoreceptor agonists. For example, adenosine will oppose β-mediated tachycardia and lipolysis. This phenomenon is translated functionally as an "antiadrenergic" effect. The physiologic relevance of this effect is not entirely clear, but some studies suggest that adenosine is more effective in reducing heart rate during isoproterenol-induced tachycardia than in the baseline state or during atropine-induced tachycardia [2].

PRESYNAPTIC EFFECTS OF ADENOSINE ON EFFERENT NERVES AND GANGLIONIC TRANSMISSION

Adenosine inhibits the release of neurotransmitters through putative presynaptic A_1 receptors in both the brain and the periphery. This is true of practically all neurotransmitters studied, including norepinephrine and acetylcholine. Blockade of forearm adenosine receptors with intrabrachial theophylline potentiates sympathetically mediated forearm vasoconstriction, suggesting that endogenous adenosine inhibits noradrenergic neurotransmission *in vivo* in humans.

A few studies have investigated the effects of adenosine on ganglionic neurotransmission, and most of them show an inhibitory effect. Adenosine inhibits the release of acetylcholine presynaptically and blocks calcium current postsynaptically in ganglia.

ADENOSINE AND CENTRAL AUTONOMIC REGULATION

Adenosine acts as a neuromodulator within the central nervous system, mostly through interaction with A_1 and A_{2A}

receptors. Of particular relevance to this review are its actions on brainstem nuclei involved in autonomic cardiovascular regulation. In general, the central actions of adenosine result in inhibition of sympathetic tone through complex, and incompletely understood, mechanisms of action. Microinjection of adenosine into the nucleus tractus solitarii (NTS) evokes a dose-related decrease in blood pressure, heart rate, and renal sympathetic nerve activity. These effects appear to be mediated, at least partially, through A_{2A} receptors. The NTS is the site of the first synapse of afferent fibers arising from baroreceptors. The NTS provides excitatory input to the caudal ventrolateral medulla, which in turn provides inhibitory input to the rostral ventrolateral medulla (RVLM), where sympathetic activity is thought to be originated. Thus, stimulation of baroreceptor afferents (e.g., by an increase in blood pressure) activates the NTS, resulting in inhibition of the RVLM and a reduction in sympathetic tone. The effect of adenosine in the NTS is similar to that of the excitatory neurotransmitter glutamate, implying that adenosine has excitatory neuromodulatory effects on the NTS. The precise mechanisms that explain this phenomenon are not known. It has been proposed that adenosine releases glutamate within the NTS [3, 4], or blunts the release of the inhibitory neuromodulator γ-aminobutyric acid (GABA). The effects of adenosine in the NTS are also blunted by microinjection of the nitric oxide synthase inhibitor N_G-nitro-L-arginine methyl ester (L-NAME), suggesting an interaction between adenosine and nitric oxide in the NTS. Regardless of the mechanism of action, microinjections of adenosine receptor antagonists into the NTS results in blunting of the baroreflex gain, suggesting a role of endogenous adenosine on central cardiovascular regulation. A_1 and A_{2A} receptors are also found in the RVLM and may modulate neuronal activity either directly or through inhibition of GABA release [5].

NEUROEXCITATORY ACTIONS OF ADENOSINE ON AFFERENT PATHWAYS

In contrast to the "inhibitory" actions of adenosine in efferent pathways, adenosine excites a variety of afferent fibers that evoke systemic sympathetic activation including carotid body chemoreceptors, renal afferents, and myocardial and skeletal muscle afferents [3, 6]. The neuroexcitatory actions of adenosine were first recognized in animals in the early 1980s when it was found that adenosine activates arterial chemoreceptors in rats and cats and renal afferents in rats and dogs. The functional relevance of these findings, however, was not apparent until human studies were performed. The most striking effect of intravenous adenosine in humans is a dramatic stimulation of respiration and sympathetic activation. This effect is caused by carotid body chemoreceptor activation because it is observed when adenosine is injected into the aortic arch at a site proximal to the origin of the carotid arteries, but not if adenosine is injected into the descending aorta. The effects of intravenous adenosine are dramatically different if the autonomic nervous system is not involved. For example, adenosine decreases blood pressure and heart rate in patients with autonomic failure.

Pain resembling angina has been reported with intravenous and intracoronary administration of adenosine, presumably because of activation of sensory afferents. Intracoronary adenosine also elicits a pressor reflex in humans, which may be explained by activation of myocardial afferents. The few animal studies that have tested this hypothesis have yielded conflicting results, perhaps because of the confounding effects of anesthesia or because of species differences. Intrabrachial adenosine also elicits a sympathetic reflex that mimics the exercise pressor reflex—that is, the increase in blood pressure and sympathetic activation that results from activation of skeletal muscle chemoreceptor afferents during ischemic exercise (Fig. 15.1) [7]. This observation raises the possibility that adenosine is a metabolic trigger of the exercise pressor reflex. It should be noted that adenosine activates only a small percentage of muscle afferents in anesthetized cats. Also, adenosine-induced activation of skeletal muscle afferents has not been apparent in the leg in humans, but forearm exercise elicits a more potent exercise pressor reflex than leg exercise.

In summary, whereas adenosine inhibits sympathetic efferents, it activates virtually all afferent nerves that currently have been tested, including arterial chemoreceptors (in animals and humans), renal afferents (animals), and muscle afferents (humans). Adenosine may also activate cardiac afferents in humans. It appears that adenosine-induced afferent activation is greater in humans and may explain the dramatic species differences in cardiovascular responses to intravenous adenosine. The autonomic excitatory actions of adenosine clearly predominate when adenosine is given intravenously to conscious human subjects [8]. This sympathetic activation may explain the usefulness of intravenous adenosine in the triggering of neurogenic syncope during tilt [9]. It remains speculative whether endogenous adenosine plays a role in the generation of spontaneous neurogenic syncope. The adenosine receptor antagonist theophylline is used in the treatment of neurogenic syncope, but controlled studies are lacking.

INTEGRATED VIEW OF ADENOSINE AND CARDIOVASCULAR AUTONOMIC REGULATION

The neuroexcitatory actions of adenosine would seem at odds with its postulated protective role, which heretofore has been assigned to its "inhibitory" effects. We postulate,

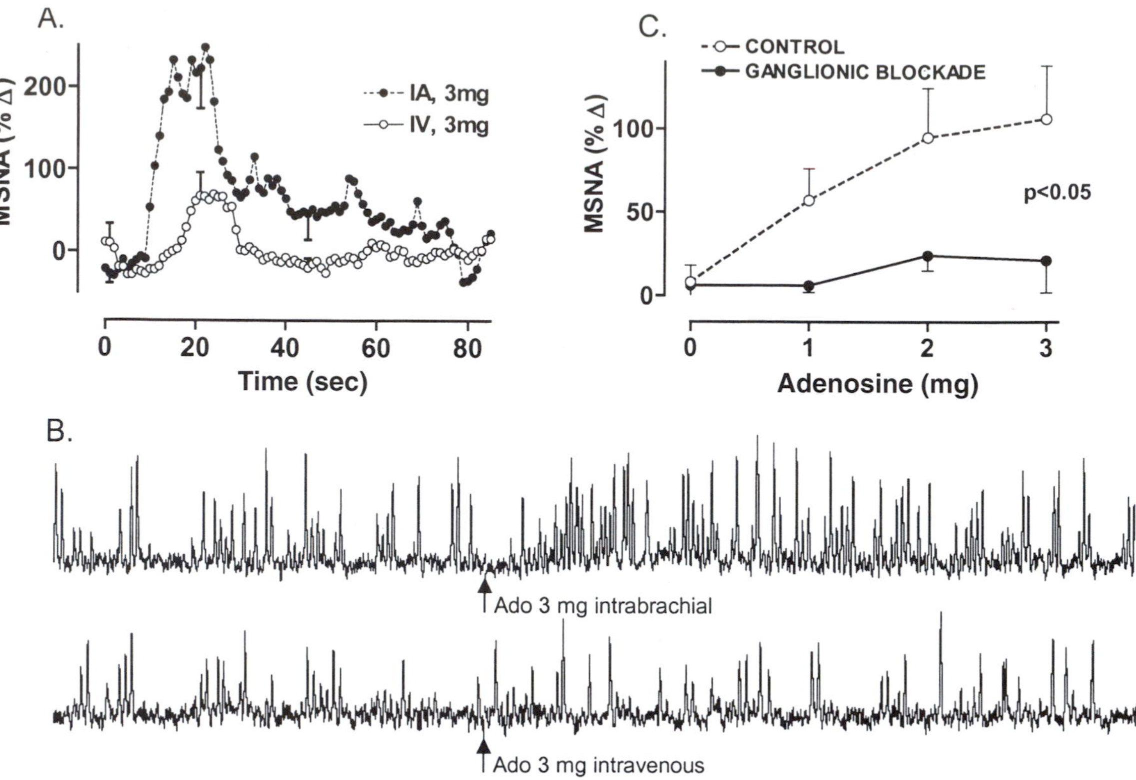

FIGURE 15.1 Activation of forearm muscle afferents by adenosine. **A**, The time course of systemic sympathetic activation, measured as muscle sympathetic nerve activity (MSNA) in the lower leg, induced by 3 mg adenosine injected either into the brachial artery (IA) or into the antecubital vein (IV). **B**, Representative tracings of MSNA before and after injection of adenosine. **C**, A dose response of intrabrachial adenosine on MSNA before and during axillary ganglionic blockade that interrupts forearm afferent pathways.

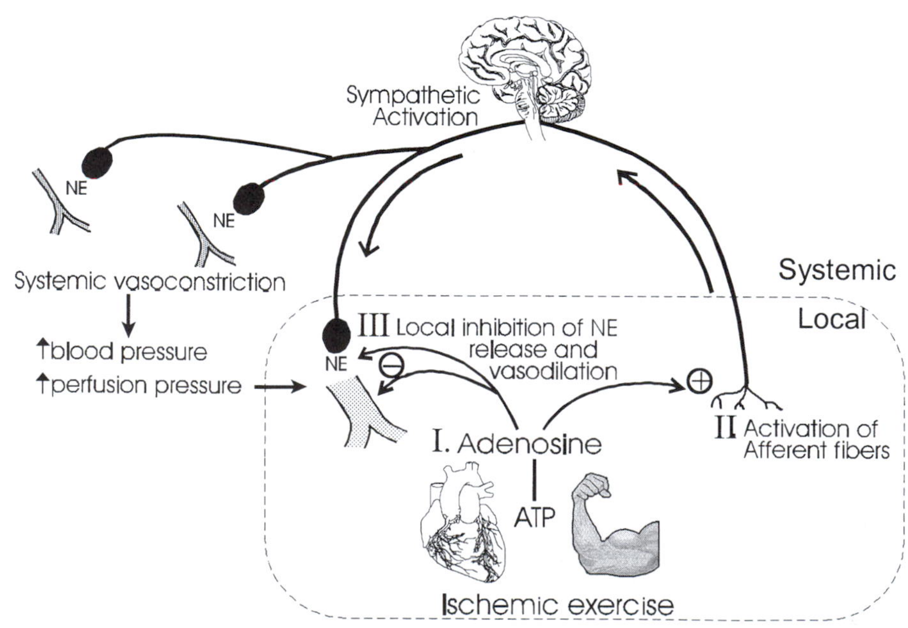

FIGURE 15.2 Postulated modulation by adenosine of autonomic cardiovascular regulation.

however, that the neuroexcitatory actions of adenosine work in tandem with its inhibitory effects to provide protection against ischemia. This framework is presented in Figure 15.2.

I. Interstitial levels of adenosine are elevated under conditions of increased metabolic demand (exercise) and decreased energy supply (ischemia), reaching physiologically relevant concentrations.

II. Adenosine then activates sensory afferent fibers that produce pain and muscle or myocardial afferents (metaboreceptors) that trigger an ischemic pressor reflex. Pain sensation is a primordial defense mechanism that signals the individual to stop exercising. Sympathetic activation leads to systemic vasoconstriction, increase in blood pressure, and improved perfusion pressure.

III. This systemic vasoconstriction would be deleterious to the ischemic organ if not for the simultaneous local inhibitory actions of adenosine, which produce vasodilation and inhibit norepinephrine release. These actions are, for the most part, circumscribed to the local ischemic tissue so that it is protected from sympathetically mediated vasoconstriction while it benefits from the improved perfusion pressure.

We propose, therefore, that the excitatory actions of adenosine work in tandem with its inhibitory effects to provide local protection against ischemia, even at the expense of the rest of the organism. Furthermore, we propose that adenosine provides a link between local mechanisms of blood flow autoregulation and systemic mechanisms of autonomic cardiovascular regulation, heretofore thought to work independent from each other. The individual components of this integrative postulate have been proven, but this hypothesis as a whole has not been tested. In particular, the sympatholytic effect of adenosine on sympathetically mediated vasoconstriction has not been proven *in vivo*. This would require the selective adenosine receptor antagonists that currently are not clinically available.

In summary, adenosine has both inhibitory and excitatory effects on the different components of the autonomic arc. We propose that these seemingly contradictory functions work in tandem to ensure tissue protection against ischemia.

References

1. Biaggioni, I. 1992. Contrasting excitatory and inhibitory effects of adenosine in blood pressure regulation. *Hypertension* 20:457–465.
2. Kou, W. H., K. C. Man, R. Goyal, S. A. Strickberger, and F. Morady. 1999. Interaction between autonomic tone and the negative chronotropic effect of adenosine in humans. *Pacing Clin. Electrophysiol.* 22:1792–1796.
3. Biaggioni, I., and R. Mosqueda-Garcia. 1995. Adenosine in cardiovascular homeostasis and the pharmacological control of its activity. In *Hypertension: Pathophysiology, managements and diagnosis*, ed. J. Laragh and B. M. Brenner, 1125–1140. New York: Raven Press.
4. Phillis, J. W., T. J. Scislo, and D. S. O'Leary. 1997. Purines and the nucleus tractus solitarius: Effects on cardiovascular and respiratory function. *Clin. Exp. Pharmacol. Physiol.* 24:738–742.
5. Spyer, K. M., and T. Thomas. 2000. A role for adenosine in modulating cardio-respiratory responses: A mini-review. *Brain Res. Bull.* 53:121–124.
6. Middlekauff, H. R., A. Doering, and J. N. Weiss. 2001. Adenosine enhances neuroexcitability by inhibiting a slow postspike afterhyperpolarization in rabbit vagal afferent neurons. *Circulation* 103:1325–1329.
7. Costa, F., A. Diedrich, B. Johnson, P. Sulur, G. Farley, and I. Biaggioni. 2001. Adenosine, a metabolic trigger of the exercise pressor reflex in humans. *Hypertension* 37:917–922.
8. Biaggioni, I., T. J. Killian, R. Mosqueda-Garcia, R. M. Robertson, and D. Robertson. 1991. Adenosine increases sympathetic nerve traffic in humans. *Circulation* 83:1668–1675.
9. Shen, W. K., S. C. Hammill, T. M. Munger, M. S. Stanton, D. L. Packer, M. J. Osborn, D. L. Wood, K. R. Bailey, P. A. Low, and B. J. Gersh. 1996. Adenosine: Potential modulator for vasovagal syncope. *J. Am. Coll. Cardiol.* 28:146–154.

16 Acetylcholine and Muscarinic Receptors

B. V. Rama Sastry
Department of Pharmacology
Vanderbilt University
Nashville, Tennessee

David Robertson
Vanderbilt University Medical Center
Clinical Research Center
Nashville, Tennessee

Acetylcholine (ACh) is synthesized by choline acetyltransferase, a soluble cytoplasmic enzyme that catalyzes the transfer of an acetyl group from acetylcoenzyme A to choline. The activity of choline acetyltransferase is much greater than the maximal rate at which ACh synthesis occurs. Choline acetyltransferase inhibitors have little effect to alter the level of this bound ACh. ACh is stored in a bound form in vesicles. Choline must be pumped into the cholinergic neuron, and the action of the choline transporter is the rate-limiting step in ACh synthesis. The choline uptake system with a high affinity for choline has been identified and designated CHT1.

On the arrival of an action potential in the cholinergic neuron terminal, voltage-sensitive calcium channels open and ACh stores are released by exocytosis to trigger a postsynaptic physiologic response. The release of ACh can be blocked by botulinum toxin, the etiologic agent in botulism. Fortunately, botulinum toxin has been used to treat an astonishing array of movement disorders and other conditions, including hyperhidrosis. Unfortunately, it requires local injection, but is often effective for weeks or months.

Much of the ACh released into the synapse is transiently associated with ACh receptors. This action is terminated by the rapid hydrolysis of ACh into choline and acetic acid. The transient, discrete, localized action of ACh is, in part, because of the great velocity of this hydrolysis. The choline liberated locally by acetylcholinesterase can captured by CHT1 (the high-affinity system described earlier) and resynthesized into ACh.

In addition to acetylcholinesterase (true cholinesterase), which is found near cholinergic neurons and in red blood cells (but not in plasma), there is also a nonspecific cholinesterase (pseudocholinesterase or butyrylcholinesterase) that is present in plasma and in some organs but not in the red blood cell or the cholinergic neuron.

Polymorphisms in pseudocholinesterase can result in a marked deficiency. One in 3000 people is a homozygote for the most common functionally abnormal variant: dibucaine-resistant pseudocholinesterase. Cholinergic nerve activity in such individuals is normal, but some drugs such as succinylcholine (used during anesthesia), which are normally broken down by pseudocholinesterase, are poorly metabolized by this variant enzyme. These patients may have prolonged muscle paralysis from succinylcholine.

ACETYLCHOLINE SYNTHESIS AND METABOLISM: DRUG MECHANISMS

Cholinergic neurotransmission can be modified at several sites, including:

a. Precursor transport blockade	Hemicholinium
b. Choline acetyltransferase inhibition	No clinical example
c. Promote transmitter release	Choline, black widow spider venom (latrotoxin)
d. Prevent transmitter release	Botulinum toxin
e. Storage	Vesamicol prevents ACh storage
f. Cholinesterase inhibition	Physostigmine, neostigmine
g. Receptors	Agonists and antagonists

ACETYLCHOLINE RECEPTORS

ACh is the postganglionic neurotransmitter in the parasympathetic nervous system. It is also the preganglionic neurotransmitter for *both* the sympathetic and parasympathetic nervous system, and it is important at nonautonomic sites. For example, ACh is the neurotransmitter by which motor nerves stimulate skeletal muscle and also the neurotransmitter at many sites in the brain and spinal cord.

As might be expected for an ancient and ubiquitous neurotransmitter, a variety of ACh (cholinergic) receptor types have emerged in evolution. The most important classification depends on their responsiveness to the agonist drugs muscarine and nicotine, and this distinction is so crucial that the terms muscarinic receptor (M) and nicotinic receptor (N) are used rather than cholinergic receptor.

Muscarinic receptors are located in the following:

- Tissues innervated by postganglionic parasympathetic neurons,
- *Presynaptic* noradrenergic and cholinergic nerve terminals,
- Noninnervated sites in vascular endothelium, and
- The central nervous system.

Nicotinic receptors are located in the following:

- Sympathetic and parasympathetic ganglia,
- The adrenal medulla,
- The neuromuscular junction of the skeletal muscle, and
- The central nervous system.

There are at least five subtypes of muscarinic receptors: referred to as M_1, M_2, M_3, M_4, and M_5. They mediate their effects through G proteins coupled to phospholipase C ($M_{1,3,5}$) or to potassium channels ($M_{2,4}$). After activation by classical or allosteric agonists, muscarinic receptors can be phosphorylated by a variety of receptor kinases and second messenger–regulated kinases. Phosphorylated muscarinic receptor subtypes can interact with beta-arrestin and presumably other adaptor proteins as well. For this reason, the various muscarinic signaling pathways may be differentially altered, leading to desensitization of a particular signaling pathway, receptor-mediated activation of the mitogen-activated protein kinase pathway downstream, or long-term potentiation of muscarinic-mediated phospholipase C stimulation. Agonist activation of muscarinic receptors may also induce receptor internalization and down-regulation. Unfortunately, there are currently few truly *subtype*-specific muscarinic agonists and antagonists of clinical use.

Studies in knockout mice have helped to elucidate the role of muscarinic receptor subtypes in a number of physiologic domains. The M_1 receptors modulate neurotransmitter signaling in cortex and hippocampus. The M_3 receptors are involved in exocrine gland secretion, smooth muscle contractility, pupil dilation, food intake, and weight gain. The role of the M_5 receptors involves modulation of central dopamine function and the tone of cerebral blood vessels. M_2-subtype receptors mediate muscarinic agonist-induced bradycardia, tremor, hypothermia, and autoinhibition of release in several brain regions. M_4 receptors modulate dopamine activity in motor tracts and act as inhibitory autoreceptors in the striatum.

In Sjögren syndrome, a systemic illness characterized by dryness of eyes, mouth, and other tissues, and sensory and autonomic neuropathy, antibodies to muscarinic receptors of the M_3 subtype have been reported in most of a small group of subjects, in whom the Sjögren syndrome is primary or secondary to other rheumatologic diseases. Whether such antibodies are a cause of some of the manifestations of Sjögren syndrome or a consequence of it requires further study.

There are at least two subtypes of nicotinic receptors, referred to as N_M and N_N. This distinction is clinically important. The N_M nicotinic receptor mediates skeletal muscle stimulation, whereas the N_N nicotinic receptor mediates stimulation of the ganglia of the autonomic nervous system, for which reason agonists and antagonists at the latter site are sometimes called ganglionic agonists and ganglionic blockers. (Nicotinic neurotransmission is discussed in chapter 17 of this Primer.)

MUSCARINIC AGONISTS

ACh itself is rarely used clinically because of its rapid hydrolysis after oral ingestion and rapid metabolism after intravenous administration. Fortunately, a number of congeners with resistance to hydrolysis (methacholine, carbachol, and bethanechol) are available, and bethanechol has the additional favorable property of an overwhelmingly high muscarinic (vs nicotinic) specificity. There are also several other naturally occurring muscarinic agonists such as muscarine, arecoline, and pilocarpine.

The pharmacologic effects of ACh and other muscarinic agonists can be seen in the following section. All these effects are parasympathetically mediated except sweat gland function, which is the unique sympathetic cholinergic category, much beloved by examination writers; these nerves are sympathetic because of their thoracolumbar origin and are cholinergic because they release ACh.

MUSCARINIC AUTONOMIC EFFECTS OF ACETYLCHOLINE

Iris sphincter muscle	Contraction (miosis)
Ciliary muscle	Contraction (near vision)
Sinoatrial node	Bradycardia
Atrium	Reduced contractility
Atrioventricular node	Reduced conduction velocity
Arteriole	Dilation (through nitric oxide)
Bronchial muscle	Contraction
Gastrointestinal motility	Increased
Gastrointestinal secretion	Increased
Gallbladder	Contraction
Bladder (detrusor)	Contraction
Bladder (trigone, sphincter)	Relaxation
Penis	Erection (but not ejaculation)
Sweat glands	Secretion
Salivary glands	Secretion
Lacrimal glands	Secretion
Nasopharyngeal glands	Secretion

Bethanechol is used (rarely) to treat gastroparesis, because it stimulates gastrointestinal motility and secretion. It also is useful in patients with autonomic failure, in whom modest improvement in gastric emptying and constipation may occur, but at a cost of some cramping abdominal discomfort. If gastric absorption is impaired, subcutaneous administration is sometimes used. Especially with intravenous administration, hypotension and bradycardia may occur. Bethanechol also is used to treat urinary retention if physical obstruction (e.g., prostate enlargement) is not the cause. This agent also occasionally is used to stimulate salivary gland secretion in patients with xerostomia, which entails the dry mouth, nasal passages, and throat occurring in Sjögren syndrome, and in some cases of traumatic or radiation injury. In rare cases, high doses of bethanechol appear to have caused myocardial ischemia in patients with a predisposition to coronary artery spasm; therefore, chest pain in a patient taking bethanechol should be taken seriously.

Pilocarpine is more commonly used than bethanechol to induce salivation, and also is used for various purposes in ophthalmology. It is especially widely used to treat open-angle glaucoma, for which a topical (ocular) preparation is available. Intraocular pressure is decreased within a few minutes after ocular instillation of pilocarpine. It causes contraction of the iris sphincter, which results in miosis (small pupils), and contraction of the ciliary muscle, which results in near (as opposed to distant) focus of vision. Pilocarpine possesses the expected side effect profile, including increased sweating, asthma worsening, nausea, hypotension, bradycardia (slow heart rate), and occasionally hiccups.

Methacholine often is used to provoke bronchoconstriction during diagnostic testing of pulmonary function. Elicitation of significant bronchoconstriction with inhaled methacholine challenge sometimes leads to the diagnosis of reactive airways disease (asthma) in patients with little baseline abnormality in pulmonary function.

MUSCARINIC ANTAGONISTS

The classical muscarinic antagonists are derived from plants. The deadly nightshade (*Atropa belladonna*), a relative of the tomato and potato, belongs to the Solanceae family, many of whose members contain atropinelike compounds. Jimson weed (*Datura stramonium*) is even more widespread than the deadly nightshade. The tiny dark seeds from the jimson weed pod are sometimes ingested for their hallucinogenic effect, a central side effect of atropinelike substances. Henbane (*Hyoscyamus niger*) contains primarily scopolamine and *hyoscine*.

Some plants of the Solancea family grow well in poor, rocky soil, whereas tomatoes grow poorly in these locations. The grafting of tomato plant stalks onto the root systems of these plants yields an unusually productive "tomato" that bears well even in dry weather, resulting in abundant large red tomatoes. Unfortunately, if the grafting is not done properly, alkaloids may enter the tomato fruit, creating the so-called happy tomatoes. Tachycardia and hallucinations (as well as more life-threatening problems) may ensue when such tomatoes are eaten.

Side effects of muscarinic antagonists include constipation, xerostomia (dry mouth), hypohidrosis (decreased sweating), mydriasis (dilated pupils), urinary retention, precipitation of glaucoma, decreased lacrimation, tachycardia, and decreased respiratory secretions.

Clinically, atropine is used for increasing heart rate during situations in which vagal activity is pronounced (e.g., vasovagal syncope). It is also used for dilating the pupils. Its most widespread current use is in preanesthetic preparation of patients; in this situation, atropine reduces respiratory tract secretions, thus facilitating intubation. It probably also has some efficacy as a bronchodilator. Ipratropium is marketed for maintenance therapy in chronic obstructive pulmonary disease. It has a long half-life.

Pirenzepine shows selectivity for the M_1 muscarinic receptor. Because of the importance of this receptor in mediating gastric acid release, M_1 antagonists such as pirenzepine help patients with ulcer disease or gastric acid hypersecretion. However, antihistamines and proton pump inhibitors are more useful and more widely used for this purpose.

References

1. Van Koppen, C. J., and B. Kaiser. 2003. Regulation of muscarinic acetylcholine receptor signaling. *Pharmacol. Ther.* 98:197–220.
2. Okuda, T., and T. Haga. 2003. High-affinity choline transporter. *Neurochem. Res.* 28:483–488.
3. Bymaster, F. P., D. L. McKinzie, C. C. Felder, and J. Wess. 2003. Use of M1-M5 muscarinic receptor knockout mice as novel tools to delineate the physiological roles of the muscarinic cholinergic system. *Neurochem. Res.* 28:437–442.
4. Waterman, S. A., T. P. Gordon, and M. Rischmueller. 2000. Inhibitory effects of muscarinic receptor autoantibodies on parasympathetic neurotransmission in Sjögren's syndrome. *Arthritis Rheum.* 43:1647–1654.
5. Caulfield, M. P., and N. J. Birdsall. 1998. International Union of Pharmacology. XVII. Classification of muscarinic acetylcholine receptors. *Pharmacol. Rev.* 50:279–290.
6. Higgins, C. B., S. F. Vatner, and E. Braunwald. 1973. Parasympathetic control of the heart. *Pharmacol. Rev.* 25:119–155.
7. Wellstein, A., and J. F. Pitschner. 1988. Complex dose-response curves of atropine in man explained by different functions of M_1- and M_2-cholinoceptors. *Naunyn Schmiedebergs Arch. Pharmacol.* 338:19–27.
8. Gomeza, J., L. Zhang, E. Kostenis, C. Felder, F. Bymaster, J. Brodkin, H. Shannon, B. Xia, C. Deng, and J. Wess. 1999. Enhancement of D_1 dopamine receptor-mediated locomotor stimulation in M_4 muscarinic acetylcholine receptor knockout mice. *Proc. Natl. Acad. Sci. USA* 96:10483–10488.
9. Köppel, C. 1993. Clinical symptomatology and management of mushroom poisoning. *Toxicology* 31:1513–1540.
10. Brown, J. H., and P. Taylor. 2001. Muscarinic receptor agonists and antagonists. In *Goodman and Gilman's the pharmacological basic of therapeutics*, ed. J. G. Hardman, and L. E. Limbird, 155–173. New York: McGraw-Hill.
11. Ferguson, S. M., and R. D. Blakely. 2004. Controlling choline uptake by regulating the choline transporter. *Molecular Interventions* 4: 22–37.

17

Nicotinic Acetylcholine Receptors

Structure and Functional Properties

Palmer Taylor
Department of Pharmacology
School of Medicine
School of Pharmacy and Pharmaceutical Sciences
University of California, San Diego
La Jolla, California

Nicotinic acetylcholine receptors are members of a large superfamily of ligand-gated ion channel receptors that include the 5-hydoxytryptamine$_3$ (5-HT$_3$), glycine, and γ-aminobutyric acid (GABA) families of receptors. Less closely related are the ligand-gated ion channels that respond to the excitatory amino acids and adenosine [1, 2]. Because of the abundance of nicotinic receptors in the electric fish and findings showing that peptide toxins that block motor activity bind to subtypes of nicotinic receptor with high affinity and selectivity, the nicotinic receptor was the first pharmacologic receptor to be purified and the cDNA encoding its subunits cloned. Appropriately, the nicotinic receptor became the prototype for the ligand-gated ion channel family.

STRUCTURAL CONSIDERATIONS

Nicotinic receptors assemble as pentamers of individual subunits. Assembly occurs in a precise manner and order such that the assembled subunits encircle an internal membrane pore and the extracellular vestibule leading to the pore. The replicated pattern of front to back assembly of subunits ensures that identical subunit interfaces are formed from the pentameric assembly of identical subunits. Moreover, the amino acid residues found at homologous positions in the receptors with heteromeric subunit assemblies should occupy the same position in three-dimensional space (Fig. 17.1).

Each subunit is believed to encode a protein with four transmembrane spans. The amino-terminal ~210 amino acids lie in the extracellular domain; this is followed by three tightly threaded transmembrane spans. A relatively large cytoplasmic loop is found between transmembrane spans 3 and 4 with a short carboxyl terminus winding up on the extracellular side. The overall structure has been detailed in a series of electron microscopy imaging studies (Fig. 17.2) and reveals a large extracellular domain, a wide-diameter vestibule on the extracellular side, and the gorge constriction region controlling the gating function to exist within the transmembrane-spanning region [3]. Rapid and slow binding of ligands appear to induce shape changes within the receptor structure that may be reflective of the individual conformational states [1–3].

More recently, a soluble protein, termed the acetylcholine binding protein, exported from glial cells of the fresh water snail has been shown to bind acetylcholine and many of the classical nicotinic agonists and antagonists [4, 5]. Homologous proteins also have been found in other invertebrate species. This protein, with identical subunits of slightly more than 200 amino acids, is composed of residues with homology to the amino-terminal, extracellular domain of family of nicotinic receptors. Its structural characterization by x-ray crystallography (Fig. 17.3) shows it to be pentameric and to contain an arrangement of amino acid residues consistent with findings from a large number of protein modification and site-specific mutagenesis studies conducted with acetylcholine receptors isolated from neuronal and muscle systems [5, 6]. The binding protein is homomeric, and its five binding sites reside at the five subunit interfaces with the binding site determinants residing on both of the proximal subunit surfaces forming the subunit interface. The ligands bind from an outer radial direction and appear to be lodged behind a loop that appears to contain selective binding determinants and proximal cysteines at or near its tip (see Fig. 17.3). Hence, consistent with other proteins that exhibit homotropic cooperativity, the binding protein and the nicotinic receptors have their binding sites located at the subunit interfaces.

SUBTYPE DIVERSITY OF NICOTINIC RECEPTORS

The receptor from skeletal muscle and its homologous forms in the fish electric organ consist of four distinct subunits, where the pentamer has two copies of the α subunit and one copy of β, γ, and δ subunits. When muscle becomes innervated, the γ subunit is replaced by an ε subunit. Within

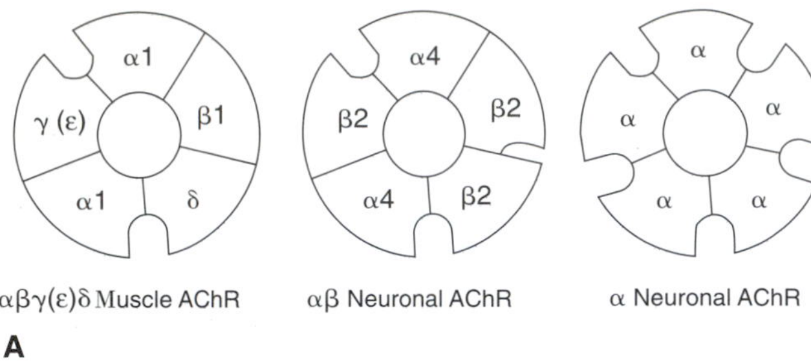

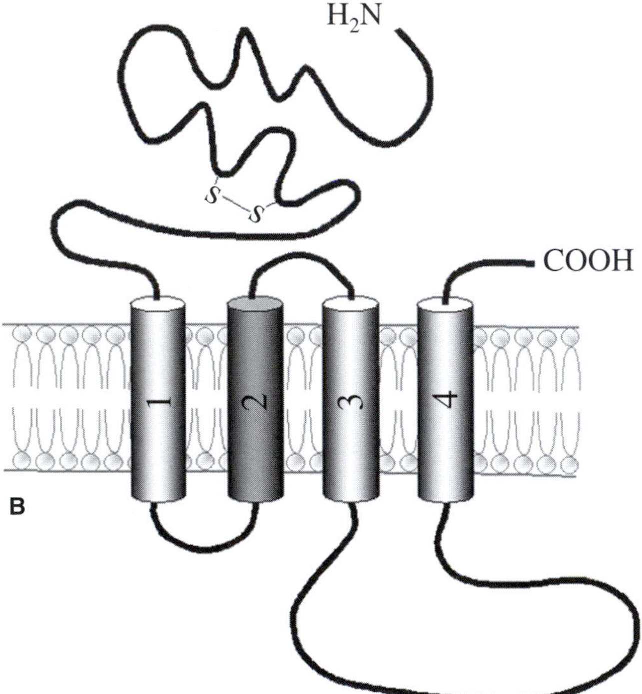

FIGURE 17.1 Structure of the nicotinic acetylcholine receptor. **A**, Arrangement of receptor subunits as pentamers in muscle and neuronal receptors. The muscle receptor exists as a pentamer with two copies of α and one copy of β, γ, and δ, as seen for the receptor found in embryonic muscle. The binding sites as designated are found at the αγ and αδ interfaces. In the case of the innervated receptor in skeletal muscle, an ε subunit of different composition replaces γ at the same position. Two types of neuronal receptors are shown: the heteromeric type is thought to have two copies of α, where α is α2, α3, α4, or α6, and three copies of β, where β can be β2, β3, or β4. The α5 subunit is thought to substitute for a β subunit at one of the nonbinding positions. The homomeric neuronal receptors are made up of pentamers of α7, α8, α9, and α10. The possibility that these α subunits can form heteromeric subtypes with each other or with certain β subunits remains open, but not proven. **B**, Threading pattern of the α-carbon chain of the subunits of the nicotinic receptor. The first ~210 amino acids form virtually the entire extracellular domain, contain the residues on the primary and complementary subunit interfaces forming the binding site determinants, and govern the subunit assembly process. Transmembrane span 2 segments from the five subunits form the inner perimeter of the channel and are involved in the ligand gating. The other transmembrane segments contribute to the structural integrity of the receptor. The extended segment between transmembrane spans 3 and 4 forms the bulk of the cytoplasmic domain.

TABLE 17.1 Nicotinic Acetylcholine Receptor Subunits

	Composition			Assembly
Muscle		α1, β1, γ, δ, ε		$\alpha_2\beta\gamma\delta$ or $\alpha_2\beta\varepsilon\delta$
Neuronal	α2	α6	β2	Various pentameric
	α3	α7	β3	assemblies of α
	α4	α8	β4	and β or α alone
	α5	α9		
		α10		

this pentameric structure, the two binding sites exist at the αδ and αγ(ε) subunit interfaces. Opposing faces of the homologous α and the γ, δ, or ε subunits make up the binding site.

The subunit compositions of the receptors expressed in the nervous system are far more complex where nine different α subtypes and three different β subtypes are found (Table 17.1). The α subtypes have been defined as those containing vicinal cysteines on a loop on which reside several binding site determinants. All α subunits, except α5, use the face with the vicinal cysteines to form the binding site. The β subunits that lack this sequence, and presumably the α5 subunit, use the opposite or complementary face to form the binding site (see Fig. 17.1).

The α subunits α2, α3, α4 and α6 combine with certain β subunits, mainly β2 and β4, to form pentameric receptors. The α5 subunit has the capacity to substitute for a β subunit in the pentameric assembly. Typically, it is thought that two of the neuronal α subunits assemble with three β subunits. Hence, typical stoichiometries would be $\alpha_2\beta_3$ or $\alpha_2\alpha5_1\beta_2$, where the generic α subtypes are usually α3 or α4, and the β subtypes are β2 or β4. Each of these heteromeric receptors would have two binding sites. Receptors composed of α7 through α10 subunits appear as functional homomeric entities where five copies of a single subunit confer function, when assembled. However, formation of functional homomeric receptors does not preclude the possibility that α7 can also partner with other subunits.

Although the assembly patterns of the neuronal nicotinic receptor subunits are diverse, only certain combinations yield functional receptors, and particular combinations seem to be prevalent within regional areas of the nervous system. For example, pentamers of α3β4 are prevalent in ganglia of the autonomic nervous system, α4β2 is most prevalent in the central nervous system, and α7 appears widely distributed [6].

ELECTROPHYSIOLOGIC EVENTS ASSOCIATED WITH RECEPTOR ACTIVATION

Currently, all of the nicotinic receptors that are well characterized are cationic channels. Thus, their activation causes

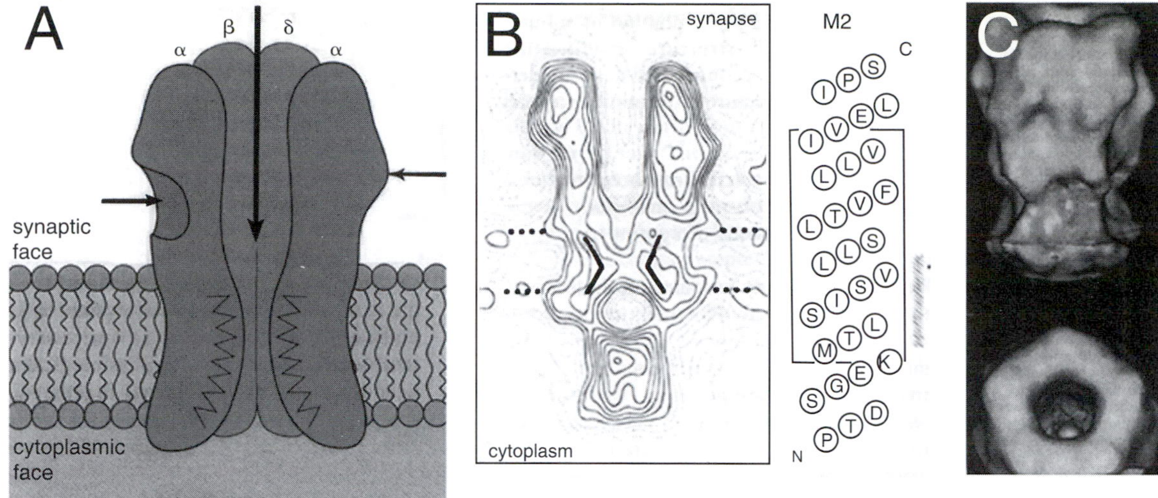

FIGURE 17.2 Overall dimensional characteristics of the nicotinic receptor. Image reconstruction of electron micrographs shows the receptor to be some ~140 Å in length and perpendicular to the membrane. Its diameter is 80 to 90 Å and contains a large central channel on the membrane surface. Rapid and prolonged exposure to acetylcholine followed by rapid freezing has yielded distinctive structures for the agonist bound, unligated, and desensitized states of the receptor [3, 6]. **A**, Arrangements of subunits with γ removed. *Vertical arrow* shows the cation path; *horizontal arrows* show the two binding sites. **B**, Electron densities of the receptor. The *solid angles* show the position of the M2 transmembrane span. **C**, Space filling model of the receptor. **Top**, View from the outer perimeter; the *darkened area* shows the transmembrane span. **Bottom**, View toward the extracellular membrane face showing the channel vestibule. (Adapted from Unwin, N. Nicotinic acetylcholine receptor at 9 Å resolution. *J. Mol. Biol.* 229:1101–1124, 1993.)

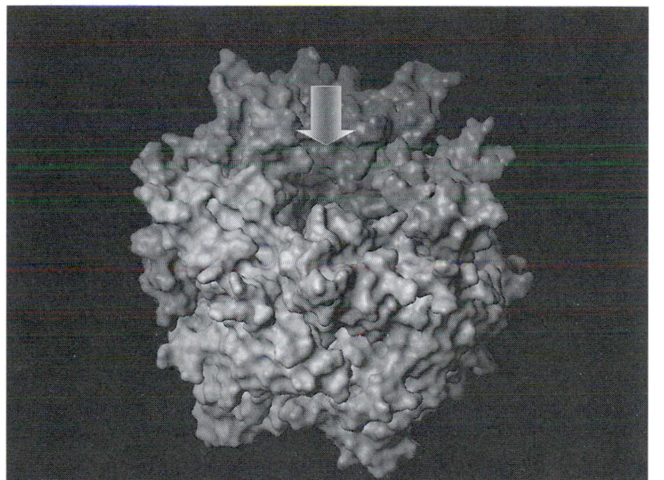

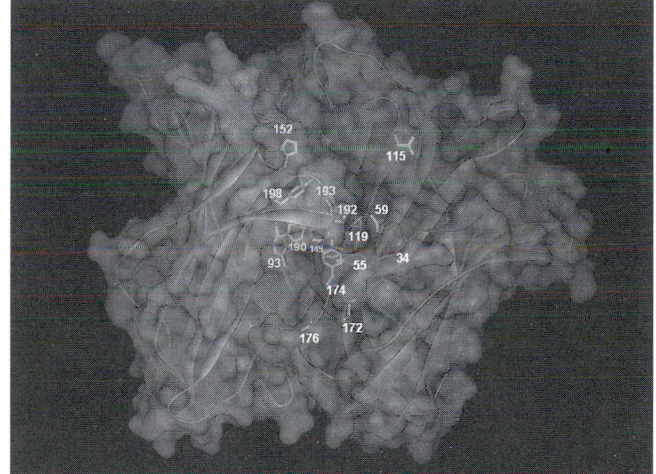

FIGURE 17.3 X-ray crystallographic structure of the acetylcholine binding protein. The structure was produced from crystallographic coordinates of Sixma and colleagues [4, 5]. Surfaces are represented as Connolly surfaces. **Left**, Colors are used to delineate the subunit interfaces in the homomeric pentamer. The vestibule on the extracellular surface that represents the entry to the internal channel in the receptor is shown by the *arrow*. **Right**, A single subunit interface. Note the residues that have been found to be determinants in the binding of agonists and alkaloid and peptidic antagonists to the receptor. Hence, the numbers (yellow, α subunit; white, γ subunit) delineate the probable binding surface(s) for large and small antagonists. These residues come from seven distinct segments of amino acid sequence in the subunit, as determined from extensive mutagenesis and labeling studies [6]. (See Color Insert)

an increase in cation permeability, which results in a depolarization. They differ substantially with respect to the permeabilities of the open channel state to Na^+ and Ca^{2+}. Na^+ permeability is most effective in initiating a rapid depolarization, whereas Ca^{2+} permeability could serve as an intrinsic activating function in cell signaling or in effecting an excitation step. However, depolarization per se through an increase in Na^+ permeability also can mobilize Ca^{2+} through voltage-sensitive Ca^{2+} channels. Typically postsynaptic nicotinic receptors, such as those found in ganglia and the neuromuscular junction, function through the simultaneous occupation of the receptor by more than a single agonist molecule. Agonist association and the ensuing channel opening reveals positive cooperativity in ligand binding. These rapid binding events cause channel opening to occur in a millisecond timeframe. Several openings and closings may occur during the short interval of agonist occupation, and the intrinsic efficacy of an agonist may be related to whether the ligand–receptor complex favors an open or closed state.

With continuous exposure to agonists, most receptors desensitize. Desensitization confers a receptor state wherein the agonist has a high affinity, but the receptor is locked in a closed channel state. Desensitization may provide an additional means by which temporal responses to an agonist can be regulated.

Antagonists may be competitive or noncompetitive. Competitive antagonists show binding that is mutually exclusive with agonists and exhibit a surmountable block of the receptor in which the dose–response curve to the agonist is shifted rightward in a parallel fashion. Occupation by a single antagonist molecule is sufficient to block function. Noncompetitive antagonists typically block the channel through which ions pass in the open state of the receptor. In the case of ganglionic nicotinic receptors, trimethaphan is a competitive agonist, whereas hexamethonium and mecamylamine are noncompetitive, therein blocking channel function.

DISTRIBUTION OF NICOTINIC RECEPTORS

Nicotinic receptors have a wide distribution in the central and peripheral nervous systems. In innervated skeletal muscle they are found in high densities localized at the endplate. Also, certain motor neurons may contain receptors at the presynaptic nerve ending to control release. In ganglia, the primary nicotinic receptor is found on the postsynaptic dendrite and nerve cell body. Others may exist presynaptically to control release from the presynaptic nerve ending. In the central nervous system, one finds that the majority of receptors are presynaptic or prejunctional. As such, they control the release of other transmitters, or in the case of acetylcholine, they play an autoreceptor role. Presynaptic nicotinic receptors found in the spinal cord and in higher centers of the brain have a functional role in modulating central control of autonomic function and sensory to autonomic control of reflexes and other functions.

References

1. Changeux, J.-P., and S. J. Edelstein. 1998. Allosteric receptors after 30 years. *Neuron* 21:959–980.
2. Karlin, A. 2002. Emerging structures of nicotinic acetylcholine receptors. *Nat. Rev. Neurosci.* 3:102–114.
3. Unwin, N., A. Miyazawa, J. Li, and Y. Fujyoshi. 2002. Activation of the nicotinic acetylcholine receptor involves a switch in conformation of the alpha subunits. *J. Mol. Biol.* 319:1165–1176.
4. Brejc, K., W. J. van Dijk, R. V. Klaasen, M. Shuurmans, J. van der Oost, A. B. Smit, and T. K. Sixma. 2001. Crystal structure of an acetylcholine binding protein reveals the ligand binding domain of nicotinic receptors. *Nature (London)* 411:269–276.
5. Sixma, T., and A. B. Smit. 2003. Acetylcholine binding protein: A secreted glial protein that provides a high-resolution model for the extracellular domain of pentameric ligand-gated ion channels. *Annu. Rev. Biophys. Biomol. Struct.* 32:311–334.
6. Clementi, F., D. Fornasi, and C. Gotti, eds. 2000. Neuronal nicotinic receptors. In *Handbook of Experimental Pharmacology, Vol. 144*, 821. Berlin: Springer-Verlag.

18 Acetylcholinesterase and Its Inhibitors

Albert Enz
Novartis Pharma AG
Nervous System Research
Basel, Switzerland

Acetylcholine (ACh) is an endogenous neurotransmitter at cholinergic synapses and at neuroeffector junctions in the central and peripheral nervous systems. The actions of ACh are mediated through nicotinic and muscarinic cholinergic receptors, which transduce signals through distinct mechanisms. To keep actions within the central nervous system and at peripheral nerve terminals localized and accessible for subsequent stimulations, ACh must be destroyed or inactivated at or near the site of its release, preferably with high velocity. The destruction of ACh at such sites is accomplished by the enzyme acetylcholinesterase (AChE). AChE is present in all parts of cholinergic neurones, in the vicinity of cholinergic synapses and in a variety of other tissues. It is also highly concentrated at neuromuscular junctions. AChE regulates the precision of nerve firing, enabling some nerve cells to fire as rapidly as 1000 times per second without overlap of the neural impulses.

MECHANISM OF ACTION

The enzyme AChE hydrolyzes ACh into choline and acetic acid. This hydrolysis reaction is preceded by a nucleophilic attack at the carbonyl carbon, by acylating the enzyme, and by liberating choline. This leads for some microseconds to an acetylated enzyme before the hydrolysis takes place, the acetate is released, and AChE is reactivated (Fig. 18.1). On the basis of interaction studies between the enzyme and various substrates and inhibitors, a hypothetical catalytic model for the cholinesterase (ChE) was elaborated. The active center in AChE has been assigned to contain two principal subsites: a negatively charged anionic site and the esteratic site containing the crucial residues. The existence of additional binding sites of AChE has been predicted, such as one hydrophilic region or peripheral anionic sites where cationic ligands bind to perform conformation changes of the enzyme. The multiple binding sites of AChE for reversible ligands are causal to the different inhibition mechanisms obtained with different classes of AChE inhibitors [2].

This model was substantiated by the pioneer work of Sussman and colleagues published in 1991 that elucidated the first X-ray structure of AChE from *Torpedo californica* (Fig. 18.2) [3].

ACETYLCHOLINESTERASE INHIBITORS

The mechanism of AChE inhibition can be either reversible, by a complete blockade of the active site by the substrate, or quasi-irreversible, by a covalent reaction between the substrate and a serine residue within the active site, thereby inactivating the catalytic ability of the enzyme. On the basis of their chemical structure, AChE inhibitors can be classified into the following three broad classes: the mono- and bis-quaternary amines, the carbamates, and the organophosphates [4] (Table 18.1).

Competitive inhibition takes place by blocking the access of the substrate at the active site (tacrine, edrophonium); noncompetitive inhibition occurs by binding to the peripheral site (propidium, gallamine). The bis-quaternary ligands decamethonium and BW284c51 bind across both active and peripheral sites.

The longest known and most widely used inhibitor is the natural alkaloid physostigmine. This carbamoylates the serine residue of the active site, slowing down the acyl-enzyme hydrolysis reaction compared with the acetylated enzyme. Organophosphorus compounds, such as diisopropyl fluorophosphate, are potent inhibitors of AChE and are used both as agricultural insecticides and as nerve gases in chemical warfare. These compounds react with the active site serine and form a stable covalent phosphoryl–enzyme complex [4, 5].

PHARMACOLOGIC ACTIONS OF ACETYLCHOLINESTERASE INHIBITION

Inhibition of AChE potentiates the effects of neuronal cholinergic stimulation at cholinoceptive cells of the central nervous system, at cholinergic synapses of the autonomic nervous system, at neuromuscular junctions, at autonomic ganglia, and at adrenal medulla (Table 18.2). The extent of the observed effects depends on the inhibitor applied and

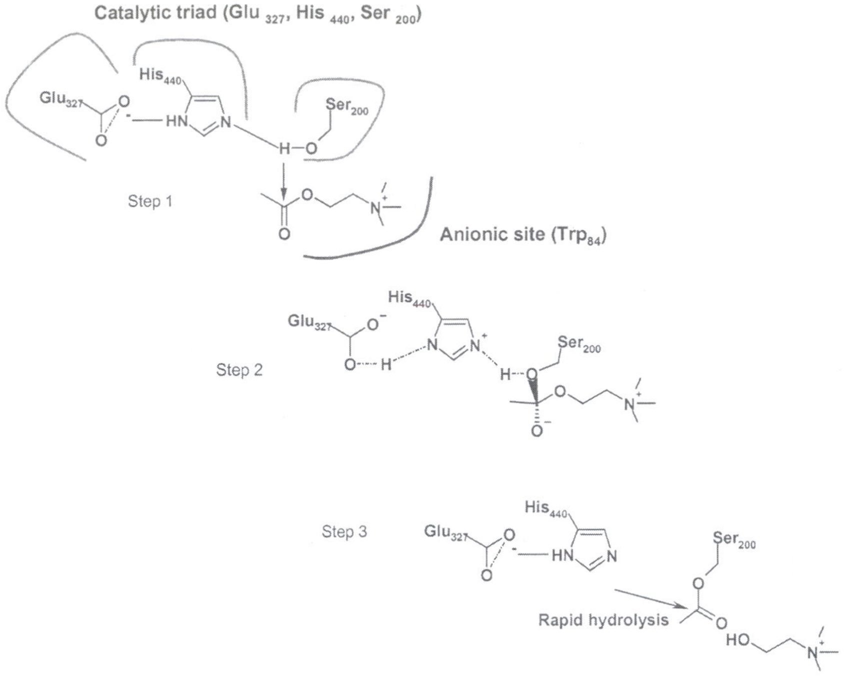

Catalytic triad (Glu $_{327}$, His $_{440}$, Ser $_{200}$)

Step 1

Anionic site (Trp_{84})

Step 2

Step 3

Rapid hydrolysis

FIGURE 18.1 Mechanism of acetylcholine (ACh) hydrolysis by acetylcholinesterase (AChE). AChE contains a "catalyptic triad" in the active site formed by a serine (Ser_{200}), a histidine (His_{440}), and a glutamic acid (Glu_{327}). Ser_{200} activated by His_{440} and Glu_{327} forms a nucleophilic attack on the carbonyl group of ACh (step 1) and the quaternary transition state (step 2) decomposes, resulting in the intermediate acetyl enzyme (step 3). Hydrolysis of the acetyl enzyme reactivates the enzyme. (See Color Insert)

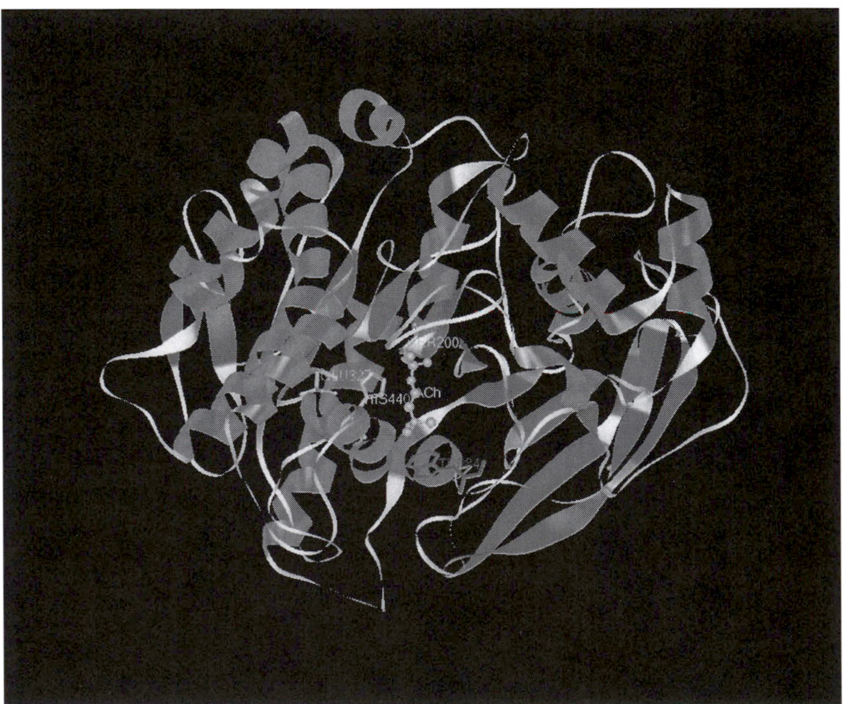

FIGURE 18.2 Ribbon scheme of the three-dimensional structure of acetylcholinesterase (AChE) from *Torpedo californica. Light blue arrows* represent β-strands, and *red coils* represent α-helices. The side chains of the catalytic triad (Ser_{200}, His_{440}, and Glu $_{327}$) and the peripheral site (Trp_{84}) in the active site gorge are indicated as stick figures. Acetylcholine (ACh) docked manually is represented in *yellow* as ball stick figure. Source: PDB ID: 2ACE (Sussman et al. 1991). (See Color Insert)

TABLE 18.1 Classification of Cholinesterase Inhibitors into Three Classes Based on Their Chemical Structures Including Some Examples

Class	General Formula	Examples
Mono-quaternary amines	R1, R2, R3, R4 on N^+	Edrophonium
Bis-quateranary amines	R_2', R_1', R_2'—N^+—$R_4^{5,55}$—N^+—R_2^{55}, R_1^{55}, R_2^{55}	Ambenonium
Carbamates	R—N—C(=O)—O—R′	Physostigmine Neostigmine
Organophospates and phosphonates	R1, R2, O, X on P R1 and R2: e.g. alkoxy or alkoxy or alkyl groups X: leaving groups e.g. fluorine, thiocholine	Isofluorophate (DFP) Parathion

the route of exposure or administration. Whereas some inhibitors act only peripherally (i.e., compounds that do not cross the blood–brain barrier such as the mostly charged molecules (quaternary compounds), other inhibitors act at both peripheral and central sites (i.e., lipophilic substances, including carbamates) [6].

CLINICAL APPLICATIONS OF ANTICHOLINESTERASES

Glaucoma is a disease characterized by increasing intraocular pressure that results in damage of the optic nerve. Anticholinesterases produce miosis and are therefore, by

TABLE 18.2 Summary of Effects of Cholinesterase Inhibitors in Humans

System or tissue	Physiological or pharmacological effects
Central nervous system	Tremor, anxiety, restlessness disrupted memory, confusion, convulsions, desynchronization of EEG, sleep disturbances, coma, circulatory and respiratory depression.
Cardiovascular	Bradycardia, decreased cardiac output, hypotension.
Respiratory	Bronchoconstriction, paralysis of respiratory muscles, increased bronchial secretions.
Digestive	Salivation, increased tone and motility in gut, abdominal cramps, diarrhea, defecation, pancreatic and intestinal secretions.
Urinary	Incontinence, increased urinary frequency.
Skeletal muscle	Paralysis, fasciculations, muscle weakness.
Visual	Lacrimation, miosis, accomodative spasm, blurred vision.
Skin	Sweating.

All the well-known side effects from these agents are cholinergic in nature due to the prolonged availability of ACh.

improving outflow facility, useful in glaucoma. AChE inhibitors such as neostigmine can be used in the treatment of atony of the urinary bladder and of adynamic ileus resulting from surgery.

A large number of drugs such as tricyclic antidepressants, phenothiazines, and antihistamines are known to exert anticholinergic (antimuscarinic) toxicity. Anticholinesterase agents, such as physostigmine, can be used as antidotes during acute intoxication with these drugs [7].

Myasthenia gravis is characterized by an impaired cholinergic neurotransmission at skeletal muscles. Symptoms including ptosis and diplopia, ultimately leading to respiratory paralysis depending on the muscles involved, also can be treated with anticholinesterase drugs. The most common drugs in therapeutic use are pyridostigmine and neostigmine, which both are devoid of central effects [8].

CHOLINESTERASE INHIBITORS AND ALZHEIMER'S DISEASE

Centrally acting ChE inhibitors gained new attractiveness once for this class of compounds. Symptomatic improvements have been reported in this age-related increasing disease. A central feature of Alzheimer's disease is chronic and progressive neurodegeneration characterized symptomatically by progressive deterioration of activities of daily living, behavioral disturbances, and cognitive loss. Currently, it is accepted that an impaired cholinergic function in the brain is causally linked with the symptomatology of Alzheimer's disease. Together with a decline in cholinergic neurotransmission, in Alzheimer's disease a substantial reduction in the choline acetyltransferase, the enzyme responsible for the synthesis of ACh, and a subsequent decline in the level of ACh in the brain is present. Currently, the only successful treatment concept that results in a significant symptomatic benefit in Alzheimer patients is ChE inhibitors [9]. ChE inhibitors with brain specificity slow the inactivation of ACh after synaptic release, thereby prolonging central ACh activity. Currently, the four ChE inhibitors—tacrine, donepezil, rivastigmine, and galanthamine—have been approved and the latter three are in wide clinical use. There are differences among these compounds with regard to their mechanism of inhibition and their selectivity toward AChE and a second esterase, butyrylcholinesterase. Donepezil and galanthamine exclusively inhibit AChE, whereas the other compounds inhibit both AChE and butyrylcholinesterase. Such a dual action could, as currently hypothesized on the basis of preclinical data, contribute to a more efficacious treatment seen in the clinic [10].

References

1. Taylor, P., and J. H. Brown. 1994. Acetylcholine. In *Basic neurochemistry*, II, ed. G. J. Siegel, B. W. Agranoff, R. W. Albers, and P. B. Molinoff, pp. 231–260. New York: Raven Press.
2. Quinn, D. M. 1993. Acetylcholinesterase: Enzyme structure, reaction dynamics, and virtual transition states. *J. Am. Chem. Soc.* 115: 10,477–10,482.
3. Sussman, J. L., M. Harel, F. Frolow, C. Oefner, A. Goldman, L. Toker, and I. Silman. 1991. Atomic structure of acetylcholinesterase from *Torpedo californica*: A prototypic acetylcholine-binding protein. *Science* 253:872–879.
4. Fukuto, T. R. 1990. Mechanism of action of organophosphorus and carbamate insecticides. *Environ. Health Perspect.* 87:245–254.
5. El Yazal, J., S. N. Rao, A. Mehl, and W. Slikker, Jr. 2001. Prediction of organophosphorus acetylcholinesterase inhibition using three-dimensional quantitative structure-activity relationship (3D-QSAR) methods. *Toxicol. Sci.* 63:223–232.
6. Taylor, P., and J. H. Brown. 2001. Anticholinesterase agents. In *Goodman & Gilman's the pharmacological basis of therapeutics*, 10th ed., ed. J. G. Hardman, L. Limbird, and A. G. Gilman, 175–189. New York: McGraw-Hill.
7. Nilsson, E. 1982. Physostigmine treatment in various drug-induced intoxications. *Ann. Clin. Res.* 14:165–172.
8. Drachman D. B., R. N. Adams, L. F. Josifex, and H. S. G. Self. 1982. Functional activities of autoantibodies to acetylcholine receptors and the clinical severity of myasthenia gravis. *N. Eng. J. Med.* 307:769–775.
9. Weinstock, M. 1999. Selectivity of cholinesterase inhibition: Clinical implications for the treatment of Alzheimer's disease. *CNS Drugs* 12:307–323.
10. Ballard, C. G. 2002. Advances in the treatment of Alzheimer's disease: Benefits of dual cholinesterase inhibition. *Eur. Neurol.* 47:64–70.

19

Amino Acid Neurotransmission

William Talman
Department of Neurology
University of Iowa and Veterans Affairs Medical Center
Iowa City, Iowa

As detailed in earlier chapters, the autonomic nervous system is highly organized from its peripheral receptors to the terminals of visceral efferents. Afferent nerve fibers from mechanoreceptors and chemoreceptors originate in neurons of autonomic ganglia. Those cells project into the central nervous sytem, where signals are processed and, through actions of converging peripheral and central inputs, are integrated into meaningful autonomic responses to simple and complex stimuli. Amino acids acting as putative neurotransmitters may play a role in signal transduction at each level of this system.

This chapter briefly outlines participation of three representative amino acids—the excitatory amino acid glutamate, and inhibitory amino acids GABA and glycine—in transmitting signals that modulate sympathetic output of one well-defined cardiovascular reflex: the baroreceptor reflex. Depending on the brain region under consideration, evidence for this involvement varies considerably. In no region can it be said that all criteria have been met to establish any one of these amino acids as a transmitter at a particular synapse, but significant data have developed over the past two decades to suggest that each agent may contribute to varying degrees at different sites.

Although none of the three amino acids has been implicated in mechanoreceptor or chemoreceptor transduction at the level of the peripheral receptor, some evidence suggests that glutamate transmission may be involved in the periphery. Specifically, glutamate binding sites are present on nodose ganglion neurons and are transported from the nodose ganglion toward the aortic arch [1]. Thus, both receptors that bind glutamate and aortic baroreceptors may be found in close proximity. In addition, neurons within the nodose ganglion are activated by their exposure to glutamate and its analogs.

Each of the three putative transmitters is present in the nodose ganglion, but neurochemical evidence suggests that of the three only γ-aminobutyric acid (GABA) and glutamate may be released from baroreceptor afferent fibers in the nucleus tractus solitarii (NTS), the primary site of termination of those and other visceral afferent fibers of the vagus and glossopharyngeal nerves. At this important site, each amino acid potentially may modulate cardiovascular activity. However, an agonist's actions alone are not sufficient evidence to support a role for the agent as a transmitter at a specific synapse. Another important criterion is the ability of selective antagonists to block effects of natural activation of that synapse. In the NTS, glutamate has met this criterion.

Numerous studies have confirmed that the baroreceptor reflex may be blocked by antagonists to glutamate receptors in the NTS. Thus, although glutamate and other agents, including glycine, may produce cardiovascular responses like those of baroreceptor reflex activation, only blockade of glutamate receptors leads to nearly total blockade of the baroreceptor reflex itself [2]. It would seem then that glutamate, whose receptors are found in the NTS [3], may be a transmitter of primary afferents in the reflex. That it may also be involved in other cardiovascular reflexes is suggested by pressor responses produced by injecting it into discrete regions of NTS where chemoreceptor reflex transmission predominates or into larger regions of NTS in unanesthetized animals [4]. Evidence from such studies supports a role for the amino acid in transmission of chemoreceptor reflexes, as well as baroreceptor reflexes at the level of NTS. Attenuation of the chemoreceptor reflex by injection of glutamate antagonists into the NTS further supports its participation in that reflex. It is likely that glutamate exerts its cardiovascular actions through NTS by interacting with other transmitters in the region. One particularly intriguing interaction is between glutamate and nitric oxide systems in NTS [5], but glutamate is clearly colocalized with other putative transmitters as well. GABA, conversely, may also be released from vagal, possibly baroreceptor, afferents, but its release into NTS does not produce a cardiovascular effect like that of baroreceptor reflex activation. Instead, it may inhibit baroreceptor reflex neurons in the NTS. Whether directly involved in cardiovascular reflex transmission, GABA and also glycine have been shown to participate in integration of signals coming into NTS. It is possible that the former is derived from peripheral afferents and from projections of other central nuclei, whereas glycine, which apparently is not released from vagal afferents, may arise from local interneurons or from other central nuclei. Like GABA, it participates in modulating responses of neurons in NTS to multiple incoming signals.

In addition, glycine also indirectly activates local neurons by initiating release of the excitatory agent acetylcholine from nerve terminals in NTS [6].

The baroreceptor reflex pathway continues beyond NTS with rostral and caudal projections to cardiovascular nuclei in the ventral medulla. More rostrally axons project directly to the rostral ventrolateral medulla (RVLM), which plays an important role in tonic maintenance of blood pressure. With activation of those fibers, there is sympathoexcitation, apparently caused by release of glutamate into the RVLM. Activation of the more caudal projection also apparently leads to release of glutamate, but, in this case, the excitatory effect is manifest on GABAergic neurons that project from the caudal ventrolateral medulla to the RVLM. Thus, their activation reduces blood pressure by inhibiting sympathoexcitatory cells on which they terminate. The mechanisms that favor activation of one pathway that is sympathoexcitatory versus another that is sympathoinhibitory are not known, but clearly other input to the RVLM may also integrate function in that nucleus during well defined behaviors.

For example, activation of the lateral hypothalamus, which may elicit a behavioral response, leads to activation of glutamate receptors on neurons in the RVLM [7]. Resulting increased sympathetic nerve activity tends to increase blood pressure. This glutamatergic input to the RVLM provides an important integrative function by overriding the inhibitory influence of baroreceptor reflex activation that would otherwise occur with increased blood pressure associated with the behavior.

Well before any role had been found for either GABA or glutamate in the RVLM, potential involvement of glycinergic transmission had already been suggested. Initially, glycine was applied to the ventral surface of the medulla, where it elicited reductions in blood pressure. Thus, a depressor function was ascribed to it within the general region of the rostral ventral medulla. However, it is now clear that glycine may elicit either depressor or pressor responses depending on the site at which it is injected into the rostral ventral medulla. The mechanism of its differing actions and the origin of glycine terminals in the region is still not known.

Completing the central portion of the sympathetic limb of the baroreceptor reflex, neurons in the RVLM project to the intermediolateral column of the spinal cord, where sympathetic preganglionic fibers originate. Glutamate may play an important role at this site also. Released from descending fibers from the medulla, it affects maintenance of sympathetic tone or increases sympathetic activity in response to stimuli. GABA and glycine, likewise, may participate in modulating sympathetic activity at the level of the intermediolateral column and may be colocalized with each other or with other more classic neurotransmitters in terminals within the region.

Clearly, each of these amino acids may contribute to regulation of cardiovascular function in normal animals, but they may also be part of derangements that lead to hypertension in experimental animals. Their importance is supported by shifts in sensitivity to GABA and glutamate injected into central nuclei in the spontaneously hypertensive rat model of genetic hypertension.

References

1. Lewis, S. J., M. Cincotta, A. J. M. Verberne, B. Jarrott, D. Lodge, and P. M. Beart. 1987. Receptor autoradiography with [^{3}H] L-glutamate reveals the presence and axonal transport of glutamate receptors in vagal afferent neurons of the rat. *Eur. J. Pharmacol.* 144:413–415.
2. Gordon, F. J., and W. T. Talman. 1992. Role of excitatory amino acids and their receptors in bulbospinal control of cardiovascular function. In *Central neural mechanisms in cardiovascular regulation, vol. 2.,* ed. G. Kunos, and J. Ciriello, 209–225. New York: Birkhauser.
3. Ashworth-Preece, M. A., F. Chen, B. Jarrott, and A. J. Lawrence. 1999. Visualisation of AMPA binding sites in the brain stem of normotensive and hypertensive rats. *Brain Res.* 834(1–2):186–189.
4. Machado, B. H., and L. G. H. Bonagamba. 1992. Microinjection of L-glutamate into the nucleus tractus solitarii increases arterial pressure in conscious rats. *Brain Res.* 576:131–138.
5. Talman, W. T., L. Wellendorf, D. Martinez, S. Ellison, X. Li, M. D. Cassell, and H. Ohta. 1994. Glycine elicits release of acetylcholine from the nucleus tractus solitarii in rat. *Brain Res.* 650:253–259.
6. Sun, M. K., and P. G. Guyenet. 1986. Hypothalamic glutamatergic input to medullary sympathetoexcitatory neurons in rats. *Am. J. Physiol.* 251:798–810.
7. Talman, W. T., D. Nitschke Dragon, H. Ohta, and L.-H. Lin. 2001. Nitroxidergic influences on cardiovascular control by NTS: A link with glutamate. *Ann. N Y Acad. Sci.* 940:169–178.

20 Peptidergic Neurotransmission

Graham J. Dockray
Physiological Laboratory
University of Liverpool
Liverpool, United Kingdom

Until the mid-1970s, it was generally thought that hormones, which included regulatory peptides, worked in a quite different way from neurotransmitters. Clear examples were recognized of functions that were regulated by both hormones and autonomic neurons (e.g., stimulation of gastric and pancreatic secretion by gut hormones and by vagal efferent neurons), but the two control systems were considered complementary. It then became clear that regulatory peptides, some of which were related to gut hormones, were also produced in neurons including those of the autonomic nervous system [1].

Events mediated by autonomic neurons that cannot be readily attributable to cholinergic or adrenergic transmission have been appreciated for decades. Recognition of the importance of these events is reflected in the widespread use of the generic term "nonadrenergic, noncholinergic" (NANC) transmission. There are many potential mediators of different NANC phenomena including nitric oxide (NO), purinergic transmitters, and serotonin. However, the biologically active peptides are by far the largest and most diverse group of putative NANC transmitters, and the term "peptidergic transmission" is used to describe the relevant mechanisms. Putative peptide transmitters frequently act in concert with classical transmitters and other NANC transmitters [2, 3].

FAMILIES OF PEPTIDE TRANSMITTERS

Peptide transmitters belong to families on the basis of their common amino acid sequences. These are considered to have evolved by a process of gene duplication and divergence—for example, the group that includes vasoactive intestinal polypeptide (VIP) and pituitary adenylate cyclase activating peptide (PACAP), and the neuropeptide Y (NPY) and peptide YY (PYY) family. Different family members may be expressed in neurons, endocrine, or other cell types [4].

GENERIC FEATURES OF PEPTIDERGIC TRANSMISSION

Biosynthesis

Neuropeptides are synthesized initially as large precursor molecules at the endoplasmic reticulum in the neuronal cell soma. Rapid cleavage of an NH_2-terminal signal peptide leaves the so-called propeptide, which traverses the Golgi complex and is sequestered at the *trans*-Golgi network in dense-cored secretory vesicles (Fig. 20.1). During passage through the Golgi complex and in secretory vesicles, the propeptide is usually modified to generate the final secretory product—for example, by endopeptidase and exopeptidase cleavage by enzymes of the prohormone convertase family and by carboxypeptidase E, and by COOH-terminal amination, glycosylation, Tyr-sulfation, or Ser-phosphorylation. These processes often vary among cell types expressing the same gene and may not be completely efficient in any particular cell type, so that mixtures of structurally related peptides all derived from the same precursor may be secreted.

Storage and Release

Golgi-derived vesicles containing neuropeptides are distinct from small clear synaptic vesicles that contain classical transmitters such as noradrenaline and acetylcholine. The latter are generated close to their site of release, and their loading into secretory vesicles depends on reuptake mechanisms at the plasma membrane and transport across the vesicle membrane. Comparable processes do not occur for peptide transmitters, the stores of which are replaced only by the generation of new vesicles at the level of the Golgi complex. The exocytosis of both synaptic and dense-cored vesicles depends on increased intracellular calcium, although at least in some cases, peptide release is associated with higher frequency stimulation.

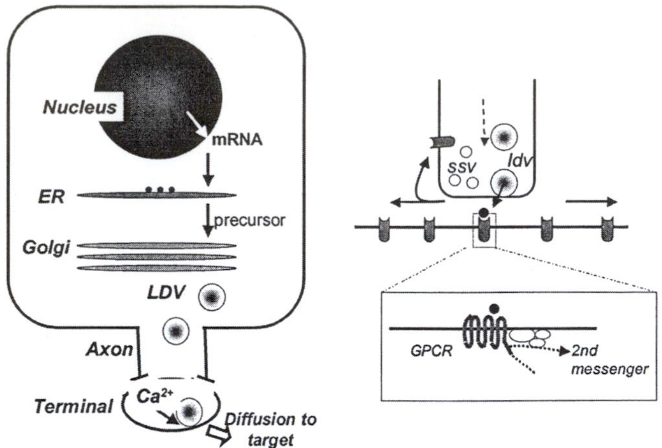

FIGURE 20.1 Schematic representation of the events involved in production of neuropeptide transmitters. **Left**, In the neuronal cell soma, the steps of transcription, mRNA nuclear export, and mRNA translation at the rough endoplasmic reticulum (ER) give rise to peptide transmitter precursors (propeptides). The latter pass through the Golgi and are sequestered in Golgi-derived large dense-cored vesicles (ldv) that pass along the nerve axon to sites of release. **Right**, Neuropeptides are released from Golgi-derived dense-cored vesicles (ldv) and act at G protein–coupled receptors (GPCR), which may be either postjunctional or prejunctional. Small synaptic vesicles (ssv) may release classical autonomic transmitters at the same sites.

Receptors

The targets of neuropeptide transmitters are characteristically G protein–coupled receptors (GPCRs). These may be postjunctional or prejunctional. There need not be a close morphologic relationship between the release site and target cell, and peptide transmitters are often considered to act over greater distances than classical autonomic transmitters. Stimulation of GPCRs activates heterotrimeric G proteins that work through diverse patterns of second messengers, including control of cyclic adenosine monophosphate, intracellular Ca^{2+}, protein kinase C, mitogen-activated protein kinase, and phosphatidyl inositol-3-kinase cascades. Families of GPCRs may exhibit differential selectivity for different related peptides. Naturally occurring and synthetic nonpeptide ligands, both agonists and antagonists, have been identified for a number of the peptide-regulated GPCRs.

Degradation

After their secretion, peptide transmitters either diffuse away from the target or are degraded to smaller peptides and amino acids by proteases in the extracellular fluid. These processes appear to be relatively slow so that peptide transmitters act over longer periods than classical transmitters. Some relevant peptidases have been characterized including endopeptidase 24.11, which cleaves many small peptide transmitters.

CHEMICAL CODING

Different patterns of expression of neuropeptide genes frequently occur in neuronal populations utilizing the same classical transmitter. These patterns, sometimes called "chemical coding," make it possible to identify subpopulations of cells within the group as a whole [5]. Importantly, changes in the pattern of expression of neuropeptide-encoding genes may occur after nerve section, damage, or inflammation, so that the neurochemical phenotype of a neuron is not an unambiguous code [2].

OVERVIEW OF PEPTIDES IN THE AUTONOMIC NERVOUS SYSTEM

The diversity in peptide distribution among species and among autonomic neurons innervating similar structures can be striking [6]. However, there are also good examples of conserved expression and function (Table 20.1). Thus,

TABLE 20.1 Common Autonomic Neuropeptide Transmitters

Peptide family	Main members	Receptors	Representative action
VIP	VIP, PHI, PACAP	PAC1, VPAC1, VPAC2	Relaxation of smooth muscle, stimulation of intestinal secretion
Tachykinins	SP, NKA	NK-1, NK-2, NK-3	Vasodilation, contraction of gut smooth muscle
NPY	NPY	Y-1 to Y-6	Vasoconstriction, inhibition of noradrenaline release
Opioids	Enk, dynorphin	-μ, -δ, -κ	Prejunctional inhibition in ENS
Galanin	Galanin	GAL-1, GAL-2	Contraction of gut smooth muscle
Somatostatin	Som	SSTR1-3	Inhibition of epithelial cell function
CGRP	CGRP	CGRP	Vasodilator
Cholecystokinin	CCK	CCK-1, CCK-2	Contraction of gallbladder, secretion of pancreatic enzymes

CCK, cholecystokinin; CGRP, calcitonin gene–related peptide; Enk, enkephalin; ENS, enteric nervous system; GAL, galanthamine hydrobromide; NK, neurokinin; NKA, neurokinin A; NPY, neuropeptide Y; PACAP, pituitary adenylate cyclase activating peptide; PHI, peptide histidine isoleucine amide; SP, substance P; VIP, vasoactive intestinal polypeptide.

postganglionic parasympathetic neurons serving a number of visceral structures express VIP and PACAP, and these peptides are thought to contribute to nerve-mediated secretion (e.g., in pancreas) and to vasodilation. Similarly, postganglionic sympathetic neurons supplying blood vessels frequently express NPY, which is a vasoconstrictor and also acts prejunctionally to inhibit noradrenaline release [6]. A particularly impressive array of neuropeptide-encoding genes is expressed in the enteric nervous system, where there are complex patterns of colocalization of different neuropeptides and classical transmitters [5]. Across a range of mammalian species, the tachykinin substance P occurs in enteric cholinergic neurons stimulating smooth muscle contraction, and VIP occurs in enteric neurons that also act through NO and perhaps adenosine triphosphate to inhibit smooth muscle. Finally, peptidergic transmitters, notably substance P and calcitonin gene–related peptide, are well recognized to be produced in afferent neurons and to mediate some of the peripheral responses to stimulation of these neurons [3, 7].

References

1. Dockray, G. J. 1988. Regulatory peptides and the neuroendocrinology of gut-brain relations. *Q. J. Exp. Physiol.* 73:703–727.
2. Hokfelt, T., C. Broberger, Z. Q. Xu, V. Sergeyev, R. Ubink, and M. Diez. 2000. Neuropeptides: An overview. *Neuropharmacology* 39:1337–1356.
3. Lundberg, J. M. 1996. Pharmacology of cotransmission in the autonomic nervous system: Integrative aspects on amines, neuropeptides, adenosine triphosphate, amino acids and nitric oxide. *Pharmacol. Rev.* 48:113–178.
4. Dockray, G. J., and J. H. Walsh. 1994. Regulatory peptide systems of the gut: An introductory essay. In *Gut peptides*, ed. J. H. Walsh and G. J. Dockray, 1–9. New York: Raven Press.
5. Furness, J. B. 2000. Types of neurons in the enteric nervous system. *J. Auton. Nerv. Syst.* 81:87–96.
6. Gibbins, I. L., and J. L. Morris. 2000. Pathway specific expression of neuropeptides and autonomic control of the vasculature. *Regul. Pept.* 93:93–107.
7. Holzer, P. 1998. Neural emergency system in the stomach. *Gastroenterology* 114:823–839.

21 Leptin Signaling in the Central Nervous System

Kamal Rahmouni
University of Iowa
Cardiovascular Center
Iowa City, Iowa

William G. Haynes
University of Iowa
Cardiovascular Center
Iowa City, Iowa

Allyn L. Mark
University of Iowa
Cardiovascular Center
Iowa City, Iowa

Historically, the importance of the central nervous system in the regulation of energy homeostasis derived from the clinical observation of excessive subcutaneous fat in patients with pituitary tumors. The role of the hypothalamus in body energy storage was later established using discrete lesions or surgical transection of neural pathways [1]. For years, it was postulated that to control body fat stores, the brain must receive afferent input in proportion to the current level of body fat. The identification in 1994 of leptin [2], the ob gene product, provided powerful support for the concept of a feedback loop between the periphery and the brain for energy homeostasis (Fig. 21.1). Leptin, a 167–amino acid protein secreted by adipocytes, circulates in proportion to the adipose tissue mass. This hormone relays a satiety signal to the hypothalamus after entering the brain by a saturable-specific transport mechanism. Leptin gene expression and secretion are increased by overfeeding, a high-fat diet, insulin, and glucocorticoids, and it is decreased by fasting and sympathetic nerve activation.

The severe obesity and the hyperphagia caused by the absence of leptin in rodents and humans make it clear that this hormone is fundamental for the control of body weight and food intake. Leptin promotes weight loss by reducing appetite and by increasing energy expenditure through stimulation of sympathetic nerve activity (see Fig. 21.1). The effect of leptin on the sympathetic nervous system is an important aspect in the regulation of energy homeostasis and several other physiologic functions. Leptin also is involved in regulation of glucose metabolism, sexual maturation and reproduction, the hypothalamic-pituitary-adrenal system, thyroid and growth hormone axes, angiogenesis and lipolysis, hematopoiesis, immune or proinflammatory responses, and bone remodeling [3]. It also appears to contribute in the regulation of cardiovascular function and may be implicated in the pathophysiology of obesity-associated hypertension [4]. Leptin regulates most of these functions by its action in the hypothalamus.

CENTRAL NEURAL ACTION OF LEPTIN

Leptin Receptor

The leptin receptor is a single transmembrane protein belonging to the cytokine receptor superfamily. Because of alternative splicing of the mRNA, at least six leptin receptor isoforms have been identified (designated Ob-Ra to Ob-Rf). Five isoforms (Ob-Ra to Ob-Rd and Ob-Rf) differ in the length of their intracellular domain [5, 6], whereas Ob-Re, which lacks the transmembrane domain, is a soluble form of the receptor. The Ob-Rb form encodes the full receptor, including the long intracellular domain, which contains all the motifs necessary to stimulate the intracellular machinery involved in leptin signaling. Leptin exerts its effects through interaction with this Ob-Rb form of the leptin receptor in specific classes of neurons. The Ob-Rb isoform is expressed in several hypothalamic nuclei, including the arcuate nucleus, ventromedial hypothalamus, paraventricular nucleus, and dorsomedial hypothalamus [5, 7]. The high levels of the short intracellular domain forms in the choroid plexus may act to transport leptin across the brain barrier [6].

INTRACELLULAR MECHANISMS OF LEPTIN SIGNALING

The leptin receptor signals through the Janus kinase/signal transducer and activator of transcription (JAK/STAT) pathway [5, 7]. On leptin stimulation, intracellular JAK proteins are activated, which, in turn, activate by phosphorylation the cytoplasmic STAT proteins. Phosphorylated STAT proteins translocate to the nucleus and stimulate transcription of target genes (Fig. 21.2).

The leptin receptor has divergent signaling capacities as its activation modulates the activity of different intracellu-

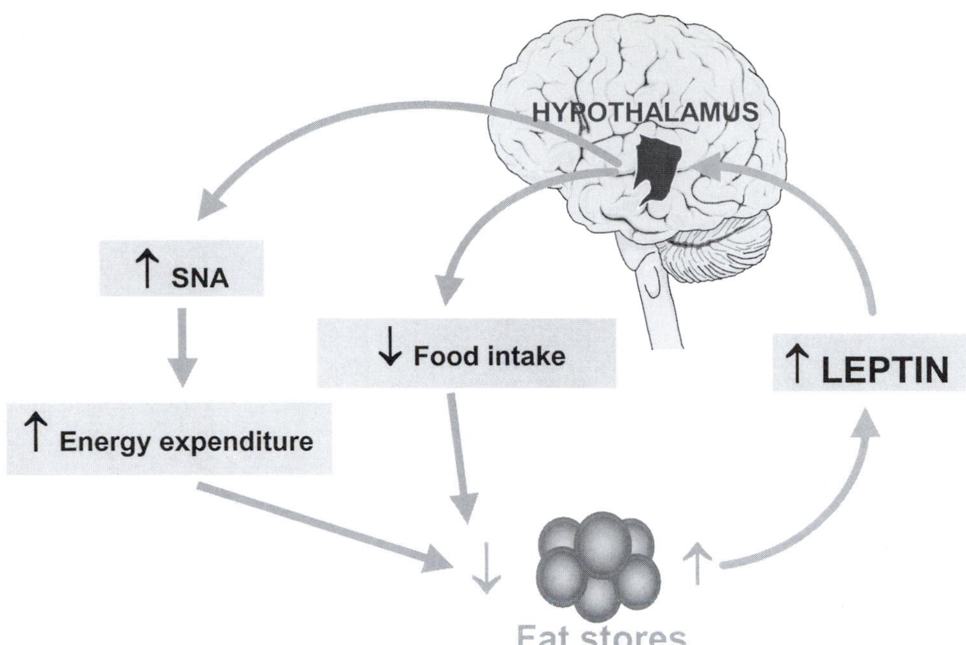

FIGURE 21.1 Role of leptin in the negative loop regulating body weight. Leptin is secreted by the adipocyte and circulates in the blood in concentrations proportional to fat mass content. Action of leptin on its receptor present in the hypothalamus inhibits food intake and increases energy expenditure through stimulation of sympathetic nerve activity (SNA). This leads to decreased adipose tissue mass and body weight.

lar enzymes, including mitogen-activated protein kinase, phosphoinositol 3 kinase, type 3 phosphodiesterase, insulin receptor substrate protein, and protein kinase C. These different intracellular pathways might mediate some central neural effects of leptin. For example, leptin-induced hyperpolarization of subsets of hypothalamic neurons that occurs within minutes of application is mediated by phosphoinositol 3 kinase (see Fig. 21.2) [7].

SITE OF LEPTIN ACTION IN THE BRAIN

The arcuate nucleus is considered as the major site of transduction of the afferent input from circulating leptin into a neuronal response [1, 7, 8]. This is supported by the decrease in food intake induced by local injection of leptin in this area, and the inability of central neural administration of leptin to affect food intake or sympathetic nerve activity after the arcuate nucleus has been destroyed. Other brain areas innervated by the arcuate nucleus neurons, such as the paraventricular nucleus and lateral hypothalamus, are considered downstream neurons of second order in the pathways regulating neuronal activity by leptin [1, 7].

INTERACTION OF LEPTIN AND NEUROPEPTIDES IN THE HYPOTHALAMUS

After activation of leptin receptors in the central nervous system, the signal is transduced by a series of integrated neuronal pathways that regulate endocrine and autonomic function. Several hypothalamic neuropeptides, monoamines, and other transmitter substances have emerged as candidate mediators of leptin action in the brain. Two classes of neurons account for leptin sensitivity in the brain: those activated (catabolic pathway, represented essentially by proopiomelanocortin neurons) and those inhibited (anabolic pathway, represented principally by the neuropeptide Y [NPY] neurons) (Fig. 21.3) [7].

Neuropeptide Y

NPY, a 36–amino acid peptide, is the most potent orexigenic (promote increased energy intake) peptide activated by decreases in leptin [9]. In the hypothalamus, NPY is synthesized by neurons of the arcuate nucleus and is secreted from their terminals in the paraventricular nucleus and lateral hypothalamus. Injection of NPY into the cerebral ventricles or direct hypothalamic administration increases food intake and promotes obesity [7]. Levels of NPY are dramatically increased in the hypothalamus of leptin-deficient mice. Moreover, leptin inhibits NPY gene expres-

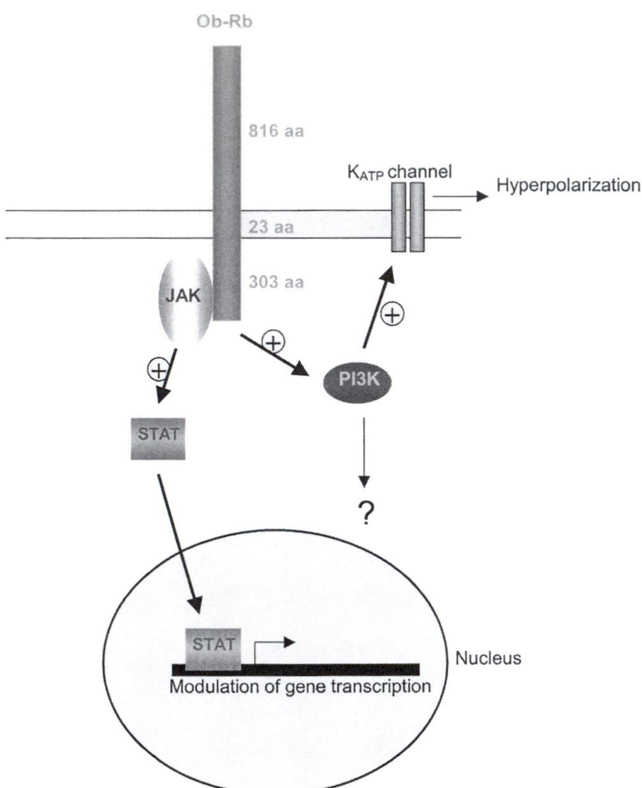

FIGURE 21.2 The long form of leptin receptor (Ob-Rb) and the intracellular mechanisms involved in leptin signaling. Leptin modulate the transcription of target genes through the Janus kinase/signal transducer and activator of transcription (JAK/STAT) pathway. Phosphoinositol 3 kinase (PI3K) seems to mediate leptin-induced hyperpolarization of hypothalamic neurons, and perhaps other actions of leptin.

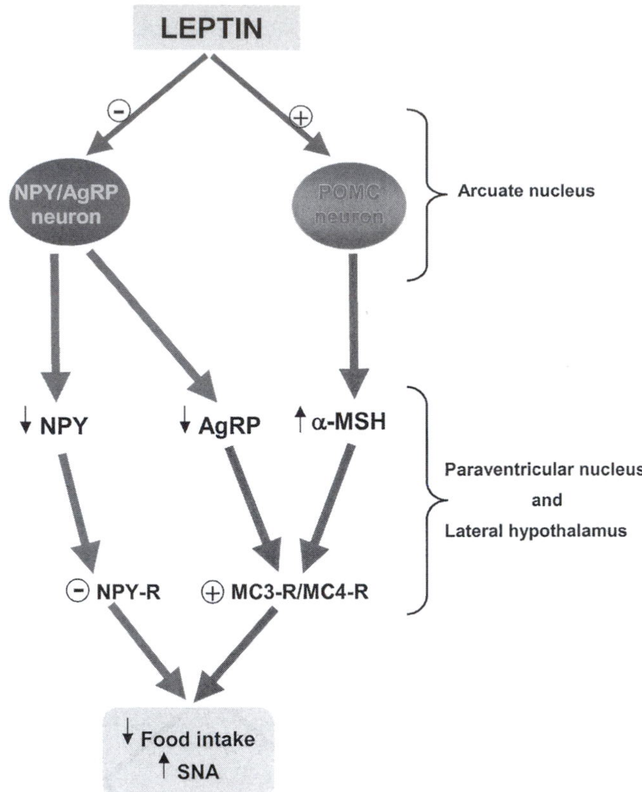

FIGURE 21.3 Interaction of leptin with neuropeptide Y (NPY)/agouti-related protein (AgRP)- and proopiomelanocortin (POMC)-containing neurons in the hypothalamic arcuate nucleus. Increased action of leptin inhibits the NPY/AgRP anabolic pathway and stimulates the POMC catabolic pathway, leading to decrease in food intake and increase in sympathetic nerve activity (SNA). MC3-R, melanocortin-3 receptor; MC4-R, melanocortin-4 receptor; α-MSH, α-melanocyte–stimulating hormone. (See Color Insert)

sion, and knockout of the NPY gene reduces the obesity and other endocrine alterations resulting from chronic leptin deficiency in ob/ob mice by about 50% [9].

Melanocortin System

There is strong evidence that many of leptin's actions are mediated by stimulation of the melanocortin system [9, 10]. The melanocortins are peptides that are processed from the polypeptide precursor proopiomelanocortin, which is produced by neurons in the arcuate nucleus of the hypothalamus and the nucleus of the tractus solitarius. Proopiomelanocortin neurons are known to express the leptin receptor, and leptin binding leads to the secretion of α-melanocyte–stimulating hormone, which in turn binds to a number of a family of melanocortin receptors. Five melanocortin receptors (MC-1R to MC-5R) have been identified. MC-3R and MC-4R are highly expressed in the central nervous system [9]. The critical role for MC-4R in energy balance was demonstrated by target disruption of the *MC-4R* gene that induces hyperphagia and obesity in mice [8, 9].

Antagonism of a central melanocortin receptor also is important in the regulation of energy homeostasis [7–10]. This concept emerged with the discovery of production within the hypothalamic neuron of a potent and selective antagonist of MC-3R and MC-4R. This molecule known as agouti-related peptide (AgRP) is expressed only in the arcuate nucleus of the hypothalamus by the same neurons that express NPY. The expression levels of AgRP are upregulated by fasting and by leptin deficiency.

Other Mediators

The complicated nature of leptin signaling pathways may be suggested from the essentially normal phenotype of NPY knockout mice [9], despite the potent stimulatory effects of NPY on food intake and body weight. This suggests that there are complementary and/or overlapping effector systems that compensate for the absence of NPY. Subsequently, other candidate molecules that can mediate the effects of leptin have been identified (Table 21.1)

TABLE 21.1 List of Neuropeptide and Monoamine Candidate Mediators in the Transduction of Leptin Action in the Central Nervous System

Catabolic molecules	Anabolic molecules
Proopiomelanocortin and derived peptides	Neuropeptide Y
Corticotrophin releasing factor	Agouti-related peptide
Cocaine-and amphetamine-regulated transcript	Melanin-concentrating hormone
Urocortin	Hypocritin 1 and 2/Orexin A and B
Neurotensin	Galanin
IL-1β	Noradrenaline
Glucagon-like peptide 1	
Oxytocin	
Neurotensin	
Serotonin	
Dopamine	

Adapted from Schwartz, M. W., S. C. Woods, D. Porte, Jr., R. J. Seeley, and D. G. Baskin. 2000. Central nervous system control of food intake. *Nature* 404:661–671.

[7, 10]. For example, leptin-dependent sympathetic activation to brown adipose tissue appears to be mediated by corticotrophin-releasing factor, because the sympathoexcitatory effect of leptin to this tissue was substantially inhibited by pretreatment with the corticotrophin-releasing factor receptor antagonist [4].

CONCLUSION

Energy balance is a highly regulated phenomenon, and the importance of the central nervous system in this regulation of energy homeostasis is well established. The centers of regulation of food intake and body weight are located in the hypothalamus. The discovery of leptin has illuminated this field of neuroscience. This hormone constitutes the signal from adipose tissue that acts in the hypothalamus to complete the feedback loop that regulates appetite and energy expenditure. The identification of the leptin receptor and its site of action in the hypothalamus have resulted in striking progress in dissecting the hypothalamic circuitry that regulates energy homeostasis. Despite the lack of many pieces of this puzzle, the network of the hypothalamic pathways that control energy balance is rapidly being defined.

References

1. Elmquist, J. K., C. F. Elias, and C. B. Saper. 1999. From lesions to leptin: Hypothalamic control of food intake and body weight. *Neuron* 22:221–232.
2. Zhang, Y., R. Proenca, M. Maffei, M. Barone, L. Leopold, and J. M. Friedman. 1994. Positional cloning of the mouse obese gene and its human homologue. *Nature* 372:425–432.
3. Wauters, M., R. V. Considine, and L. F. Van Gaal. 2000. Human leptin: From an adipocyte hormone to an endocrine mediator. *Eur. J. Endocrinol.* 143:293–311.
4. Rahmouni, K., W. G. Haynes, and A. L. Mark. 2002. Cardiovascular and sympathetic effects of leptin. *Curr. Hypertens. Rep.* 4:119–125.
5. Heshka, J. T., and P. J. Jones. 2001. A role for dietary fat in leptin receptor, OB-Rb, function. *Life Sci.* 69:987–1003.
6. Tartaglia, L. A. 1997. The leptin receptor. *J. Biol. Chem.* 272: 6093–6096.
7. Schwartz, M. W., S. C. Woods, D. Porte, Jr., R. J. Seeley, and D. G. Baskin. 2000. Central nervous system control of food intake. *Nature* 404:661–671.
8. Kalra, S. P., M. G. Dube, S. Pu, B. Xu, T. L. Horvath, and P. S. Kalra. 1999. Interacting appetite-regulating pathways in the hypothalamic regulation of body weight. *Endocr. Rev.* 20:68–100.
9. Inui, A. 2000. Transgenic approach to the study of body weight regulation. *Pharmacol. Rev.* 52:35–61.
10. Flier, J. S., and E. Maratos-Flier. 1998. Obesity and the hypothalamus: Novel peptides for new pathways. *Cell* 292:437–440.

22 Nitrergic Neurotransmission

Jill Lincoln
Autonomic Neurosciences Institute
Department of Anatomy and Developmental Biology
University College London
London, United Kingdom

Nitric oxide (NO) is one of the most recent substances to be proposed to act as a neurotransmitter in the autonomic nervous system and is very different from the classical neurotransmitters, noradrenaline and acetylcholine. NO is a free radical and potentially very toxic. It passes freely through membranes and, thus, cannot be stored in vesicles for release during an action potential. In addition, it cannot act in a stereospecific way on postjunctional receptors on the target membrane to produce a response. Therefore, new pharmacological approaches have had to be developed to prove that NO is a neurotransmitter. It is now known that NO does act as a neurotransmitter wihin the autonomic nervous system, particularly within the parasympathetic and enteric nervous systems. It is synthesized by the neuronal isoform of nitric oxide synthase (nNOS) in a highly regulated, Ca^{2+}-dependent, manner. NO relaxes smooth muscle by activating soluble guanylate cyclase, which increases cGMP levels. Nitrergic neurotransmission has been demonstrated in the gastrointestinal, urogenital, and cardiovascular systems and is particularly important in the control of penile erection and of sphincteric regions in the gastrointestinal tract. Loss of nitrergic neurotransmission has also been implicated in a variety of pathological conditions.

SYNTHESIS OF NITRIC OXIDE

NO is synthesized by the enzyme nitric oxide synthase (NOS), which can exist in three isoforms. The isoform involved in nitrergic neurotransmission in the autonomic nervous system is known as neuronal (nNOS) or type I NOS. The other sources of NO are endothelial NOS in the endothelium of blood vessels and inducible NOS, which is produced as part of an immune response. nNOS is a highly complex enzyme (Fig. 22.1A) that exists as a dimer, in which each monomer consists of two enzymes in one. One end, the reductase domain, produces electrons during the conversion of reduced nicotinamide adenine dinucleotide phosphate (NADPH) to NADP. The electrons are passed along the enzyme by flavin cofactors until they reach the oxygenase domain. An important region, the calmodulin-binding region, links the two domains. In the oxygenase domain there is a heme-binding site. In the presence of electrons, heme and O_2, L-arginine is converted to citrulline, resulting in NO synthesis. At resting concentrations of Ca^{2+} within the nerve, nNOS is inactive [1].

MECHANISMS OF NITRERGIC NEUROTRANSMISSION

The process of nitrergic neurotransmission is represented schematically in Figure 22.1B, together with the pharmacologic tools that have been used to demonstrate this process. During an action potential, intracellular concentrations of Ca^{2+} increase resulting in the binding of calmodulin to nNOS and activation of the enzyme. Thus, in contrast with classical neurotransmitters, it is the synthesis rather than the release of the neurotransmitter that is coupled with the action potential. Nitrergic neurotransmission can be inhibited by Ca^{2+} chelators and calmodulin antagonists. Once activated, nNOS converts L-arginine to citrulline and NO. The most important step in demonstrating nitrergic neurotransmission has been the development of L-arginine analogs that can inhibit NO synthesis in a stereospecific manner. Analogs such as N^G-nitro-L-arginine methyl ester (L-NAME) or N^G-monomethyl-L-arginine (L-NMMA) can inhibit nitrergic neurotransmission, whereas the D-analogs are ineffective. In addition, the effects of such nNOS inhibitors can be reversed by application of L-arginine but not D-arginine.

NO cannot be stored but reaches the postjunctional target by diffusion. Drugs have been developed that act as NO donors (e.g., *S*-nitroso-*N*-acetyl-D,L-penicillamine), and these have demonstrated that exogenous NO can mimic the effects of nitrergic neurotransmission. The half-life of NO is short, and there is no need for any specific mechanism to inactivate it (unlike classical neurotransmitters). NO reacts

a) Neuronal NOS

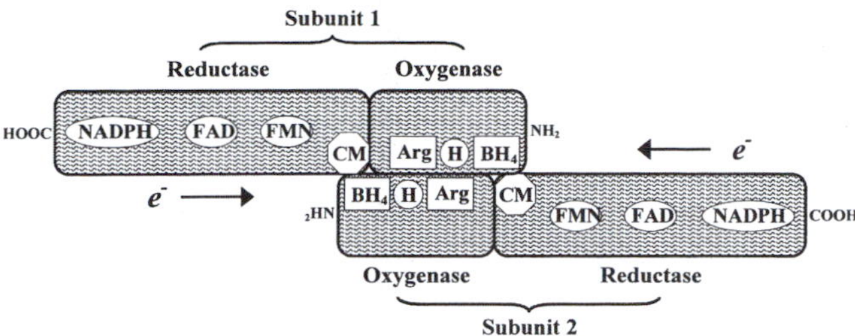

b) Nitrergic Neurotransmission

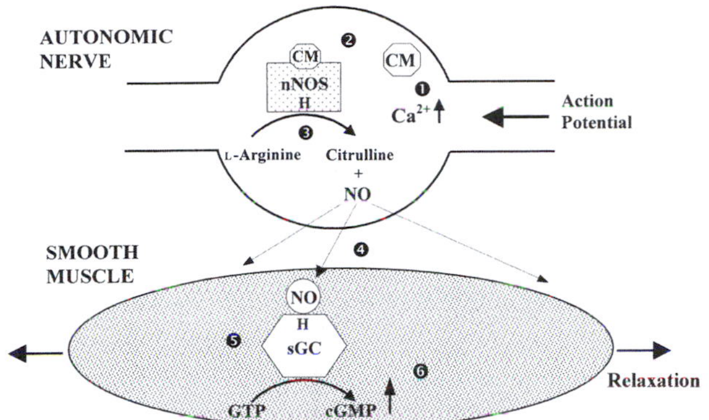

FIGURE 22.1 Schematic representation of (**A**) neuronal nitric oxide synthase (nNOS) and (**B**) the processes involved in nitrergic neurotransmission. **A**, nNOS consists of a dimer with two identical subunits joined in a head-to-head configuration. Each subunit has a reductase domain where electrons (e^-) are produced from the oxidation of reduced nicotinamide adenine dinucleotide phosphate (NADPH) and transported by flavin adenine dinucleotide (FAD) and flavin mononucleotide (FMN). Synthesis of nitric oxide (NO) is carried out during the conversion of L-arginine to citrulline in the presence of heme and O_2 in the oxygenase domain. Tetrahydrobiopterin (BH_4) plays several roles in catalysis including the promotion of dimerization. When bound to Ca^{2+}, calmodulin (CM) promotes the transfer of electrons from one domain to the other and activates NO synthesis. **B**, Nitrergic neurotransmission consists of six steps, each of which can be influenced by different types of agents: (1) an action potential increases Ca^{2+}—inhibited by Ca^{2+} chelators; (2) Ca^{2+} binds to CM, which enables it to bind to nNOS and activate the enzyme—inhibited by calmodulin antagonists; (3) L-arginine is converted to citrulline and NO—inhibited by L-analogs of L-arginine that bind to nNOS but do not act as a substrate; (4) NO diffuses out of the nerve into the target smooth muscle—hemoglobin and reactive species such as superoxides react with NO preventing its actions; (5) NO interacts with heme (H) on soluble guanylate cyclase (sGC) activating the enzyme—sGC inhibitors inhibit effects of nitrergic neurotransmission; (6) increased cyclic guanosine monophosphate (cGMP) levels lead to relaxation of smooth muscle—mimicked by cGMP analogues, inhibited by phosphodiesterases, potentiated by phosphodiesterase inhibitors.

with hemoglobin or other reactive species such as superoxide anions, both of which inhibit neurotransmission or the response to NO donors, or both. There is still some controversy as to whether NO comes out of the nerve as free NO or as a thiol derivative that subsequently breaks down to NO to produce a response in the target. Once NO enters the postjunctional smooth muscle cell, it produces a response by interacting with the enzyme soluble guanylate cyclase (sGC); indeed, sGC has been described as the "intracellular receptor" for NO. NO binds to the heme group on sGC, resulting in the activation of the enzyme and production of increased levels of cyclic guanosine monophosphate (cGMP), which causes relaxation of smooth muscle. Thus, drugs that inhibit sGC can inhibit the response to stimulation of nitrergic transmission and to NO donors, and cGMP analogs can mimic the response. Drugs that inhibit the breakdown of cGMP by phosphodiesterases can potentiate nitrergic neurotransmission, and this forms the basis of clinical therapy, such as Viagra in impotence. Once the physiologic stimulus of the action potential has ended, Ca^{2+} levels in the nerve return to low resting levels and NO synthesis stops. Thus, the amount of NO synthesized in autonomic nerves does not reach toxic levels [1, 2].

NITRERGIC NEUROTRANSMISSION IN THE AUTONOMIC NERVOUS SYSTEM AND PATHOLOGIC IMPLICATIONS

NO, itself, is difficult to detect or measure. However, the capacity to synthesize NO can be readily demonstrated in the autonomic nervous system either by immunohistochemical localization of nNOS or by NADPH diaphorase histochemistry, which uses the electrons produced in the reductase domain of nNOS to convert nitroblue tetrazolium to a blue formazan product that can be visualized. nNOS has been localized in both sympathetic and parasympathetic preganglionic neurons; but, in postganglionic neurones, it is largely restricted to the parasympathetic nervous system, where it is commonly colocalized with vasoactive intestinal polypeptide or acetylcholine. In addition, nNOS is particularly prominent in the enteric nervous system, where it is localized in the myenteric and submucosal plexuses [1, 3]. Functional studies have demonstrated nitrergic neurotransmission throughout the cardiovascular, urogenital, respiratory, and gastrointestinal systems (Table 22.1) [1, 3–6]. NO can function either to cause direct inhibition of smooth muscle or as a neuromodulator by inhibiting excitatory transmission. It is probable that NO also can regulate secretion, but the precise mechanisms for this have yet to be clearly defined.

NO was first discovered as an autonomic neurotransmitter in the bovine retractor penis muscle, and NO is currently

TABLE 22.1 Summary of Selected Regions Where There Is Functional Evidence from *In Vitro* Pharmacological Studies that NO Acts as an Autonomic Neurotransmitter

Region	Response to nitrergic neurotransmission *in vitro*[a]	
Cardiovascular System		
Cerebral arteries	↓ *	acetylcholine modulates NO synthesis
Mesenteric artery	↓	inhibition of sympathetic excitation
Renal artery	↓	inhibition of sympathetic excitation
Saphenous artery	↓	
Hepatic portal vein	↓	
Uterine artery	↓ *	
Urinary Tract		
Urethra	↓ *	
External urethral sphincter	↓	
Bladder trigone	↓	little evidence for transmission in detrusor
Genital Tract		
Bovine retractor penis muscle	↓	
Corpus cavernosum	↓ *	
Prostate	↓ *	may also be involved in secretion
Uterus	↓ *	tonic inhibition
Respiratory Tract		
Trachea		inhibition of cholinergic excitation
Airway smooth muscle	↓ *	inhibition of cholinergic excitation
Gastrointestinal Tract		
Oesophagus	↓ *	
Lower Oesophageal sphincter	↓ *	
Sphincter of oddi	↓	
Stomach	↓ *	
Pyloric sphincter	↓	
Duodenum	↓	inhibition of excitatory transmission
Ileum	↓ *	tonic inhibition
Ileocolonic junction	↓ *	
Colon	↓ *	and rebound excitation?
Internal anal sphincter	↓ *	

[a] ↓ indicates that the response to nitrergic neurotransmission and/or to NO donors is relaxation of smooth muscle. * indicates that evidence has been obtained from experiments on human tissue as well as other species.

accepted as the major parasympathetic neurotransmitter mediating penile erection. Decreased nitrergic neurotransmission has been demonstrated in erectile tissue in diabetes and has been implicated in the development of impotence [4]. In the lower urinary tract, NO may contribute to relaxation of the urethra alongside other inhibitory neurotransmitters [4, 5]. nNOS has been demonstrated in perivascular nerves supplying many blood vessels. The most detailed evidence for parasympathetic nitrergic vasodilation has been found in cerebral vessels where NO and acetylcholine are both released from the same nerves. In addition, acetylcholine may regulate NO synthesis by modulating Ca^{2+} influx into the nerves [6]. Thus, cotransmission and neuromodulation also form part of nitrergic mechanisms. NO synthesized in the enteric nervous system causes relaxation throughout the gastrointestinal tract, but it may be of particular functional significance in sphincteric regions [1, 3]. A notable feature of knockout mice with targeted deletion of nNOS is the presence of gross distension of the stomach, which is similar to infantile pyloric stenosis, in which reduced nitrergic neurotransmission has been found. Similarly, reduced nNOS activity or impaired nitrergic neurotransmission has been reported in achalasia and severe idiopathic constipation, disorders of the gastroesophageal junction, and anal sphincter, respectively [1, 3].

References

1. Lincoln, J., C. H. V. Hoyle, and G. Burnstock, G. 1997. *Nitric oxide in health and disease.* Cambridge, UK: Cambridge University Press.
2. Gibson, A., and E. Lilley. 1997. Superoxide anions, free-radical scavengers and nitrergic neurotransmission. *Gen. Pharmacol.* 28:489–493.
3. Rolle, U., L. Nemeth, and P. Puri. 2002. Nitrergic innervation of the normal gut and in motility disorders of childhood. *J. Pediatr. Surg.* 37:551–567.
4. Burnett, A. L. 1995. Nitric oxide control of lower genitourinary tract functions: A review. *Urology* 45:1071–1083.
5. Mumtaz, F. H., M. A. Khan, C. S. Thompson, R. G. Morgan, and D. P. Mikhailidis. 1999. Nitric oxide in the lower urinary tract: Physiological and pathological implications. *BJU Int.* 85:567–578.
6. Lee, T. J. F., J. Liu, and M. S. Evans. 2001. Cholinergic-nitrergic transmitter mechanisms in the cerebral circulation. *Microsc. Res. Tech.* 53:119–128.

23 Serotonin Receptors and Neurotransmission

Elaine Sanders-Bush
Department of Pharmacology
Vanderbilt University
Nashville, Tennessee

Charles D. Nichols
Department of Pharmacology
Vanderbilt University
Nashville, Tennessee

Serotonin (or 5-hydroxytryptamine [5-HT]) is a neurotransmitter and a circulating hormone. Serotoninergic neurons in the brain synthesize and store serotonin at axon terminals, where it is released and interacts with cell-surface receptors on adjacent neurons. The action of serotonin is terminated by reuptake into presynaptic terminal mediated by the serotonin transporter or by metabolism by monoamine oxidase. Of the 14 different receptor subtypes, most generate intracellular messengers by coupling to G proteins and modulate, rather than mediate, fast neurotransmission. This multitude of receptors explains the variety of actions of serotonin in normal and abnormal states and provides ample opportunity for drug development for treatment of brain diseases.

LOCALIZATION

Serotonin, or 5-HT, is a simple indoleamine (Fig. 23.1), which was discovered more than five decades ago. Since then, 5-HT has been shown to function as a neurotransmitter in the central nervous system (CNS) and also as circulating hormone [1]. The principal source of circulating 5-HT is the intestinal enterochromaffin cells, where 5-HT is synthesized, stored, and released into the bloodstream. 5-HT in blood is concentrated in platelets by an active transport mechanism. In the pineal gland, 5-HT is converted by a two-step process to melatonin (5-methoxy-*N*-acetyltryptamine), a hormone that regulates ovarian function and has been implicated in the control of biologic rhythms. The brain 5-HT–containing neurons are localized in raphe nuclei of the brainstem, which project diffusely throughout the brain and spinal cord.

SYNTHESIS AND METABOLISM

The pathway of synthesis is common throughout the body. 5-HT is synthesized from tryptophan, an essential amino acid obtained in the diet. 5-HT synthesis requires the action of two synthetic enzymes, as illustrated.

SYNTHETIC PATHWAY

Tryptophan $\xrightarrow[1]{}$ 5-hydroxytryptophan $\xrightarrow[2]{}$ 5-HT

1. tryptophan hydroxylase—rate limiting.
2. 5-hydroxytrytophan decarboxylase—generates 5-HT as end product

Tryptophan hydroxylase, the rate-limiting enzyme, is not saturated under normal conditions, rendering 5-HT levels sensitive to changes in blood tryptophan. This translates into the remarkable finding that brain levels of this neurotransmitter can be regulated by the dietary intake of tryptophan. Clinical studies of the role of 5-HT in behavior and drug action often have used a tryptophan-free diet to decrease brain 5-HT and, by inference, evaluate its role in a particular behavior or drug effect.

METABOLIC PATHWAY

5-HT $\xrightarrow[1]{}$ 5-hydroxyindole acetic acid (5-HIAA)

1. monoamine oxidase (MAO)

The principal metabolism of 5-HT is mediated by the ubiquitous enzyme, MAO, to form an inactive product, 5-HIAA. 5-HIAA is subsequently secreted in the cerebrospinal fluid and urine. MAO is a family of mitochondrial enzymes that metabolize all biogenic amines.

NEUROTRANSMISSION

In the CNS, the entire pathway of synthesis and metabolism exists at axon terminals; MAO is also highly expressed in adjacent cells. The life cycle of 5-HT at the synapse is illustrated in Figure 23.2. Both synthetic enzymes are present in the presynaptic terminal. Newly synthesized 5-HT is accumulated in synaptic vesicles to protect it from degradation by MAO. Uptake into vesicles is mediated by the vesicular monoamine transporter (VMAT). Stored 5-HT is released from synaptic vesicles by a complex series of

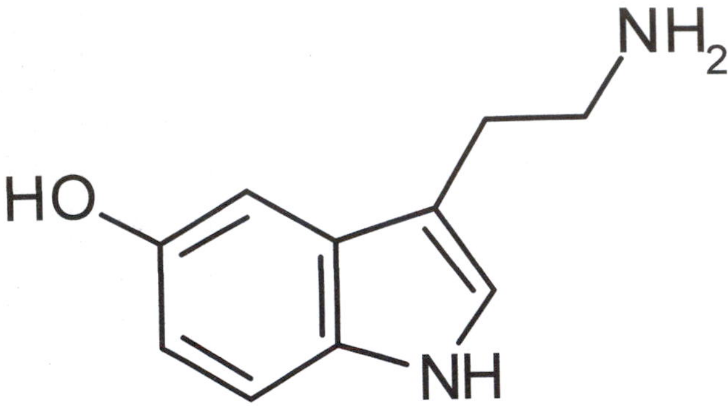

FIGURE 23.1 The chemical structure of serotonin (5-hydroxytryptamine [5-HT]).

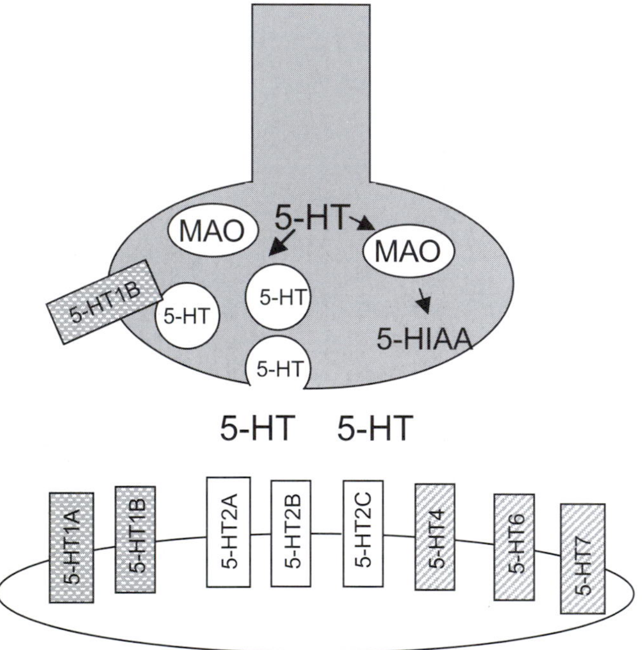

FIGURE 23.2 Schematic of serotonin (5-hydroxytryptamine [5-HT]) nerve terminal. Newly synthesized 5-HT is stored in synaptic vesicles to avoid metabolism to 5-hydroxyindole acetic acid (5-HIAA) by mitochondrial monoamine oxidase (MAO). Released 5-HT interacts with receptors on the postsynaptic membrane or on autoreceptors presynaptically. The principal mechanism of inactivation is reuptake into presynaptic terminal by the 5-HT transporter.

phosphorylation-dependent protein–protein interactions initiated by the influx of calcium. Once released, 5-HT is inactivated by MAO in the synaptic cleft or its action is terminated by reuptake into the presynaptic terminal by the 5-HT transporter (SERT). Once in the presynaptic terminal, 5-HT is either accumulated in synaptic vesicles through VMAT or metabolized by MAO.

The two transporters in 5-HT nerve terminals, VMAT and SERT, belong to different gene families and have markedly different properties. SERT is a sodium-dependent carrier that translocates 5-HT into the presynaptic nerve terminal. VMAT is driven by a proton gradient; it is promiscuous, present in 5-HT and catecholamine vesicles. SERT is expressed exclusively in serotoninergic neurons in the CNS and also is found in the enteric nervous system and in blood platelets. Platelets are devoid of 5-HT synthetic enzymes; transport into platelets by SERT is responsible for the high level of 5-HT found in platelets.

RECEPTORS

5-HT in the synaptic cleft interacts with postsynaptic receptors localized at the postsynaptic membrane or on the presynaptic terminal. The 14 serotonin receptors were reclassified in 1994 [2] and are currently grouped into 7 families (Table 23.1). All but one are members of the superfamily of G protein–coupled receptors (GPCRs), which are predicted to span the plasma membrane seven times, with the N-terminus on the outside of the cell and the C-terminus intracellularly [3]. The intracellular loops and C-terminal tail interact directly with G proteins (Fig. 23.3). As illustrated in Figure 23.2, most of the G protein–coupled 5-HT receptors are localized on postsynaptic membranes and modulate neurotransmission through second messenger pathways. In contrast, the 5-HT$_3$ receptor is a multimeric 5-HT–gated cation channel; it is primarily localized on presynaptic terminals of nonserotoninergic neurons, where it regulates the release of other neurotransmitters such as acetylcholine.

GPCRs generate intracellular second messengers such as cyclic adenosine monophosphate and calcium and stimulate or inhibit various kinases and phosphatases, which, in turn, regulate proteins by changes in their phosphorylation state [4]. Therefore, these receptors act as neuromodulators, modulating other receptors and ion channels that mediate fast neurotransmission. The 5-HT$_3$ receptor is the only 5-HT receptor that gates ions, hence, directly altering membrane potential. The other 5-HT receptors indirectly modify the membrane potential by regulating voltage-gated ion channels (such as Ca^{2+} or K^+ channels) or ligand-gated ion channels (such as glutamate receptors). For example, presynaptic 5-HT$_{1B}$ receptors inhibit N-type calcium channels through G protein, thereby decreasing 5-HT release. This receptor and other G protein–coupled 5-HT receptors are expressed on the presynaptic terminals of other neurotransmitter releasing neurons; these so called heteroreceptors inhibit or potentiate neurotransmitter release at these synapses. Thus, the possibilities of neurotransmitter crosstalk are numerous and widespread.

PHARMACOLOGY AND ROLE IN DISEASE

The large number of receptors translates into a complex pharmacology and a myriad of targets for drug development.

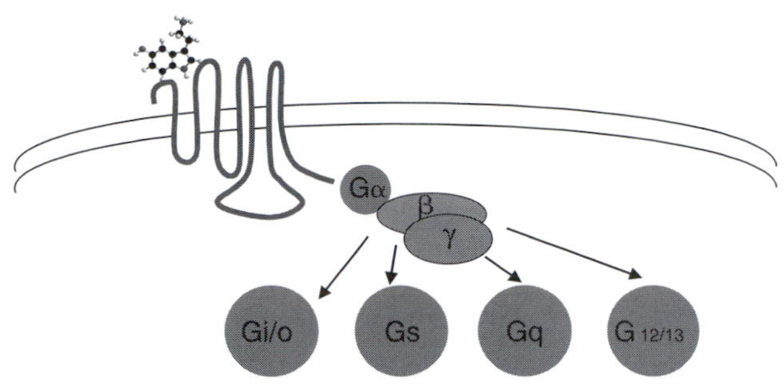

FIGURE 23.3 Serotonin (5-hydroxytryptamine [5-HT]) receptors couple to multiple G proteins. G proteins are classified on the basis of their α subunits. 5-HT receptors have been definitively shown to couple to four different families of G proteins. (See Color Insert)

Specific drugs do exist, but they are rare. The drugs listed in Table 23.1 are at least 50-fold more potent at their primary target, which translates into reasonable specificity *in vivo*. (For more information about pharmacologic properties, access the extensive database at http://pdsp.cwru.edu/pdsp.htm.) Serotonin plays a role in a myriad of behaviors [5]. Recent advances in genetically modified mice have advanced our understanding of the role of specific receptors in behaviors and drug actions [6].

The clinically available drugs that target 5-HT neurotransmission (Table 23.2) have a range of disease targets and varying degrees of specificity. Citalopram, for example, is a highly specific inhibitor of 5-HT transporter with three orders of magnitude lesser affinity for secondary targets

TABLE 23.1 Serotonin Receptor Subtypes and Pharmacology

Recept or Family	Subtype	Transduction pathway	Pharmacology: agonist	Pharmacology: antagonist
5-HT_1	5-HT_{1A}	Inhibition of Adenylate Cyclase ($G_{\alpha i/o}$)	8-OH-DPAT	WAY100635
	5-HT_{1B}		Anpirtoline	SB 224289
	5-HT_{1D}		PNU-142633	BRL15572
	5-HT_{1E}		LY344864	
	5-HT_{1F}			
5-HT_2	5-HT_{2A}	Activation of Phospholipase Cβ ($G_{\alpha q}$)	DOI	MDL100907
	5-HT_{2B}		DOI	LY 266097
	5-HT_{2C}		DOI	SB 221284
5-HT_3		Ligand-gated ion channel	m-CPBG	Ondansetron
5-HT_4		Activation of adenylate cyclase ($G_{\alpha s}$)	Cisapride	SB 203186
5-HT_5	5-HT_{5A}	Inhibition of adenylate cyclase ($G_{\alpha i/o}$)		
	5-HT_{5B}			
5-HT_6		Activation of adenylate cyclase ($G_{\alpha s}$)		SB 271046
5-HT_7		Activation of adenylate cyclase ($G_{\alpha s}$)	8-OH-DPAT	SB 258741

5-HT, 5-hydroxytryptamine; CNS, central nervous system; MAO, monoamine oxidase; 5-HTAA, 5-hydroxyindole acetic acid; VMAT, vesicular monoamine transporter; SERT, serotonin transporter; GPCR, G protein–coupled receptor.

TABLE 23.2 Clinically Available 5-Hydroxytryptamine Drugs

Target	Action	Clinical use	Examples
MAO	Antagonist	Major depressive illness	Tranylcypromine
5-HT transporter	Antagonist	Major depressive illness, panic attacks	Fluoxetine, citalopram
5-HT_{1A} receptor	Agonist (partial)	Anxiety	Buspirone
5-HT_{1D} receptor	Agonist	Migraine	Sumatriptan
5-HT_2 receptor	Antagonist	Migraine	Methysergide
5-HT_{2A} receptor	Antagonist	Schizophrenia	Clozapine, risperidone
5-HT_3 receptor	Antagonist	Chemotherapy-induced nausea	Ondansetron
5-HT_4 receptor	Agonist	Gastroesophageal reflux disease	Cisapride

5-HT, 5-hydroxytryptamine; MAO, monoamine oxidase.

(catecholamine transporters). Conversely, tranylcypromine blocks the degradation of serotonin, dopamine, and norepinephrine equally well. One of the most exciting areas of current research deals with genetic variations in 5-HT receptor and transporter genes and their association with human diseases, such as schizophrenia and major depressive illness. Research has focused on more common genetic alterations referred to as single-nucleotide polymorphisms (SNPs) and, although inconsistent, the early results suggest that SNPs in serotonin-related genes may be associated with disease symptoms and drug response [7].

References

1. Sanders-Bush, E., and S. E. Mayer. 2001. 5-Hydroxytryptamine (Serotonin): Receptor agonists and antagonists. In *The pharmacological basis of therapeutics,* ed. J. G. Hardman, L. E. Limbird, and A. G. Gilman, 15–34. New York: McGraw-Hill.
2. Hoyer, D., D. E. Clarke, J. R. Fozard, P. R. Hartig, G. R. Martin, E. J. Mylecharane, P. R. Saxena, and P. P. Humphrey. 1994. International Union of Pharmacology classification of receptors for 5-hydroxytryptamine (serotonin). *Pharmacol. Rev.* 46:157–203.
3. Kroeze, W. K., and B. L. Roth. 1998. The molecular biology of serotonin receptors: Therapeutic implications for the interface of mood and psychosis. *Biol. Psychiatry* 44:1128–1142.
4. Aghajanian, G. K., and E. Sanders-Bush. 2002. Serotonin. In *Neuropsychopharmacology: The fifth generation of progress,* ed. K. L. Davis, D. Charney, J. T. Coyle, and C. Nemeroff, 15–34. Philadelphia: Lippincott Williams & Wilkins.
5. Lucki, I. 1998. The spectrum of behaviors influenced by serotonin. *Biol. Psychiatry* 44:151–162.
6. Murphy, D. L., C. Wichems, Q. Li, and A. Heils. 1999. Molecular manipulations as tools for enhancing our understanding of 5-HT neurotransmission. *Trends Pharmacol. Sci.* 20:246–252.
7. Hariri, A. R., V. S. Mattay, A. Tessitore, B. Kolachana, F. Fera, D. Goldman, M. F. Egan, and D. R. Weinberger. 2002. Serotonin transporter genetic variation and the response of the human amygdala. *Science* 297:400–403.

24 Antidepressant-Sensitive Norepinephrine Transporters
Structure and Regulation

Randy D. Blakely
Center for Molecular Neuroscience
Vanderbilt University
Nashville, Tennessee

Chemical signaling at central and peripheral noradrenergic synapses is terminated through reuptake of released norepinephrine (NE) [1]. The protein executing this activity, the antidepressant-sensitive NE transporter (NET), has been cloned from multiple species, including humans [2]. The human NET (hNET) gene encodes a 617–amino acid polypeptide believed to span the plasma membrane 12 times with intracellular NH_2 and COOH termini (Fig. 24.1). Expression of the original hNET isolate confers antidepressant-sensitive NET on non-neuronal cells [2]. During biosynthesis, hNET protein is N-glycosylated at sites on a large extracellular loop situated between transmembrane domains (TMDs) 3 and 4, and the protein is subsequently trafficked to the plasma membrane [3]. Although hNET glycosylation is not known to be regulated, this modification enhances catalytic function and protein stability [4]. Once inserted in the plasma membrane, hNET is exposed to the transmembrane sodium gradient that the transporter uses to catalyze NE uptake. Extracellular chloride also facilitates uptake of NE and intracellular potassium may offer further stimulation, although evidence that potassium is countertransported is lacking. In addition, hNET supports NE-gated channel states that may allow NE to translocate hNET at high rates when synaptic concentrations are increased [5]. To take advantage of this possibility, NETs would need to be enriched at synaptic sites. Studies with NET-specific antibodies revealed a marked enrichment at varicosities [6, 7] consistent with this possibility.

Additional hNET splice variants have been identified at the mRNA level, predicting additional NET species with altered COOH termini [8]. Whereas related, though not identical, mRNA variants have been identified in rat brain [9] and bovine adrenal [10], evidence of splice variant protein expression currently is lacking. Recent heterologous expression studies incorporating these variants reveal significantly disrupted maturation and surface trafficking [11], raising doubt as to their functional relevance, at least as monomers. In this regard, although a single hNET cDNA can confer NE transport activity, multiple hNET proteins may assemble together as an oligomeric complex. Indeed, dimer or higher order complexes have been documented for the closely related dopamine transporter (DAT) [12] and serotonin transporter (SERT) [13] and their presence for hNET would offer an explanation for genetic NET deficiency exhibited by subjects with only a single mutant *hNET* gene [14]. Mouse models of genetic NET deficiency are currently available and support a contribution of transporter expression to presynaptic NE homeostasis, extracellular NE clearance, and psychostimulant action [15].

Studies conducted over the past few years have revealed that NET and related transporters are subject to rapid regulation including changes in transporter surface expression and intrinsic catalytic activity [16–19]. This regulatory potential is believed to involve both transporter phosphorylation and the regulated associations of accessory proteins. Thus, NETs have been found to complex with the catalytic subunit of protein phosphatase 2A (PP2Ac) [16], the SNARE protein syntaxin 1A [7], and the scaffolding protein PICK1 [20]. The NH_2 terminus of hNET supports syntaxin 1A associations, whereas the transporter's COOH terminal PDZ domain is required for PICK1 binding. Protein kinase C activators disrupt syntaxin and PP2Ac associations, stimulation that also leads to NET internalization. PP2Ac also appears to be required for alterations in hNET catalytic activity triggered by insulin and mitogen-activated protein kinase–linked pathways [18]. Possibly, trafficking and catalytic function are coregulated through kinase-dependent mechanisms. Although these are early days in molecular studies of NET regulation, it is already clear that NE clearance capacity is likely to involve multiple regulatory proteins that localize, stabilize, and activate NETs (Fig. 24.2). They may also influence the tendency of NETs to support catecholamine efflux when ion gradients are perturbed because they can be in ischemic insults. Finally, successful assimilation of these proteins into a regulatory model of NE inactivation should offer new opportunities to manipulate NET in cardiovascular and mental disorders, including depression, in which altered noradrenergic signaling has been recognized.

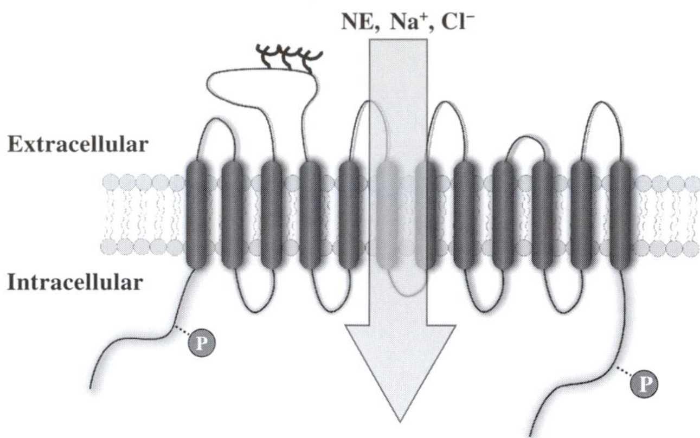

FIGURE 24.1 Norepinephrine transporters (NETs). Depicted is the 12-transmembrane topology predicted for the NET protein, bearing three N-glycosylated residues on the second extracellular loop. The cytoplasmic NH_2 and COOH termini bear multiple consensus sites for Ser/Thr phosphorylation. Norepinephrine (NE) is depicted as cotransported with Na^+ and Cl^-, which provide the energy for uptake of catecholamine into the presynaptic terminal.

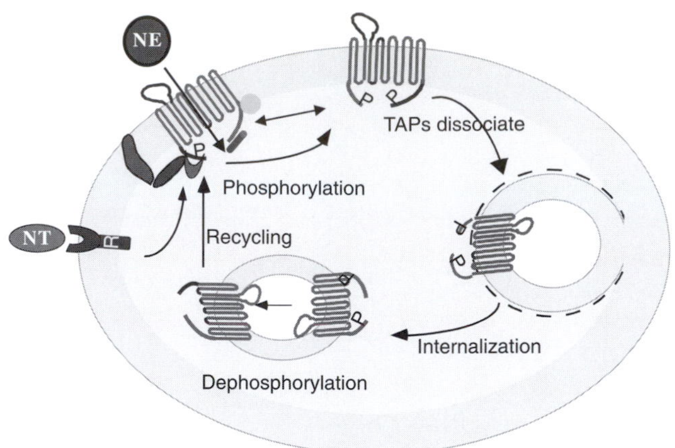

FIGURE 24.2 Norepinephrine transporter (NET) regulation. Illustrated is a cycle for the regulated trafficking of NET proteins. NETs are depicted in complex with multiple associated proteins that may stabilize the transporter at the plasma membrane. Stimuli linked to receptor activation by other neurotransmitters, hormones, or cytosolic second messengers influence the stability of the NET-associated protein complex and enhance NET phosphorylation. In parallel with or as a result of such stimulation, NET proteins internalize leaving reduced presynaptic norepinephrine (NE) transport capacity. NETs can recycle to the plasma membrane, a process that likely occurs at basal rates but which may also may be linked to regulatory stimuli.

Acknowledgments

R.D. Blakely gratefully acknowledges the NIMH and NHLBI for their support of studies on NET genetics and regulation.

References

1. Iversen, L. L. 1978. Uptake processes for biogenic amines. In *Handbook of psychopharmacology,* 3rd ed., ed. L. L. Iversen, S. D. Iverson, and S. H. Snyder, 381–442. New York: Plenum Press.
2. Pacholczyk, T., R. D. Blakely, and S. G. Amara. 1991. Expression cloning of a cocaine- and antidepressant-sensitive human noradrenaline transporter. *Nature* 350:350–354.
3. Melikian, H. E., J. K. McDonald, H. Gu, G. Rudnick, K. R. Moore, and R. D. Blakely. 1994. Human norepinephrine transporter: Biosynthetic studies using a site-directed polyclonal antibody. *J. Biol. Chem.* 269:12290–12297.
4. Melikian, H. E., S. Ramamoorthy, C. G. Tate, and R. D. Blakely. 1996. Inability to N-glycosylate the human norepinephrine transporter reduces protein stability, surface trafficking, and transport activity but not ligand recognition. *Mol. Pharmacol.* 50:266–276.
5. Galli, A., R. D. Blakely, and L. J. DeFelice. 1998. Patch-clamp and amperometric recordings from norepinephrine transporters: Channel activity and voltage-dependent uptake. *Proc. Natl. Acad. Sci. USA* 95:13260–13265.
6. Savchenko, V., U. Sung, and R. D. Blakely. 2003. Cell surface trafficking of the antidepressant-sensitive norepinephrine transporter revealed with an ectodomain antibody. *Mol. Cell Neurosci.* 24(4):1131–1150.
7. Sung, U., S. Apparsundaram, A. Galli, K. M. Kahlig, V. Savchenko, S. Schroeter, M. W. Quick, and R. Blakely. 2003. A regulated interaction of syntaxin 1A with the antidepressant-sensitive norepinephrine transporter establishes catecholamine clearance capacity. *J. Neurosci.* 23(5):1697–1709.
8. Pörzgen, P., H. Bönisch, R. Hammermann, and M. Brüss. 1998. The human noradrenaline transporter gene contains multiple polyadenylation sites and two alternatively spliced C-terminal exons. *Biochi. et Biophys. Acta.* 1398:365–370.
9. Kitayama, S., T. Ikeda, C. Mitsuhata, T. Sato, K. Morita, and T. Dohi. 1999. Dominant negative isoform of rat norepinephrine transporter produced by alternative RNA splicing. *J. Biol. Chem.* 274:10731–10736.
10. Burton, L. D., A. G. Kippenberger, B. Lingen, M. Brüss, H. Bönisch, and D. L. Christie. 1998. A variant of the bovine noradrenaline transporter reveals the importance of the C-terminal region for correct targeting to the membrane and functional expression. *Biochem. J.* 330:909–914.
11. Bauman, P. A., and R. D. Blakely. 2002. Determinants within the C-terminus of the human norepinephrine transporter dictate transporter trafficking, stability, and activity. *Arch. Biochem. Biophys.* 404: 80–91.
12. Hastrup, H., A. Karlin, and J. A. Javitch. 2001. Symmetrical dimer of the human dopamine transporter revealed by cross- linking Cys-306 at the extracellular end of the sixth transmembrane segment. *Proc. Natl. Acad. Sci. USA* 98:10055–10060.
13. Kilic, F., and G. Rudnick. 2000. Oligomerization of serotonin transporter and its functional consequences. *Proc. Natl. Acad. Sci. USA* 97:3106–3111.
14. Shannon, J. R., N. L. Flattem, J. Jordan, G. Jacob, B. K. Black, I. Biaggioni, R. D. Blakely, and D. Robertson. 2000. Orthostatic intolerance and tachycardia associated with norepinephrine transporter deficiency. *N. Engl. J. Med.* 342:541–549.
15. Xu, F., R. R. Gainetdinov, W. C. Wetsel, S. R. Jones, L. M. Bohn, G. W. Miller, Y. M. Wang, and M. G. Caron. 2000. Mice lacking the norepinephrine transporter are supersensitive to psychostimulants. *Nat. Neurosci.* 3:465–471.
16. Bauman, A. L., S. Apparsundaram, S. Ramamoorthy, B. E. Wadzinski, R. A. Vaughan, and R. D. Blakely. 2000. Cocaine and antidepressant-sensitive biogenic amine transporters exist in regulated complexes with protein phosphatase 2A. *J. Neurosci.* 20:7571–7578.
17. Blakely, R. D., and A. L. Bauman. 2000. Biogenic amine transporters: Regulation in flux. *Curr. Opin. Neurobiol.* 10:328–336.

18. Apparsundaram, S., U. Sung, R. D. Price, and R. D. Blakely. 2001. Trafficking-dependent and -independent pathways of neurotransmitter transporter regulation differentially involving p38 mitogen-activated protein kinase revealed in studies of insulin modulation of norepinephrine transport in SK-N-SH cells. *J. Pharmacol. Exp. Ther.* 299: 666–677.
19. Zahniser, N. R., and S. Doolen. 2001. Chronic and acute regulation of Na+/Cl− dependent neurotransmitter transporters: Drugs, substrates, presynaptic receptors, and signaling systems. *Pharmacol. Ther.* 92: 21–55.
20. Torres, G. E., W. D. Yao, R. R. Mohn, H. Quan, K. Kim, A. I. Levey, J. Staudinger, and M. G. Caron. 2001. Functional interaction between monoamine plasma membrane transporters and the synaptic PDZ domain-containing protein PICK1. *Neuron* 30:121–134.
21. Hahn, M. K., D. Robertson, and R. D. Blakely. 2003. A mutation in the human norepinephrine transporter gene (SLC6A2) associated with orthostatic intolerance disrupts surface expression of mutant and wild-type transporters. *J. Neurosci.* 23:4470–4478.

P A R T III

PHYSIOLOGY

25 Cardiac and Other Visceral Afferents

John C. Longhurst
Department of Medicine
University of California, Irvine
Irvine, California

Visceral afferents subserve an important warning mechanism: alerting the organism to both physiologic and pathophysiologic changes in the local environment. Physiologically, visceral afferents provide information about the function of abdominal and thoracic organ systems, including visceral organs of digestion and excretion, and the lungs and heart, allowing for reflex responses that typically aid in the normal function of these systems. Pathophysiologically, these sensory nerves provide a warning system—for example, to alert the organism to the presence of injury or conditions that can lead to injury. Thus, they assist both in normal function and to maintain homeostasis. The reflex arc includes the afferent or sensory limb, central neural integration, and efferent motor system innervating effector organs. This chapter focuses on afferent fibers present in the vagus and sympathetic (spinal) pathways that respond to mechanical and chemical alterations in the environment, and the resulting reflex responses highlighting the condition of ischemia. Ischemia is relevant to all visceral organs because it can lead to irreversible cell death and dysfunction and, hence, constitutes an important condition associated with cardiovascular disease. Stimulation of visceral sensory nerves leads to important cardiovascular reflex responses mediated by the autonomic nervous and humoral systems.

ANATOMIC FRAMEWORK

Finely myelinated and unmyelinated afferent pathways, including Aβ, Aδ, and C fibers, innervating either unspecialized dense, diffuse, or bare nerve endings, form the afferent pathway of visceral cardiovascular reflexes (Table 25.1) [1]. The nerve endings typically are located within the interstitial space and respond to mechanical or chemical events, or both. Afferents ascend to the central nervous system (CNS) through either the vagus or sympathetic (spinal, e.g., spinothalamic and spinoreticular) pathways. A number of nuclei in the thalamus, hypothalamus, midbrain, and medulla, including the nucleus tractus solitarii, caudal and rostral ventral lateral medulla, parabrachial nucleus, paraventricular nucleus periaqueductal gray, lateral tegmental field, dorsal motor nucleus of the vagus, and nucleus ambiguus, among others, help to integrate input from visceral afferents before directing them toward sympathetic and vagal autonomic motor fibers that distribute outflow to cardiovascular effector organs. This reflex arc forms the pathway for visceral reflexes concerned with regulation of the cardiovascular system.

AFFERENT STIMULI

Visceral afferent fibers responsive to mechanical stimuli can be classified as either high or low threshold, with the high-threshold endings serving as nociceptors [2, 3]. Low-threshold mechanosensitive receptors respond to changes in stress or strain and provide information relevant to digestion (gut) or cardiac filling or function (cardiac venoatrial, atrial, and ventricular). For example, cardiac atrial receptors, located mainly in the venoatrial junctions, that are innervated by myelinated afferents that course through the vagus trunk, respond to changes in balloon distension involving modest changes in volume but high tensions [4]. Many ventricular mechanosensitive C-fibers appear to respond to changes in end-diastolic volume (i.e., stretch) rather than systolic pressure (i.e., compression) [4]. The differences in responsiveness likely are related to the location of the endings of these afferents. Sensory nerves that respond to changes in stress or strain in the gastrointestinal tract largely course through the vagus nerves and appear to be concerned with transmission of information related to digestion rather than cardiovascular function.

Many of the high-threshold mechanosensitive endings also respond to chemical events and, hence, are at least bimodal in their sensitivity. A number of chemical stimuli activate these endings, depending on the organ in which they are situated and the condition imposed [5]. For example, ischemia causes the production and release of a number of chemical mediators, including protons, kinins, serotonin, histamine, cyclooxygenase and lipoxygenase products, reactive oxygen species, such as hydroxyl radicals, among other species (Fig. 25.1). Each mediator either primarily stimulates these high-threshold afferent endings or sensitizes them to the action of other chemical mediators. Other chemical

TABLE 25.1 Classification of Afferent Fibers from Abdominal Viscera

Fiber type	Cross-sectional diameter (μm)	Conduction velocity (m/sec)	Terminal ending	Effective stimulus
Aβ (myelinated)	6–12	20–84	Pacinian corpuscle	Vibration
Aδ (finely myelinated)	2–6	3–30	Unknown, bare nerve endings	Vibration, pulse pressure, contraction, distension, chemicals, noxious stimuli
C (unmyelinated)	0.3–1.5	0.3–2.5	Unknown, bare nerve endings	Strong mechanical stimuli, chemicals, noxious stimuli

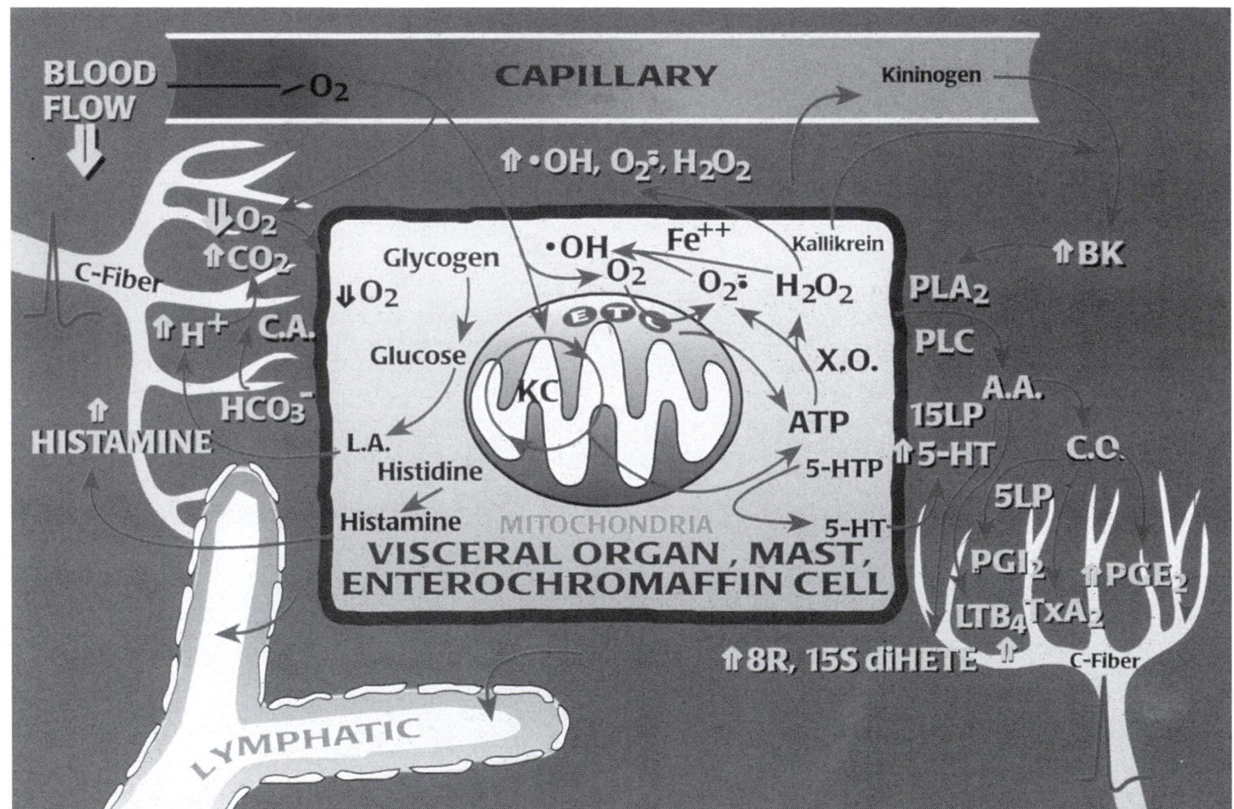

FIGURE 25.1 Chemical pathways involved in activation of visceral afferents during ischemia and reperfusion. Capillary, lymphatic, prototypic parenchymal cell, and two afferent (C-fibers) nerve endings are shown. Ischemia and reperfusion activate pathways that lead to changes in PCO_2; protons (H^+); histamine; arachidonic acid cleavage products through 5, and 15 lipoxygenase pathways including leukotriene B_4 (LTB_4) and 8R, 15S-dihydroxyicosa (5E-9,11,13Z) tetraenoic acid (*8R, 15S*-diHETE), respectively; and cyclooxygenase (COX) pathway products, including thromboxane A_2 (TxA_2), and prostaglandins I_2 and E_2 (PGI_2, PGE_2); 5-hydroxytryptamine (5-HT), or serotonin; bradykinin (BK) and reactive oxygen species, including superoxide ($O_2^{\cdot-}$) and hydroxyl radicals (COH) and hydrogen peroxide (H_2O_2). 5-HTP, 5-hydroxytryptamine; CA, carbonic anhydrase; ECT, electron transport chain in the mitochondria; Fe^{2+}, ferrous iron; HCO_3G, bicarbonate; KC, Krebs cycle; LA, lactic acid; O_2, oxygen; PLA_2, phospholipase A_2; PLC, phospholipase C. (Modified with permission from Longhurst J. C. 1995. Chemosensitive abdominal visceral afferents. In *Proceedings: Visceral pain symposium*, ed. G. F. Gebhard, 99–132. Seattle: IASP Press.)

changes occurring with ischemia, which are associated with activation of central and peripheral chemoreceptors, such as hypoxia and hypercapnia, are not important stimuli of chemosensitive abdominal or thoracic (cardiac) visceral sensory nerve endings. This differential sensitivity has led to use of the term *chemosensitive* visceral receptors to distinguish them from the arterial chemoreceptors.

The sources of many of these mediators are the parenchymal cells of the organ (e.g., cardiac myocytes) [6]. Also, circulating precursors or enzymes that initiate cascades leading to the production of mediators, such as kinins, which form an important source together with blood elements, such as platelets, have been shown to play a critical role in the production and release of mediators during ischemia and

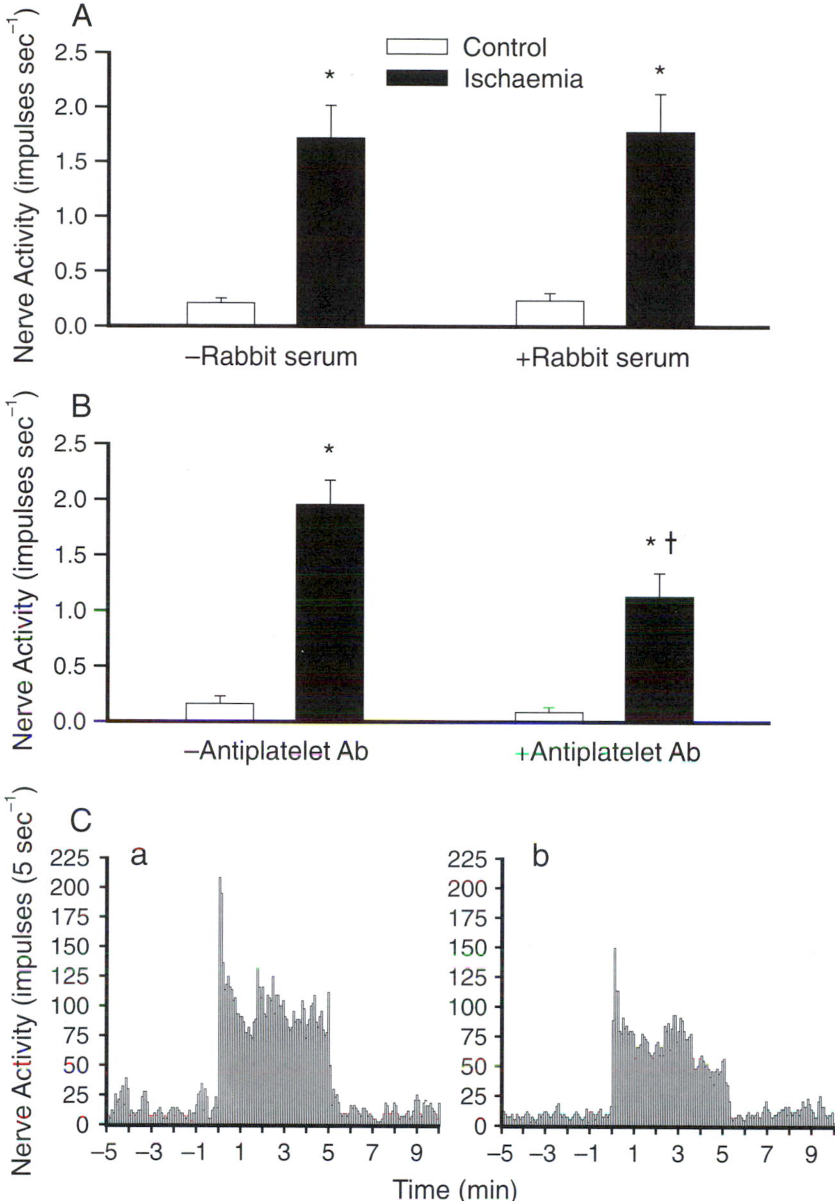

FIGURE 25.2 Responses of ischemically sensitive cardiac ventricular afferents to repeated ischemia before and after treatment with rabbit serum (**A**), exposure to a polyclonal rabbit antiplatelet antibody (**B**), and composite histogram of responses of eight afferents to a 5-minute period of regional coronary artery occlusion to induce ischemia before (*a*) and after (*b*) treatment with the antiplatelet antibody (**C**). *Asterisk* indicates significant difference ($P < 0.05$), comparing control with ischemia, and † indicates significant difference in response to ischemia, comparing before and after treatment with antibody. (Reproduced with permission from Fu L.-W., and J. C. Longhurst. 2002. Role of activated platelets in excitation of cardiac afferents during myocardial ischemia in cats. *Am. J. Physiol. Heart Circ. Physiol.* 282:H100–H109.)

reperfusion. Platelets aggregate at the site of injury of arterial endothelium after rupture of an atherosclerotic plaque or after occlusion of a coronary artery. Activated platelets release serotonin, histamine, and thromboxane A_2, each of which independently or in combination may activate cardiac sympathetic afferent endings (Fig. 25.2).

Some mediators, like adenosine, remain controversial with regard to their role in stimulating afferent endings during ischemia [4]. Some reports, consisting mainly of reflex studies in larger species, such as the dog, suggest that adenosine mediates autonomic reflexes that influence renal function. Other studies, such as in the cat, suggest that

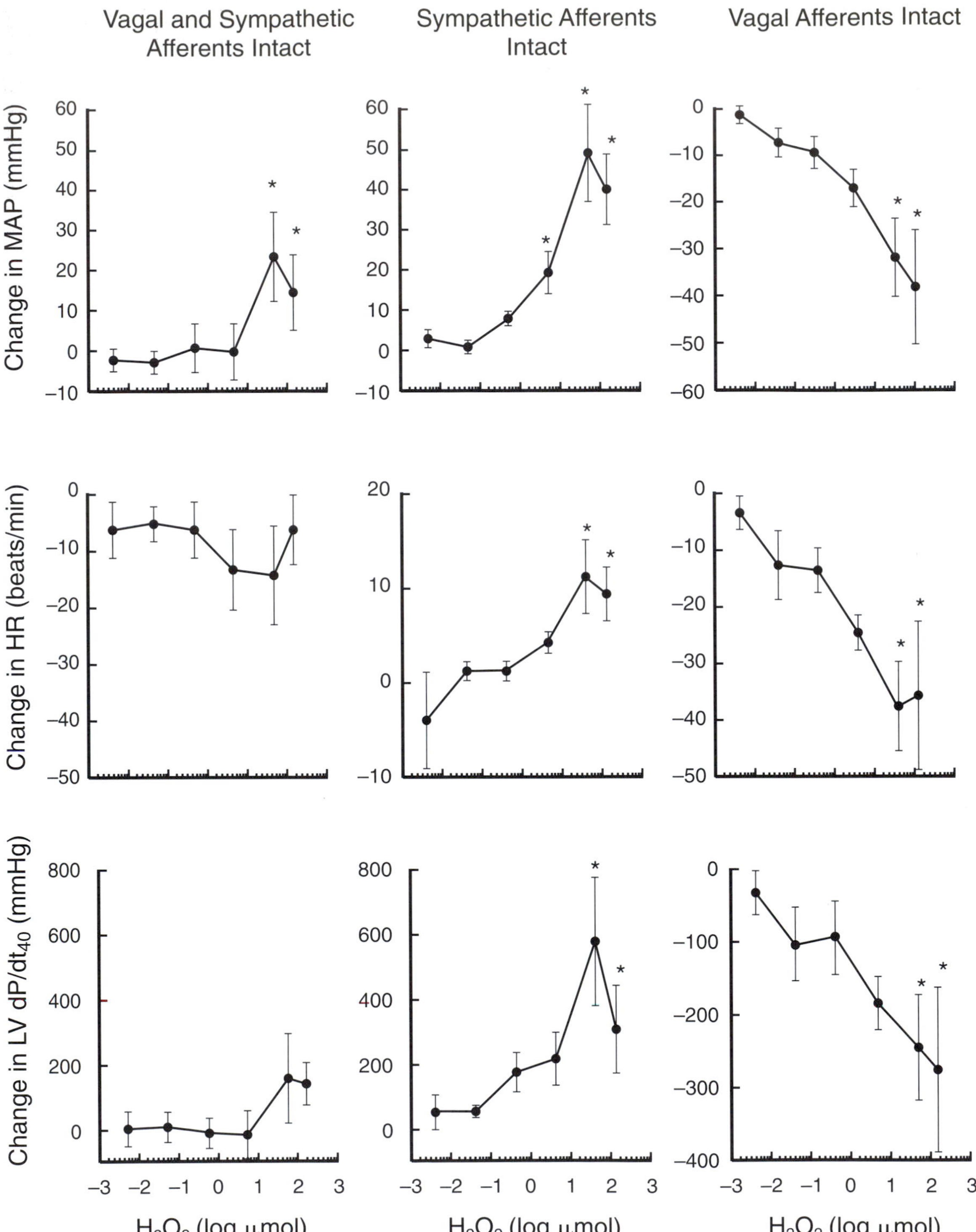

FIGURE 25.3 Reflex blood pressure, heart rate, and contractile responses to graded doses of hydrogen peroxide (H_2O_2) applied to the cardiac epicardium with afferent pathways intact (*left*) and following transection of cervical vagus nerves leaving sympathetic afferents intact (*center*) or removal of T_1–T_4 sympathetic ganglia leaving the vagal afferent pathways intact (*right*). *Asterisk* significantly from saline control, $P < 0.05$. (Reproduced with permission from Huang, H. S., G. L. Stahl, and J. C. Longhurst. 1995 Cardiac-cardiovascular reflexes induced by hydrogen peroxide in cats. *Am. J. Physiol.* 268:H2114–H2124.)

adenosine is ineffective in stimulating ischemically sensitive afferents, either during ischemia or when administered in large (pharmacologic) concentrations in the absence of ischemia.

AUTONOMIC REFLEX RESPONSES TO VISCERAL AFFERENT ACTIVATION

Cardiovascular reflex responses evoked by stimulation of visceral afferents can be divided broadly into two types: those that consist of cardiovascular inhibition and those that lead to reflex excitation (Fig. 25.3). For the most part, stimulation of vagal afferents, whose pathways travel with parasympathetic nerves, causes reflex inhibition, including decreased heart rate, blood pressure, and myocardial contractility, as a result of withdrawal of sympathetic neural tone to the heart and blood vessels. Conversely, stimulation of sympathetic afferents that travel centrally through sympathetic nerves and spinal pathways leads to reflex cardiovascular excitation, including increases in heart rate, blood pressure, and myocardial performance, caused mainly by increased sympathetic efferent activity and, to a small extent, withdrawal of parasympathetic tone to the heart. Cardiovascular reflex responses originating from the heart consist of either reflex inhibitory or excitatory responses, or, more often, a combination of the two. For example, stimulation of the posterior–inferior and inner regions of the wall of the left ventricle, either in animal preparations or during myocardial ischemia in patients, results in reflex bradyarrhythmias and hypotension. Conversely, stimulation of the anterior and superficial regions of the wall of the left ventricle leads to reflex tachyarrhythmias and hypertensive responses. Frequently, however, both vagal and sympathetic afferent pathways are stimulated concomitantly, and the resulting reflex reflects a mixed response often consisting of a small increase (and less commonly a small decrease) in blood pressure (see Fig. 25.3) as a result of a neural occlusive response occurring in the CNS, in regions that include the nucleus tractus solitarii [7].

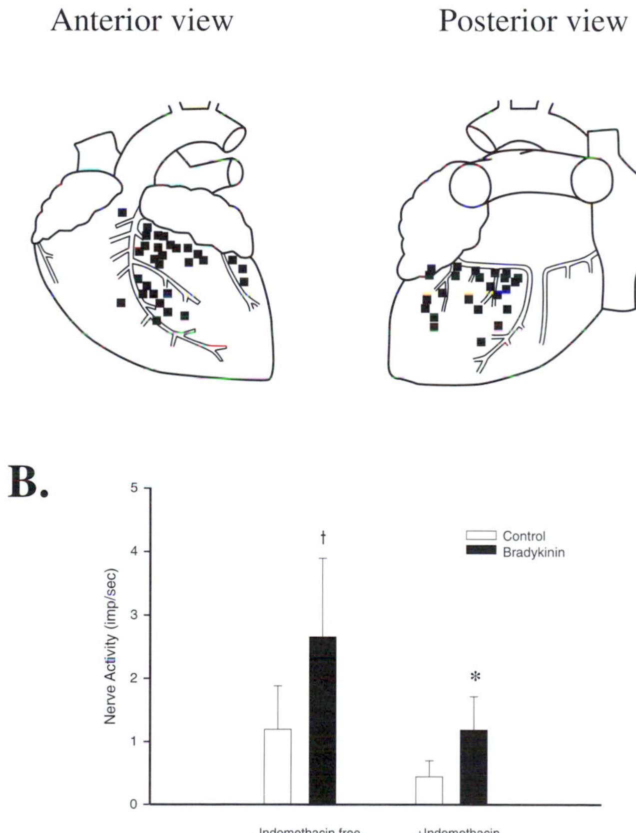

FIGURE 25.4 Location of ischemically sensitive cardiac endings on anterior and posterior surfaces of left and right ventricles (**A**). Influence of inhibition of cyclooxygenase system with indomethacin on response of these afferents to application of bradykinin to epicardial surface of the heart (**B**). The increased activity in response to bradykinin (†, $P < 0.05$) was reduced by indomethacin (*asterisk*, $P < 0.05$). (Modified with permission from Tjen-A-Looi S. C., H. L. Pan, and J. C. Longhurst. 1998. Endogenous bradykinin activates ischaemically sensitive cardiac visceral afferents through kinin B_2 receptors in cats. *J. Physiol.* 510:633–641.)

Although stimulation of cardiac afferents can lead to reflex cardiovascular depression or excitation, stimulation of abdominal visceral afferents more commonly leads to reflex stimulation because spinal pathways from this region predominate. Thus, stimulation of chemosensitive, mechanosensitive, and polymodal receptors in the mesenteric region and a number of abdominal organs activate spinal pathways that result in increased heart rate, myocardial contractility, and arteriolar constriction in several regional circulations, including the coronary system [1, 5]. Vagal afferent pathways from the abdominal region appear to reflexly regulate digestive organ function rather than the cardiovascular system.

In addition to cardiovascular regulation, stimulation of visceral afferents can cause a number of other important reflex events. For example, stimulation of cardiac vagal afferents during myocardial ischemia can lead to relaxation of the stomach, the antecedent of nausea and vomiting that frequently accompanies inferior myocardial infarctions [4, 6]. Stimulation of sympathetic afferents in the heart or abdominal region frequently leads to pain. Hence, many of the high-threshold visceral sympathetic afferents function as nociceptors [3].

PATHOLOGIC ALTERATIONS OF VISCERAL AFFERENTS

In addition to ischemia, there are a number of conditions that activate visceral afferents. For example, inflammatory states typically lead to the production of a number of chemical (and sometimes mechanical) changes, including increases in kinins, activation of the cyclooxygenase and lipoxygenase systems, and enhanced formation of reactive oxygen species. Interestingly, some chemical mediators appear to act as primary stimuli, whereas others either sensitize (e.g., prostaglandin E_2; Fig. 25.4) or modulate (e.g., leukotriene B_4) the sensory nerve endings to the action of the primary stimulus. Other clinical conditions, like hypertension or heart failure, modify the responsiveness of nerve endings in the atria or ventricles. Hypertension may do this by altering the mechanical substrate in which the endings are located. Heart failure may do this by altering the sensitivity of the nerve ending to mechanical or chemical events.

References

1. Longhurst, J. C. 1984. Cardiovascular reflexes of gastrointestinal origin. In *Physiology of the intestinal*, ed. A. P. Shepherd, and D. N. Granger, 165–178. New York: Raven Press.
2. Longhurst, J. C. 1991. Reflex effects from abdominal visceral afferents. In *Reflex control of the circulation,* ed. I. H. Zucker, and J. P. Gillmore, 551–577. Caldwell, NJ: Telford Press.
3. Pan, H.-L., and J. C. Longhurst. 1996. Ischaemia-sensitive sympathetic afferents innervating the gastrointestinal tract function as nociceptors in cats. *J. Physiol.* 492:841–850.
4. Longhurst, J. C. 1984. Cardiac receptors: Their function in health and disease. *Prog. Cardiovasc. Dis.* XXVII:201–222.
5. Longhurst, J. C. 1995. Chemosensitive abdominal visceral afferents. In *Proceedings: Visceral pain symposium*, ed. G. F. Gebhard, 99–132. Seattle: IASP Press.
6. Longhurst, J. C., S. Tjen-A-Looi, and L.-W. Fu. 2001. Cardiac sympathetic afferent activation provoked by myocardial ischemia and reperfusion: mechanisms and reflexes. *Ann. NY Acad. Sci.* 940:74–95.
7. Tjen-A-Looi, S., A. Bonham, and J. Longhurst. 1997. Interactions between sympathetic and vagal cardiac afferents in nucleus tractus solitarii. *Am. J. Physiol.* 272:H2843–H2851.
8. Fu, L.-W., and J. C. Longhurst. 2002. Activated platlets contribute to stimulation of cardiacafferents during ischemia in cats: Role of 5-HT_3, receptors. *J. Physiol.* 544.3:897–912.

26 Skeletal Muscle Afferents

Marc P. Kaufman
Division of Cardiovascular Medicine
Departments of Internal Medicine and Human Physiology
University of California at Davis
Davis, California

Skeletal muscle afferents, when stimulated by exercise, cause important reflex autonomic responses. In particular, stimulation of these afferents evokes reflex increases in sympathetic activity, decreases in parasympathetic activity, and increases in α-motoneuronal discharge to respiratory muscles. These reflex increases in autonomic and α-motoneuron discharge cause cardioacceleration, vasoconstriction, airway dilation, and increases in cardiac contractility and minute volume of ventilation [1]. The constellation of cardiovascular and respiratory responses evoked by the stimulation of skeletal muscle afferents has been termed the exercise pressor reflex [2].

The obvious purpose of the exercise pressor reflex is to deliver oxygenated blood to metabolically active tissues (i.e., the exercising muscles) and to remove carbon dioxide and hydrogen ions from these tissues. In addition, the exercise pressor reflex contributes significantly to the increase in cardiac output evoked by dynamic exercise. Furthermore, the reflex increases sympathetic discharge to the vascular beds of dynamically exercising muscles [3], an effect that partly counters the increase in vascular conductance, which, in turn, is caused by the increase in muscle metabolism. The exercise pressor reflex also plays an important role during static exercise. Specifically, it functions to increase the perfusion pressure of working muscles whose arterioles are mechanically constricted by the increases in intramuscular pressure that arise during sustained contraction.

Skeletal muscle is innervated by five types of afferents. The first afferent is the primary muscle spindle (group Ia), whose afferent fiber is thickly myelinated; in cats, it conducts impulses between 72 and 120 meters per second [4]. The primary muscle spindle is stimulated by stretch and is inhibited by shortening, such as that which occurs during muscle twitch. The second type is the Golgi tendon organ (group Ib), whose afferent fiber also is thickly myelinated; in cats, it also conducts impulses between 72 and 120 meters per second [4]. The Golgi tendon organ responds vigorously to muscle shortening and weakly to stretching. The third type is the secondary muscle spindle (group II), whose afferent fiber is myelinated and, in cats, conducts impulses between 31 and 71 meters per second [4]. The discharge properties of secondary muscle spindles are similar to those of primary spindles, except that secondary spindles do not display dynamic sensitivity to muscle stretch, whereas primary spindles do. The fourth type is the group III (Aδ) afferent, which has a free ending and whose afferent fiber is thinly myelinated, conducting impulses, in cats, between 2.5 and 30 meters per second [1]. Group III endings are frequently found in connective tissue (i.e., collagen), such as that found near the junction of skeletal muscle and tendon [5]. The fifth type is the group IV (C) afferent, which also has a free ending, but whose afferent fiber is unmyelinated, conducting impulses in cats at less than 2.5 meters per second [1]. Group IV endings are frequently found in the walls of small vessels, including arterioles, venules, and lymphatics [5].

The afferent limb of the exercise pressor reflex is composed of group III and IV afferents (Fig. 26.1), which together are called thin fiber afferents. Groups Ia, Ib, and II play no role in evoking this reflex [1, 6]. Consequently, the remainder of this chapter focuses solely on the discharge properties of group III and IV muscle afferents. Particular attention will be paid to the mechanical and metabolic stimuli that cause these thin fiber afferents to discharge during muscular contraction.

In general, group III muscle afferents display a greater sensitivity to mechanical stimuli than do group IV muscle afferents. For example, most group III afferents respond to muscle stretch, a pure mechanical stimulus, whereas most group IV afferents do not [1]. Likewise, most group III afferents respond to non-noxious and often gentle probing of their receptive fields, whereas most group IV afferents do not. Group IV afferents usually require vigorous and often noxious squeezing of the muscle to discharge them [1]. In addition, many group III afferents respond to static contraction by discharging a burst of impulses with a latency of less than 1 second, whereas some group IV afferents may respond to static contraction by discharging an impulse or

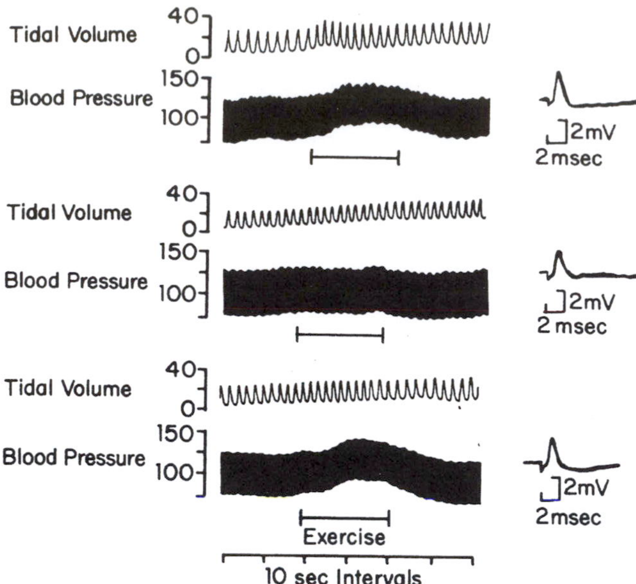

FIGURE 26.1 The exercise pressor reflex is evoked by the stimulation of thinly myelinated (group III) and unmyelinated (group IV) muscle afferents. Each panel shows tidal volume, arterial pressure, and dorsal root compound potentials. **Top**, Static contraction (signaled by the bracket) before topical application of lidocaine to the L7-S1 dorsal roots. **Middle**, Static contraction 3.5 minutes after application of lidocaine. Note that static contraction had no effect on arterial pressure or ventilation, yet the A wave of the compound action potential was, for the most part, unaffected by the blockade. **Bottom**, Static contraction after the lidocaine was washed from the spinal cord. Note the restoration of the pressor and ventilatory responses to contraction. (From McCloskey, D. I., and J. H. Mitchell. 1972. Reflex cardiovascular and respiratory responses originating in exercising muscle. *J. Physiol.* 224:173–186.)

two with a latency of about 2 or 3 seconds, but the great majority of their response comes after the muscle has been contracting for at least 5 seconds. Finally, group III afferents synchronize their discharge in response to repetitive twitch contraction, whereas group IV afferents do not [1].

Both groups III and IV afferents respond to exogenous chemical stimuli injected into the arterial supply of skeletal muscle [1]. These chemical stimuli include lactic acid, prostaglandins, bradykinin, and potassium [1]. The finding that group III afferents respond to both mechanical and chemical stimuli has led some investigators to classify them as polymodal. Nevertheless, a significantly greater percentage of group IV afferents respond more to contraction when the arterial supply to the working muscles is occluded than when it is not occluded (i.e., the working muscles are freely perfused) [1]. These findings have led to the conclusion that group IV afferents respond to metabolic stimuli arising in an exercising muscle and that these C-fiber afferents signal the central nervous system that muscle blood flow is not adequate to its metabolic needs.

Exercise physiologists often perceived the exercise pressor reflex as a mechanism that attempts to correct a mismatch between blood supply and demand in exercising muscles. Consequently, they paid little attention to mechanoreceptor (i.e., group III afferents) contributions to this reflex. Recently, however, blockade of mechanoreceptor channels in muscle with gadolinium has shown that the pressor component of the exercise pressor reflex was reduced by more than half [7] in decerebrate cats (Fig. 26.2). This finding raised the possibility that group III afferents play an important role in evoking the reflex.

Finally, although thin fiber muscle afferents were known to respond to static (i.e., tetanic) contraction, their response to a true form of exercise remained in doubt. This concern was eliminated when both group III and IV afferents were found to respond to dynamic exercise induced by stimulation of the mesencephalic locomotor region in decerebrate cats (Figs. 26.3 and 26.4) [8–10]. Moreover, these thin fiber afferents responded to dynamic exercise at a relatively low level of oxygen consumption (25% of maximal).

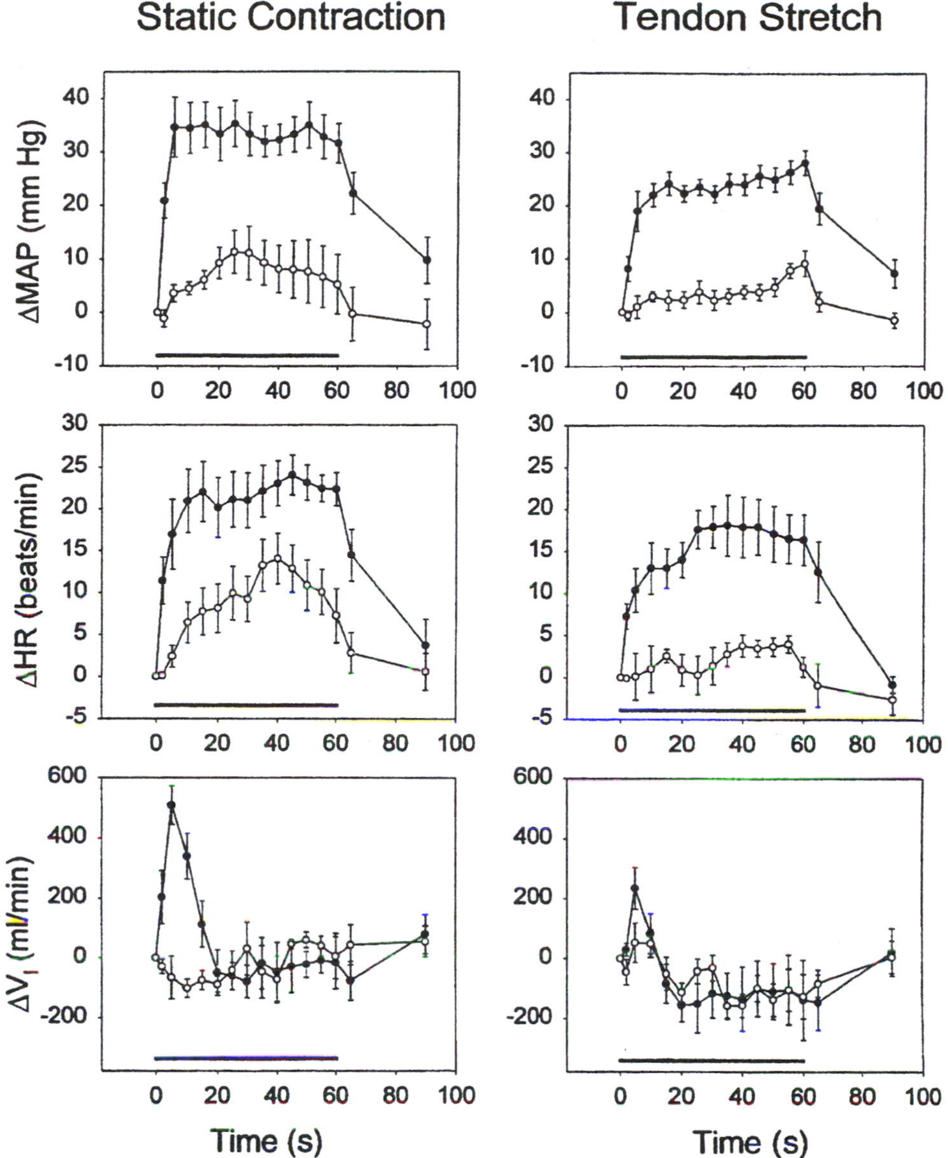

FIGURE 26.2 Time course of pressor, cardioaccelerator, and ventilatory responses to static contraction (**left**) and tendon stretch (**right**) before (*filled circle*) and 60 minutes after (*open circle*) gadolinium injection into the femoral artery (n = 7). *Circles* represent means, and *brackets* represent ± SE. Circles at time zero represent baseline (i.e., before the maneuver). First circle after time zero represents the mean 2 seconds after either contraction or tendon stretch started, and every circle afterward represents the mean at 5-second intervals starting from time zero. Time period when the muscle were contracted or stretched is represented by the *filled horizontal bar*. During contraction and stretch, all means for change in mean arterial pressure (ΔMAP) and change in heart rate (ΔHR) before gadolinium injection were significantly greater ($P < 0.05$) than their corresponding means 60 minutes after gadolinium injection. Also, during contraction, means for the change in minute volume of inspiratory ventilation (ΔV_I) at 2, 5, 10, and 15 seconds before gadolinium were significantly greater ($P < 0.05$) than corresponding means 60 minutes after gadolinium injection. During stretch, however, only the mean ΔV_I value at 5 seconds before gadolinium was significantly greater ($P < 0.05$) than its corresponding mean 60 minutes later. (From Hayes, S. G., and M. P. Kaufman. (2001). Gadolinium attenuates exercise pressor reflex in cats. *Am. J. Physiol.* 280:H2153–H2161.)

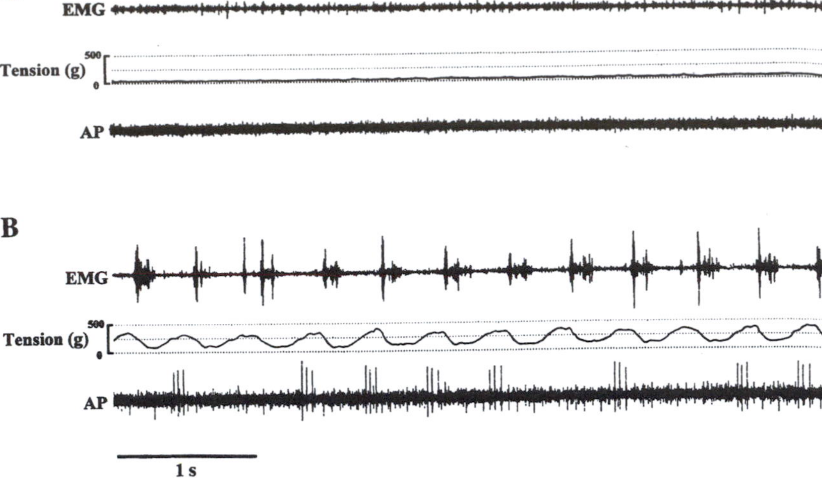

FIGURE 26.3 Response of group III afferent (conduction velocity = 20.3 m/sec) to dynamic exercise of left triceps surae muscles induced by stimulation of the mesencephalic locomotor region (MLR). **A**, Before stimulation of MLR. Traces from top to bottom are electromyograph (EMG) from right gastrocnemius muscle, tension from left triceps surae muscles, and action potentials (APs) before stimulation of MLR. Note that group III afferent was silent while cat was at rest. **B**, Response of group III afferent to dynamic exercise. Note that group III afferent discharged in synchrony with contractions of triceps surae muscles. (From Adreani, C. M., J. M. Hill, and M. P. Kaufman. 1997. Responses of group III and IV muscle afferents to dynamic exercise. *J. Appl. Physiol.* 86:1811–1817.)

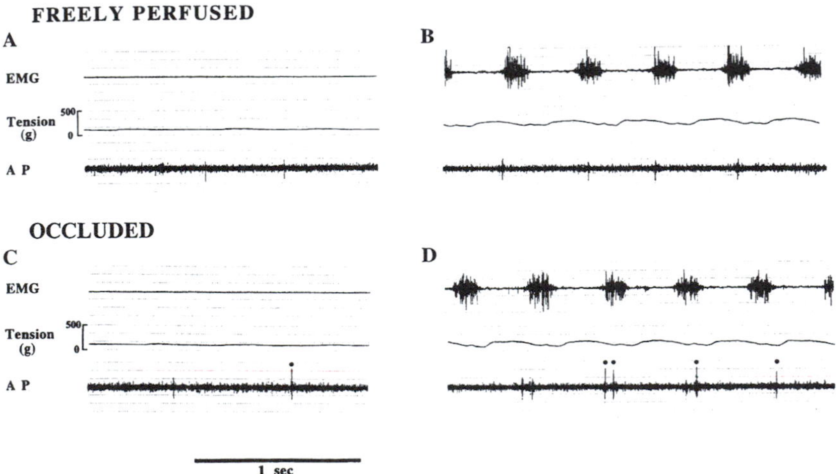

FIGURE 26.4 Original trace of two group IV afferents (unmarked action potentials [APs] have a conduction velocity [CV] = 2.4 m/sec; AP with • have a CV = 1.7 m/sec) with femoral artery freely perfused (**A** and **B**) and with femoral artery occluded (**C** and **D**). Afferent with unmarked AP responded to exercise whether femoral artery was occluded or was freely perfused. Afferent with AP marked by (•) did not discharge when femoral artery was freely perfused but did discharge during rest and exercise when femoral artery was occluded. (From Adreani, C. M., and M. P. Kaufman. 1998. Effect of arterial occlusion on responses of group III and IV afferents to dynamic exercise. *J. Appl. Physiol.* 84:1827–1833.)

References

1. Kaufman, M. P., and H. V. Forster. 1996. Reflexes controlling circulatory, ventilatory and airway responses to exercise. In *Exercise: Regulation and integration of multiple systems*, ed. L. B. Rowell, 381–447. New York: Oxford University Press.
2. Mitchell, J. H., M. P. Kaufman, and G. A. Iwamoto. 1983. The exercise pressor reflex: Its cardiovascular effects, afferent mechanisms, and central pathways. *Ann. Rev. Physiol.* 45:229–242.
3. Victor, R. G., S. L. Pryor, N. H. Secher, and J. H. Mitchell. 1989. Effects of partial neuromuscular blockade on sympathetic nerve responses to static exercise in humans. *Circ. Res.* 65:468–476.
4. Matthews, P. B. C. 1972. *Mammalian muscle receptors and their central actions*. London: Edward Arnold.
5. von During, M., and K. H. Andres. 1990. Topography and ultrastructure of group III and IV nerve terminals of cat's gastrocnemius-soleus muscle. In *The primary afferent neuron: A survey of recent morpho-functional aspects*, ed. W. Zenker and W. L. Neuhuber, 35–41. New York: Plenum.
6. McCloskey, D. I., and J. H. Mitchell. 1972. Reflex cardiovascular and respiratory responses originating in exercising muscle. *J. Physiol.* 224:173–186.
7. Hayes, S. G., and M. P. Kaufman. (2001). Gadolinium attenuates exercise pressor reflex in cats. *Am. J. Physiol.* 280:H2153–H2161.
8. Pickar, J. G., J. M. Hill, and M. P. Kaufman. 1994. Dynamic exercise stimulates group III muscle afferents. *J. Neurophysiol.* 71:753–760.
9. Adreani, C. M., J. M. Hill, and M. P. Kaufman. 1997. Responses of group III and IV muscle afferents to dynamic exercise. *J. Appl. Physiol.* 86:1811–1817.
10. Adreani, C. M., and M. P. Kaufman. 1998. Effect of arterial occlusion on responses of group III and IV afferents to dynamic exercise. *J. Appl. Physiol.* 84:1827–1833.

27 Entrainment of Sympathetic Rhythms

Michael P. Gilbey
Department of Physiology
University College London
London, United Kingdom

SYMPATHETIC RHYTHM

The term "sympathetic rhythm" describes the moment to moment waxing and waning in amplitude (signal strength) of population activity recorded from whole sympathetic nerves that contain thousands of fibers. Such rhythms are commonly observed in the discharges of preganglionic and postganglionic nerves regulating heart and blood vessels. Rhythm is frequently only an emergent property of population activity; that is, the discharges of single neurons sampled from the population may not necessarily demonstrate rhythmicity, however, the tendency for subpopulations of neurons to discharge action potentials almost coincidentally but intermittently gives rise to rhythmicity in aggregate activity. Although Adrian and colleagues described rhythmic activity in the first published recordings of mammalian sympathetic nerves (1932), underlying mechanism(s) and possible functional significance are still uncertain [1–4].

CARDIAC- AND RESPIRATORY-RELATED RHYTHMS

The most common sympathetic rhythms are cardiac- (pulse-) and respiratory-related. With regard to respiratory rhythm, two components can be distinguished: one associated with central respiratory activity and another dependent on afferent activity related to pulmonary ventilation (e.g., from pulmonary stretch receptors and baroreceptors) [5, 6].

MECHANISMS UNDERLYING RHYTHMS

Two major hypotheses have been proposed to account for the appearance of cardiac- and respiratory-related rhythms in sympathetic discharges.

Phasic Inputs Generate Rhythms

The classic view holds that these rhythms are imposed on sympathetic discharge by "external" inputs. In the case of the cardiac-related rhythm, an increase in baroreceptor discharge during systole is considered to inhibit tonic excitatory drive to sympathetic nerves, thereby giving rise to waxing and waning of sympathetic discharges [4]. A similar mechanism is proposed for rhythms related to pulmonary ventilation cycles where activation of lung stretch and baroreceptors afferents, for example, may cause periodic inhibition of activity (independent of the central respiratory rhythm-generating network) [5, 6]. Concerning central respiratory-related rhythms, it is suggested that elements within the central respiratory network provide excitatory or inhibitory inputs, or both, to central networks providing tonic drive to sympathetic nerves [5, 6]. In addition, Richter and colleagues [7] have argued for the existence of a common cardiorespiratory network.

Entrainment of Rhythms

The observation of a non–respiratory-related and non–cardiac-related sympathetic rhythm ("10-Hz" rhythm: Green and Heffron, 1967; see 1, 4) provided the first indication that sympathetic rhythms might not arise exclusively from phasic inputs to tonic sympathetic tone–generating networks. Some 8 years later, Taylor and Gebber observed that sympathetic rhythms with a frequency similar to heart rate persisted after baroreceptor denervation [see 1, 4]. Thus, the idea developed that cardiac-related rhythms in sympathetic nerve discharge are a consequence of the entrainment of central oscillator(s) within the brainstem (i.e., that central networks driving sympathetic outflow may be intrinsically capable of generating their own rhythms). Here, phasic baroreceptor input acts as a forcing input that can entrain a central oscillator. Consequently, in the absence of, or with reduced, baroreceptor activity, there is a continuous phase shift between cardiac cycle and sympathetic rhythm resulting from lack of entrainment [1, 2, 4]. There is evidence also supporting the hypothesis that respiratory-related rhythm in sympathetic discharges arises from oscillator(s) other than those responsible for central respiratory rhythm [8]. First, in vagotomized anesthetized animals, a "slow" rhythm in the range of central respiratory rhythm has been observed during central apnea (indicated by absence of rhythmic phrenic discharge). Second, "slow" rhythms in the discharges of pairs of sympathetic nerves at the frequency of central respiratory drive have been observed to remain correlated after mathematical removal of the component of these signals common to phrenic nerve activity (an indicator of central respiratory drive)—that is, "theoretical removal of central respiratory drive." Third, locking ratios other than 1 : 1 can be observed between rhythmic phrenic and sympathetic discharge (e.g., 2 : 1, 3 : 1, and 2 : 3). It is also apparent that afferents activated during pulmonary ventilation can act as an entraining force [3].

HOW MANY CENTRAL OSCILLATORS?

Zhong and colleagues [8] have provided evidence that separate oscillators, capable of coupling, may drive activity to different sympathetic nerves: they noted from paired nerve recordings that rhythmic discharges of similar frequency could be but were not obligatorily phase-locked, and their variation in amplitude was not necessarily proportionate. In addition, the observations of Gilbey and colleagues [3, 9] have raised the intriguing possibility that activity of sympathetic neurons regulating the same target may be influenced by a family of weakly coupled or uncoupled oscillators, and that their degree of synchronization is influenced by inputs related to lung inflation, central respiratory drive, various afferents (e.g., somatic and baroreceptor), and possibly arousal state.

FUNCTIONAL SIGNIFICANCE

Whatever mechanism(s) lie behind the generation of sympathetic rhythms, their characteristic phasic nature indicates coordination of neuronal discharges. Whereas it is clear why coordinated phasic discharges are required in locomotor and respiratory motor control, the need for patterning and synchronization in sympathetic motor control of heart and blood vessels is not readily apparent. With regard to neuroeffector transmission, many rhythms will be filtered out (i.e., a sympathetic rhythm >1 Hz will not lead to a 1-Hz vasomotion) as the time constant for response is ~2 seconds [1, 3, 4].

It has been suggested that coordination may be particularly easy to achieve between oscillating neural networks. Barman and Gebber [1] have suggested, on the basis of experimental observation, that coupled sympathetic oscillators may be important in the generation of differential patterns of sympathetic activity to blood vessels of muscle, skin, and viscera associated with behavioural alerting. Furthermore, the observations on entrainment of sympathetic rhythms indicate that, when appropriate, sympathetic and respiratory networks may "bind" together to form a highly coordinated "supernetwork" [3].

There are also many indications that pattern and synchrony coding are used in addition to rate coding in various nervous system functions [3]. At the level of the single neuron, pattern of firing appears important in determining probability of transmitter release, synaptic plasticity, types of transmitter released, and receptors activated. In these ways, firing pattern probably influences ganglionic and neuroeffector transmission [3, 4, 10]. Synchrony may be important because it favors summation, which increases the efficacy of transmission and also can have longer-term influences on synaptic and neuroeffector function. Synchrony, therefore, may enhance ganglionic transmission by increasing the probability of summation of weak inputs and improve neuroeffector control by coordinate activation of postjunctional receptors [3, 4]. Consequently, if as suggested by Gilbey and co-workers [3] a population of neurons regulating a single target is influenced by a family of oscillators, their dynamic and graded synchronization through variable entrainment could lead to the modulation of target organ function.

References

1. Barman, S. M., and G. L. Gebber. 2000. "Rapid" rhythmic discharges of sympathetic nerves: Sources, mechanisms of generation, and physiological relevance. *J. Biol. Rhythm* 15:365–379.
2. Gebber, G. L. 1990. Central determinants of sympathetic nerve discharge. In *Central regulation of autonomic functions*, ed. A. D. Loewy and K. M. Spyer, 126–144. New York: Oxford University Press.
3. Gilbey, M. P. 2001. Multiple oscillators, dynamic synchronization and sympathetic control. *Clin. Exp. Pharmacol. Physiol.* 28:130–137.
4. Malpas, S. C. 1998. The rhythmicity of sympathetic nerve activity. *Prog. Neurobiol.* 56:65–96.
5. Habler, H. J., W. Janig, and M. Michaelis. 1994. Respiratory modulation in the activity of sympathetic neurones. *Prog. Neurobiol.* 43:567–606.
6. Koepchen, H.-P., D. Klussendorf, and D. Sommer. 1981. Neurophysiological background of central neural cardiovascular-respiratory coordination: Basic remarks and experimental approach. *J. Auton. Nerv. Syst.* 3:335–368.
7. Richter, D. W., K. M. Spyer, M. P. Gilbey, E. E. Lawson, C. R. Bainton, and Z. Wilhelm. 1991. On the existence of a common cardiorespiratory network. In *Cardiorespiratory and motor coordination*, ed. H.-P. Koepchen, and T. Huopaniemi, 118–130. Berlin: Springer-Verlag.
8. Zhong, S., S. Y. Zhou, G. L. Gebber, and S. M. Barman. 1997. Coupled oscillators account for the slow rhythms in sympathetic nerve discharge and phrenic nerve activity. *Am. J. Physiol.* 272:R1314–R1324.
9. Staras, K., H. S. Change, and M. P. Gilbey. 2001. Resetting of sympathetic rhythm by somatic afferents causes post-reflex coordination of sympathetic activity in rat. *J. Physiol. (Lond.)* 533:537–545.
10. Karila, P., and J. P. Horn. 2000. Secondary nicotinic synapses on sympathetic B neurons and their putative role in ganglionic amplification of activity. *J. Neurosci.* 20:908–918.

28 Sexual Function

John D. Stewart
Montreal Neurological Hospital
Montreal, Quebec, Canada

Sexual function is controlled by the complex integrated activity of the central nervous system (supraspinal and spinal) and the autonomic and somatic components of the peripheral nervous system. Penile and clitoral engorgement is a central part of this process, brought about by vascular dilatation of the cavernosal tissues. The most important mediator of this is nitric oxide (NO) released from non-adrenergic noncholinergic (NANC) nerves. Other nerves, neurotransmitters, and modulators play contributory roles. Glandular secretion and semen ejaculation are the other neurally mediated components of the sexual act.

The physiologic events of the sexual act are mediated by the integrated activities of the central and peripheral somatic and autonomic nervous systems. Despite the obvious anatomic differences between male and female individuals, many of the physiologic sexual responses are similar: arousal, erectile tissue engorgement and detumescence, glandular secretion, and contraction of smooth and striated muscles.

PERIPHERAL STRUCTURES

The erectile tissue of the penis and clitoris consists of the corpora cavernosa. These comprise many blood-filled spaces called lacunae [1, 2]. The walls of the lacunae are the trabeculae, which, like blood vessels, consist of smooth muscle and fibroelastic tissue. Within each cavernosum lies a cavernosal artery, which gives off numerous helicine arteries that open directly into the lacunae. Small veins lie among the lacunae and drain into the deep dorsal vein of the penis (or clitoris). The striated muscles of the perineum—the bulbospongiosus and ischiocavernosus muscles—contribute to the maintenance of erections in some species and are important for ejaculation.

CENTRAL NERVOUS SYSTEM

The parts of the central nervous system involved in sexual responses are a central brain network, descending and ascending pathways, and the lower spinal cord.

The central network remains poorly understood; information is based primarily on data from animals. The hypothalamus (particularly the paraventricular nucleus) and limbic pathways play a key role in erection. However, many structures are involved: prefrontal cortex, hippocampus, amygdala, midbrain, pons, and medulla [3, 4]. Descending pathways include the bulbospinal and other pathways. Ascending pathways such as the spinothalamic tract transmit tactile and other such stimuli centrally. The distal spinal cord contains the cell bodies of the sympathetic and parasympathetic nerves and also Onuff's nucleus—the origin of the motor fibers to the muscles of the perineum.

Three sets of peripheral nerves are involved [1, 3, 5]: (1) thoracolumbar sympathetic nerves, (2) sacral parasympathetic nerves, and (3) pudendal somatic nerves. The sympathetic and parasympathetic nerves join to form the pelvic plexus. From this arise adrenergic, cholinergic, and NANC nerves. These innervate erectile tissue, nonerectile smooth muscle, glandular tissue, and blood vessels. The pudendal somatic nerves supply the bulbocavernosus and ischiocavernosus muscles and contain the sensory nerves of the genitalia.

PHYSIOLOGIC EVENTS

Penile erection and clitoral engorgement result from the integrated activity in the vasomotor nerves that modify the flow of blood in the erectile tissues and its drainage. Relaxation of the smooth muscle of the cavernosal and helicine arteries and of the cavernosal trabeculae are the key physiologic changes. These occur from both active relaxation of the smooth muscle walls and a reduction in their tonically contracted state.

The most important neurotransmitter mediating these changes is NO. This is derived from two sources: (1) directly from NANC parasympathetic nerves and (2) indirectly from the endothelium lining the cavernosal sinusoids and blood vessels in response to cholinergic stimulation. The former is the more important. NO activates guanylate cyclase, which induces the formation of intracellular cyclic guanosine monophosphate. This, in turn, produces relaxation of vascular and trabecular smooth muscle in the corpora cavernosa.

Noradrenergic nerves release norepinephrine that acts on α_1 receptors to cause arterial and trabecular smooth muscle contraction, thereby maintaining flaccidity; a reduction in this activity contributes to erection.

Other neurotransmitters and neuromodulators that are probably involved in these responses include vasoactive intestinal peptide, other peptides, adenosine triphosphate, and endothelin.

Emission of semen occurs by smooth muscle contraction in the epididymis, vas deferens, seminal vesicles, and the prostate gland. This deposits spermatozoa and seminal fluid into the proximal urethra. Contraction of bladder neck sphincters prevents backflow of semen into the bladder (retrograde ejaculation). These events are principally mediated by the sympathetic nerves. Ejaculation consists of the semen being rapidly transmitted down the urethra and released in spurts. This is accomplished by rhythmic contractions of the bulbocavernosus, ischiocavernosus, and periurethral striated muscles supplied by the pudendal nerve.

References

1. de Groat, W. C., and W. D. Steers. 1990. Autonomic regulation of the urinary bladder and sexual organs. In *Central regulation of autonomic functions*, ed. A. D. Loewy and K. M. Spyer, 310–333. New York: Oxford University Press.
2. Lue, T. F., and E. Tanagho, 1988. Functional anatomy and mechanism of penile erection. In *Contemporary management of impotence and infertility*, ed. E. Tanagho, T. Lue, and T. McClure. Baltimore: Williams and Wilkins.
3. Giuliano, F., and O. Rampin. 2000. Central neural regulation of penile erection. *Neurosci. Biobehav. Rev.* 24:517–533.
4. Rampin, O., and F. Giuliano. 2001. Brain control of penile erection. *World J. Urol.* 19:1–8.
5. Steers, W. D. 2000. Neural pathways and central sites involved in penile erection: Neuroanatomy and clinical implications. *Neurosci. Biobehav. Rev.* 24:507–516.

29

Gastrointestinal Function

Michael Camilleri
Mayo Clinic
Rochester, Minnesota

Proper function of the gastrointestinal tract is essential for the orderly digestion, absorption, and transport of food and residue. Digestion requires secretion of endogenous fluids from the salivary glands, stomach, pancreas, and small bowel to facilitate intraluminal breakdown of foods; fluids, electrolytes, and smaller building blocks of the macronutrients are then absorbed, leaving nondigestible residue to be excreted [1].

The motor activity of the gut is one of the integrated functions that is essential for the normal assimilation of food. Gut motility facilitates the transport of nutrients, brings together digestive enzymes and their substrates, temporarily stores content, particularly in the distal small bowel and right colon, for optimal absorption, and finally, excretes nondigestible residue by defecation in a well-coordinated function under voluntary control. The extrinsic autonomic nervous system is critically important for almost all secretory and motor functions in the digestive tract (Fig. 29.1).

SALIVARY SECRETION

Presentation of food to the mouth and olfactory stimulation trigger afferent nerves that stimulate secretory centers in the medulla. These reflexly stimulate efferent fibers along parasympathetic and sympathetic pathways: parasympathetic fibers course along the facial nerve to sublingual and submaxillary glands, and the glossopharyngeal nerve to the parotid gland. Synapse with postganglionic fibers occurs in or near the glands. Sympathetic fibers reach the salivary glands through the cervical sympathetic trunk, but the brainstem centers are unclear. Parasympathetic efferents stimulate secretion; sympathetic fibers serve to cause contraction of myoepithelial cells on the duct.

The human salivary glands secrete 0.5–1.0 liter saliva per day at a maximal rate of 4 ml/min. Saliva facilitates speech, lubricates food for swallowing, and contains the amylase ptyalin, which begins the digestion of starch. Bicarbonate in saliva neutralizes noxious acidic ingesta.

GASTRIC SECRETION

Gastric secretion is stimulated by the act of eating (cephalic phase) and the arrival of food in the stomach (gastric phase). Arrival of the food in the intestine also controls gastric secretion (intestinal phase). The secreted fluid contains hydrochloric acid, pepsinogen, intrinsic factor, bicarbonate, and mucus. Gastric secretion of acid and pepsinogen follows stimulation of oral and gastric vagal afferents. Efferent vagal pathways synapse with submucous plexus neurons, which innervate secretory cells through several important bioactive molecules including gastrin, histamine, and somatostatin. In the stomach, there is some digestion of carbohydrate and protein, but little absorption except for some fat-soluble substances. The mucus-bicarbonate layer protects the stomach lining from autodigestion by acid.

PANCREATICOBILIARY SECRETION

Pancreatic juice consists of alkaline (chiefly bicarbonate) fluid and enzymes; 200–800 mL is produced each day. The enzymes trypsin, lipase, and amylase are essential for digestion of most of the protein, fat, and carbohydrate in the meal. The pancreas consists of exocrine and endocrine portions: bicarbonate and fluid are secreted by ductular cells, chiefly under the influence of secretin; enzymes are produced by acinar cells in response to vagal stimulation of intrapancreatic cholinergic neurons. Recent data suggest that cholecystokinin (CCK), which is released from the duodenal mucosal enteroendocrine cells after chemical stimulation by food, activates pancreatic enzyme secretion by stimulating vagal afferents.

BILE

Bile is continuously secreted by the liver as two fractions: the bile salt-independent fraction, controlled by secretin and

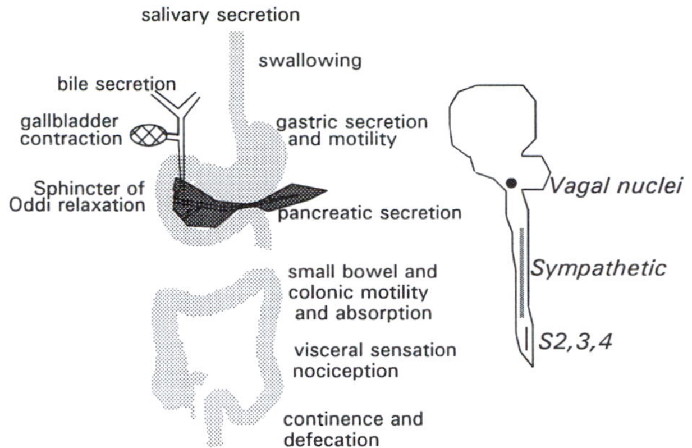

FIGURE 29.1 Gastrointestinal physiology: functions under extrinsic autonomic control.

CCK, is similar to pancreatic juice; the bile salt–dependent fraction contains bile salts. Bile flow is controlled by storage in the gallbladder and by the sphincter of Oddi. Postprandially, the gallbladder contracts under vagal and CCK stimulation, and the basal sphincter tone within the ampulla of Vater falls to allow bile to enter the duodenum. There is evidence for interdigestive cycling of pancreaticobiliary secretion that is synchronous with the main phases of the gut's cyclical migrating motor complex (*vide infra*).

INTESTINAL SECRETION AND ABSORPTION

The small bowel produces about 5 liters of fluid per day during the equilibration of osmotic loads induced by ingested nutrients and during intraluminal digestion. Yet, most of the 7 liters entering the digestive tract each day is reabsorbed (about 80% in small bowel, 20% in colon) during the organized flow of chyme through the small bowel and colon, thereby ensuring a stool weight less than 200 g/day in health. Water and electrolyte fluxes are generally independent of extrinsic neural control; conversely, the submucosal plexus is increasingly recognized as a key factor influencing mucosal blood flow and enterocyte function.

Absorption of macronutrients and micronutrients is generally determined by concentration gradients or active carrier-mediated, energy-requiring transport processes. These are indirectly influenced by the autonomic nervous system through its effects on the secretion of salivary, gastric, and pancreaticobiliary juices and by the motor processes of mixing and delivery of substrate to sites of preferential absorption—for example, B_{12} to the ileum.

CONTROL OF GUT MOTILITY

The function of the gastrointestinal smooth muscle is intimately controlled by release of peptides and transmitters by the intrinsic (or enteric) nervous system; modulation of the latter input arises in the extrinsic autonomic nerves, the craniospinal (vagus, and S2, S3, and S4 nerves) parasympathetic excitatory input, and the thoracolumbar sympathetic outflow, which is predominantly inhibitory to the gut, but excitatory to the sphincter (Fig. 29.2). Gastrointestinal smooth muscle forms an electrical syncytium whereby the impulse that induces contraction of the first muscle cell results in efficient transmission to a sheet of sequentially linked cells in the transverse and longitudinal axes of the intestine. The pacemaker of the intestinal muscle syncytium is the network of interstitial cells of Cajal, which serve to coordinate contraction circumferentially and longitudinally along the gut [2, 3].

In several species, including humans, the enteric nervous system is formed of a series of ganglionated plexuses, such as the submucosal (Meissner), myenteric (Auerbach), deep muscular (Cajal), mucosal, and submucosal plexuses. Together these enteric nerves number almost 100 million neurons; this number is roughly equivalent to the number of neurons in the spinal cord.

At the level of the diaphragm, the vagus nerve consists predominantly of afferent fibers. Thus, the classical concept that preganglionic vagal fibers synapse with a few motor neurons is not tenable, in view of the overwhelmingly larger number of effector cells that would need to be innervated by the smaller number of preganglionic nerves. The current concept (Fig. 29.3) is that each vagal command fiber supplies an integrated circuit that is hardwired in the intestinal wall and results in a specific motor or secretory response [4]. These hardwired circuits in the enteric nervous system are also important in many of the automated responses of the gut, such as the peristaltic reflex, which persist even in a totally extrinsically denervated intestine. The enteric nerves also control pacemaker activity. Pacemakers located on the greater curve of the gastric corpus and the duodenal bulb "drive" the maximum intrinsic frequency of contractions: 3 per minute in the stomach and 12 per minute in the small intestine. As in the heart, malfunction of the pacemaker with the greatest frequency results in "take over" of pacemaker function by the region with the next greatest intrinsic contractile frequency. Derangement of the extrinsic neural control of the gastrointestinal smooth muscle forms the basis for disorders of motility encountered in clinical practice, such as diabetic gastroparesis and anal incontinence after obstetric trauma. Other diseases result from disorders of enteric neural function including achalasia or Hirschsprung's disease.

NORMAL GASTROINTESTINAL MOTOR FUNCTION

Swallowing involves chewing of food, transfer from the oral cavity to the hypopharynx, ejection of the bolus into the

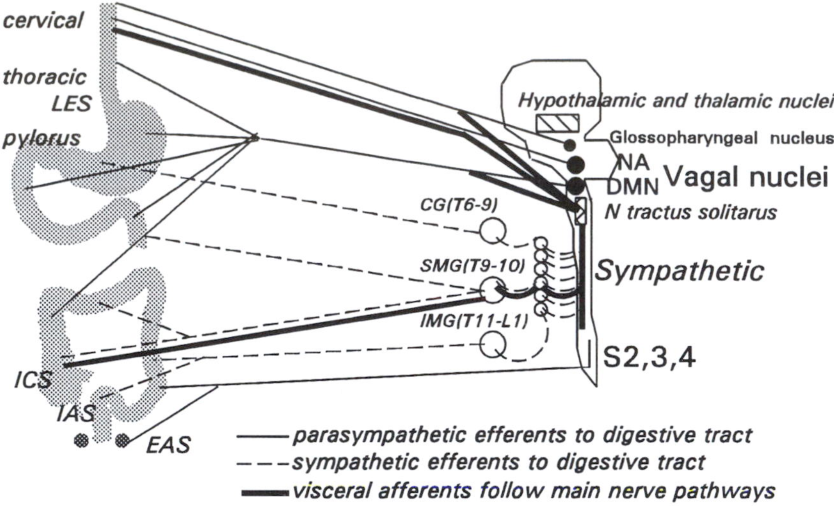

FIGURE 29.2 Neural pathways with sympathetic and parasympathetic nervous systems to the gastrointestinal tract.

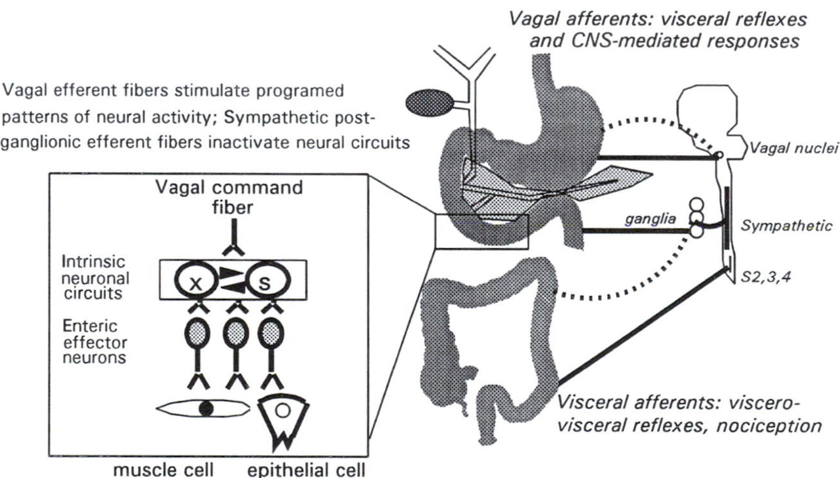

FIGURE 29.3 Integration between extrinsic and intrinsic (or enteric) neural control. Hardwired programs controlling such functions of peristalsis are modulated by efferents in the vagus and sympathetic nerves, which also contain afferent fibers mediating visceral sensation, nociception, and reflex responses.

esophagus, and esophageal peristalsis. The lower esophageal sphincter relaxes at the onset of the swallowing reflex and remains open for a period of about 8 seconds until the bolus passes through the entire esophagus. Then the sphincter contracts to prevent gastroesophageal reflux. Reflux also is prevented by the positive intraabdominal pressure that occludes the short intraabdominal portion of the esophagus. Extrinsic neural control reaches the esophagus through efferent pathways in the glossopharyngeal (upper esophagus) and vagus nerves.

The motor functions of the stomach and small bowel differ greatly between the fasting and postprandial periods. During fasting, cyclical motor events sweep through the stomach and small bowel and are associated with similarly cyclical secretion from the biliary tract and pancreas. The cyclical motor activity is called the interdigestive migrating motor complex; this consists of a phase I of quiescence, phase II of intermittent pressure activity, and phase III or the activity front when contractions of the maximal frequency typical of each region (3 per minute in stomach, 12 per minute in the small bowel) sweep through the gut like a housekeeper, transporting nondigestible residue, products of digestion, and epithelial debris toward the colon for subsequent excretion. The pacemaking functions, cyclical motor

Resting

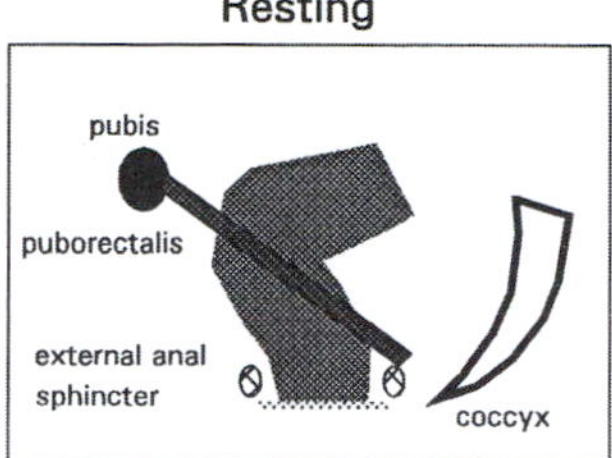

Straining

pubis
puborectalis
external anal sphincter
coccyx

Relaxation of puborectalis
Straightening of rectoanal angle
Relaxation of external anal sphincter

Rectoanal Angle

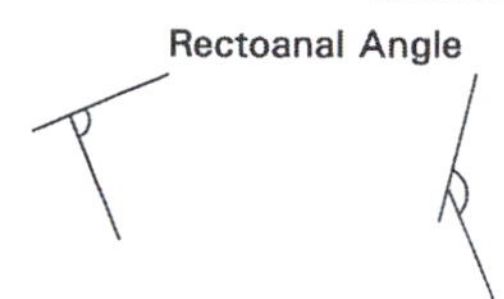

FIGURE 29.4 Dynamics of normal defecation. Note the straightening of the rectoanal angle by relaxation of the puborectalis to facilitate evacuation.

activity, and peristalsis are essentially controlled by intrinsic neural pathways, but they can be modulated by extrinsic nerves.

Postprandially, this cyclical activity is abolished, and the different regions of the gut subserve specific functions. Tonic contractions in the gastric fundus result in the emptying of liquids; antral contractions sieve and triturate solid food and propel particles that are less than 2 mm in size from the stomach. Irregular, frequent contractions in the postprandial period serve to mix food with digestive juices in the duodenum and jejunum and to propel it aborally. The duration of small bowel transit is on average about 3 hours, and the ileum is a site of temporary storage of chyme, allowing salvage of nutrients, fluids and electrolytes, that were not absorbed upstream. Residues are finally discharged from the ileum to the colon in bolus transfers that probably result from prolonged propagated contractions or reestablished interdigestive cyclical motor activity. The vagus nerve is critically important in efferent control of the fed phase; splanchnic and vagal afferents convey signals from the gut to the prevertebral ganglia, spinal cord, and brain to evoke reflex responses and coordinate secretory and motor functions.

In the dog, the colon also demonstrates cyclical activity, but this is less understood than in the small bowel. The proximal colon (ascending and transverse regions) stores solid residue. The ascending colon has variable patterns of emptying: relatively linear, or constant; intermittent; or sudden mass movements. The descending colon is mainly a conduit, and the rectosigmoid functions as a terminal reservoir leading to the call to defecate and empty under voluntary control.

Defecation results from a well-coordinated series of motor responses (Fig. 29.4). The rectoanal angle is maintained relatively acute by the puborectalis muscle sling or pelvic floor, and this is important to maintain continence. For defecation to occur, this sling relaxes, thereby opening the rectoanal angle to allow a straighter rectal conduit; the anal sphincters are inhibited by parasympathetic (S2, S3, S4) input; and intracolonic pressure increases predominantly by an increase in intraabdominal pressure associated with straining. In contrast, continence is maintained by contraction of the puborectalis (parasympathetic S2, S3, S4), contraction of the internal sphincter (sympathetic lumbar colonic nerves), and contraction of the external sphincter (pudendal nerve).

References

1. Davenport, H. W. 1982. *Physiology of the digestive tract*, 5th ed. St. Louis: Year Book Medical Publisher.
2. Camilleri, M. 1997. Autonomic regulation of gastrointestinal motility. In *Clinical autonomic disorders: Evaluation and management*, 2nd ed., ed. P. A. Low, 135–145. Philadelphia: Lippincott-Raven.
3. Camilleri, M. 1995. Gastrointestinal motor mechanisms and motility: Hormonal and neural regulation. In *Gastrointestinal tract and endocrine system*, ed. M. V. Singer, R. Ziegler, and G. Rohr, 237–253. Dordrecht, The Netherlands: Kluwer Publishers.
4. Cooke, H. J. 1989. Role of "little brain" in the gut in water and electrolyte homeostasis. *FASEB. J.* 3:127–138.

30 Regulation of Metabolism

Robert Hoeldtke
Division of Endocrinology
West Virginia University
Morgantown, West Virginia

Epinephrine, the adrenal medullary hormone, and norepinephrine, the sympathetic neurotransmitter, have multiple effects on intermediary metabolism, most of which act synergistically to mobilize stored fuels. In addition to direct effects on target organs (primarily liver, adipose, and muscle), catecholamines act on the pancreatic islets where they regulate the secretion of insulin and glucagon. The most important effect on the islet is to suppress insulin secretion by α-adrenergic mechanisms. Thus, the direct catabolic effects of catecholamines are amplified by their suppression of the predominant anabolic hormone: insulin.

CATECHOLAMINES AND GLUCOSE METABOLISM

Catecholamines activate β-adrenergic receptors in the liver and stimulate hepatic glucose production by multiple mechanisms. Glycogenolysis and gluconeogenesis are enhanced, whereas glycogen synthesis is inhibited. In addition to stimulating the entry of glucose into the bloodstream, catecholamines decrease plasma glucose clearance by both direct (β) and indirect (α) adrenergic mechanisms as illustrated in Figure 30.1. These multiple catecholamine effects are synergistic insofar as they all serve to increase plasma glucose concentrations. These mechanisms become physiologically important in the setting of hypoglycemia, the classical stimulus to epinephrine secretion by the adrenal medulla. Thus, the autonomic activation associated with hypoglycemia serves the ultimate purpose of mobilizing endogenous substrates for glucose production and increasing glucose concentrations in the bloodstream so that central nervous system demand for its obligatory fuel can be met.

The autonomic mechanisms for correcting hypoglycemia are well established; nevertheless, glucose counter-regulation remains intact in adrenalectomized patients and in those subjected to combined (α plus β) adrenergic blockade. This is because the glucagon response to hypoglycemia, which has effects similar to those of epinephrine, is preserved. Glucose counter-regulation, therefore, only becomes compromised when there is failure of both glucagon secretion and adrenergic responses. This commonly occurs in the setting of diabetes, in which a single hypoglycemic event may suppress all counter-regulatory responses to subsequent hypoglycemic events for at least 24 hours, the syndrome of hypoglycemia-associated autonomic failure [1]. Patients with type 1 diabetes are especially vulnerable to severe hypoglycemia because most lose their ability to secrete glucagon during the first decade of their illness. They, therefore, become dependent on adrenergic mechanisms for counter-regulation, which often are inadequate in patients with long-standing disease and autonomic neuropathy [2].

CATECHOLAMINES AND FAT METABOLISM

Catecholamines act directly on adipose tissue to stimulate fat breakdown. This is a β_1-adrenergic effect involving adenyl cyclase–mediated activation of hormone-sensitive triacylglycerol lipase, the enzyme that cleaves triglyceride in adipose tissue into fatty acids and glycerol. Insulin inhibits catecholamine-induced lipolysis; thus, catecholamine-mediated suppression of insulin secretion is synergistic with the direct catecholamine effects on adipose tissue.

Locally released norepinephrine is probably more important than circulating catecholamines in regulating lipolysis. In patients with diabetic ketoacidosis, however, circulating catecholamines become high enough to stimulate both lipolysis and ketogenesis.

CATECHOLAMINES AND THERMOGENESIS

Obligatory thermogenesis (basal metabolic rate) is regulated by thyroid hormones, whereas facultative thermogenesis (total heat production minus basal) is regulated by the adrenergic nervous system predominantly through β_3-adrenoreceptors. Cold exposure and exercise stimulate the adrenergic nervous system and thereby enhance facultative thermogenesis. The increase in heat production associated with eating (dietary-induced thermogenesis) cannot be fully attributed to the energy cost of digestion, absorption, and metabolism of nutrients. Food ingestion activates the

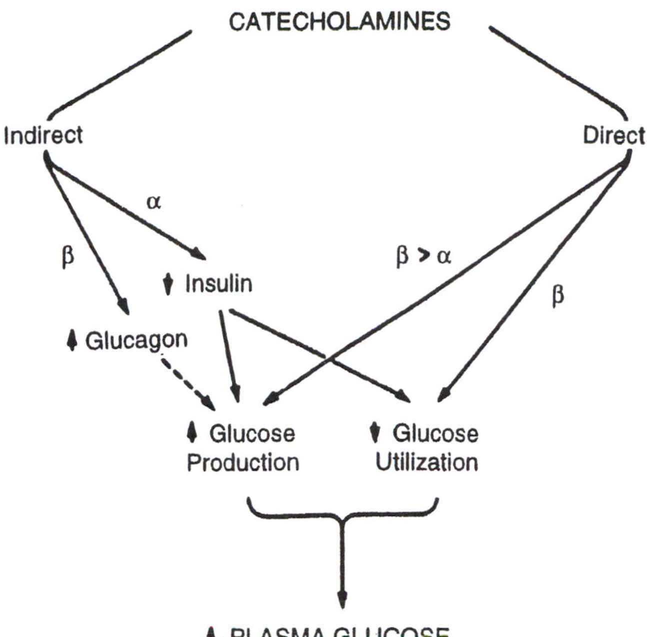

FIGURE 30.1 Mechanisms for catecholamine-induced increments in plasma glucose concentrations.

sympathetic nervous system, stimulates thermogenesis, and may serve to protect against obesity.

INSULIN AND AUTONOMIC FUNCTION

Fasting suppresses the activity of the sympathetic nervous system, whereas overeating is stimulatory [3, 4]. These considerations have suggested that insulin mediates these nutritional effects because it stimulates sympathetic activity. This theory has been controversial because studies of the effects of insulin on plasma catecholamines have yielded inconsistent results [5, 6]. Moreover, it has been argued that insulin's stimulation of sympathetic activity is a nonspecific response to its vasodilator effects. Microneurographic studies, however, have confirmed that insulin stimulates muscle sympathetic nerves and documented this at doses of insulin that do not cause vasodilation. These findings have supported the hypothesis that hyperinsulinemia and sympathetic activation promote the development of hypertension in patients with type 2 diabetes and obesity. Increased spillover of norepinephrine into the renal veins has been documented in patients with insulin resistance, although this may reflect an effect of increased leptin rather than hyperinsulinemia. In either case, activation of renal sympathetic neurons probably explain the sodium retention and hypervolemia that characterize the hypertension associated with obesity. Sympathetic activation may also lead to left ventricular hypertrophy and increased cardiac output. Thus, it appears that many of the cardinal physiologic disturbances associated with obesity are linked to activation of the sympathetic nervous system. It remains uncertain, however, whether the latter is a consequence of hyperinsulinemia or some other obesity-related metabolic disturbance.

References

1. Cryer, P. E. 1994. Banting Lecture. Hypoglycemia: The limiting factor in the management of IDDM. *Diabetes* 43:1378–1389.
2. Hoeldtke, R. D., and G. Boden. 1994. Epinephrine secretion, hypoglycemia unawareness, and diabetic autonomic neuropathy. *Ann. Intern. Med.* 120:512–517.
3. Rocchini, A. P., J. Key, D. Bondie, R. Chico, C. Moorehead, V. Katch, and M. Martin. 1989. The effects of weight loss on the sensitivity of blood pressure to sodium in obese adolescents. *N. Engl. J. Med.* 321:580–585.
4. Landsberg, L. 1999. Role of the sympathetic adrenal system in the pathogenesis of the insulin resistance syndrome. *Ann. NY Acad. Sci.* 892:84–90.
5. Hausberg, M., A. L. Mark, R. P. Hoffman, C. A. Sinkey, and E. A. Anderson. 1995. Dissociation of sympathoexcitatory and vasodilator actions of modestly elevated plasma insulin levels. *J. Hypertens.* 13: 1015–1021.
6. Esler, M. 2000. The sympathetic system and hypertension. *Am. J. Hypertens.* 13:99S–105S.

31 The Sweat Gland

Phillip A. Low
Department of Neurology
Mayo Clinic
Rochester, Minnesota

ANATOMY AND FUNCTION OF THE SWEAT GLAND

Type

There are two types of sweat glands: eccrine and apocrine. The eccrine sweat glands are simple tubular glands that extend down from the epidermis to the lower dermis. The lower portion is a tightly coiled secretory apparatus consisting of two types of cells. The apocrine gland is a dark basophilic cell that secretes mucous material, and the eccrine sweat gland is a light acidophilic cell that is responsible for the passage of water and electrolytes. Differences between the two types of glands are described in Table 31.1. Apocrine sweat glands are found in the axilla, the anogenital zone, the areola of the nipple, and the external auditory meatus.

Density and Distribution

Eccrine sweat glands are of greater interest in neuroscience, and the rest of the description focuses on eccrine sweat glands. It weighs about 30–40 μg each [1]. It first appears in the 3.5-month-old fetus in the volar surface of the hands and feet. Eccrine glands show area differences with the greatest density in the palms and soles. They vary in density from $400/mm^2$ on the palm to about $80/cm^2$ on the thigh and upper arm. The total numbers are approximately 2 to 5 million. Male and female individuals have the same number of sweat glands. However, the size and volume secreted by each gland is about 5 times greater in males [2].

Surrounding the secretory cells are myoepithelial cells whose contraction is thought to aid the expulsion of sweat. These glands receive a rich supply of blood vessels and sympathetic nerve fibers, but they are unusual in that sympathetic innervation is largely cholinergic. The full complement of eccrine glands develops in the embryonic state [3]; no new glands develop after birth.

Physiology of Sweat Glands

The physiology of human sweat response is known from the detailed *in vitro* studies of Sato [4]. Acetylcholine secretion results in the production of an ultrafiltrate (isotonic) by the secretory coil. Directly collected sweat samples yield Na^+ and K^+ values identical with plasma. Reabsorption of sodium ions by the eccrine sweat duct results in hypotonic sweat, confirmed in directly collected sweat samples from proximal duct (Na^+: 20–80 mM; K^+: 5–25 mM; [1]). Extracellular Ca^{2+} is important because removal of periglandular Ca^{2+} with EGTA completely inhibits sweat secretion, whereas Ca ionophore A23187 strongly and persistently stimulates sweating [1]. Magnesium ions appear to be unimportant.

Function

The major function of the sweat gland in humans is thermoregulatory. There are a number of factors that affect the sweat response (Table 31.2). With repeated episodes of profuse sweating, the salt content of the sweat progressively declines. In the individual acclimatized to a hot climate, the salt content is reduced, probably reflecting an increase of mineralocorticoids in response to thermal stress [3]. The sweat gland is prone to atrophy and hypertrophy. Repeated stimulation results in a several-fold increase in the size and function of the gland.

Diffuse loss or absence of sweat can be caused by absence of sweat glands or widespread denervation. Heat intolerance can be a major problem, especially in young patients with widespread anhidrosis, for example, in the condition chronic idiopathic anhidrosis [5].

INNERVATION OF SWEAT GLAND

Innervation of the sweat gland is mainly by sympathetic postganglionic cholinergic fibers. In isolated human eccrine

TABLE 31.1 Comparison of Eccrine with Apocrine Sweat Gland

Parameter	Eccrine	Apocrine
Size	Relatively small	Large
Duct	Long and thin	Short and thick
Ductal opening	Skin surface (near hair)	Directly into upper follicular canal
Secretory coil	Small external diameter Very narrow lumen	Large external diameter Wide lumen
Cell type	Secretory (clear); dark myoepithelial	Columnar secretory; myoepithelial
Intercellular canaliculi	Present	Absent
Development	Present at birth	Present at birth
Pharmacology	Cholinergic ≫ β-adrenergic ≫ α-adrenergic	Cholinergic = β-adrenergic
Sweat secret rate	Continuous high	Intermittent variable
Secretory product	Serous	Milky protein-rich

TABLE 31.2 Factors That Affect the Sweat Responses

Parameter	Comments
Factors that **increase** the sweat response	
Mental stress	Greatest effect on palmar, sole, and axillary sites
Exercise rehydration	Precedes increase in core temperature Decreases core temperature
Male sex	Greater sweat gland volume
Race	Blacks > whites but difference is quite small
Acclimatization	Increased gain (sweating/temperature change); reduced sweat sodium content
Circadian rhythm	Higher in PM
Seasonal variation	Greater response in winter
Alcohol and drugs	Cutaneous vasodilatation; reduced hypothalamic set-point
Factors that **reduce** the sweat response	
Skin pressure	Mechanoreceptor stimulation; inhibition of local sympathetic efferents
Hydromeiosis	Water on skin surface reduces sweating rate
Dehydration	Reduced skin blood flow
Hyperosmolarity	Reduced skin blood flow
Cold stimulus	Inhibition of sudomotor activity

sweat gland regulation, the regulation of sweating is cholinergic and muscarinic, being completely inhibited by atropine [1]. Sudomotor function is metabolically active; it is inhibited by cold, involves active transport, and is inhibited by metabolic inhibitors. Microtubules may be important because vinblastine strongly, but reversibly, inhibits sweating. Endogenous cyclic adenosine monophosphate (cAMP) appears to be the second messenger, because theophylline by phosphodiesterase inhibition markedly increases the sweat response. The muscarinic receptor subtype is M_3 [6].

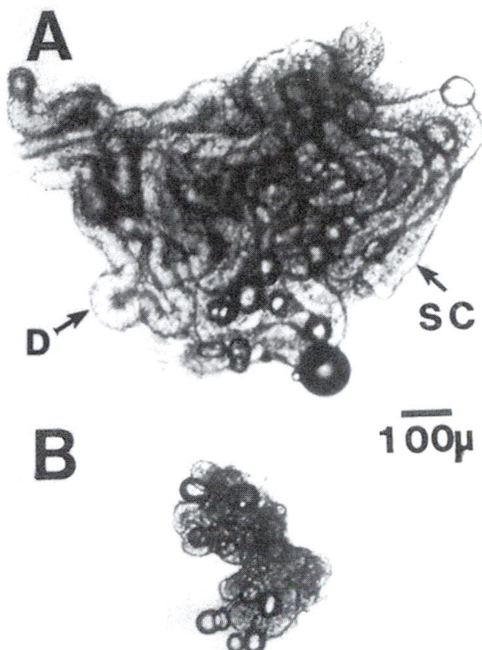

FIGURE 31.1 Human eccrine sweat gland from a normal subject (**A**) and a patient with chronic idiopathic anhidrosis (**B**). There is marked sweat gland atrophy secondary to disuse. D, duct; SC, secretory coil. (Reprinted with permission from Sato, K. 1997. Normal and abnormal sweat gland function. In *Clinical autonomic disorders: Evaluation and management*, ed. P. A. Low, 97–108. Philadelphia: Lippincott-Raven.)

The prostaglandin E_1 has a sudorific effect *in vitro* comparable to ACh and was thought to act through cAMP. Histochemical labeling studies show prominent innervation with vasoactive intestinal polypeptide and calcitonin gene–related peptide fibers and presence of substance P and tyrosine hydroxylase fibers [7].

There is, however, dual innervation with a loose network of catecholamine-containing nerves around sweat glands. Innervation of human sweat glands show similarities to rat and mouse sweat glands. In rodents, innervation is initially completely adrenergic followed by an adrenergic to cholinergic switch during development [8]. It is not known if such a switch occurs in humans during development or with neuropathy and fiber regeneration. There are a number of observations that suggest adrenergic innervation increases with certain diseases. The human sweat gland responds to intradermal and intraarterial adrenaline (10% of cholinergic) [9]. There is evidence of both α-adrenergic (blocked by dibenamine) and β-adrenergic mechanism (blocked by propranolol, but not phentolamine). Prominent hyperhidrosis and adrenergic sensitivity occurs in certain neuropathies and complex regional pain syndrome type I (CRPS I), suggesting increased sympathetic innervation. Indeed, the postganglionic sympathetic neuron has been shown to enhance adrenergic sweating in CRPS I [10]. *In vitro* studies suggest the following rank order of sudorific effect ACh > epinephrine ($\alpha + \beta$) $\approx$ isoproterenol (β) > phenylephrine (α).

Denervation

Denervation of sweat glands occurs in preganglionic lesions (such as spinal cord injury or multiple system atrophy) or postganglionic lesions (as in the autonomic neuropathies). The size and function of the sweat gland under these circumstances undergoes dramatic atrophy (Fig. 31.1 [4]). Another mechanism of injury is that of trans-synaptic degeneration of postganglionic axons that could occur with chronic preganglionic lesions. There is also evidence that in early or mild neuropathy affecting the feet there is excessive forearm response, suggesting hypertrophy. The postganglionic sweat response progressively fails with increasing age [11]. The sweat loss is associated with a loss of cholinergic unmyelinated fiber stained with the panaxonal marker PGP9.5 and acetylcholinesterase [12].

In summary, the eccrine sweat gland is an important appendage, which subserves thermoregulation. Its absence results in heat intolerance. Alterations in its function provide important clues to the status of the autonomic nervous system.

References

1. Sato, K., and F. Sato. 1983. Individual variations in structure and function of human eccrine sweat gland. *Am. J. Physiol.* 245:R203–R208.
2. Ogawa, T., and P. A. Low. 1997. Autonomic regulation of temperature and sweating. In *Clinical autonomic disorders: Evaluation and management*, ed. P. A. Low, 83–96. Philadelphia: Lippincott-Raven.
3. Kuno, Y. 1956. *Human perspiration*. Springfield, IL: Charles C. Thomas.
4. Sato, K. 1997. Normal and abnormal sweat gland function. In *Clinical autonomic disorders: Evaluation and management*, ed. P. A. Low, 97–108. Philadelphia: Lippincott-Raven.
5. Low, P. A., and J. G. McLeod. 1997. Autonomic neuropathies. In *Clinical autonomic disorders: Evaluation and management*, ed. P. A. Low, 463–486. Philadelphia: Lippincott-Raven.
6. Torres, N. E., P. J. Zollman, and P. A. Low. 1991. Characterization of muscarinic receptor subtype of rat eccrine sweat gland by autoradiography. *Brain Res.* 550:129–132.
7. Low, P. A., and W. R. Kennedy. 1997. Cutaneous effectors as indicators of abnormal sympathetic function. In *Autonomic innervation of the skin*, Vol. 12, ed. J. L. Morris and I. L. Gibbins, 165–212. Amsterdam: Harwood Academic Publishers.
8. Landis, S. C. 1988. Neurotransmitter plasticity in sympathetic neurons. In *Handbook of chemical neuroanatomy: The peripheral nervous system*, Vol. 6, ed. A. Björklund, T. Hökfelt, and C. Owman, 65–115. Amsterdam: Elsevier.
9. Sato, K. 1973. Sweat induction from an isolated eccrine sweat gland. *Am. J. Physiol.* 225:1147–1152.
10. Chemali, K. R., R. Gorodeski, and T. C. Chelimsky. 2001. Alpha-adrenergic supersensitivity of the sudomotor nerve in complex regional pain syndrome. *Ann. Neurol.* 49:453–459.
11. Low, P. A. 1997. The effect of aging on the autonomic nervous system. In *Clinical autonomic disorders: Evaluation and management*, ed. P. A. Low, 161–175. Philadelphia: Lippincott-Raven.
12. Abdel-Rahman, T. A., K. J. Collins, T. Cowen, and M. Rustin. 1992. Immunohistochemical, morphological and functional changes in the peripheral sudomotor neuro-effector system in elderly people. *J. Auton. Nerv. Syst.* 37:187–197.

32

Temperature Regulation

Mikihiro Kihara
Department of Neurology
Kinki University School of Medicine
Osaka, Japan

Junichi Sugenoya
Department of Physiology
Aichi Medical University
Aichi, Japan

Phillip A. Low
Department of Neurology
Mayo Clinic
Rochester, Minnesota

Homeotherms, including humans, can regulate their body temperature by controlling the rates of heat production and heat loss. Heat is continuously produced in the body, primarily by visceral organs and muscles. To maintain a constant body temperature, heat loss must exactly balance heat production. At high environmental temperature, there is reduced heat loss from skin surface; body temperature would become increased and this, in turn, enhances heat loss activity such as cutaneous vasodilatation or sweating. Body temperature regulation depends on the integrated activities of the autonomic nervous system, centered predominantly in the hypothalamus.

CENTRAL INTEGRATION

The human thermoregulatory system is outlined in Figure 32.1. The preoptic and anterior hypothalamus (PO/AH) are assumed to be the brain structures most responsible for body temperature regulation [1]. There are two types of thermosensitive neurons in PO/AH: warm-sensitive and cold-sensitive neurons. These neurons are sensitive to changes in brain temperature. The PO/AH neurons also integrate the thermal signals that arise at these neurons (brain temperature) and the skin (skin temperature). Body (core) temperature is regulated with reference to the set-point temperature, which is determined as a temperature at which the signal rate of the warm-sensitive and the cold-sensitive neurons balance (set-point theory). The set-point temperature is not fixed, but it is altered dynamically by various nonthermal signals that arise at various homeostatic regulatory systems [2]. In the case of fever, which is induced by pyrogen, activities of warm-sensitive neurons decrease, whereas those of cold-sensitive neurons increase [3], resulting in an upward shift of the set-point. Thus, the body temperature is regulated around an increased set-point (Fig. 32.2). Similarly, an upward shift of set-point is induced by the action of progesterone [4]. Conversely, thyrotropin-releasing hormone (TRH) elicits a downward shift of the set-point temperature [5], but, interestingly, TRH fails to produce such a downshift in patients with Parkinson's disease [6]. Alcohol ingestion may also induce a downward shift of the set-point temperature (see Fig. 32.2), as is evidenced by a profuse sweating during drinking. During slow wave sleep, the set-point also is decreased. Thus, thermoregulation is modulated by other homeostatic regulatory systems. The convergence of nonthermal signals to PO/AH neurons is evidenced in animals by the abundant neuronal connections from other hypothalamic or extrahypothalamic regions [7].

EFFECTOR MECHANISMS

Effector mechanism to maintain thermoregulation comprises autonomic and behavioral regulation. Behavioral regulation is phylogenetically older and plays a major role for many poikilotherms to respond to various temperature environments, whereas autonomic regulation has evolved only in birds and mammals [1]. Autonomic thermoregulation involves the control of shivering, nonshivering thermogenesis, cutaneous blood flow, sweat secretion, and piloerection. Thermoregulatory behavior, conversely, involves such behaviors as seeking shelter, changing posture, clothing, adjusting artificial heating or cooling, and occurs in response to temperature perceptions and emotional feelings of thermal comfort or discomfort. Behavioral reactions to heat and cold modify the relation between the organism and its environment, and thereby may contribute to reducing the costs for autonomic thermoregulation.

SHIVERING

Shivering is the involuntary contraction of skeletal muscle to increase the production of heat. Shivering thermogenesis is functionally an autonomic (involuntary) phenomenon, although it is mediated by somatic motor nerves. Shivering is a major thermogenetic response in humans, except in neonates, in whom shivering mechanisms are immature. The center of control for shivering is assumed to be in the posterior hypothalamus. The efferent pathway travels through tegmentum, the pons, the lateral part of the medullary reticular formation, and rubrospinal tracts [8].

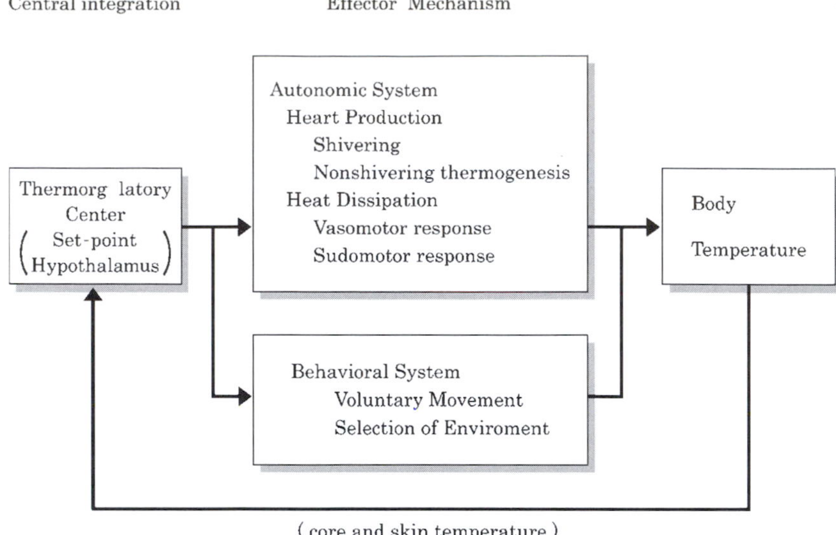

FIGURE 32.1 Outline of the human thermoregulatory system.

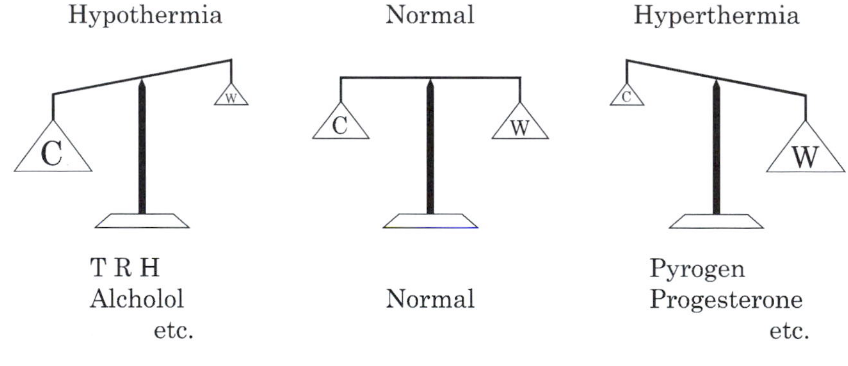

FIGURE 32.2 Concept of thermoregulatory set point as being a balance between activities or warm-sensitive (W) and cold-sensitive (C) neurons.

NONSHIVERING THERMOGENESIS

Nonshivering thermogenesis is metabolic heat production. Metabolic heat production is dependent on sympathetic and sympathoadrenal systems. Thermogenesis produced by sympathetic activity can be distinguished from that produced by the sympathoadrenal system. The sympathoadrenal system stimulates hepatic glycogenolysis and glyconeogenesis and modulates pancreatic insulin and glucagons release [8]. Sympathetic nerves, however, can also directly affect metabolic activity. In humans, brown adipose tissue is the most important site for nonshivering thermogenesis during the perinatal period. With increasing age, however, the amount of brown adipose tissue decreases. In small animals, α_1-receptors of brown adipose tissue increase in number when acclimatized to cold [9].

VASOMOTOR RESPONSE

In most areas of the body surface, the counteraction between neurogenic mechanisms (vasoconstrictor and possibly sudomotor or vasodilator) and local vasodilator actions (vasodilator metabolites, vasoactive peptides, and the direct effects of temperature) determines vascular insulation in skin tissues. Sympathetic vasoconstrictor tone is marked in the limbs, and the inhibition of this tone induces generalized vasodilatation (passive vasodilatation). Vasoconstrictor fibers supplying the skin are (nor)adrenergic and release neuropeptide Y as a cotransmitter. Vasodilatation, however, may also be produced by vasodilator peptides such as vasoactive intestinal polypeptide or calcitonin gene–related peptide that are released from cholinergic sudomotor nerves during sweating (active vasodilatation) [10]. It is not still clear whether vasodilator fibers are present in the human skin. Arteriovenous anastomosis, which is present abundantly in the palms, ears, and soles, is innervated densely by the sympathetic vasoconstrictor system and is responsible for remarkable increases in cutaneous blood flow at the extremities. In a cool environment, the arteriovenous anastomoses close, leading to a reduced blood flow in the distal part of the extremities. In addition, superficial cutaneous veins constrict, resulting in a redirection of blood to deep veins, the venae comitantes. Because these veins run close to the limb arteries, a countercurrent heat exchange system operates between the veins and arteries. Thus, the heat conveyed from the body core is largely restored to the core before it reaches the hands or feet, which is the major part of heat loss. In a warm environment, arteriovenous anastomoses open and superficial veins dilate, enhancing the removal of heat from venous blood at skin surface. Finger blood flow begins to increase at a lower ambient temperature than does toe blood flow [1].

SUDOMOTOR RESPONSE

Sweat glands are conventionally classified to apocrine and eccrine glands, on the basis of their secretory processes. The latter glands are distributed all over the body surface, and those except the palm and the sole are involved in thermoregulation. Sympathetic postganglionic cholinergic innervation of the eccrine sweat gland plays a major role in thermoregulatory heat loss in humans [1]. Sudomotor neurons are activated during body heating and are inhibited during body cooling. Sudomotor neurons also are activated transiently by various mental stimuli. There are topographic differences in the regional distribution of the 2 to 5 million eccrine sweat glands in human skin [11]. In spontaneous thermoregulatory sweating, sweat is discharged in a pulsatile fashion with irregular rhythm, the rate ranging from several to more than 20 times per minute. These sweat expulsions reflect the burst activity of the postganglionic sudomotor neuron. Accordingly, sweat expulsions appear synchronously all over the body surface except the palm and the sole, and their rate is highly related to the ambient temperature or the body temperature [1].

References

1. Ogawa, T., and P. A. Low. 1997. Autonomic regulation of temperature and sweating. In *Clinical autonomic disorders*, 2nd ed., ed. P. A. Low, 83–96. Philadelphia: Lippincott-Raven.
2. Hori, T., and T. Katafuchi. 1998. Cell biology and the functions of thermosensitive neurons in the brain. In *Progress in brain research*, ed. H. S. Sharma and J. Westman, 9–23. Amsterdam: Elsevier.
3. Eisenmann, J. S. 1969. Pyrogen-induced changes in thermosensitivity of septal and preoptic neurons. *Am. J. Physiol.* 216:330–334.
4. Nakayama, T., M. Suzuki, and N. Ishizuka. 1975. Action of progesterone on preoptic thermosensitive neurons. *Nature* 258:80.
5. Sugenoya, J., M. Kihara, T. Ogawa, A. Takahashi, T. Mitsuma, and Y. Yamashita. 1988. Effects of thyrotropin releasing hormone on human sudomotor and cutaneous vasomotor activities. *Eur. J. Appl. Physiol.* 57:632–638.
6. Kihara, M., Y. Kihara, T. Tukamoto, Y. Nishimura, H. Watanabe, and R. Hanakago. 1993. Assessment of sudomotor dysfunction in early Parkinson's disease. *Eur. Neurol.* 33:363–365.
7. Chiba, T., and Y. Murata. 1985. Afferent and efferent connections of the medical preoptic area in the rat: A WGA-HRP study. *Brain Res. Bull.* 14:261–272.
8. Collins, K. J. 1993. The autonomic nervous system and the regulation of body temperature. In *Autonomic failure*, ed. R. Banister and C. J. Mathias, 212–230. Oxford: Oxford University Press.
9. Raasmaja, A., N. Mohell, and J. Nedergaard. 1985. Increased alpha-adrenergic receptor density in brown adipose tissue of cold-acclimated rats and hamsters. *Eur. J. Pharmacol.* 106:489–498.
10. Benarroch, E. E. 1997. Postganglionic sympathetic outflow and its clinical evaluation. In *Central autonomic network*, ed. E. E. Benarroch, 139–168. New York: Futura Publishing Company.
11. Kihara, M., R. D. Fealey, and J. D. Schmelzer. 1995. Sudomotor dysfunction and its investigation. In *Handbook of autonomic nervous system dysfunction*, ed. A. D. Korczyn, 523–533. New York: Marcel Dekker.

33 Autonomic Control of Airways

Peter J. Barnes
Department of Thoracic Medicine
National Heart and Lung Institute
London, United Kingdom

Airway nerves regulate the caliber of the airways and control airway smooth muscle tone, airway blood flow, and mucus secretion.

OVERVIEW OF AIRWAY INNERVATION

Three types of airway nerve and several neurotransmitters are recognized (Table 33.1):

- Parasympathetic nerves that release acetylcholine (ACh),
- Sympathetic nerves that release norepinephrine, and
- Afferent (sensory) nerves whose primary transmitter may be glutamate.

In addition to these classical transmitters, multiple neuropeptides have now been localized to airway nerves and may have potent effects on airway function. Several neural mechanisms are involved in the regulation of airway caliber, and abnormalities in neural control may contribute to airway narrowing in diseases, such as asthma and chronic obstructive pulmonary disease (COPD), contributing to the symptoms and possibly to the inflammatory response. There is a close interrelation between inflammation and neural responses in the airways, because inflammatory mediators may influence the release of neurotransmitters through activation of sensory nerves leading to reflex effects and through stimulation of prejunctional receptors that influence the release of neurotransmitters [1]. In turn, neural mechanisms may influence the nature of the inflammatory response, either reducing inflammation or exaggerating the inflammatory response.

AFFERENT NERVES

At least three types of afferent fibers have been identified in the lower airways (Fig. 33.1).

Slowly Adapting Receptors

Myelinated fibers associated with smooth muscle of proximal airways are probably slowly adapting (pulmonary stretch) receptors that are involved in reflex control of breathing and in the cough reflex.

Rapidly Adapting Receptors

Aδ myelinated fibers in the epithelium show rapid adaptation. Rapidly adapting receptors (RARs) account for 10–30% of the myelinated nerve endings in the airways. These endings are sensitive to mechanical stimulation and to protons, low chloride solutions, histamine, cigarette smoke, ozone, serotonin, and prostaglandin $F_{2\alpha}$, although it is possible that some responses are secondary to the mechanical distortion produced by bronchoconstriction.

C-Fibers

There is a high density of unmyelinated (C-fibers) in the airways, which contain neuropeptides, including substance P (SP), neurokinin A (NKA), and calcitonin gene–related peptide (CGRP). They are selectively stimulated by capsaicin and also activated by bradykinin, protons, hyperosmolar solutions, and cigarette smoke.

Cough

Cough is an important defense reflex that may be triggered from either laryngeal or lower airway afferents [2]. Both RAR and C-fibers may mediate the cough reflex, which may be sensitized in inflammatory diseases by the release of mediators, including neurotrophins [3].

Neurogenic Inflammation

Activation of C-fibers may result in the antidromal release of neuropeptides, such as SP, NKA, and CGRP (Fig. 33.2). This may increase inflammation in the airways in asthma and COPD, although the role of neurogenic inflammation has been debated [4].

CHOLINERGIC NERVES

Cholinergic nerves are the major neural bronchoconstrictor mechanism in human airways and are the major determinant of airway caliber.

Cholinergic Efferents

Cholinergic nerve fibers arise in the nucleus ambiguus in the brainstem and travel down the vagus nerve and synapse in parasympathetic ganglia that are located within the airway wall. From these ganglia short postganglionic fibers travel to airway smooth muscle and submucosal glands and release ACh that acts on muscarinic receptors (Fig. 33.3).

Muscarinic Receptors

Three subtypes of muscarinic receptor are found in human airways [5]. M1 receptors are localized to parasympathetic ganglia and facilitate neurotransmission. M2 receptors serve as feedback inhibitory receptors on postganglionic nerves (and may be defective in asthma), whereas M3 receptors mediate the bronchoconstrictor and mucus secretory effect of ACh.

TABLE 33.1 Neurotransmitters in the Airways

Neurotransmitter	Receptors	Airway smooth muscle	Mucus secretion	Airway vessels
Acetylcholine	M3	Constrict	Increase	Dilate
Norepinephrine	α_1	No effect	No effect	Constrict
Epinephrine	β_2	Dilate	Increase	No effect
Nitric oxide	GMP	Dilate	Increase	Dilate
VIP	VIP	Dilate	Increase	Dilate
Substance P	NK_1, NK_2	Constrict	Increase	Dilate

GMP, guanosine monophosphate; NK, neurokinin; VIP, vasoactive intestinal polypeptide.

Cholinergic Reflexes

Reflex cholinergic bronchoconstriction may be activated by afferent receptors in the larynx or lower airways. Cholinergic reflexes are exaggerated in asthma and COPD because of increased responsiveness to ACh.

Anticholinergics in Airway Disease

Muscarinic antagonists (anticholinergics), such as ipratropium and tiotropium, cause bronchodilatation in airway disease through the relief of intrinsic cholinergic tone [6]. They are the bronchodilators of choice in COPD treatment, but they are less effective than β_2-adrenergic agonists in asthma in which several other bronchoconstrictor mechanisms are operative.

BRONCHODILATOR NERVES

Neural bronchodilator mechanisms exist in airways and there are considerable species differences.

Sympathetic Nerves

Sympathetic innervation of human airways is sparse and there is no functional evidence for direct innervation of airway smooth muscle, although sympathetic nerves regulate bronchial blood flow and to a lesser extent mucus secretion (Fig. 33.4). Adrenergic tone in the airways is primarily regulated by circulating epinephrine.

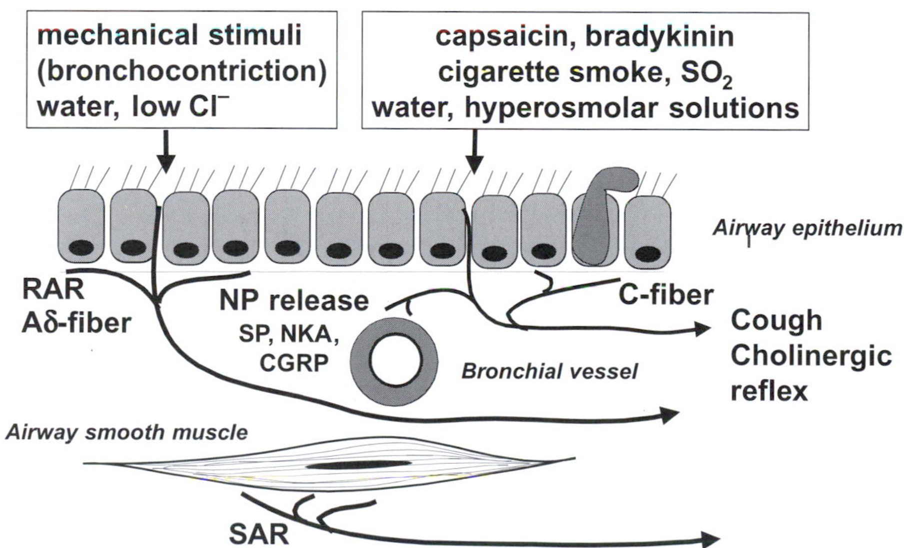

FIGURE 33.1 Afferent nerves in airways. Slowly adapting receptors (SARs) are found in airway smooth muscle, whereas rapidly adapting myelinated receptors (RARs) and unmyelinated C-fibers are present in the airway mucosa. CGRP, calcitonin gene–related peptide; NKA, neurokinin A; NP, neuropeptide; SP, substance P.

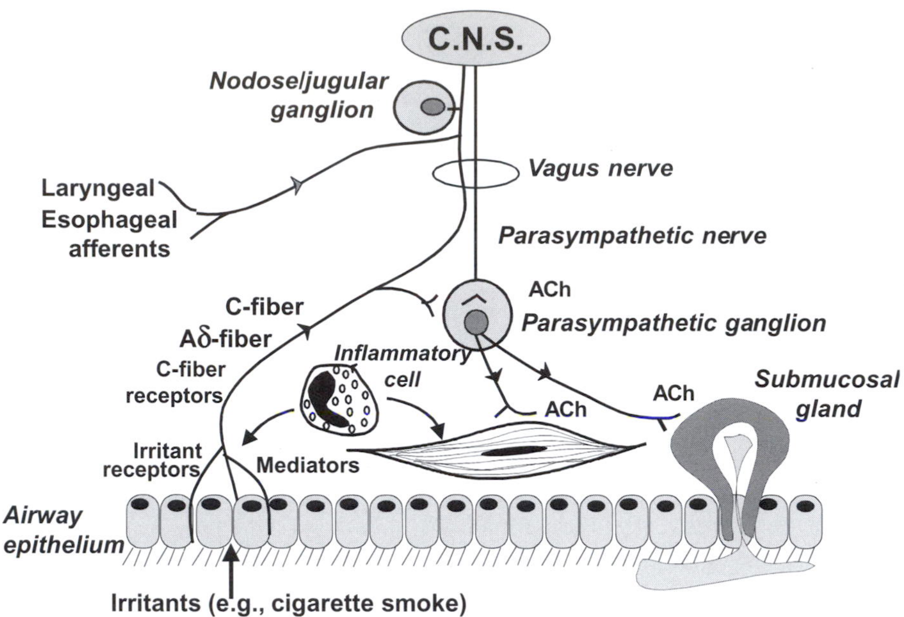

FIGURE 33.2 Neurogenic inflammation. Possible neurogenic inflammation (axon reflex) in asthmatic airways through retrograde release of peptides from sensory nerves through an axon reflex. Substance P (SP) causes vasodilatation, plasma exudation, and mucus secretion, whereas neurokinin A (NKA) causes bronchoconstriction, enhanced cholinergic reflexes, and calcitonin gene–related peptide (CGRP) vasodilatation.

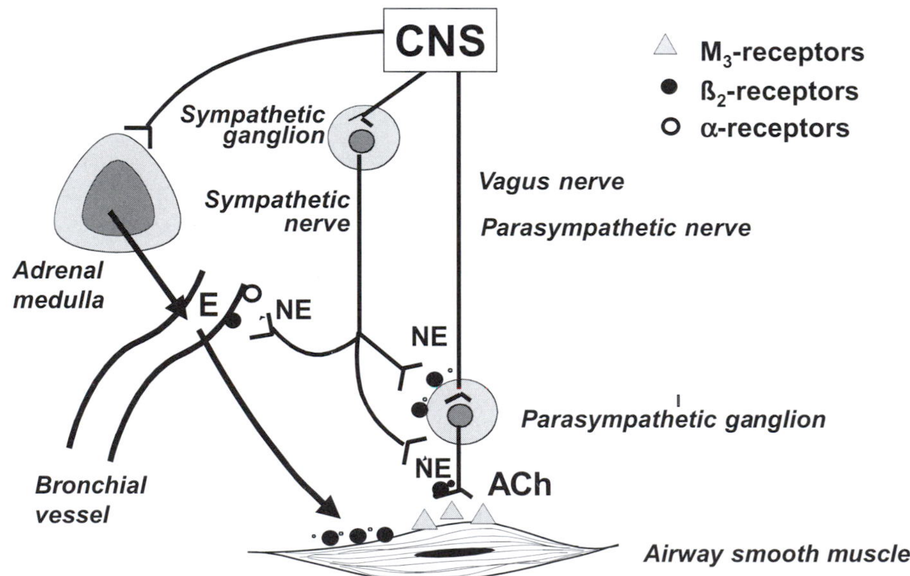

FIGURE 33.3 Cholinergic control of airway smooth muscle. Preganglionic and postganglionic parasympathetic nerves release acetylcholine (ACh) and can be activated by airway and extrapulmonary afferent nerves. E, epinephrine; NE, norepinephrine.

Inhibitory Nonadrenergic Noncholinergic Nerves

The bronchodilator nerves in human airways are nonadrenergic noncholinergic, and the major neurotransmitter is nitric oxide (NO). Neuronal NO synthase is expressed mainly in cholinergic neurons.

NEUROPEPTIDES

Multiple neuropeptides have been localized to nerves in the respiratory tract and function as cotransmitters of classical autonomic nerves to fine-tune airway function [7, 8]. Vasoactive intestinal peptide and related peptides act as bronchodilators and vasodilators, whereas neuropeptide Y is

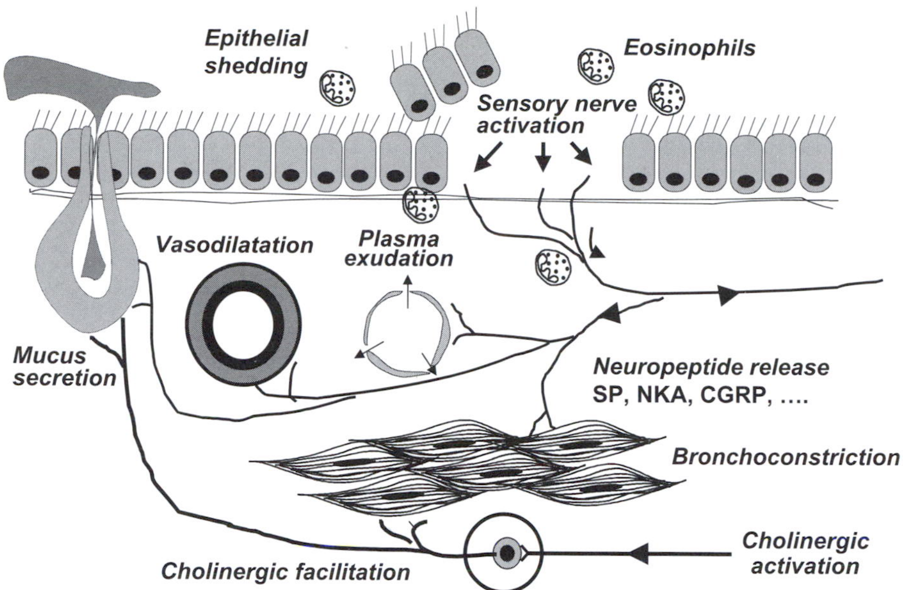

FIGURE 33.4 Adrenergic control of airway smooth muscle. Sympathetic nerves release norepinephrine (NE), which may modulate cholinergic nerves at the level of the parasympathetic ganglion or postganglionic nerves, rather than directly at smooth muscle in human airways. Circulating epinephrine (E) is more likely to be important in adrenergic control of airway smooth muscle. CGRP, calcitonin gene–related peptide; NKA, neurokinin A; SP, substance P.

a bronchoconstrictor and vasoconstrictor. The neuropeptides in sensory nerves (SP, NKA, and CGRP) act as bronchoconstrictors and also increase mucus secretion and inflammation in the airways [9].

NEURAL CONTROL OF AIRWAYS IN DISEASE

Autonomic control of airways may be abnormal and contribute to the pathophysiology in several airway diseases.

Asthma

Neural mechanisms contribute to the pathophysiology of asthma is several ways [10, 11]. Several triggers activate reflex cholinergic bronchoconstriction and the cough reflex may be sensitized by inflammatory mediators, including neurotrophins. The role of neurogenic inflammation and neuropeptides, however, remains uncertain.

Chronic Obstructive Pulmonary Disease

The structural narrowing of the airways in COPD means that the normal vagal cholinergic tone has a relatively greater effect on caliber than in normal airways for geometric reasons. Cholinergic mechanisms are the only reversible component of COPD and may contribute to the mucus hypersecretion of chronic bronchitis.

References

1. Barnes, P. J. 1992. Modulation of neurotransmission in airways. *Physiol. Rev.* 72:699–729.
2. Widdicombe, J. 2002. Neuroregulation of cough: Implications for drug therapy. *Curr. Opin. Pharmacol.* 2:256–263.
3. Carr, M. J., D. D. Hunter, and B. J. Undem. 2001. Neurotrophins and asthma. *Curr. Opin. Pulm. Med.* 7:1–7.
4. Barnes, P. J. 2001. Neurogenic inflammation in the airways. *Respir. Physiol.* 125:145–154.
5. Barnes, P. J. 1993. Muscarinic receptor subtypes in airways. *Life Sci.* 52:521–528.
6. Jacoby, D. B., and A. D. Fryer. 2001. Anticholinergic therapy for airway diseases. *Life Sci.* 68:2565–2572.
7. Barnes, P. J., J. Baraniuk, and M. G. Belvisi. 1991. Neuropeptides in the respiratory tract. I. *Am. Rev. Respir. Dis.* 144:1187–1198.
8. Barnes, P. J., J. Baraniuk, and M. G. Belvisi. 1991. Neuropeptides in the respiratory tract. II. *Am. Rev. Respir. Dis.* 144:1391–1399.
9. Joos, G. F., P. R. Germonpre, and R. A. Pauwels. 2000. Role of tachykinins in asthma. *Allergy* 55:321–337.
10. Barnes, P. J. 1995. Is asthma a nervous disease? *Chest* 107:119S–124S.
11. Undem, B. J., and M. J. Carr. 2002. The role of nerves in asthma. *Curr. Allergy Asthma Rep.* 2:159–165.

34 Autonomic Control of Cardiac Function

Kleber G. Franchini
Department of Internal Medicine
State University of Campinas
Campinas, Brazil

Allen W. Cowley, Jr.
Department of Physiology
Medical College of Wisconsin
Milwaukee, Wisconsin

The autonomic neural regulation of cardiovascular function is of great importance for survival. The centrally orchestrated sympathetic and parasympathetic neural pathways enable the cardiovascular system to optimize its delivery of blood flow to specific regions of the organism to satisfy the requirements of different physiologic and behavioral stimuli such as eating, sleeping, and the many conditions of exercise and stress to which the body is subjected. It has long been recognized that each of the components of the cardiovascular system can operate and respond independently of neural and hormonal control systems. The classical example for this was the demonstration by Starling early in the twentieth century that an isolated heart is capable of increasing its stroke volume simply by increasing the volume preload into the right ventricle. Thus, when a greater amount of blood returns to the heart under conditions such as exercise, the heart is intrinsically capable of increasing its workload and responding with an increase of cardiac output. It is recognized, however, that this intrinsic length–tension mechanism of the cardiac muscle is only capable of increasing cardiac output from resting levels of about 5 liters per minute in humans to a maximum permissive pumping level of about 13 liters per minute. This is far less than the maximum permissive pumping level of normal individuals who can achieve levels of nearly 20 liters per minute during sustained exercise. The optimum levels of cardiac pumping ability can be achieved only in the presence of increased contraction force and an increased heart rate brought about through the coordinated activities to the sympathetic and parasympathetic nervous system as described later.

Although blood flow to many regions of the systemic circulation may be regulated by local mechanisms (autoregulation) independent of the nervous system, optimization of blood flow to the various regions of the body cannot be achieved without complex sensors, central coordination, and effectors of the autonomic nervous system. This includes stressors such as exercise; underwater submersion; high altitudes; temperature stress such as fever, frost bite, and hypothermia; hypotensive hemorrhage; systemic hypertension; congestive heart failure; and emotional behavior such as excitement and aversion.

AUTONOMIC NERVES INNERVATING THE MAMMALIAN HEART

The classical view of autonomic control of cardiac function presumes a dual regulation by both divisions of extrinsic cardiac nerves. In general, the sympathetic nerves to the heart are facilitatory, whereas the parasympathetic (vagus) nerves are inhibitory. Efferent neurons projecting to the heart originate in intrathoracic or cervical sympathetic ganglia. Postganglionic axons originating in those ganglia run parallel with coronary vessels and innervate the sinoatrial (S-A) and atrioventricular (A-V) node, the conduction system, the myocardial fibers, and the coronary vessels. The parasympathetic neurons originated within the medulla of the brainstem relay at ganglia of the epicardial neural plexus, mainly located at the A-V groove within 0.25–0.5 mm of the epicardial surface. These regions are densely innervated by cardiac intrinsic neurons, which include short postganglionic parasympathetic neurons, among others. Abundant nerve terminals from the postganglionic vagal fibers innervate the region of the S-A and A-V nodes, but a small to moderate number of cholinergic nerves, compared with many adrenergic nerves, are distributed within the atrial and ventricular myocardium.

Cardiac neurons actually constitute an intrinsic plexus that retains the ability to act independently when severed from their efferent inputs. These intrinsic neurons are organized in multiple aggregates and neural interconnections, localized to discrete atrial and ventricular regions. Among these distinct ganglionated plexuses that constitute what is now recognized as the intrinsic cardiac nervous system, preferential control of specific cardiac functions has been identified. For example, the ganglionic plexus of the right atrial neurons have been associated primarily, but not exclusively, with the control of sinoatrial nodal function. The ganglion of the inferior vena cava–inferior atrial plexus neurons primarily, but not exclusively, are involved with control of A-V nodal function. Moreover, the intrinsic cardiac plexus also contains the somata of afferent neurons, some of which project axons to central neurons, mainly through the vagus and nerves that conduct efferent sympathetic fibers.

Cardiac intrinsic plexus contain a heterogeneous population of neurons and fibers capable of synthesizing or responding to several different neurotransmitters and neuropeptides, besides the classical norepinephrine and acetylcholine. Enzymes involved in the synthesis of nitric oxide, dopamine, and norepinephrine exist within cardiac ganglia. Techniques of immunohistochemistry have also revealed the presence of vasoactive intestinal peptide (VIP), substance P, somatostatin, and neuropeptide Y (NPY) immunoreactivity within cardiac intrinsic neurons. Receptor characterization studies suggest not only cholinergic but also β-adrenergic, serotonergic, and purinergic receptors on these neurons. Furthermore, electrophysiologic studies show that neurons within cardiac ganglia respond to application of cholinergic, adrenergic, histaminergic, purinergic, and peptidergic agonists, and antagonists. This diverse neuronal and neurotransmitter composition of cardiac intrinisic neurons suggests potentially complex neuronal processing within cardiac ganglia. Although the function of intrinsic neurons in cardiac function remains largely unknown, it has been proposed that they are important for the maintenance of adequate cardiac output, particularly in disease states such as myocardial ischemia. Intrinsic cardiac neurons of chronically decentralized canine hearts also were shown to display spontaneous activity capable of being modulated by cardiac mechanoreceptors.

Mammalian heart displays regionality in the distribution of autonomic innervation. The general distribution of nerves throughout selected regions of endocardium, myocardium, and epicardium has been assessed quantitatively by immunofluorescent staining for the general neural marker PGP 9.5 (neuron-specific cytoplasmic protein); these studies reveal a gradient in the endocardium from right to left sides, with a significantly higher density of immunostained nerves being found in the right ventricular and right atrial endocardium compared with that of the left-sided chambers. An atrial to ventricular gradient also has been characterized with significantly higher density of PGP 9.5–immunoreactive nerves in the myocardium of the right atrium, followed by left atrium, and then the left and right ventricles, which possess a similar, but much lower, density of nerves. In contrast, the epicardial innervation of both left and right ventricles displayed a greater percentage of immunostained nerve area than that of the right and left atria. The complex neural network of these cardiac tissues is composed of numerous nerve trunks (diameter, 10–25 um), together with varicose and nonvaricose nerve fibers (diameter, 1–6 um). Large nerve trunks were abundant within the epicardial plexus, especially in the epicardial tissue of the left ventricle (diameter, 40–160 um).

Nerves marked positively for acetylcholinesterase (AChE-positive) are the predominant neural subtype observed throughout the endocardium, myocardium, and epicardium. The density and pattern of distribution of these nerves, however, vary within and between the endocardial, myocardial, and epicardial tissues, and also between the chambers of the heart. AChE-positive nerves of the endocardial plexus display a right to left gradient in density that was absent from both the myocardial and epicardial tissues.

Sympathetic efferent fibers display tyrosine hydroxylase (TH) immunoreactivity and immunoreactivity for NPY. TH and NPY immunoreactivity show a subpopulation of ganglion cell bodies in the atrial epicardial plexus, and particularly in the ganglia of the atrioventricular groove. Endocardial TH and NPY-immunoreactive nerves also display a right to left gradient in density, whereas in the epicardial tissues they display a ventricular to atrial gradient in density. The right ventricular endocardium possesses a significantly greater percentage stained area of TH and NPY-immunoreactive nerves than the other chambers, but this is significantly less than the percentage stained area of AChE-positive nerves observed in the same endocardial region. Similar proportions of TH and NPY-immunoreactive nerves were observed throughout the myocardial tissues, ranging from 35 to 40% of the total innervation.

Besides AChE and TH, cardiac neurons and fibers also show immunoreactivity for other neurotransmitters such as calcitonin gene–related peptide (CGRP), somatostatin, substance P, and VIP, with currently largely unknown fuction.

The conduction system is differentially innervated as visualized by the general marker PGP 9.5. The rank order in relative neural density is transitional atrioventricular node, sinus node and atrioventricular penetrating bundle, left bundle branch, and right bundle branch. Rank order corrected by PGP 9.5–immunoreactive innervation throughout the conduction system has been reported as AChE (60–70%), TH and NPY (25–35%), CGRP (8–19%), somatostatin (<13%), and VIP. Substantial proportion of AchE-positive innervation within the conduction system is intrinsic in origin. The large TH-positive fibers are probably postganglionic efferent nerves.

There is histochemical evidence for the existence of dual adrenergic and cholinergic innervation of coronary arteries and arterioles, which have been shown to play a role in the fine control of coronary circulation.

MYOCARDIAL NERVE TERMINALS

Terminal ramifications of nerves are found in the myocardium, especially in relation to sinoatrial and atrioventricular nodes, and the outer layer of coronary arteries and arterioles. Three main types of axon varicosities can be distinguished in the myocardium. (1) Typical cholinergic varicosities that enclose small (diameter, 30–60 nm) clear vesicles containing acetylcholine, as well as a few large granular vesicles and numerous mitochondria. There is no recognizable thickening on the axolemma or on the sarcolemma of nearby cardiac myocytes, which are separated by variable gap ranging from 20 to 100 nm. (2) Noradrenergic terminals enclose small granular vesicles (30–60 nm) containing norepinephrine, large granular vesicles, and mitochondria. Like cholinergic terminals, there are no presynaptic or postsynaptic membrane thickenings in these terminals, and the gap between the terminal and the nearest myocyte may be as much as 100 nm. (3) Noncholinergic, nonadrenergic terminals are characterized by their content of densely packed mitochondria and no small vesicles of the clear or granular variety.

THE AUTONOMIC NERVOUS SYSTEM AND CARDIAC FUNCTION

Sympathetic and parasympathetic divisions of the autonomic nervous system play a major role in the regulation of cardiac performance. In general, the sympathetic nerves to the heart are facilitatory, whereas the parasympathetic (vagus) nerves are inhibitory. The kinetics of the two autonomic divisions differ substantially. The vagal effects develop rapidly, often within one heartbeat, and they decay nearly as quickly. Hence, the vagus nerves can exert beat-by-beat control of cardiac function. Conversely, the onset and decay of the sympathetic effects are much more gradual; only small changes are affected within the time of one cardiac cycle. When both autonomic systems act concomitantly, the effects are not additive algebraically, but complex interactions prevail. Such interactions may be mediated either prejunctionally or postjunctionally with respect to the neuroeffector junction.

The resting activity of the sympathetic postganglionic neurons is determined by the interaction between intrinsic rhythms generated in the central nervous system and the cyclic inputs from various afferent signaling pathways. Under different conditions, the activity may be influenced by inputs from a variety of peripheral reflexes and from central areas involved in the coordination of the cardiovascular responses to complex behaviors. Tonic and reflex activity of sympathetic efferents results in release of norepinephrine and other neurotransmitters such as NPY and adenosine triphosphate. Norepinephrine is responsible for most of the postsynaptic sympathetic effects on cardiac function, which include the positive inotropic and chronotropic effects, and coronary vasoconstriction. During stimulation of the cardiac sympathetic nerves, the heart rate and cardiac contraction begin to increase after a latent period of 1–3 seconds, approaching a steady-state level in about 30 seconds. After cessation of stimulation, the return toward the control level takes place much more gradually than at the onset of stimulation. The slow return of the heart rate and cardiac contraction to the normal levels after cessation of the sympathetic stimulation is related to the relatively slow rate of metabolism of norepinephrine by the cardiac tissue.

Sympathetic activation also enhances the contractile activity and the diastolic relaxation of the left ventricle. Radioligand binding techniques have shown that both β_1- and β_2-adrenergic receptors coexist in the heart. Physiologic studies indicate that β_1 receptors are predominantly related to the inotropic response, whereas both β_1 and β_2 receptors are linked to the chronotropic response. In the heart, the α-adrenergic receptors are almost exclusively of the α_1 subtype, and their stimulation usually causes a modest inotropic effect by increasing transarcolemmal calcium influx. In coronary vessels, the α_1-receptor stimulation causes vasoconstriction, but usually this effect is overshadowed by the simultaneous increase in the oxygen consumption that stimulates local mechanisms to increase blood flow. As illustrated in Figure 34.1, β-adrenergic receptors are members of a large multigene family of the G protein–coupled receptors, which have a secondary structure consisting of seven transmembrane-spanning domains and transduce signal through a G protein (G_S). The positive inotropic effect of the sympathetic nervous system is partially mediated by an increase in voltage-gated Ca^{2+} current. This increase is generally attributed to a β-adrenergic, receptor-stimulated, cyclic adenosine monophosphate (cAMP)–dependent phosphorylation of calcium channels. The positive effects of β-adrenergic stimulation on heart rate are related to a stimulation of the slow calcium

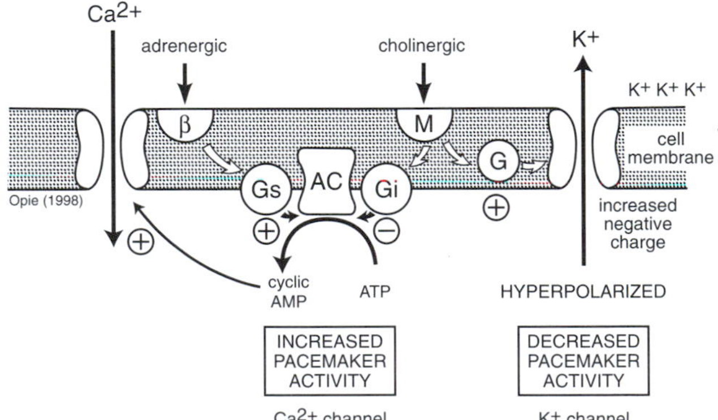

FIGURE 34.1 A simplified scheme of sarcolemma-related receptors and channels. The two receptors shown are the β-adrenergic receptor and the cholinergic muscarinic (M_2 receptor), the latter for acetylcholine (ACh). *Left*, The β-adrenergic receptor is coupled to adenylate cyclase through the activated G protein subunit α_S-guanosine triphosphate (GTP). Consequent formation of cyclic adenosine monophosphate (cAMP) activates calcium channel to increase calcium entry. Activity of adenylate cyclase can be decreased by the inhibitory subunits of the ACh-associated G protein (α_1; β-γ). Also note activation of ACh-operated potassium channel through β-γG and phospholipase A_2. (Reprinted with permission from Opie, L. H. 1998. *The heart. Physiology: From cell to circulation*, 3rd ed. Philadelphia: Lippincott-Raven Publishers.)

channel by the increased intracellular cAMP on the S-A and A-V node, bundle of His, and Purkinje fibers.

Under normal conditions, cardiac parasympathetic neurons fire in synchrony with the cardiac cycle, because of an excitatory input arising from peripheral baroreceptors. They also can be excited powerfully by inputs arising from peripheral chemoreceptors, cardiac receptors, and trigeminal receptors. Vagus activation releases acetylcholine and VIP in the heart. Although VIP may exert some presynaptic effect on the autonomic transmission, the parasympathetic influence on cardiac function occurs predominantly through the binding of acetylcholine to muscarinic receptors. As illustrated in Figure 34.1, muscarinic receptors are also members of the G protein–coupled receptors and the M_2 receptor is the isoform most frequently found in the heart. Acetylcholine binding to the muscarinic receptors stimulates the G_i protein to combine with guanosine triphosphate (GTP), which, in turn, inhibits adenylate cyclase activity. These events result in the decrease of intracellular cAMP, which is apparently responsible for the negative inotropic effect of acetylcholine, through the inhibition of the calcium current.

Muscarinic receptors are also directly and importantly coupled to specific sarcolemmal potassium channels ($I_{K, Ach}$) apparently by G_i or G_0. Acetylcholine-induced opening of potassium channels results in membrane hyperpolarization that occurs within 100 msec of the initiation of vagal stimulation. This leads to a longer period for the membrane potential of S-A node to reach the activation threshold for spontaneous firing (Fig. 34.2).

The net effect of cholinergic activation is a decrease in the heart rate because of a decrease in the excitability of the pacemaker cells and a decrease in the conductivity of intracardiac conduction pathways. The chronotropic response depends on the timing of the vagal stimuli relative to the phase of cardiac cycle. This phase dependency related to repetitive vagal stimulation confers a peculiar characteristic to each stimulation such that the stimuli tend to entrain the S-A nodal pacemaker cells and coordinate the automatic activity of diverse cell clusters within the S-A node. The changes in heart rate produced by vagal stimuli appear after a brief latent period, reach a steady-state response within a few beats, and decay rapidly back to the control level once stimulation is discontinued. This rapid decay is attributed to the large quantities of AChE present in close proximity to the automatic cells in the S-A node. Electrophysiologic studies have revealed that the initial prolongation of the cardiac cycle length evoked by brief vagal stimulus is a result of prolongation of the S-A conduction time rather than a true reduction in firing rate of automatic cells of S-A node. Vagal stimulation also reduces the contractile force of myocardial cells of left and right ventricles and atria.

One of the most dramatic illustrations of the parasympathetic efferents of the cardiovascular system related to stress is associated with the diving reflex. Head submersion activates the trigeminal afferents and chemoreceptors and simultaneously elicits a potent sympathetic and parasympathetic activation. The sympathetic activation increases vascular resistance in all organs, except in the heart and in the brain. The potent cardiac-vagal activation elicits an intense bradycardia and a decrease in cardiac contraction, which allows a reduction in energy demand by the heart in a situation of precarious oxygen availability.

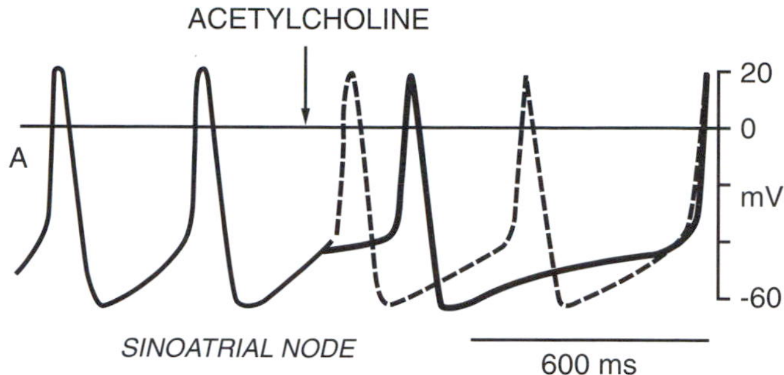

FIGURE 34.2 Mechanism for sinus bradycardia in response to increased vagal tone. At the terminal neurons of vagus, acetylcholine (ACh) is released, which acts on the muscarinic receptor to stimulate the intracellular protein G, which, in turn, opens the activation gate of $I_{K,ACh}$. The result is flow of potassium current and hyperpolarization, and a longer time is needed to reach the activation threshold for spontaneous firing of the nodal action potential. The result is a sinus bradycardia. (Reprinted with permission from Opie, L. H. 1998. *The heart. Physiology: From cell to circulation*, 3rd ed. Philadelphia: Lippincott-Raven Publishers.)

INTERACTIONS BETWEEN SYMPATHETIC AND PARASYMPATHETIC NERVES

The tonic vagal inhibitory effects on the heart oppose the facilitatory influence of the sympathetic nerve. Changes in heart rate and A-V nodal conduction result not simply from individual additive increases or decreases in sympathetic or vagal nerve activity, but from opposing variations in the tone of these branches of the autonomic nervous system. Although antagonism between the two divisons is a well-known phenomenon, other, more complex interactions may occur. For example, simultaneous activation of sympathetic nerve fibers may exaggerate or blunt cardiovascular responses to parasympathetic activity, depending on the circumstances. Functional interactions between both branches of cardiac autonomic nervous efferents have been demonstrated to occur through presynaptic interneuronal and postsynaptic intracellular mechanisms. Interneuronal interactions occur between the terminal postganglionic vagal and sympathetic fibers, which often lie in close apposition to each other in the heart. Acetylcholine liberated at vagal endings is able to reduce the quantity of norepinephrine released at the sympathetic terminals at any given level of sympathetic neural activity. In addition, NPY released by sympathetic activation may exert inhibitory influence on vagal cholinergic transmission. At the postsynaptic level, the interactions occur through effects on the sarcolemmal membrane receptor sites. Activation of β-adrenergic and muscarinic receptors influence ionic currents, adenylate cyclase activity, and changes in the concentrations of cAMP, cyclic GMP, and other cellular processes. These are generally counter-regulatory responses and are not generally understood at this time.

References

1. Crick, S. J., M. N. Sheppard, S. Y. Ho, and R. H. Anderson. 1999. Localisation and quantitation of autonomic innervation in the porcine heart. I. Conduction system. *J. Anat.* 195:341–357.
2. Crick, S. J., R. H. Anderson, S. Y. Ho, and M. N. Sheppard. 1999. Localisation and quantitation of autonomic innervation in the porcine heart. II. Endocardium, myocardium and epicardium. *J. Anat.* 195:359–373.
3. Chow, L. T. C., S. S. M. Chow, R. H. Anderson, and J. A. Gosling. 2001. Autonomic innervation of the human cardiac conduction system: Changes from infancy to senility—an immunohistochemical and histochemical analysis. *Anat. Rec.* 264:169–182.
4. Levy, M. N., and P. J. Martin. 1979. Neural control of the heart. In *Handbook of physiology, Section 2: The cardiovascular system*, Vol. 1, ed. R. M. Berne, N. Sperelakis, and S. R. Geiger. Bethesda, MD: American Physiological Society.
5. Vatner, S. F. 1992. Sympathetic mechanisms regulating myocardial contractility in conscious animals. In *The heart and cardiovascular system: Scientific foundations*, 2nd ed., ed. H. A. Fozzard, et al. New York: Raven Press.
6. Schwinn, D. A., M. Caron, and R. Lefkowitz. 1992. The beta-adrenergic receptors as a model for molecular structure-function relationship in G-protein coupled receptors. In *The heart and cardiovascular system: Scientific foundations,* 2nd ed., ed. H. A. Fozzard, et al. New York: Raven Press.
7. Opie, L. H. 1998. *The heart. Physiology: From cell to circulation,* 3rd ed. Philadelphia: Lippincott-Raven Publishers.

35 Neurogenic Control of Blood Vessels

Kleber G. Franchini
Department of Internal Medicine
State University of Campinas
Campinas, Brazil

Allen W. Cowley, Jr.
Department of Physiology
Medical College of Wisconsin
Wisconsin, Milwaukee

The small arteries with thick muscular walls and diameters of 250 μm or less and the arterioles are responsible for the major resistance to blood flow in the circulatory system. Normally these vessels are maintained in a state of functional constriction (vascular tone) determined by the interaction between intrinsic (myogenic tone) and extrinsic (neurotransmitters, hormones, autacoids, and products of metabolism) factors. Myogenic tone is a property of arteriolar smooth muscle that is independent of any other influence and is the reference tone for the control of vascular resistance by extrinsic factors. A complex interaction between these factors allows the circulatory system to accomplish the requirements for increased or decreased blood flow to different organs during various physiologic situations.

Neurogenic mechanisms occupy a central position in the normal regulation of vascular tone. The importance of the contribution of neurogenic mechanisms to baseline vascular tone is apparent by the decrease of nearly 50 mm Hg in mean arterial pressure after pharmacologic blockade of the α-adrenergic receptors or surgical sympathectomy in normal subjects or animals. In addition, neurogenic mechanisms, by coordinating the degree of transient changes in vascular tone in many regions and organs, enable the rapid redistribution of blood flow to areas functionally important to specific activities. This redistribution of blood flow, coordinated by a combination of centrally driven autonomic nerve activity and its modulation by cardiovascular receptors (mainly the arterial baroreceptors), allows, for example, a person to stand up after awakening without exhibiting hypotension and syncope. In exercise, it enables optimization of skeletal muscle blood flow by diverting cardiac output away from the splanchnic and renal circulation.

Less apparent but by no means less important for circulatory homeostasis is the regulation of venous capacity by neurogenic mechanisms. By controlling the venous tone, neurogenic mechanisms control the systemic blood volume distribution—a critical mechanism in the regulation of venous return to the heart, and thereby in the regulation of cardiac output. Most of the blood in the body is contained in the veins (approximately 70%) and venules, which are relatively flaccid and of larger diameter when compared with arteries and arterioles at normal distending pressures. Smooth muscle lines the wall of much of the venous system, and its volume can be altered by sympathetic venoconstriction.

Finally, although neurogenic mechanisms predominantly have vasoconstrictor function through noradrenergic terminals, vasodilator neurogenic mechanisms play an essential role in more restricted areas such as those supplied by cranial and sacral nerves from the parasympathetic division of the autonomic nervous system.

SYMPATHETIC COMPONENT

The sympathetic division is by far the most important division influencing both the whole-body hemodynamics and the local vascular tone in many areas. The activity of sympathetic neurons usually elicits vasoconstriction roughly proportional to the level of neural activity. This vasoconstriction is determined by various combinations of norepinephrine, neuropeptides, and purines. However, there are some species, including humans, in which stimulation of sympathetic fibers directed to vessels of skeletal muscles causes vasodilatation that is blocked by atropine. When this type of fiber is stimulated, the responses are transient and confined to arterioles. In addition, adrenergic influence may also produce vasodilatation when β_2–adrenergic receptors instead of α_1-adrenergic receptors are the mediators of norepinephrine released by the adrenergic terminals.

Sympathetic Fibers

The sympathetic innervation of the vascular system is divided into different groups on the basis of the particular bed and its reflex responses. Physiologically, these different groups do not function as one; rather, the activity of the neurons in each pathway is governed separately. Blood flow to the skin, for example, is regulated separately from blood flow to the skeletal muscles or to abdominal organs. Discrete neuronal phenotypes can be distinguished in prevertebral ganglia on the basis of electrophysiologic properties, neurochemistry, or morphology.

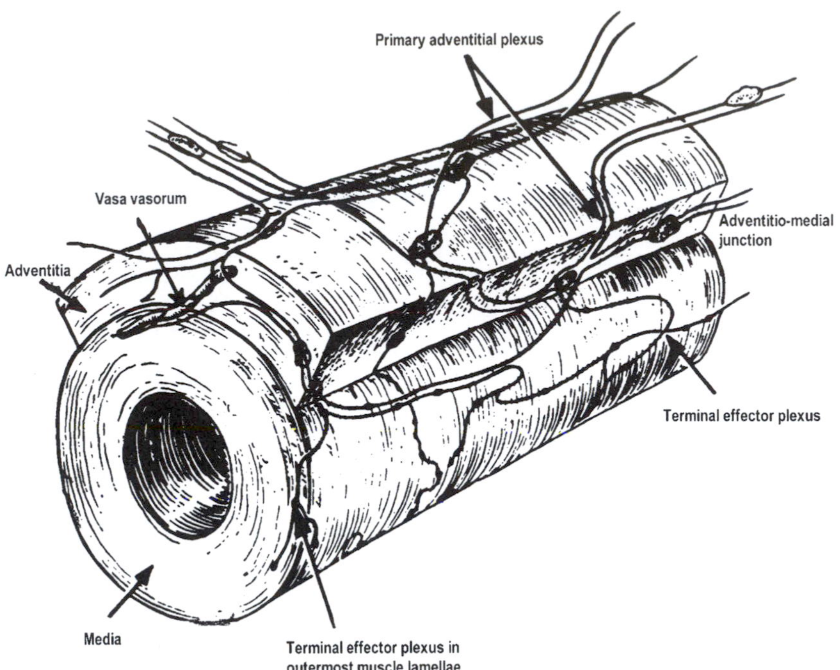

FIGURE 35.1 Arrangement of vascular neuroeffector apparatus. Postganglionic autonomic nerves ramify into small bundles forming a primary plexus, which is located in loose adventitia. Bundles give rise to varicosed fibers forming terminal effector plexus, located on surface of medial layer. (Reprinted with permission from Verity, M. A. 1971. Morphologic studies of the vascular neuroeffector apparatus. In *Physiology and pharmacology of vascular neuroeffector systems*, ed. J. A. Bevan, R. F. Furchgott, R. A. Maxwell, and A. A. Somlyo, 2–12. Basel, Switzerland: Karger.)

Neuroeffector Junction

The postganglionic autonomic nerves innervating blood vessels ramify into small bundles, which form a primary plexus located in the loose adventitia of the blood vessels. The autonomic nerve bundles form the terminal effector plexus located on the medial layer where they approach the surface of smooth muscle cell and establish neuromuscular contact (Fig. 35.1). These nerves end in strings of varicosities (~1 μm in extent and separated by 2–4 μm) entirely devoid of Schwann cell sheathes from which the transmitter is released on arrival of the nerve impulse. Compared with central synaptic clefs, which are not wider than 20 nm, the peripheral neuroeffector units are generally no closer than 100 nm in distance to the membrane of the smooth muscle cells. It is now known that the sympathetic axon varicosities commonly form structurally specialized neuromuscular junctions with vascular smooth muscle cells of most resistance arteries and some small veins (Fig. 35.2). Neuromuscular junctions, defined as axon varicosities containing synaptic vesicles, closely apposed to the outer surface of smooth muscle cells, with only a single layer of basal lamina intervening between axon and muscle membranes, were identified in all three species. Junctions are also found in most vessels less than 1 mm in diameter with a frequency ranging from 8000 to 150,000 junctions/mm^2 smooth muscle surface, the number generally increasing with decreasing arterial diameter. These small arteries are primarily, but not exclusively, muscular rather than elastic.

Neurotransmitters of Sympathetic Component

Neurotransmitters are stored in vesicles at the neuroeffector junction. Norepinephrine is the classical neurotransmitter released from sympathetic nerve terminals during sympathetic discharge and produces vasoconstriction by activating α-adrenoceptors located on vascular smooth muscles. Most of the norepinephrine contained in adrenergic nerves is stored in granular vesicles. Two types of granular vesicles—small and large dense-cored vesicles, both storing norepinephrine—have been identified by separation by density gradient electron microscopy. Norepinephrine is believed to be stored in the vesicles in a complex with adenosine triphosphate (ATP), but the vesicles also contain enzymes involved in norepinephrine synthesis, such as dopamine β-hydroxylase, and proteins, such as chromogranin. It is currently widely accepted that the ATP released together with norepinephrine from sympathetic nerves may act as a sympathetic cotransmitter together with norepinephrine. The concentration of norepinephrine in the nerve cell body is on the order of 10–100 μg/g wet weight and

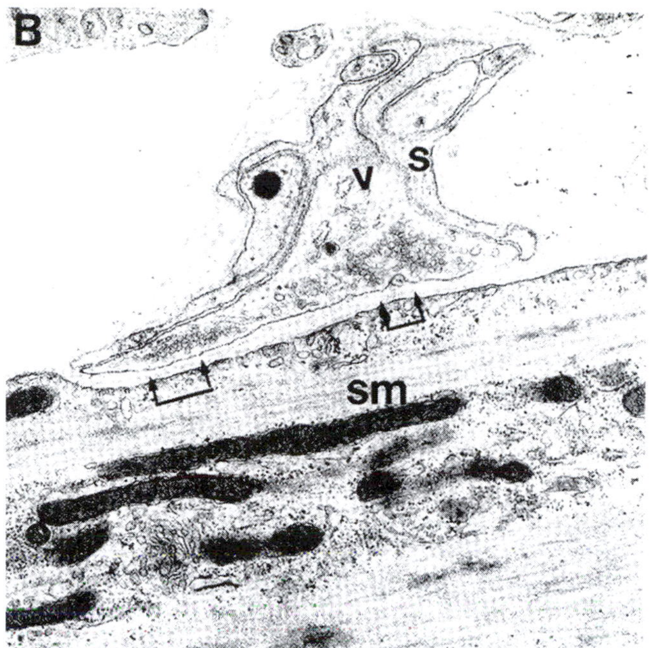

FIGURE 35.2 Electron micrograph of sympathetic neuromuscular junction. A varicosity has formed a flange extending along the surface of a smooth muscle cell of a rabbit ear artery. (Reprinted with permission from Luff, S. E. 1996. Ultrastructure of sympathetic axons and their structural relationship with vascular smooth muscle. *Anat. Embryol.* 193:515–531, 1996; Secaucus, NJ: Springer-Verlag New York, Inc.)

amine synthesis and storage occurs in this part of the neuron, where turnover has been calculated as 1–5 hours. A varicosity-forming contact with vascular smooth muscle cells contains from 500 to 1500 synaptic vesicles, and the norepinephrine concentration in each synaptic vessel has been estimated to be about 2.4 M.

In addition to norepinephrine, neuropeptide Y (NPY) and galanin also are found in sympathetic nerve fibers. Subcellular fragmentation experiments suggest that NPY, galanin, and norepinephrine are colocalized in large dense-core vesicles. NPY elicits a pressor response after intravenous administration or release by the sympathetic terminals. In certain blood vessels, the vasoconstrictor potency of NPY is 25 times greater than norepinephrine on a molar basis. In addition, a prominent action of NPY is to potentiate the postjunctional contractile effect of norepinephrine and that of other vasoactive agents.

Release of Transmitter and Effector Action

The variations in distance between adrenergic nerve terminals and smooth muscle cells vary depending on vessel size and location (Table 35.1). In the smallest arterioles and venules, only one or two muscle cells may be present, but in large arteries, the media thickness may be as great as 500 μm or more. The concentration of norepinephrine in the

TABLE 35.1 Distance between Autonomic Nerve Terminals and Smooth Muscular Media Layer in Arterial Vessels

Blood vessel	External diameter (μm)	Neuromuscular interval (nm)
Precapillary arteriole	~20	20
Renal cortex arteriole	25–35	200–400
Pancreatic arteriole	20–50	<400
Coronary arteriole	~50	300–700
Auricular artery	~1500	~500
Mesenteric artery	100–200	~500
Pulmonary artery	>5000	~2000

Reprinted with permission from Verity, M. A. 1971. Morphologic studies of the vascular neuroeffector apparatus. In *Physiology and pharmacology of vascular neuroeffector systems,* ed. J. A. Bevan, R. F. Furchgott, R. A. Maxwell, and A. P. Somlyo, 2–12. Basel, Switzerland: Karger.

Note that mean neuromuscular interval roughly parallels vessel diameter.

extracellular space has been difficult to estimate during nerve activation, but in extracellular spaces where the axon varicosity is at close contact to the vascular smooth muscle, it appears to be on the order of 10^{-6} to 10^{-5} g/ml. Only a small fraction of the cells in the vascular musculature is directly innervated by autonomic nerves; therefore it appears that individual smooth muscle cells probably are electrically and mechanically coupled. Gap junctions have been identified between the opposing membranes between adjacent smooth muscles that offer pathways for low electrical resistance and electrical coupling between adjacent muscle cells.

Released norepinephrine binds to lipoprotein sites called receptors on the vascular smooth muscle membrane where the vasoconstrictor response is initiated. Norepinephrine is removed from the junctional cleft by active reuptake, by the neuronal cell membrane (active carrier coupled to Na^+, K^+, and adenosine phosphatase), and by leakage into the capillaries. Nearly 80% of the norepinephrine released is incorporated back into the nerve terminal for storage. The amount that is spilled into the capillaries, if widespread, can serve as a rough index of total sympathetic nervous activity.

NPY is released together with norepinephrine and ATP, although there is preferential release of NPY with higher frequencies and intermittence of stimulation. Release of NPY from vasoconstrictor neurons occurs *in vivo* in response to moderate or intense, but not mild, reflex activation of sympathetic pathways. The three major sympathetic cotransmitters—norepinephrine, ATP, and NPY—each have been demonstrated to contribute to sympathetic vasoconstriction, although the relative contribution of each varies between vascular beds and segments. Although norepinephrine seems to be responsible more for the fast phase of vasoconstriction, NPY mediates the slow phase of vasoconstriction through Y1 receptors.

PARASYMPATHETIC COMPONENT

The cranial and sacral nerves of the parasympathetic nervous system also regulate the vascular tone, and their activity results in vasodilatation because of the combined action of acetylcholine, vasoactive intestinal peptide (VIP), and nitric oxide (NO). It is generally accepted that cholinergic nerves contain predominantly small agranular vesicles (35–60 nm). However, a few large granular vesicles with a dense core usually also are present. Cholinergic fibers originating in the craniosacral-parasympathetic outflow are known to supply arterioles in the brain, heart, erectile tissue of the genitalia, and various glands in the gastrointestinal tract. Although the role played by these vasodilator fibers is generally unknown, their importance in contributing to hyperemia in the engorgement of erectile tissue in the genitalia is well established. However, the parasympathetic nervous system does not appear to participate in any significant way in the major homeostatic reflexes contributing to the vascular tone.

Despite its high endogenous concentration in cerebral blood vessels, acetylcholine is not the transmitter for vasodilation in this region. Acetylcholine exhibits a negligible direct effect on vascular smooth muscle tone, possibly because of its low synaptic concentration and the wide synaptic distance. In fact, the direct effect of exogenous acetylcholine on cerebral vascular smooth muscle is a constriction rather than a dilation. Results from pharmacologic studies have demonstrated that NO, but not acetylcholine, mediates the major component of neurogenic vasodilation. In this context, NO synthase and choline acetyltransferase have been found to coexist in the parasympathetic ganglion and perivascular nerves in cerebral blood vessels of several species. More recently, acetylcholine and NO have been shown to corelease from the same cholinergic-nitrergic nerves, and it has been shown that acetylcholine acts as a presynaptic transmitter in modulating NO release. The exact mechanism of this presynaptic cholinergic modulation of NO-mediated vasodilation, however, is not clarified.

Parasympathetic neurons also contain VIP, which together with NO contribute to vasodilation of head and pelvic nerve. It is currently known that there is almost universal coexistence of VIP with acetylcholine and NO synthase in vasodilator neurons innervating the major distributing arteries in the head and pelvis. VIP was the first neuropeptide found colocalized with acetylcholine in cranial vasodilator neurons, and it can be detected in perivascular nerve fibers supplying most of the major arteries and many veins in the head. Furthermore, VIP is strongly expressed in pelvic vasodilator neurons of many species and in cholinergic sympathetic vasodilator neurons innervating skeletal muscle arteries. Vasodilator neurons that synthesize VIP also contain structurally unrelated peptides, including NPY, dynorphins, enkephalin, galanin, somatostatin, and calcitonin gene–related peptide, but their function remains unknown.

NEURAL CONTROL OF VEINS

Veins appear to be innervated by α-adrenergic fibers of the sympathetic nervous system only. It is important to recognize that the two regions in the human cardiovascular system that contain the most capacity to store volume (high-capacitance regions) are the splanchnic and cutaneous venous beds. These venous beds are also the most richly innervated, particularly the larger veins in these regions, which contain the major fraction of the total blood volume, whereas the smaller venules are sparsely innervated. There is evidence that active sympathetic vasoconstriction of veins participates in the regulation of ventricular filling pressure. Reflex-induced increase in venous tone in compensation for mild hemorrhage in dogs appears to account for about one third of the reduction in venous capacitance, whereas another third appears to be accounted for by passive venous collapse and another third by transcapillary fluid shifts. Such assessments have been difficult to make in human subjects, and it can only be assumed that active control of venous tone is of at least as great importance and probably greater, given the responses required of the veins to upright posture and heat stress.

DIFFERENTIAL VASOMOTOR CONTROL

The concept originally put forward by Cannon in 1915, that the entire sympathetic nervous system is activated *en masse* so as to produce uniform outflow, had to be modified over the past several decades. There are significant regional variations in the responsiveness of arterioles to sympathetic activity. There are a number of factors that enable the nervous system to provide differential vasomotor control among organs. One important factor is that the density of α-adrenergic innervation varies from organ to organ. Innervation to arterioles is especially dense in vessels supplying skin, splanchnic organs, skeletal muscle, kidneys, and adipose tissue. Veins in the splanchnic and cutaneous circulation are heavily innervated, whereas veins deep in the limbs are sparsely innervated. Second, sensitivity of vascular smooth muscle to norepinephrine varies from region to region, in part because of the density of α-adrenergic receptor sites. Third, there is heterogeneity of α-adrenergic receptors among organs. Fourth, neuronal reuptake of norepinephrine differs from region to region. Fifth, structure and vascular size vary among tissues and contribute to the heterogeneity of responses to changes in sympathetic stimulation. In small vessels with small junctional clefts, the actions of released norepinephrine can be more localized.

Regional variations in the responsiveness of arterioles to sympathetic activity also result from variations in regional levels of basal myogenic tone. It is well recognized that the level of myogenic tone varies among different organs, being greatest in the heart, brain and skeletal muscle, and less in the kidneys. Vasoconstrictor sympathetic nerves increase resistance above vascular basal tone by active vasoconstriction, but can only decrease vascular resistance below basal tone by so-called passive dilatation. Thus, in regions with high basal tone (e.g., skeletal muscle), which receive a tonic sympathetic vasoconstrictor outflow, considerable vasodilatation can be achieved by withdrawal of resting sympathetic tone. In contrast, in regions that have low basal tone (e.g., kidneys), minimal vasodilatation can be achieved by withdrawal of sympathetic tone.

It is important to recognize that blood flow is closely linked to the rate of metabolism in active vascular beds such as skeletal muscle, cerebral and coronary. An increase in metabolic activity in these beds normally results in an autoregulatory vasodilatation of blood vessels in these beds, which overrides sympathetic neural control.

Release of endogenous vasoactive substances (autacoids) such as NO, eicosanoids, histamine, kinins, adenine nucleotides, and locally produced vasodilator metabolites all can counteract sympathetic vasoconstriction and contribute to regional modulations of vascular sympathetic responses.

Finally, it must be recognized that circulating humoral agents can both impede and potentiate the response to neurogenic vasoconstrictor activity. For example, angiotensin II potentiates the effects of norepinephrine, whereas vasodilator substances such as atrial natriuretic peptide impede the response to neurogenic vasoconstrictor activity. Thus, the sympathetic influence on regional circulations may also vary depending on the circulating levels and on regional differences in the vascular reactivity to vasoactive hormones. It is evident that all of the above factors that account for regional differences in the response to sympathetic vasoconstrictor discharge must be carefully considered when examining the contribution of sympathetic nerves to the regulation of vascular tone and regional blood flow.

References

1. Bevan, J. A., R. D. Bevan, and S. P. Duckles. 1980. Adrenergic regulation of vascular smooth muscle. In *Handbook of physiology. Section 2: The Cardiovascular System. Vol. 2. Vascular Smooth Muscle*, ed. D. F. Bohr, A. P. Somlyo, and H. V. Sparks, Jr. Bethesda, MD: American Physiological Society.
2. Luff, S. E. 1996. Ultrastructure of sympathetic axons and their structural relationship with vascular smooth muscle. *Anat. Embryol. (Berl.).* 193:515–531.
3. Christopherson, K. S., and D. S. Bredt. 1997. Nitric oxide in excitable tissues: Physiological roles and disease. *J. Clin. Invest.* 100:424–429.
4. Gibbins, I. L., and J. L. Morris. 2000. Pathway specific expression of neuropeptides and autonomic control of the vasculature. *Reg. Peptides* 93:93–107.
5. Joyner, M. J., and J. R. Halliwill. 2000. Sympathetic vasodilatation in human limbs. *J. Physiol.* 526:471–480.
6. Lee, T. J., J. Liu, and M. S. Evans. 2001. Cholinergic-nitrergic transmitter mechanisms in the cerebral circulation. *Microsc. Res. Tech.* 53:119–128.
7. Henning, R. J., and D. R. Sawmiller. 2001. Vasoactive intestinal peptide: Cardiovascular effects. *Cardiovasc. Res.* 49:27–37.
8. Joyner, M. J., and J. R. Halliwill. 2000. Sympathetic vasodilatation in human limbs. *J. Physiol.* 526:471–480.

36

Cerebral Circulation

Autonomic Influences

Peter J. Goadsby

Headache Group
Institute of Neurology
The National Hospital for Neurology and Neurosurgery
London, United Kingdom

The maintenance of cerebral perfusion is one of the fundamental goals of the autonomic nervous system. This is achieved by means of cardiovascular regulatory mechanisms designed to control perfusion pressure and the local effects of the autonomic innervation of the cerebral vessels. The classic regulatory functions of the brain circulation are perfusion autoregulation, vasoneuronal coupling, and carbon dioxide/oxygen–driven changes. Cerebral perfusion autoregulation allows vessels to adjust their lumen to maintain brain blood flow constant in the face of changes in blood pressure. Vasoneuronal coupling allows local brain blood flow to respond to metabolic needs, whereas brain circulatory responses to carbon dioxide and oxygen provide a general mechanism to control the biochemical milieu of the brain in the face of important changes in arterial blood gases. These issues are covered more generally elsewhere in specialized physiologic textbooks [1–3]. This chapter covers the neurovascular influences on the brain circulation with emphasis on the extrinsic autonomic nervous influences. Necessarily this will have a more physiologic flavor. For a more clinical perspective, information is available elsewhere in other textbooks [4, 5].

NEURAL INNERVATION OF BRAIN CIRCULATION

The neural innervation of the brain provides a means by which brain vessel caliber can be altered without changes in perfusion pressure, local metabolic needs, or arterial blood gases. The intrinsic systems consist of nerves that arise from within the brain and pass through brain substance to innervate parenchymal vessels (Table 36.1). The extrinsic systems, although arising in the brain, pass out of the brain to traverse peripheral nerves returning to innervate large intracranial and pial vessels (Table 36.2). It is the extrinsic system that is the branch of the autonomic nervous system that influences brain blood flow. The intrinsic system is detailed in Table 36.1; also, specific reviews are available elsewhere [5].

EXTRINSIC NEURAL INFLUENCES

Here the autonomic extrinsic neural influences on the cerebral circulation are reviewed. The third component of the extrinsic innervation is the sensory innervation from the trigeminal nerve: the trigeminovascular system [6]. The trigeminovascular system has important antidromic and reflex orthodromic vasodilator effects on the cerebral circulation. Its reflex connections act through the parasympathetic outflow that is detailed later in this chapter.

Sympathetic Nervous System

Anatomy of Sympathetic Nerves

It has been established by careful anatomic studies that the origin of the major part of the sympathetic innervation arises from the superior cervical ganglion. The fibers form a meshwork around the vessels. The innervation is densest for forebrain structures whose vascular supply is from the carotid system when compared with hindbrain structures, which are more usually supplied by the vertebrobasilar system. Few of the fibers that innervate these vessels pass deep into the muscularis mucosa. For the large cerebral vessels and pial vessels, these nerves arise from the superior cervical ganglion. The noradrenaline-containing nerves that appear to innervate the cerebral parenchymal vessels do not arise from the superior cervical ganglion, but do arise centrally from the major central source of noradrenaline in the pons: the nucleus locus ceruleus (see Table 36.1).

Transmitters in the Sympathetic Nervous System

The sympathetic nervous innervation of the cerebral circulation has been classically marked by its content of noradrenaline, which is now recognized to colocalize with the peptide transmitter neuropeptide Y (NPY). Sympathetic fibers containing noradrenaline course from the superior cervical ganglion along the internal carotid artery and to the

TABLE 36.1 Intrinsic Neural Innervation of the Cerebral Circulation–Implicated Structures

Structure	Effect on cerebral blood flow
Medulla	
Dorsal medullary reticular formation	+
Rostroventrolateral medulla	+
Pons	
Locus ceruleus	–
Parabrachial nucleus (medial)	–
Midbrain	
Dorsal raphe nucleus	+
Cerebellum	
Fastigial nucleus (electrical)	+
Forebrain	
Basal forebrain	+
Centromedian parafascicular thalamus	+

+, Increased cerebral blood flow; –, decreased cerebral blood flow (when the listed structure is stimulated).

TABLE 36.2 Extrinsic Innervation of the Cerebral Circulation

	Ganglia	Effect of stimulation on CBF	Transmitters/ Receptors
Sympathetic	Superior cervical	–	Noradrenaline
			NPY
Parasympathetic	Pterygopalatine		Acetylcholine
	Otic	+	VIP
	IC miniganglia		PHI (M)
			PACAP
			Helodermin
			Helospectin I and II
			NO
Trigeminal	Trigeminal	+	Substance P
			CGRP
			Amylin
			Neurokinin A
			Cholecystokinin-8
			PACAP
			Nociceptin
			NO
			VR1

CBF, cerebral blood flow; CGRP, calcitonin gene–related peptide; IC, internal carotid; NO, nitric oxide; NPY, neuropeptide Y; PACAP, pituitary adenylate cyclase–activating polypeptide; PHI (M), peptide histidine isoleucine (methionine); VIP, vasoactive intestinal polypeptide; VR1, vanilloid receptor 1.

circle of Willis, and then to the basilar artery. After superior cervical ganglionectomy noradrenaline is undetectable, whereas stimulation of perivascular nerves releases noradrenaline from the neuronal vesicles. There is a rich supply of nerves containing NPY in the adventitia and adventitia-medial border of the large cerebral vessels that is substantially eliminated by removal of the superior cervical ganglion.

Role of the Sympathetic Innervation

Cerebral arteries and arterioles constrict in response to sympathetic nerve stimulation *in vivo*. It also has been shown that the sympathetic nervous system can have trophic influences on the cerebral circulation, which further complicates the understanding of its influence here. There is evidence to suggest that the sympathetic nervous innervation plays a permissive role in cerebral autoregulatory responses. Sympathetic nerve stimulation extends the upper limit of autoregulation, whereas acute sympathectomy, α-blockade, or inhibition of the effects of NPY shift the lower limit of autoregulation toward a lower blood pressure. The pharmacologic action of NPY is to constrict cerebral vessels as potently as noradrenaline, but with a more prolonged time course. This similar, but more sustained, action of NPY may have functional implications particularly because autoregulation has a time course of seconds.

Parasympathetic Nervous System

The parasympathetic innervation represents the most powerful of the neural vasodilator influences on the cerebral circulation, and its further definition will ultimately lead to a better physiologic understanding of the brain circulation.

Anatomy of the Parasympathetic Innervation

The parasympathetic system may be characterized as arising from the superior salivatory nucleus and passing out of the central nervous system in facial (cranial nerve VII) nerve–distributing fibers through the cranial autonomic ganglia, and acting to dilate cerebral vessels almost certainly by way of a peptidergic transmitter. The terms pterygopalatine and sphenopalatine are completely equal, with the former being used in humans. In some species, including humans, there may be additional variably sized microganglia located in the wall of the internal carotid artery that contribute to this system. Fibers arising from the superior salivatory nucleus pass through the geniculate ganglion without synapsing. The fibers pass in the greater superficial petrosal nerve to the carotid plexus directly, and to the carotid artery through the sphenopalatine and otic ganglia where they synapse. Postsynaptic fibers pass into the ethmoidal nerve to innervate cerebral vessels.

Transmitters and Modulators

The parasympathetic system uses several neurotransmitter/neuromodulators that have a vasodilator action. Substances found include acetylcholine, nitric oxide, and secretin family peptides: vasoactive intestinal polypeptide (VIP), peptide histidine isoleucine (methionine; PHI/M), pituitary adenylate cyclase activating polypeptide, helodermin, and helospectin I and II.

Effect of Parasympathetic Blockade on Normal Physiology

The facial/greater superficial petrosal innervation is not involved in autoregulatory responses of the cerebral vessels. Sectioning the facial nerve does not alter autoregulation, resting cerebral blood flow, or glucose utilization. The main parasympathetic outflow ganglia, the pterygopalatine ganglion, may be ablated without any alteration of hypercapnic vasodilatation.

Effect of Direct Parasympathetic Stimulation on Cerebral Blood Flow *In Vivo*

Direct stimulation of the facial nerve in humans leads to an increase in total cranial blood flow, as does chemical stimulation of the superior salivatory nucleus. Stimulation of the facial nerve increases cerebral blood flow without altering metabolic activity as reflected by stable glucose utilization or sagittal sinus oxygen content. These responses are meditated through a classical parasympathetic ganglion because they can be blocked by hexamethonium. VIP is released when cerebral arterial nerves are stimulated. Indeed, although no antagonist to VIP is available, a specific VIP antiserum has been used to inhibit noncholinergic, nonadrenergic dilator responses in the cranial circulation resulting from both direct and distant nerve stimulation. It has been shown that facial nerve stimulation results in local cortical release of VIP, and this release is blocked by hexamethonium. Similarly, direct stimulation of the pterygopalatine ganglion leads to cerebral vasodilation that is not dependent on any change in local metabolic activity.

Possible Roles for the Parasympathetic Innervation

The parasympathetic nerves are not directly involved in the most basic cerebrovascular responses, such as hypoxic or hypercapnic vasodilatation, and they do not appear to play a role in autoregulation. There are capable, however, of eliciting vasodilation of a neurogenic, or neurovascular, nature without any associated change in brain metabolism. What role could this have? Perhaps their role is during physiologic threat, such as in ischemia, or in perceived threat as might be associated with activation of nociceptive pathways [7]. The parasympathetic system is ideally placed to be engaged to increase cerebral blood flow when ordinary metabolic driving factors are impaired. This protection may, however, be regionally variable because the posterior circulation innervation with VIP is much less than that seen anteriorly. This finding may have implications in situations in which predominantly posterior changes are reported such as migraine. It may be too narrow a perspective to consider only a vasomotor function for these nerves because there is evidence that cholinergic mechanisms can alter capillary permeability including the movement of amino acids.

References

1. Edvinsson, L., and R. Uddman. 1993. *Vascular innervation and receptor mechanisms: New perspectives.* London: Academic Press.
2. Edvinsson, L., and D. N. Krause. 2002. *Cerebral blood flow and metabolism*, 2nd ed. Philadelphia: Lippincott Williams & Wilkins.
3. Mraovitch, S., and R. Sercombe. 1996. *Neurophysiological basis of cerebral blood flow control: An introduction.* London: John Libbey and Sons.
4. Asbury, A. K., G. M. McKhann, W. I. McDonald, P. J. Goadsby, and J. C. McArthur. 2002. *Diseases of the nervous system: Clinical neuroscience and therapeutic principles,* 5th ed. Cambridge: Cambridge University Press.
5. Goadsby, P. J., and L. Edvinsson. 2002. Neurovascular control of the cerebral circulation. In *Cerebral blood flow and metabolism*, 2nd ed., ed. Edvinsson, L., and D. N. Krause, 172–188. Philadelphia: Lippincott Williams & Wilkins.
6. May, A., and P. J. Goadsby. 1999. The trigeminovascular system in humans: Pathophysiological implications for primary headache syndromes of the neural influences on the cerebral circulation. *J. Cereb. Blood Flow Metab.* 19:115–127.
7. May, A., C. Buchel, R. Turner, and P. J. Goadsby. 2001. MR-angiography in facial and other pain: Neurovascular mechanisms of trigeminal sensation. *J. Cereb. Blood Flow Metab.* 21:1171–1176.

37 High-Pressure and Low-Pressure Baroreflexes

Dwain L. Eckberg
Cardiovascular Physiology
Hunter Holmes McGuire Department of Veterans Affairs Medical Center
Richmond, Virginia

High- and low-pressure baroreflexes represent classic negative feedback mechanisms. Pressure changes alter firing of stretch-sensitive neurons located in the walls of arteries and cardiac chambers. Changes of baroreceptor input to the brain provoke changes of neural output from vagal and sympathetic motoneurons. These changes of efferent nerve activity set in motion cardiovascular adjustments that counter the pressure changes that initiated the cascade of neurologic events. Thus, baroreflex mechanisms finely tune heart rate, atrioventricular node conduction, myocardial contractility and electrophysiologic properties, and peripheral resistance on a beat-by-beat basis, and dampen the effects of environmental perturbations that arise during everyday living [1]. This chapter focuses primarily on arterial baroreceptors in healthy humans.

ANATOMY

Arterial baroreceptors are located in the adventitia of the carotid sinuses and aortic arch. Neurons thought to be baroreceptors appear in histologic sections as complex arborizations. All barosensitive neurons are tethered to surrounding structures; this coupling contributes viscoelastic properties that figure importantly in baroreceptor transduction. Afferent baroreceptor impulses travel over rapidly conducting myelinated and slowly conducting unmyelinated nerve fibers in the carotid sinus and aortic nerves to the medulla.

The experimental literature groups together (inappropriately) a variety of heterogeneous receptors located in the walls of intrathoracic vessels and the heart as cardiopulmonary baroreceptors. These receptors are distributed widely in the superior and inferior vena cavae; atria, ventricles, and coronary arteries; and pulmonary arteries and veins. Afferent fibers from cardiopulmonary receptors course with sympathetic nerves to the spinal cord and with vagus nerves to the medulla. Most myelinated afferent cardiopulmonary neurons fire with periodicities related to atrial or ventricular events; most unmyelinated afferent neurons fire sporadically, without clear relation to cardiac events [2].

Nearly all baroreceptor neurons, cardiopulmonary and arterial, converge on the same neuron pools (and on the same neurons in about 15% of cases) in the solitary tract nucleus of the medulla. Because of its position as a way station for incoming baroreceptor information, the solitary tract nucleus may be a major center for arterial and cardiopulmonary baroreflex integration [3]. Incoming baroreceptor information is carried over interneurons (with many possibilities for interactions with other neural activity, particularly that related to respiration) to vagal motoneurons in the medulla and, through the rostral ventrolateral medulla, to sympathetic motoneurons in the spinal cord.

TRANSDUCTION

Arterial baroreceptors sense distortion, not pressure. However, because the degrees of pressure and distortion usually are related closely, baroreceptor transduction is discussed in terms of pressure changes. Arterial baroreceptors are extraordinarily sensitive; they respond to changes of arterial flow that do not provoke measurable changes of pressure. (This assertion may be true, in part, because the ability of laboratory devices to transduce pressure changes is crude, relative to that of baroreceptors.) Individual receptors begin firing when some threshold pressure is exceeded, fire in proportion (i.e., nearly linearly) to further pressure increases, and reach a saturation level, above which additional increases of pressure do not provoke increases of firing.

Recordings made from families of baroreceptor neurons document a smoothly rounded threshold region—a gradual increase, rather than the abrupt onset of firing that occurs in individual baroreceptors. This appearance results because as pressure increases, more baroreceptors are recruited, and those whose firing had already commenced fire at more rapid rates. Thus, the relation between arterial pressure and multifiber baroreceptor nerve activity is sigmoid, with threshold, linear, and saturation regions. In animals, and probably also in humans, resting arterial pressure (called the operational, or set point) lies on the linear portion of this relation.

The viscoelastic coupling of baroreceptors to their surroundings exerts an important influence on their function. One manifestation of this is rate-sensitivity: rapid pressure changes elicit more rapid firing rates than slow pressure changes. Another manifestation is adaptation: firing rates are more rapid at the beginning of a step increase of pressure than they are at the end. A third manifestation is hysteresis: firing rates are greater when pressure is increasing than when pressure is returning to or below baseline levels.

METHODS FOR STUDY OF HUMAN BAROREFLEXES

Although two groups have recorded human arterial baroreceptor traffic directly (during neck surgery), virtually all that is known about human baroreflex function is derived from correlations between R-R interval (or heart rate) or sympathetic nerve activity and spontaneous or provoked changes of arterial distending pressure [1]. Such correlations usually yield a baroreflex slope (or gain) over a limited range of the linear portion of the sigmoid arterial pressure/vagal or reverse sigmoid/sympathetic response relations.

More information on baroreflex responses can be obtained when pressure changes are elicited experimentally. For example, substantial increases (amounting to tens of mmHg) can be provoked by Valsalva maneuvers (voluntary straining against a closed glottis). After release of straining, R-R interval increases can be plotted as functions of preceding arterial (usually systolic) pressures to derive baroreflex slopes and, sometimes, indications of baroreflex threshold. Bolus injections or infusions of vasoactive drugs, such as sodium nitroprusside or phenylephrine hydrochloride, can be given to provoke arterial pressure changes, and these pressure changes can be related to R-R intervals and sympathetic nerve activity. (However, it may be difficult to provoke significant changes of arterial pressure with vasoactive drug infusions in subjects who have very responsive baroreflexes.) Sequential injections of a vasodepressor followed by a vasoconstrictor agent may yield information on baroreflex thresholds and slopes in the linear range.

Finally, pressure or suction can be applied as single or repetitive pulses to a chamber strapped to the anterior neck, to modify carotid transmural pressure. This approach has two advantages: first, activity of only one barosensitive area, the carotid baroreceptors, can be modified selectively; and, second, large pressure changes (limited primarily by the subject's tolerance) can be applied. (One method [1] uses a brief 40–mmHg pressure increment, followed by a series of 15–mmHg pressure decrements, to −65 mmHg—a total change of 105 mm Hg.) Neck chamber methods have several disadvantages. Although pressure is transmitted from the chamber to internal structures in the neck reproducibly in serial applications of neck pressure or suction, it is not transmitted totally. More importantly, changes of transmural carotid pressure provoked by neck pressure or suction are opposed by reflex changes of arterial pressure sensed by aortic baroreceptors. Because all baroreceptor inputs terminate on the same solitary tract nucleus neuron pool, abrupt changes of carotid baroreceptor activity occurring simultaneously with opposing changes of aortic baroreceptor activity are discounted. For example, sustained (lasting seconds) neck pressure may alter efferent sympathetic nerve traffic for only one heart beat. (Vagal, or R-R interval, responses to carotid baroreceptor stimulation last longer than sympathetic responses.) Probably as a result of aortic baroreceptor opposition, baroreflex slopes measured during neck pressure changes are much less than baroreflex slopes measured during arterial pressure changes (which provoke parallel changes of firing in all baroreceptors).

One problem besets all methods used to estimate baroreflex gain during sustained (lasting more than 1 second) changes of baroreceptor input: because baroreflex adjustments occur so rapidly, measured arterial pressure changes represent pressure changes driving baroreceptors, less baroreflex-mediated pressure adjustments. Therefore, measured pressure changes are functions of baroreceptor stimuli rather than the stimuli themselves.

It is unlikely that noninvasive methods can alter activity of human cardiopulmonary baroreceptors selectively. A genre of literature from human and animal studies is based on the mistaken notion that experimental perturbations, such as infusions of "subpressor" doses of pressor agents, leg raising, mild hemorrhage or fluid infusion, or lower body suction, which alter pressure measured in the cardiopulmonary region (usually in the vena cavae or right atrium), but which do not alter pressure measured in arteries, are selective for cardiopulmonary receptors. The fallacy in this thinking arises from at least two mistaken notions. The first notion is that the cardiovascular system can be segmented; because this system is continuous, it is unlikely that a perturbation can be applied to one segment that does not affect all segments. The second mistaken notion is that arterial baroreceptors sense pressure; baroreceptors sense changes of dimensions, not pressure. Therefore, absence of pressure changes cannot be taken as evidence for absence of dimension changes. (This assertion is related to the fact that arterial baroreceptors are so sensitive and efficient that they can respond to changes of dimensions in baroreceptive arteries by restoring arterial pressure nearly perfectly.) Although minor levels (20 mmHg or less) of lower body suction (the prototype of experimental interventions used in humans to perturb cardiopulmonary receptors selectively) do not alter

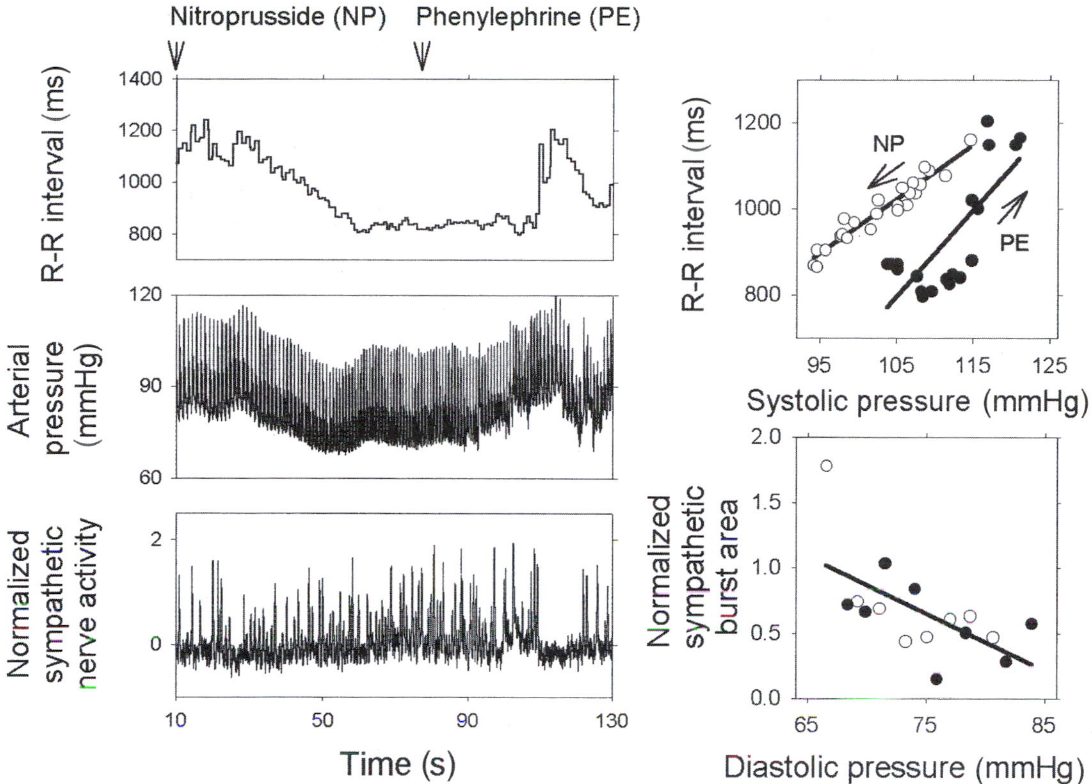

FIGURE 37.1 Vagal and sympathetic responses to sequential arterial pressure reductions and increases. (Reproduced with permission from Rudas, L., A. A. Crossman, C. A., Morillo, J. R., Halliwill, K. U. O., Tahvanainn, T. A., Kuusela, and D. L. Eckberg. 1999. Human sympathetic and vagal responses to sequential ntiroprusside and phenylephrine. *Am. J. Physiol.* 276:H1691–H1698.).

arterial pressure, they provoke major reductions of carotid artery and ascending aorta dimensions.

INTEGRATED BAROREFLEX RESPONSES

Figure 37.1 illustrates several features of integrated human baroreflex responses [4]. These data were obtained from a healthy human volunteer who was given sequential intravenous bolus injections of nitroprusside and phenylephrine. At the beginning of the recording, the reduction of arterial pressure provoked parallel reductions of R-R intervals (withdrawal of vagal restraint) and increases of muscle sympathetic nerve activity. Note that the increase of arterial pressure after the phenylephrine injection silenced muscle sympathetic nerve activity (see Fig. 37.1, bottom left, extreme right). The top right graph in Figure 37.1 documents proportionality between R-R intervals and arterial pressure and indicates that the R-R interval/systolic pressure relation is steeper when pressures are increasing than when they are decreasing (baroreflex hysteresis). The bottom right graph in Figure 37.1 documents inverse proportionality between arterial pressure and muscle sympathetic nerve activity.

Figure 37.2 shows stylized (but faithfully reproduced) muscle sympathetic nerve and R-R interval responses of a group of healthy subjects to abrupt increases or decreases of carotid baroreceptor input provoked by brief neck suction or pressure. These data illustrate several important features of human baroreflex function. First, in humans as in animals, the relation between arterial distending pressure and vagal-cardiac nerve activity is sigmoid (reverse sigmoid in the case of sympathetic nerve activity). Second, resting pressure (denoted by the closed circles in Fig. 37.2) lies on the linear portion of both relations; therefore, all arterial pressure changes elicit sympathetic and vagal neural responses. Third, in healthy young supine subjects (who were studied to obtain these data), resting arterial pressure is only slightly below the threshold for sympathetic activation. In such subjects, baseline levels of sympathetic activity are low, and small increases of arterial pressure above baseline levels silence muscle sympathetic motoneurons.

Figure 37.3 illustrates how arterial baroreceptors control vagus nerve traffic to the heart (as reflected by R-R intervals) and sympathetic nerve traffic to the large (about 40% of body mass) muscle vascular bed. During increases and decreases of arterial pressure provoked by infusions of phenylephrine and nitroprusside, sympathetic and vagal traffic varied reciprocally. At the greatest pressure (see Fig. 37.3, top), sympathetic "bursts" were absent and fluctuations of R-R intervals were maximal; and at the lowest pressure (see Fig. 37.3, bottom), sympathetic bursts were plentiful and large, and fluctuations of R-R intervals were nearly absent.

The role of baroreceptors in setting absolute levels of arterial pressure is controversial. Denervation of arterial baroreceptors leads to permanent and large lability of arterial pressure, but to only transient arterial pressure increases.

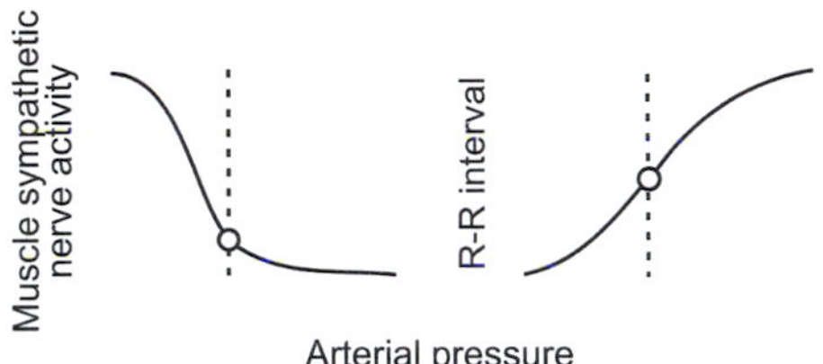

FIGURE 37.2 Average muscle sympathetic nerve and R-R interval responses of a group of healthy subjects to brief neck pressure or suction. *Open circles* indicates resting arterial pressure.

However, subsequent denervation of cardiopulmonary baroreceptors raises arterial pressure above normal levels [5].

BAROREFLEX RESETTING

Tethering of baroreceptors to surrounding structures introduces a viscoelastic element that importantly determines baroreceptor function. After the beginning of abrupt distension of a baroreceptive artery, afferent baroreceptor nerve traffic decays (or adapts) as a power function—that is, the log of baroreceptor nerve firing, plotted as a function of the log of time, is linear. After an abrupt step increase of pressure, baroreceptor firing decays to about one fourth of its peak value in less than 0.5 second. One practical implication of this is that changes of baroreceptor nerve activity provoked by sustained stimuli, such as neck suction, are likely to decline rapidly. (The experimental literature contains numerous examples of studies in which the tacit and

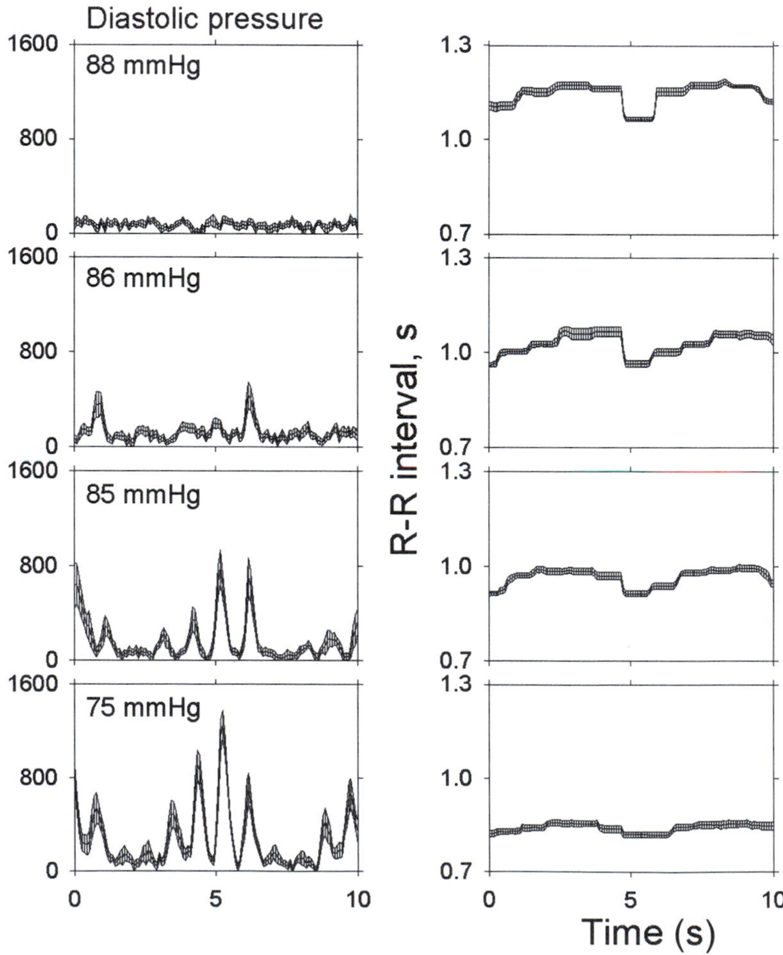

FIGURE 37.3 Average (±SEM) muscle sympathetic nerve traffic and R-R intervals of one supine healthy subject at different arterial pressures during infusions of phenylephrine (*top*), saline (*middle*), and nitroprusside (*bottom*).

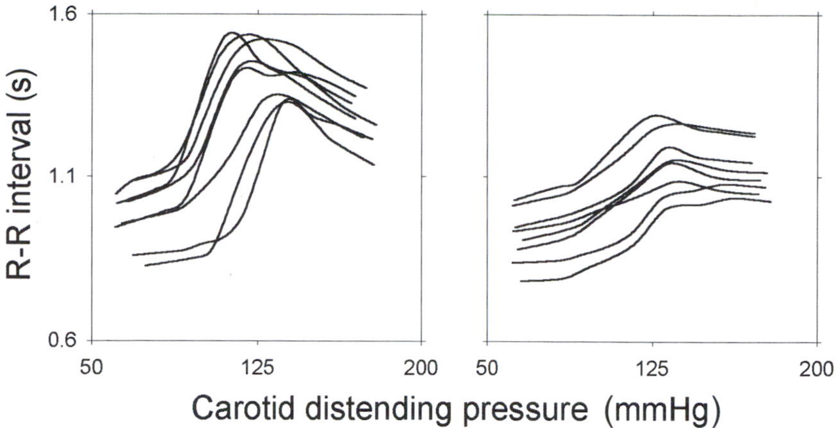

FIGURE 37.4 Average R-R interval responses to a ramped neck pressure—suction sequence of two subjects studied while awake, over 24 hours.

erroneous assumption is made that increases of baroreceptor nerve traffic are the same at the beginning as at the end of neck suction.)

The relation between arterial pressure and efferent autonomic outflow is highly fluid (Fig. 37.4). These sigmoid arterial pressure input/vagal–cardiac nerve output relations were measured in two supine subjects studied while awake, every 3 hours, for 24 hours. Shifts of the stimulus-response relations shown in Figure 37.4 occur rapidly (within tens of seconds) during experimentally induced arterial pressure changes and extend the range of pressures over which baroreflexes are operative.

CARDIOPULMONARY BAROREFLEXES

Hainsworth ably reviewed reflexes triggered by cardiac receptors [2], and Chapter 38 reviews reflexes triggered by cardiac receptors that are chemosensitive. As mentioned earlier, I am skeptical about claims that small changes of effective blood volume, such as those provoked by low levels of lower body suction, alter cardiopulmonary, but not baroreceptor, function. Nonetheless, there are several human reflex responses that seem to be initiated by cardiopulmonary receptors. One response is the human response to intracoronary injections of radiographic contrast medium. The simultaneous occurrence of bradycardia and hypotension suggests that during such injections arterial baroreflex responses are overridden. (The combination of hypotension and bradycardia also occurs during inferior left ventricular ischemia.) A second response is the marked diuresis that sometimes accompanies supraventricular tachycardias, which may represent a neurohumoral response initiated by atrial receptors.

SUMMARY

Arterial baroreflexes are prime examples of negative feedback mechanisms. Pressure changes alter stretch of barosensitive neurons, and changes of baroreceptor nerve activity trigger changes of sympathetic and vagal nerve activity and set in motion reflex adjustments that restore pressure toward baseline levels. Viscoelastic coupling of baroreceptors exerts important effects on their pressure transduction. The relation between arterial pressure and baroreflex responses is sigmoid (or reverse sigmoid in the case of sympathetic traffic), with threshold, linear, and saturation ranges. Arterial baroreflexes can be studied in humans by quantitating the effects of spontaneous or provoked changes of arterial distending pressure on sympathetic and vagal activity. Because denervation of all barosensory areas, cardiopulmonary and arterial, provokes sustained hypertension, it is likely that baroreceptors set absolute levels of arterial pressure.

References

1. Eckberg, D. L., and P. Sleight. 1992. *Human baroreflexes in health and disease*. Oxford: Clarendon Press.
2. Hainsworth, R. 1991. Reflexes from the heart. *Physiol. Rev.* 71: 617–658.
3. Mifflin, S. W., and R. B. Felder. 1990. Synaptic mechanisms regulating cardiovascular afferent inputs to solitary tract nucleus. *Am. J. Physiol.* 259:H653–H661.
4. Rudas, L., A. A. Crossman, C. A., Morillo, J. R., Halliwill, K. U. O., Tahvanainn, T. A., Kuusela, and D. L. Eckberg. 1999. Human sympathetic and vagal responses to sequential ntiroprusside and phenylephrine. *Am. J. Physiol.* 276:H1691–H1698.
5. Persson, P. 1988. Cardiopulmonary receptors in "neurogenic hypertension." *Acta. Physiol. Scand.* 133(Suppl. 570):1–53.

38 Venoarteriolar Reflex

Phillip A. Low
Department of Neurology
Mayo Clinic
Rochester, Minnesota

SKIN BLOOD FLOW

Skin is a highly complex structure with a multitude of nerve fibers and their receptors, blood vessels, sweat glands, hair follicles, sebaceous glands, and numerous other structures, all of which may be affected by vasomotor dysfunction.

There are two types of skin blood flow (SBF) that serve different purposes and have quite different morphologic substrates. Nutritive skin blood flow (SBF_n) is carried in capillaries that are 5–8 µm in diameter. These microvessels are thin walled and supply oxygen and other nutrients to tissue. Arteriovenous skin blood flow ($SBF_{A\text{-}V}$), in contrast, is carried in large-diameter (25–150 µm), low-resistance vessels that shunt blood from arterioles to venules at high flow rates and do not delivery oxygen to tissue. Instead, in human skin, $SBF_{A\text{-}V}$ shunts blood to superficial skin to enhance heat loss, serving its key role in thermoregulation. An increase of either $SBF_{A\text{-}V}$ or SBF_n increases heat conductance. Under conditions of maximal heat conductance, both $SBF_{A\text{-}V}$ and capillary flow are usually maximal. However, high heat conductance can occur with maximal $SBF_{A\text{-}V}$ and low SBF_n, suggesting that $SBF_{A\text{-}V}$ is far more important in thermoregulation. This conclusion is not surprising considering that maximal capillary flow is 19 µl/100 g/min, whereas minimal $SBF_{A\text{-}V}$ flow is 92 µl/100 g/min [1]. The major role of SBF is thermoregulatory. It also is important in the maintenance of skin nutrition, barrier function, and wound healing. SBF also affects sweat production.

VENOARTERIOLAR REFLEX

The maintenance of stable blood flow despite changes in posture of the whole subject or a limb is important. A major change in position causes a change in blood and pulse pressure and activation of arterial baroreflexes. A lesser change in position changes venous volume and activation of venous baroreflexes. When only a limb is moved, these baroreflexes are not activated. Instead, when venous transmural pressure is increased by 25 µmHg (e.g., by lowering a limb), there is a reduction in blood flow by 50%. This abrupt reduction in flow is often termed the venoarteriolar reflex [2] (Fig. 38.1). This response exists in all tissues of the limbs, including subcutaneous adipose, muscle, and skin; hence, it is an important vasoregulatory mechanism. Henriksen and coworkers [3] suggested that ~45% of the change in systemic vascular tone during upright tilt may be caused by this response, with the remaining 55% caused by reflex mechanisms elicited through baroreceptors unloading.

The existence and importance of the reflex is unquestioned, but the mechanism of this "reflex" is uncertain [4]. Investigators have attempted to define the neural pathway, citing intactness of the reflex with acute spinal blockade, but disappearing after sympathectomy [3]. They proposed an α-adrenergic mechanism because the venoarteriolar reflex was blocked or markedly reduced by local injections of phentolamine [5]. Henriksen and colleagues [2, 3] concluded that the underlying neural pathway was that of an axon reflex, and they advanced apparently convincing documentation. The response is blocked by local anesthetic without impairing vasomotion [3, 6].

More recent rigorous studies cast doubt on the role of the axon reflex. Crandall and colleagues [6] found that none of a variety of antiadrenergic drugs had a significant effect on the reflex. These findings do not support an adrenergic mechanism. Presynaptic blockade of sympathetic nerve terminals with intradermal bretylium did not affect the response, ruling out roles both for noradrenaline and any coreleased transmitter [7]. The recent studies suggest that sympathetic vasoconstrictor nerves are not required for the venoarteriolar reflex.

These recent studies are consonant with the clinical experience. The venoarteriolar reflex has been measured in the foot of patients with diabetes and is reported to be reduced in those with diabetic neuropathy [8]. However, the dissonance with other evidence of peripheral autonomic denervation has been problematic. For example, Moy and colleagues [9] compared this response with other indexes of autonomic denervation in 45 control subjects, 49 patients with diabetes, and 29 patients with other neuropathies. Results for patients whose postganglionic sudomotor axon reflex test was completely absent and who also had severe orthostatic hypotension (indicating postganglionic adrener-

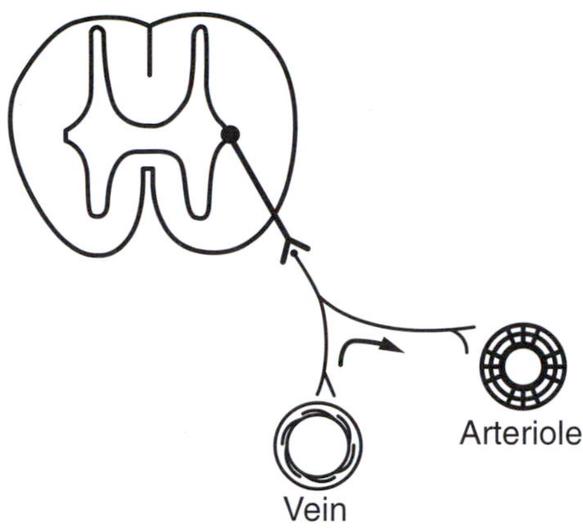

FIGURE 38.1 Presumed neural pathway of the venoarteriolar reflex.

gic failure) were not significantly different from the rest of the neuropathic group, whereas both quantitative sudomotor axon reflex test (QSART) and heart rate responses were significantly more abnormal in this subset. We concluded that the venoarteriolar reflex, although impaired in the neuropathies, is of little value as a clinical test and is a poorer test of autonomic function than the QSART or the cardiovascular heart rate tests.

Currently, there is good evidence for "reflex" venoconstriction in response to distension of veins. Neural and vascular mechanisms are involved, but evidence for an adrenergic reflex is weak.

References

1. Johnson, J. M., G. L. Brengelmann, J. R. Hales, P. M. Vanhoutte, and C. B. Wenger. 1986. Regulation of the cutaneous circulation. *Fed. Proc.* 45:2841–2850.
2. Henriksen, O. 1977. Local sympathetic reflex mechanism in regulation of blood flow in human subcutaneous adipose tissue. *Acta Physiol. Scand. Suppl.* 450:1–48.
3. Henriksen O., K. Skagen, O. Haxholdt, and V. Dyrberg. 1983. Contribution of local blood flow regulation mechanisms to the maintenance of arterial pressure in upright position during epidural blockade. *Acta Physiol. Scand.* 118, 271–280.
4. Johnson, J. M. 2002. How do veins talk to arteries? *J. Physiol.* 538:341.
5. Henriksen, O. 1991. Sympathetic reflex control of blood flow in human peripheral tissues. *Acta Physiol. Scand. Suppl.* 603:33–39.
6. Crandall C. G., M. Shibasaki, and T. C. Yen. 2002. Evidence that the human cutaneous venoarteriolar response is not mediated by adrenergic mechanisms. *J. Physiol.* 538:599–605.
7. Stephens D. P., K. Aoki, W. A. Kosiba, and J. M. Johnson. 2001. Nonnoradrenergic mechanism of reflex cutaneous vasoconstriction in men. *Am. J. Physiol. Heart Circ. Physiol.* 280:496–504.
8. Rayman, G., A. Hassan, and J. E. Tooke. 1986. Blood flow in the skin of the foot related to posture in diabetes mellitus. *Br. Med. J.* 292:87–90.
9. Moy, S., T. L. Opfer-Gehrking, C. J. Proper, and P. A. Low. 1989. The venoarteriolar reflex in diabetic and other neuropathies. *Neurology* 39:1490–1492.

39 The Cardioinhibitory Vasodepressor Reflex

Valentina Accurso
Department of Medicine
Mayo Clinic
Rochester, Minnesota

Virend K. Somers
Department of Medicine
Mayo Clinic
Rochester, Minnesota

The heart serves not only as a pump, but also as a sensory organ with both neural and endocrine functions. Stimulation of sensory nerve endings in the heart can induce potent reflex hemodynamic effects, primarily vasodilation and bradycardia. Afferents for this reflex are located predominantly in the inferoposterior wall of the left ventricle. Activation of this reflex may contribute to neurocardiogenic or vasovagal syncope and to exertional syncope in aortic stenosis [1]. The cardiac inhibitory reflex should be suspected whenever hypotension is associated with paradoxical bradycardia, such as during inferoposterior myocardial infarction.

PHYSIOLOGY

The afferent limb of the reflex consists of cardiac sensory nerve endings that originate in the atria and ventricles and travel through the vagus to the central nervous system. The sensory receptors are distributed predominantly in the ventricles and are activated by chemical agents such as veratrum alkaloids, nicotine, and phenylbiguanide (the Bezold-Jarisch reflex). Mechanical stimulation of the ventricle, either by acute increases in left ventricular pressures and inotropism or by ventricular distortion, may also elicit the reflex.

CLINICAL CONDITIONS PREDISPOSING TO ACTIVATION OF THE REFLEX

Afferents for the reflex are distributed preferentially in the inferoposterior wall of the left ventricle. Thus, in animal studies, occlusion of the circumflex coronary artery (supplying the inferoposterior left ventricle) results in hypotension and bradycardia, and no reflex skeletal muscle vasoconstriction in response to the hypotension. These reflex responses are less pronounced with occlusion of the left anterior descending artery (supplying the anterior wall). Vagotomy abolishes the reflex inhibitory response to occlusion of the circumflex artery. In humans, there is an increased incidence of bradyarrhythmias and hypotension in inferior wall infarction (70%) compared with anterior wall infarction (30%). In patients with Prinzmetal's angina, spasm of vessels supplying the inferior myocardium induces bradycardia, in contrast to tachycardia during anterior wall ischemia. After intracoronary thrombolytic therapy, patients with right coronary artery occlusion and reperfusion have a greater incidence of bradycardia and hypotension than those with left coronary reperfusion, in whom hypertension and tachycardia are more frequent. During coronary arteriography, bradycardia and hypotension are most marked during injections into a dominant right coronary artery, supplying the inferior wall of the heart.

The reflex may also be implicated in exertional syncope in patients with aortic stenosis. During exercise in normal subjects, blood pressure and heart rate increase in response to stimulation of somatic afferent receptors in skeletal muscle (Fig. 39.1). The increased blood pressure results from increased cardiac output and vasoconstriction in viscera and in nonactive muscles. In patients with aortic stenosis, leg exercise is associated with increased left ventricular end-diastolic pressure and absence of vasoconstriction in the nonexercising (forearm) muscle. Furthermore, in patients with aortic stenosis and a history of exertional syncope, paradoxic forearm vasodilation occurs during leg exercise. After valve replacement, the paradoxic forearm vasodilation is replaced by forearm vasoconstriction during exercise.

Acute hypotension occurs in about 30% of patients during hemodialysis. Possible etiologic factors include pericardial effusion and tamponade or autonomic neuropathy. However, Converse and colleagues [2] showed that patients with hypotension during dialysis often have intact sympathetic activity, but paradoxic bradycardia, vasodilation, sympathetic inhibition, and profound hypotension develop with reduction of intravascular volume. In these patients, echocardiographic studies demonstrated that hemodialysis was accompanied by progressive reduction in left ventricular end-systolic dimensions with virtual cavity obliteration before hypotensive episodes. In patients on hypotension-resistant hemodialysis, arterial pressure remained stable throughout dialysis, with progressive increases in heart rate and sympathetic activity. Thus, excessive myocardial contraction around an empty chamber, with consequent deformation of ventricular mechanoreceptors, may activate the cardiac inhibitory reflex and promote hypotension and syncope in patients on hemodialysis.

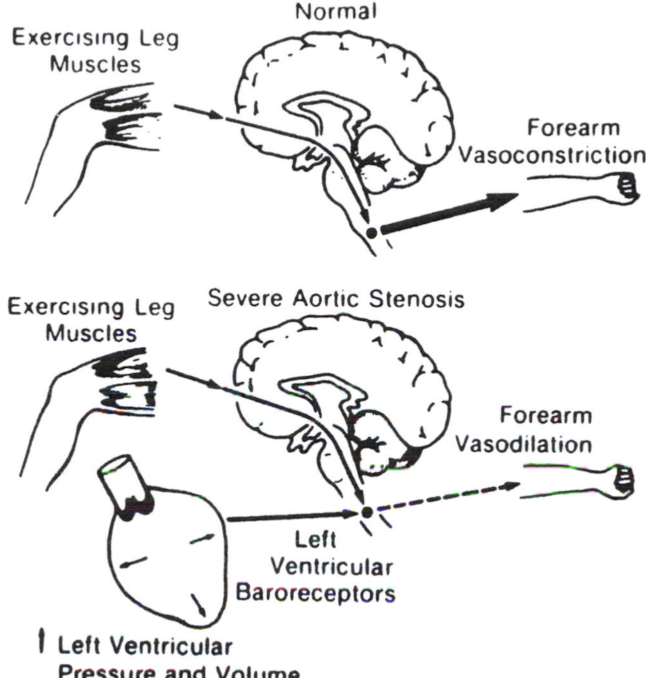

FIGURE 39.1 Schematic diagram showing effects of activation of left ventricular baroreceptors during exercise in patients with severe aortic stenosis. *Top*, Afferent impulses originating in exercising leg muscle, normally producing reflex vasoconstriction in the nonexercising forearm. *Bottom*, Increased left ventricular pressure with activation of left ventricular baroreceptors and consequent inhibition, and reversal of forearm vasoconstriction. (From Mark, A. L. 1983. The Bezold-Jarisch reflex revisited: Clinical implications of inhibitory reflexes originating in the heart. *J. Am. Coll. Cardiol.* 1:90–102, with permission).

There has been a surge of interest in the use of upright tilt as a diagnostic test in patients with recurrent neurocardiogenic or vasovagal syncope. In many of these patients, upright tilt results in hypotension with paradoxic bradycardia and syncope. Sequential atrioventricular pacing does not prevent syncope, indicating a potent vasodilator component [3]. There is marked withdrawal of efferent sympathetic nerve activity to muscle blood vessels during vasovagal syncope in humans [4] (Fig. 39.2). Prolonged upright tilt with pooling of blood in the lower extremities results in decreased cardiac filling pressure and increased myocardial contractility. This can produce activation of cardiac mechanoreceptors with consequent sympathetic withdrawal, vasodilation, bradycardia, and syncope. Release of humoral agents such as epinephrine, vasopressin, and prostaglandins potentiate this response. Tilt testing also has implicated the cardioinhibitory vasodepressor reflex in the syncope associated with blood phobia [6].

Mechanisms other than the cardiogenic cardioinhibitory vasodepressor reflex may be implicated in neurocardiogenic syncope. Vasodepressor syncope has been reported during nitroprusside infusion in a patient after heart transplantation, where ventricular vagal afferent pathways are presumably denervated. A study of patients after heart transplantation revealed that 7 of 10 patients demonstrated bradycardia and hypotension during upright tilt. In four of these patients there was no evidence of vagal efferent reinnervation [5]. Thus, left ventricular receptors alone may not completely explain all cases of simultaneous hypotension and bradycardia.

In this regard, studies indicate a possible role for humoral substances such as serotonin and nitric oxide in mediating simultaneous hypotension and bradycardia. These may act at a central neural level. During severe hemorrhagic

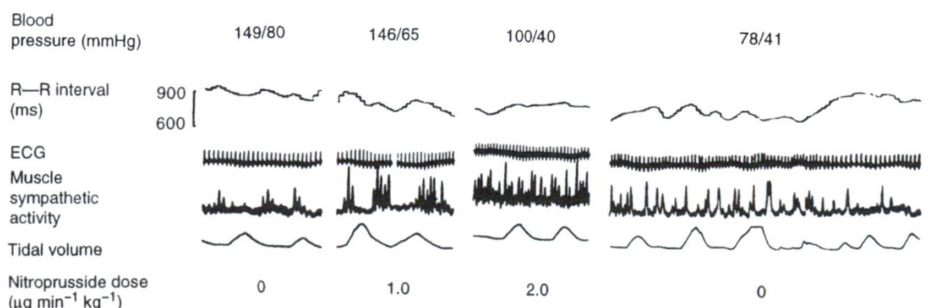

FIGURE 39.2 Vasovagal response during sodium nitroprusside infusion in a healthy subject. Initially, as arterial blood pressure decreases, muscle sympathetic nerve activity increases. Impending vasovagal syncope is accompanied by a decrease in blood pressure with simultaneous reduction in sympathetic nerve discharge. (From Eckberg, D. L., and P. Sleight. 1992. *Human baroreflexes in health and disease*, 153–215. Oxford: Clarendon Press, with permission).

hypotension in rats, paradoxic bradycardia and sympathetic withdrawal are accompanied by increased sympathetic activity to the adrenal gland. This increased adrenal nerve activity is prevented by inhibitors of serotonin synthesis. Serotonin administration into cerebral ventricles can induce hypotension, inhibition of renal sympathetic activity, and increased adrenal sympathetic activity. Thus, serotonin may act centrally to inhibit reflex sympathetic activation and serotonin antagonists may be effective in preventing vasodepressor syncope. Nitric oxide also has been reported to act as a central neurotransmitter that might inhibit sympathetic nerve activity and promote bradycardia and hypotension. The role of serotonin and nitric oxide in reflex control and the pathogenesis of neurocardiogenic syncope in humans is unclear.

References

1. Mark, A. L. 1983. The Bezold-Jarisch reflex revisited: Clinical implications of inhibitory reflexes originating in the heart. *J. Am. Coll. Cardiol.* 1:90–102.
2. Converse, Jr., R. L., T. N. Jacobsen, C. M. T. Jost, R. D. Toto, P. A. Grayburn, T. M. Obregon, F. Fouad-Tarazi, and R. G. Victor. 1992. Paradoxical withdrawal of reflex vasoconstriction as a cause of hemodialysis-induced hypotension. *J. Clin. Invest.* 90:1657–1665.
3. Sra, J. S., M. R. Jazayeri, B. Avitall, A. Dhala, S. Deshpande, Z. Blanck, and M. Akhtar. 1993. Comparison of cardiac pacing with drug therapy in the treatment of neurocardiogenic (vasovagal) syncope with bradycardia or asystole. *N. Engl. J. Med.* 328:1085–1090.
4. Wallin, B. G., and G. Sundlof. 1982. Sympathetic outflow to muscles during vasovagal syncope. *J. Auton. Nerv. Syst.* 6:287–291.
5. Fitzpatrick, A. P., N. Banner, A. Cheng, M. Yacoub, and R. Sutton. 1993. Vasovagal reactions may occur after orthotopic heart transplantation. *J. Am. Coll. Cardiol.* 21:1132–1137.
6. Accurso, V., M. Winnicki, A. Shamsuzzaman, A. Wenzel, A. Johnson, and V. K. Somers. 2001. Predisposition to vasovagal syncope in subjects with blood/injury phobia. *Circulation* 104:903–907.

40 Autonomic Control of the Kidney

Edwin K. Jackson
Center for Clinical Pharmacology
Pittsburgh, Pennsylvania

INNERVATION OF THE KIDNEY

Autonomic control of the kidney is predominantly sympathetic, and there is only scant evidence for parasympathetic innervation [1, 2]. Postganglionic sympathetic neurons densely innervate the kidneys and have varicosities on renal vascular smooth muscle cells in the interlobar, arcuate, and interlobular arteries, on afferent and efferent arterioles, on juxtaglomerular cells, and on epithelial cells in proximal tubules, thick ascending limbs of Henle's loops, distal convoluted tubules, and collecting ducts (Fig. 40.1). In this regard, the density of sympathetic varicosities is much greater on vascular structures and juxtaglomerular cells compared with renal tubular epithelial cells.

The cell bodies of renal sympathetic postganglionic neurons reside for the most part in prevertebral sympathetic ganglia including the celiac, superior mesenteric, aorticorenal, and posterior renal ganglia, as well as in a variable number of smaller renal ganglia. The axons of renal sympathetic preganglionic neurons that synapse with renal postganglionic neurons exit the thoracic (T10-T12) and lumbar (L1-L3) sympathetic trunk and reach the outlying prevertebral ganglia through the thoracic splanchnic and lumbar splanchnic nerves, respectively. Some renal preganglionic neurons have cell bodies in T4-T8 with axons that descend through the sympathetic trunk to T10-L3.

Cell bodies of premotor neurons projecting to and controlling renal sympathetic preganglionic neurons in the intermediolateral column of the spinal cord reside predominantly in the rostral ventrolateral medulla, A5 noradrenergic cell group in the caudal ventrolateral pons, the caudal raphe nuclei, and the paraventricular nucleus of the hypothalamus, with the rostral ventrolateral medulla being most critical and providing the primary tonic excitatory input to preganglionic sympathetic neurons. The premotor neurons controlling the renal sympathetic system, in turn, receive projections from a number of brain regions involved in cardiovascular and renal regulation, the most important of which is the nucleus tractus solitarius, which receives direct inputs from the peripheral arterial and cardiopulmonary baroreceptors and chemoreceptors. This arrangement allows blood volume, pressure, and composition to modulate appropriately renal function, which, in turn, corrects blood volume, pressure, and composition in an elegant negative feedback loop.

AUTONOMIC RECEPTORS IN THE KIDNEY

The basal discharge rate of renal sympathetic nerves is 0.5 to 2 Hz, and this causes the continuous basal release of the dominant neurotransmitter in the sympathetic varicosity, norepinephrine, together with lesser amounts of the cotransmitter, neuropeptide Y. Both norepinephrine and neuropeptide Y cause autoinhibition (prejunctional negative feedback) of neurotransmitter release through prejunctional α_2-adrenoceptors and Y_2 receptors, respectively. In addition, several other humoral and paracrine factors also prejunctionally modulate noradrenergic neurotransmission—for example, angiotensin II through AT_1 receptors and epinephrine through β_2-adrenoceptors, both of which facilitate renal noradrenergic neurotransmission (Fig. 40.2).

Norepinephrine acts directly on granular juxtaglomerular cells, a type of modified smooth muscle cell in afferent arterioles, to increase the rate of renin release. This effect of norepinephrine is mediated exclusively by β_1-adrenoceptors and involves the following signal transduction process: (1) activation of G_s; (2) stimulation of adenylyl cyclase; (3) increased levels of cyclic adenosine monophosphate; (4) stimulation of protein kinase A; (5) phosphorylation of proteins leading to increased H^+ translocation into renin-containing granules; (6) increased KCl/H^+ exchange; (7) osmotically driven influx of H_2O into the granule; (8) granule swelling; and (9) exocytosis of renin.

Renal artery hypotension (intrarenal baroreceptor mechanism) and decreased influx of NaCl into macula densa cells in the thick ascending limb of Henle's loop (macula densa mechanism) also stimulate renin release, and renal sympathetic nerve activation can indirectly increase renin release by activating these mechanisms secondary to changes in renal hemodynamics. Importantly, a powerful synergy exists between β_1-adrenoceptor–induced renin release and intrarenal baroreceptor and macula densa-induced renin release.

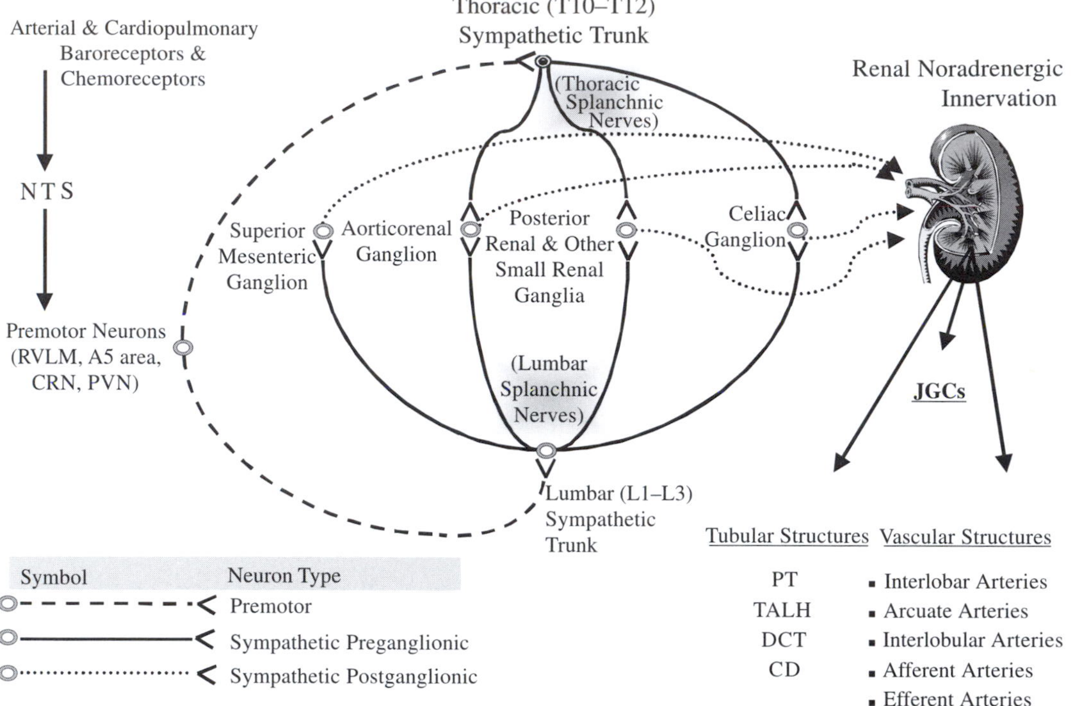

FIGURE 40.1 Diagram of efferent innervation of the kidney. A5 area, A5 noradrenergic cell group in the caudal ventrolateral pons; CD, collecting duct; CRN, caudal raphe nuclei; DCT, distal convoluted tubule; NTS, nucleus tractus solitarius; JGCs, juxtaglomerular cells; PT, proximal tubule; PVN, paraventricular nucleus of the hypothalamus; TALH, thick ascending limb of Henle's loop; RVLM, rostral ventrolateral medulla.

Norepinephrine released from renal sympathetic varicosities also acts directly on renal epithelial cells to accelerate the rate of solute and water reabsorption from the tubular lumen. This effect of norepinephrine occurs in most nephron segments, but it is particularly pronounced in the proximal tubule. Although norepinephrine directly affects epithelial cell transport, norepinephrine-induced changes in renal blood flow and glomerular filtration rate may also contribute to sympathetically induced decreases in renal excretion of electrolytes and water [3–7]. The direct effects of norepinephrine on tubular transport are mediated exclusively by α_1-adrenoceptors, which appear to engage the following signal transduction process: (1) activation of G_q; (2) stimulation of phospholipase C-β; (3) increased production of inositol trisphosphate; (4) release of intracellular calcium; (5) calcium-mediated activation of the phosphatase calcineurin; and (6) calcineurin-mediated dephosphorylation and activation of Na^+-K^+ ATPase.

Stimulation of renal sympathetic nerves profoundly decreases renal blood flow and glomerular filtration rate. These effects are mediated mostly by norepinephrine-induced activation of α_1-adrenoceptors, which mediate intense contraction of vascular smooth muscle cells leading to constriction of the renal microcirculation. The signal transduction pathway is, in part, the following: stimulation of $G_q \rightarrow$ activation of phospholipase C-β $\rightarrow$ inositol trisphosphate –induced calcium release + diacylglycerol production $\rightarrow$ activation of protein kinase C. In this regard, preglomerular microvessels appear to be more responsive to norepinephrine than are postglomerular microvessels, an imbalance that contributes to norepinephrine-induced reductions in glomerular capillary hydrostatic pressure. Norepinephrine reduces single nephron glomerular filtration rate by (1) decreasing glomerular capillary hydrostatic pressure; (2) reducing the glomerular capillary ultrafiltration coefficient by contracting mesangial cells; and (3) decreasing single nephron blood flow.

Although α_1-adrenoceptors mediate most of the renal hemodynamic effects of renal sympathetic nerve stimulation, α_2-adrenoceptors and Y_1 receptors also participate, with considerable species variation. Both α_2-adrenoceptors and Y_1 receptors may contribute to renal vasoconstriction by inhibiting adenylyl cyclase through a G_i-mediated mechanism.

Studies involving direct electrical stimulation of renal nerves support the conclusion that different frequency

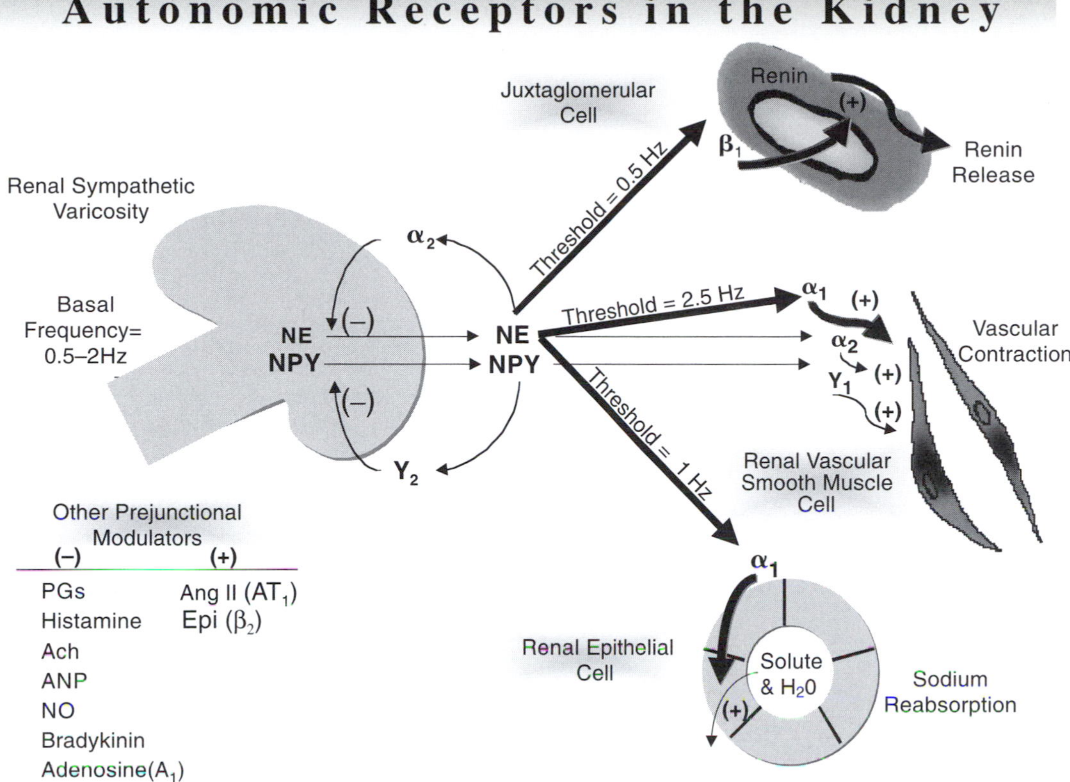

FIGURE 40.2 Summary of autonomic receptors in the kidney. α_1, α_1-adrenoceptors; A_1, A_1 adenosine receptor; Ach, acetylcholine; Ang II, angiotensin II; ANP, atrial natriuretic peptide; β_1, β_1-adrenoceptors; Epi, epinephrine; NE, norepinephrine; NO, nitric oxide; NPY, neuropeptide Y; PGs, prostaglandins; Y_1, Y_1 receptors for neuropeptide Y; Y_2, Y_2 receptors for neuropeptide Y.

threshold levels of efferent renal sympathetic nerve activity alter renin release (0.5 Hz), tubular transport (1 Hz), and renal hemodynamics (2.5 Hz). However, direct simultaneous recordings of renal sympathetic nerve activity and renal blood flow in conscious animals suggest that the full spectrum of physiologically relevant renal sympathetic nerve activity affects renal blood flow. Currently, this is an unresolved controversy.

REFLEX REGULATION OF BLOOD VOLUME

Autonomic control of the kidney enables an important renal reflex that buffers changes in blood volume and contributes to the rapid restoration of normal blood volume after a positive or negative perturbation in volume status caused by, for example, a large volume load or blood loss (Fig. 40.3). Increases in blood volume stimulate cardiopulmonary baroreceptors, particularly those in the left atrium. Stimulation of cardiopulmonary baroreceptors by an expanding blood volume increases afferent vagal signals to the nucleus tractus solitarius, which relays these incoming signals to cardiovascular centers in the brain for further integration. The net result is an inhibition of antidiuretic hormone secretion from the posterior pituitary and a reduction in efferent renal sympathetic nerve activity. The decrease in efferent renal sympathetic nerve activity decreases renin release and renal tubular epithelial transport and increases renal blood flow and glomerular filtration rate. These changes, in conjunction with decreases in antidiuretic hormone levels, markedly increase the excretion rate of NaCl and water, which accelerates the restoration of a normal blood volume. Conversely, a reduction in blood volume (e.g., by severe bleeding) increases antidiuretic hormone levels and efferent renal sympathetic nerve activity, and these changes reduce NaCl and water excretion to prevent further reductions in blood volume.

As a general rule, evolution provides multiple homeostatic mechanisms controlling physiologic parameters critical to life, and blood volume is no exception. Redundancy exists in the homeostasis of blood volume and the extent to which autonomic control of the kidney contributes to blood volume regulation depends on multiple factors such as the magnitude of blood volume, perturbation and the physiological status of other regulatory mechanisms [8].

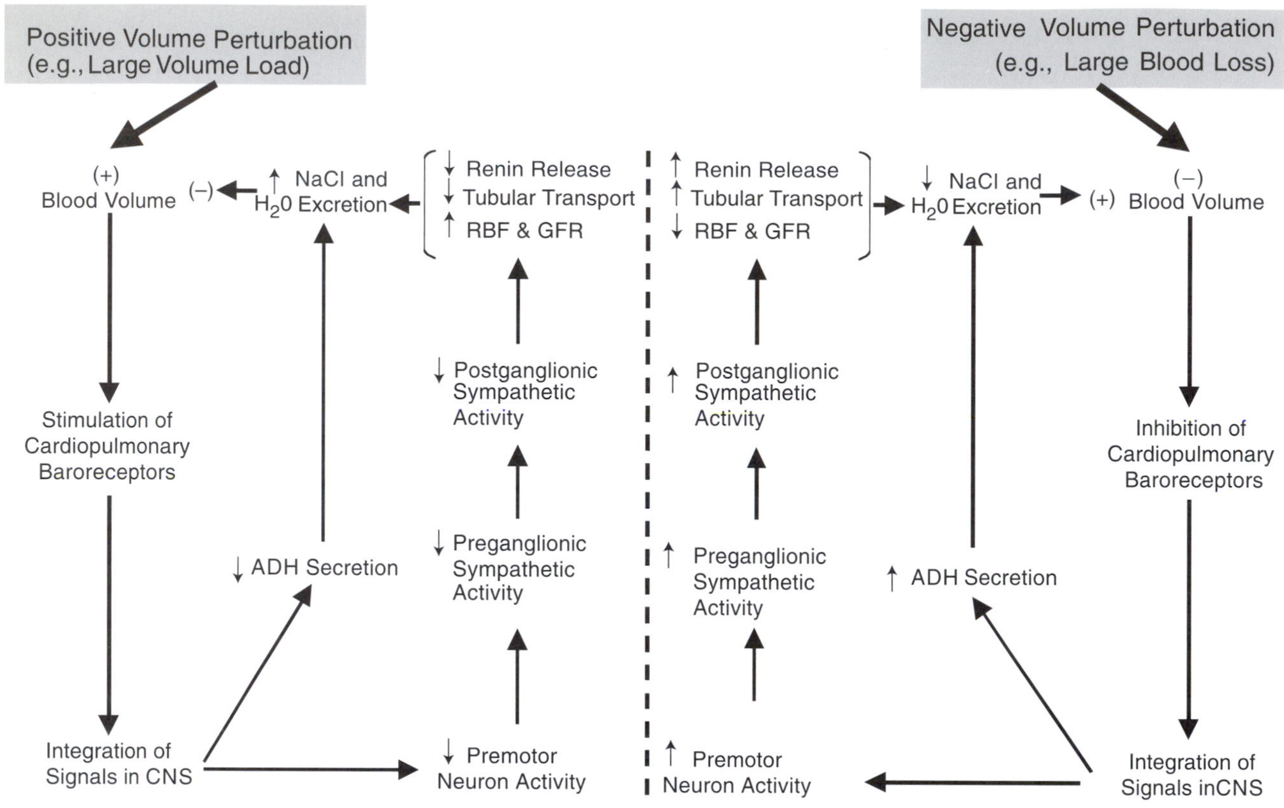

FIGURE 40.3 Reflex regulation of blood volume by the renal autonomic system. ADH, antidiuretic hormone; CNS, central nervous system; GFR, glomerular filtration rate; RBF, renal blood flow.

THE RENORENAL REFLEX

Because two kidneys regulate blood volume, pressure, and composition, it is not surprising that a mechanism exists to balance these critical tasks between the two kidneys. This mechanism is the renorenal reflex (Fig. 40.4).

Increased renal blood flow and glomerular filtration rate to one kidney results in ipsilateral increases in renal venous and pelvic pressures because of greater volumes of blood and urine, respectively, in those compartments. Pressure in the renal venous and pelvic structures activates renal mechanoreceptors residing in the major renal veins, the renal pelvis, and the corticomedullary connective tissue. Release of substance P and calcitonin gene–related peptide from afferent nerve endings, as well as local formation of prostaglandin E_2, may augment the discharge of afferent renal sensory nerves [8].

Renal afferent nerves have their cell bodies in the ipsilateral dorsal root ganglia (T10-L1), and incoming signals pass through the spinal cord to cardiovascular/renal integration centers in the central nervous system. With increased incoming afferent traffic from the ipsilateral kidney, these centers of integration command a decrease in efferent renal sympathetic nerve activity to the contralateral kidney, which results in increases in renal blood flow to and glomerular filtration by the contralateral kidney, thereby increasing the workload on the contralateral kidney. Moreover, diuresis and natriuresis by the contralateral kidney gradually decreases arterial blood pressure, which ultimately reduces the renal blood flow and glomerular filtration rate of the ipsilateral kidney. The net result is a near equal renal blood flow and glomerular filtration rate between the kidneys and, consequently, an equal sharing of the workload of maintaining a constant blood volume, pressure, and composition (see Fig. 40.4).

AUTONOMIC CONTROL OF THE KIDNEY IN PATHOPHYSIOLOGIC STATES

The relation between mean arterial blood pressure and the renal excretion rate of sodium—that is, the renal

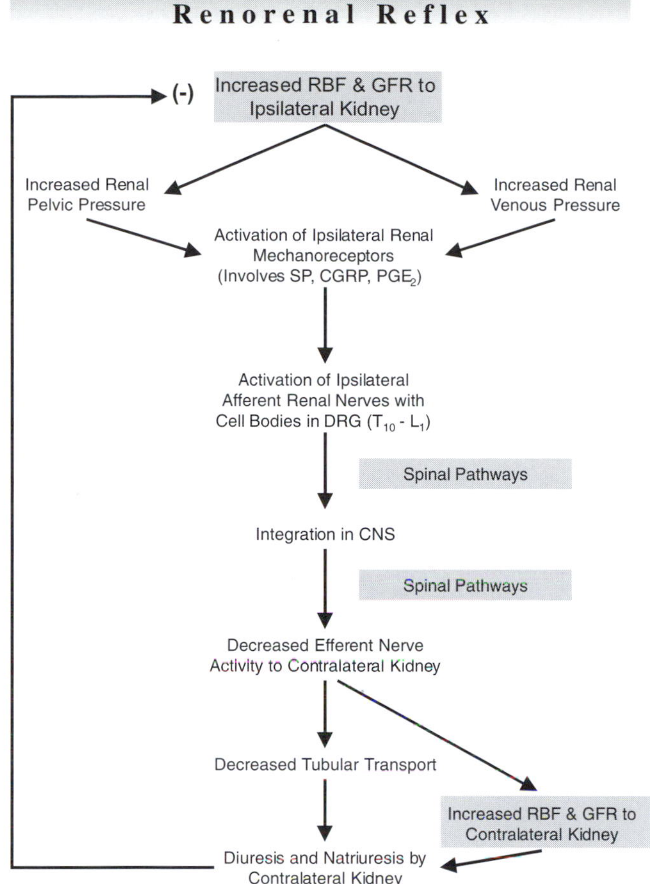

FIGURE 40.4 Shown is how the renorenal reflex distributes workload evenly between the kidneys. CGRP, calcitonin gene–related peptide; CNS, central nervous system; GFR, glomerular filtration rate; PGE_2, prostaglandin E_2; RBF, renal blood flow; SP, substance P; DRG, dorsal root ganglia.

pressure-natriuresis curve—determines long-term levels of arterial blood pressure. Increased renal efferent sympathetic nerve activity impairs renal sodium excretion and shifts the renal pressure-natriuresis curve to the right such that greater long-term levels of blood pressure are required to maintain sodium excretion in balance with sodium intake [9]. It is not surprising, therefore, that efferent renal sympathetic nerve activity contributes to the pathophysiology of hypertension [8]. Evidence for this conclusion includes: (1) complete renal denervation delays or attenuates, or both, the development of hypertension in a wide spectrum of experimental animal models; (2) efferent renal sympathetic nerve activity is usually increased in hypertension; (3) chronic low-level renal nerve stimulation or chronic intrarenal infusions of norepinephrine induce hypertension; and (4) sympatholytic drugs decrease blood pressure. It is certain, however, that the pathophysiology of hypertension is multifactorial and that efferent renal sympathetic nerves are only one among several participating mechanisms.

Renal retention of NaCl and water is a prerequisite for edema formation in congestive heart failure, hepatic cirrhosis, and nephrotic syndrome. In these pathophysiologic states, blood pressure, intravascular extracellular fluid volume, or both are often diminished, even though total extracellular fluid volume is usually expanded. These perturbations inappropriately engage an arterial baroreceptor-mediated or cardiopulmonary baroreceptor-mediated reflex increase in efferent renal sympathetic nerve activity, or both, which contributes significantly to the retention of NaCl and water and, consequently, to the edematous state. Accordingly, maneuvers that attenuate efferent renal sympathetic nerve activity—for example, head-out water immersion, bilateral lumbar sympathetic anesthetic block, and administration of sympatholytics—increase NaCl and water excretion in edema associated with heart, liver, or kidney disease [9, 10].

References

1. Barajas, L., L. Liu, and K. Powers. 1992. Anatomy of the renal innervation: Intrarenal aspects and ganglia of origin. *Can. J. Physiol. Pharmacol.* 70:735–749.
2. Luff, S. E., S. G. Hengstberger, E. M. McLachlan, and W. P. Anderson. 1992. Distribution of sympathetic neuroeffector junctions in the juxtaglomerular region of the rabbit kidney. *J. Auton. Nerv. Syst.* 40:239–253.
3. Malpas, S. C., and B. L. Leonard. 2000. Neural regulation of renal blood flow: A re-examination. *Clin. Exp. Pharmacol. Physiol.* 27: 956–964.
4. Kopp, U. C., and G. F. DiBona. 1993. Neural regulation of renin secretion. *Sem. Nephrol.* 13:543–551.
5. Moss, N. G., R. C. Colindres, and C. W. Gottschalk. 1992. Neural control of renal function. In *Handbook of physiology: Renal physiology, Vol I*, 1061–1128. Bethesda, MD: American Physiological Society.
6. DiBona, G. F. 1989. Neural control of renal tubular solute and water transport. *Miner. Electrolyte. Metab.* 15:44–50.
7. Gottschalk, C. W. 1979. Renal nerves and sodium excretion. *Annu. Rev. Physiol.* 41:229–240.
8. DiBona, G. F., and Kopp, U. C. 1997. Neural control of renal function. *Physiol. Rev.* 77:75–197.
9. Johns, E. J. 1989. Role of angiotensin II and the sympathetic nervous system in the control of renal function. *J. Hypertens.* 7:695–701.
10. DiBona, G. F. 1989. Neural control of renal function: Cardiovascular implications. *Hypertension* 13:539–548.

41 Autonomic Control of the Pupil

H. Stanley Thompson
Department of Ophthalmology
University of Iowa
Iowa City, Iowa

The iris hangs in a bath of aqueous humor. The actions of the sphincter and dilator muscles on the size of the pupil are not impeded by bulky tissue, and they are in plain view. It is not surprising that 80 to 100 years ago, at the very beginning of autonomic pharmacology, the pupil was frequently used as an indicator of drug action. In those years it was shown that parasympathetic and sympathetic neural impulses to the iris muscles could be modified by drugs at the synapses and at the effector sites, because it was at these locations that the transmission of the impulse depended on chemical mediators (Fig. 41.1). In this chapter, these well known, autonomically active drugs are grouped according to the site and their mechanism of action.

A few general cautionary words should first be said about the interpretation of pupillary responses to topically instilled drugs. There are large interindividual differences in the responsiveness of the iris to typical drugs, and this becomes most evident when weak concentrations are used. For example, 0.25% pilocarpine will produce a minimal constriction in some patients and an intense miosis in others. This means that the most secure clinical judgments stem from comparisons with the action of the drug on the other normal eye.

The general status of the patient also will influence the size of the pupils. If the patient becomes uncomfortable or anxious while waiting for the drug to act, both pupils may dilate. If the patient becomes drowsy, both pupils will constrict. Thus, if a judgment is to be made about the dilation or contraction of the pupil in response to a drug placed in the conjunctival sac, one pupil should be used as a control whenever possible [4].

PARASYMPATHOLYTIC (ANTICHOLINERGIC) DRUGS

The belladonna alkaloids occur naturally. They can be found in various proportions in deadly nightshade (*Atropa belladonna*), henbane (*Hyoscyamus niger*), and jimsonweed (*Datura stramonium*). Potions made from these plants were the tools of professional poisoners in ancient times. The word belladonna ("beautiful lady") was derived from the cosmetic use of these substances as mydriatics in sixteenth-century Venice. The mischief caused by the ubiquitous jimsonweed is typical of this group of plants. Jimsonweed has been used as a poison, has been taken as a hallucinogen, has caused accidental illness and death, and it can cause an alarming accidental mydriasis. These solanaceous plants, which are related to the tomato, potato, and eggplant, are still cultivated for medical purposes.

Atropine and **scopolamine** block parasympathetic activity by competing with acetylcholine at the effector cells of the iris sphincter and ciliary muscle, thus preventing depolarization. After conjunctival instillation of atropine (1%), mydriasis begins within about 10 minutes and is fully developed at 35 to 45 minutes; cycloplegia is complete within 1 hour. The pupil may stay dilated for several days, but accommodation usually returns in 48 hours. Scopolamine (0.2%) causes mydriasis that lasts, in an uninflamed eye, for about 2 days; it is a less effective cycloplegic than atropine.

Tropicamide and **cyclopentolate** are synthetic parasympatholytics with a relatively short duration of action. Tropicamide (1%) is an effective, short-acting mydriatic (3 to 6 hours), which results in only a transient paresis of accommodation. Compared with tropicamide, cyclopentolate (1%) seems to be a more effective cycloplegic and a slightly less effective mydriatic, especially in dark eyes; accommodation takes about half a day to return and the pupil still may not be working perfectly after more than 24 hours.

Botulinum toxin blocks the release of acetylcholine, and hemicholinium interferes with the synthesis of acetylcholine both at the preganglionic and postganglionic nerve endings, thus interrupting the parasympathetic pathway in two places. The outflow of sympathetic impulses is also interrupted by systemic doses of these drugs, because the chemical mediator in sympathetic ganglia is also acetylcholine.

PARASYMPATHOMIMETIC (CHOLINERGIC) DRUGS

Pilocarpine and **methacholine** are structurally similar to acetylcholine and are capable of depolarizing the effector

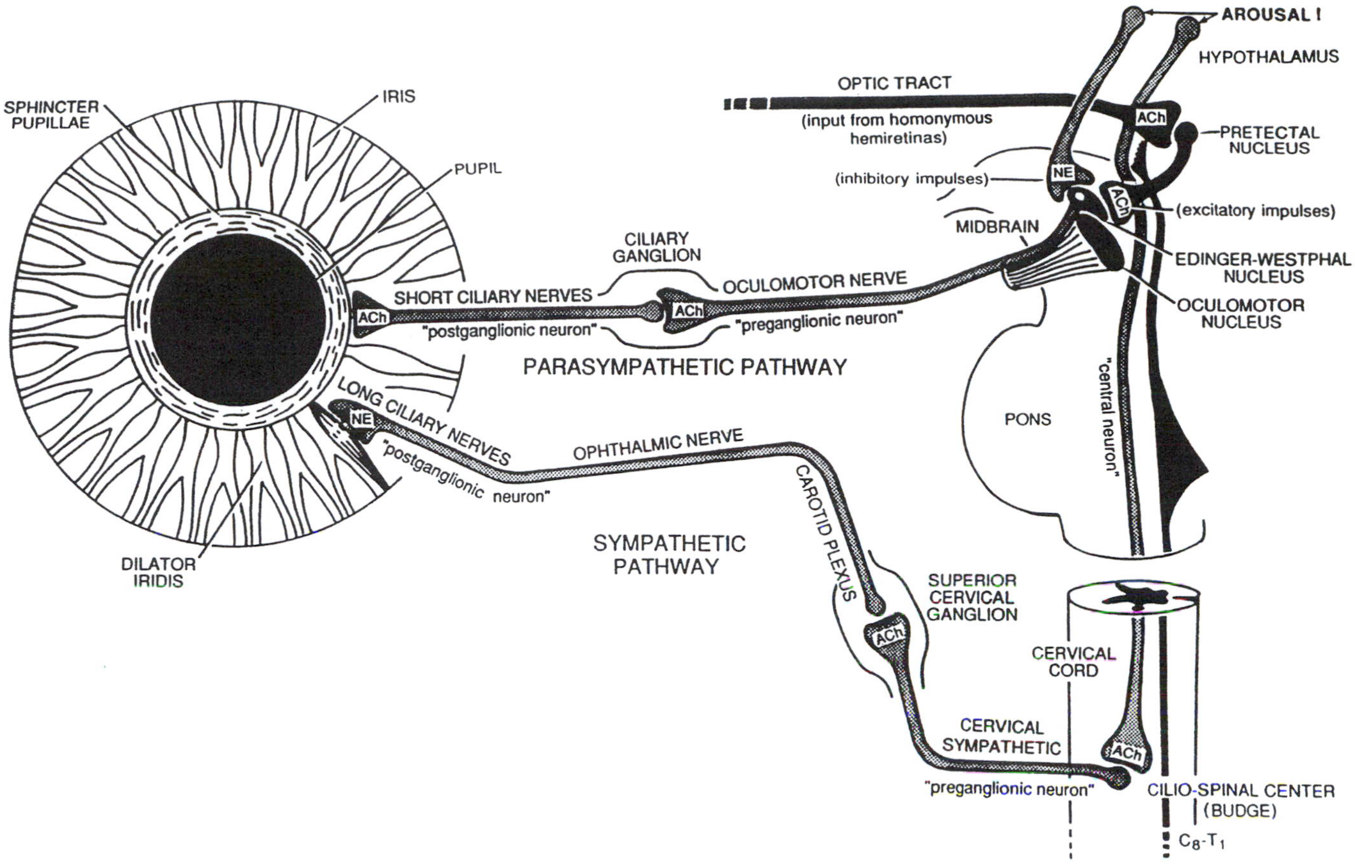

FIGURE 41.1 The innervation of the iris muscles, showing the pathways and the terminology in general use. Note that an alerting stimulus dilates the pupil in two ways, both of them with a noradrenergic step in the pathway. The alerting stimulus inhibits the iris sphincter nucleus and at the same time sends a message down to the cervical cord and the out along the cervical sympathetic pathway. This arrives at the iris about half a second after the sphincter-relaxing message and causes the radial dilator muscle to tighten, thus widening the pupil.

cell, thus causing miosis and spasm of accommodation. Methacholine is still sometimes used in a weak (2.5%) solution to test for cholinergic supersensitivity of the sphincter muscle in autonomic failure. It is being replaced by weak pilocarpine (0.1%).

Arecoline is a naturally occurring substance with an action similar to that of pilocarpine and methacholine. Its chief advantage is that it acts quickly; a 1% solution produces a full miosis in 10 to 15 minutes (compared with 20 to 30 minutes for 1% pilocarpine) [3].

Carbachol acts chiefly at the postganglionic cholinergic nerve ending to release the stores of acetylcholine. There also is some direct action of carbachol on the effector cell. A 1.5% solution causes intense miosis, but the drug does not penetrate the cornea easily and is therefore usually mixed with a wetting agent (1:3500 benzalkonium chloride).

Acetylcholine is liberated at the cholinergic nerve endings by the neural action potential and is promptly hydrolyzed and inactivated by cholinesterase. Cholinesterase, in turn, can be inactivated by any one of the many anticholinesterase drugs. These drugs either block the action of cholinesterase or deplete the stores of the enzyme in the tissue. They do not act on the effector cell directly; they just potentiate the action of the chemical mediator by preventing its destruction by cholinesterase. It follows from their mode of action that these drugs will lose their cholinergic activity once the innervation has been completely destroyed.

Physostigmine (eserine) is the classic anticholinesterase. Along the Calabar coast of West Africa, the native tribes once conducted trials "by ordeal" using a poison prepared from the bean of the plant *Physostigma venenosum.* The local name for this big bean was the "esere nut." The organic phosphate esters (echothiophate [Phospholine], isoflurophate [diisopropyl fluorophosphate], tetraethyl pyrophosphate, hexaethyltetraphosphate, parathion), many of which are in widespread use as insecticides, cause a much longer miosis than the other anticholinesterases, but even this potent effect, thought to be caused by interference with cholinesterase synthesis, can be reversed by pralidoxime chloride.

SYMPATHOMIMETIC (ADRENERGIC) DRUGS

Epinephrine stimulates the receptor sites of the dilator muscle cells directly. When applied to the conjunctiva, the 1 : 1000 solution does not penetrate into the normal eye in sufficient quantity to have an obvious mydriatic effect. If, however, the receptors have been made supersensitive by previous denervation, or if the corneal epithelium has been damaged, allowing more of the drug to get into the eye, then this concentration of epinephrine will dilate the pupil.

Phenylephrine in the 10% solution has a powerful mydriatic effect. Its action is almost exclusively a direct alpha stimulation of the effector cell. The pupil recovers in 8 hours and shows a "rebound miosis" lasting several days. A 2.5% solution is now commonly used for mydriasis. **Ephedrine** acts chiefly by releasing endogenous norepinephrine from the nerve ending, but it also has a definite direct stimulation effect on the dilator cells.

Tyramine (5%) and **hydroxyamphetamine** (1%) have an indirect adrenergic action: they release norepinephrine from the stores in the postganglionic nerve endings. According to current knowledge, that is their only effective mechanism of action.

Cocaine (5 to 10%) is applied to the conjunctiva as a topical anesthetic, a mydriatic, and a test for Horner syndrome. Its mydriatic effect is the result of an accumulation of norepinephrine at the receptor sites of the dilator cells. The transmitter substance builds up at the neuroeffector junction because cocaine prevents the reuptake of the norepinephrine back into the cytoplasm of the nerve ending. Cocaine itself has no direct action on the effector cell, it does not serve to release norepinephrine from the nerve ending, and it does not retard the physiologic release of norepinephrine from the stores in the nerve ending. Its action is indirect, it interferes with the mechanism for prompt disposition of the chemical mediator, and in this respect its action is analogous to that of the anticholinesterases at the cholinergic junction. If the nerve action potentials along the sympathetic pathway are interrupted, as in Horner syndrome, the transmitter substance will not accumulate and the pupil will not dilate. The duration of cocaine mydriasis is quite variable; it may last more than 4 hours. It does not show "rebound miosis."

Sympatholytic Drugs (Adrenergic Blockers)

Thymoxamine HCl (0.5%) and **dapiprazole** ("Rev Eyes") are α-adrenergic blockers that will reverse phenylephrine mydriasis by taking over the α-receptor sites on the iris dilator muscle.

Other Agents

Substance P affects the sphincter fibers directly and will constrict the pupil of a completely atropinized eye. The chief pupillary action of morphine is to cut off cortical inhibition of the iris sphincter nucleus in the midbrain, with resultant miosis. Topical morphine, however, even in strong solutions (5%), has a minimal miotic effect on the pupil. Nalorphine and levallorphan are antinarcotic drugs that when administered parenterally reverse the miotic action of morphine.

Intravenous heroin seems to produce miosis in proportion to its euphoric effect. In a habituated heroin user, the same dose of the drug seems to produce less pupillary constriction than in a naïve subject. Thus, given the plasma drug concentration and the size of the pupil in darkness, it should be possible to produce a measure of the degree of physical dependence in a given individual.

During the induction of anesthesia the patient may be in an excited state and the pupils are often dilated. As the anesthesia deepens, supranuclear inhibition of the sphincter nuclei is cut off and the pupils become small. If the anesthesia becomes dangerously deep and begins to shut down the midbrain, the pupils become dilated and fail to react to light.

The concentration of calcium and magnesium ions in the blood may affect the pupil. Calcium facilitates the release of acetylcholine, and when calcium levels are abnormally low, the amount of acetylcholine liberated by each nerve impulse decreases to less than the level needed to produce a postsynaptic potential, thus effectively blocking synaptic transmission. Magnesium has an opposite effect—a high concentration of magnesium can block transmission and this may dilate the pupil.

IRIS PIGMENT AND PUPILLARY RESPONSE TO DRUGS

In general, the more pigment in the iris, the more slowly the drug takes effect and the longer its action lingers. This is probably because of the drug being bound to iris melanin and then slowly released. It should be noted that there are wide individual differences in pupillary responses to topical drugs. There is probably a greater range of responses among blue eyes than there is between the average response of blue eyes and the average response of dark brown eyes. Some of these individual differences are because of corneal penetration of the drug [4].

References

1. Loewenfeld, I. E. 1993. *The pupil: Anatomy, physiology and clinical applications.* 797–826, 1255–1558. Ames: Iowa State University Press. (This fabulously thorough textbook went quickly out of print and was reprinted by Butterworth-Heinemann in 1997).
2. Thompson, H. S. 1992. The pupil. In *Alder's physiology of the eye*, 9th ed., ed. W. M. Hart, 429. St. Louis: Mosby.
3. Babikian P. V., and H. S. Thompson. 1984. Arecoline miosis [Letter]. *Am. J. Ophthalmol.* 98:514–515.
4. Kardon, R. 1998. Drop the Alzheimer's Drop Test [Editorial]. *Neurology* 50:588–591.

42 Intraocular Pressure and Autonomic Dysfunction

Karen M. Joos
Department of Ophthalmology
Vanderbilt Eye Center
Nashville, Tennessee

The ocular ciliary body produces aqueous humor that nourishes the lens and other ocular structures before exiting the eye, primarily through the trabecular meshwork in the anterior chamber or through the secondary uveal-scleral pathway (Fig. 42.1). An inadequate outflow of aqueous causes an increase of intraocular pressure (IOP). An IOP increase is a significant risk factor for the development of glaucoma. Glaucoma is defined as optic nerve damage in which there is a characteristic acquired loss of retinal ganglion cells and damage to the optic nerve. Vision loss in untreated glaucoma is progressive and permanent. Glaucoma generally is bilateral and affects the peripheral vision initially. It may also occur in patients with measured IOP within the population physiologic range of 10 to 21 mmHg. Therapy is directed at decreasing IOP.

An IOP may also become too low with folds developing in the retina and choroid (hypotony maculopathy), or fluid collecting beneath the choroid to push it upward into the vitreous cavity (choroidal detachment). This may occur after ocular surgery or in inflammatory ocular conditions. Therapy is directed at increasing the IOP.

The regulation of IOP is not well understood, but it may be partially under systemic vascular control [1]. The vascular system is influenced by myogenic tone, local metabolic changes, humoral influences, and autonomic control.

SYSTEMIC BLOOD PRESSURE AND INTRAOCULAR PRESSURE RELATION

A positive correlation has been found between systemic blood pressure and IOP in large population studies. Generally, systolic rather than diastolic blood pressure was the responsible component. This is believed to be caused by increased ultrafiltration in aqueous production. This relation occurs in multiple races and in both sexes [2–5]. The ratio of IOP/systolic blood pressure declines with age in normal populations. Increased peripheral resistance from arteriosclerosis may account for this change [2].

OCULAR BLOOD FLOW

Ocular or optic nerve head blood flow (OBF) is defined with reference to systemic and IOP variables:

$$\begin{aligned} \text{OBF} &= \text{mean ocular perfusion pressure/resistance} \\ &= (2/3 \text{ diastolic blood pressure} + 1/3 \text{ systolic blood pressure} - \text{IOP})/\text{resistance} \end{aligned}$$

From this equation it can be determined that a decrease in blood pressure or an increase in IOP can decrease OBF unless blood pressure and IOP change concurrently or autoregulation is intact to alter resistance. Autoregulation occurs over a physiologic range of pressures. The system can be overcome with extreme changes. For example, normal human OBF autoregulation can be overwhelmed by a marked acute increase of IOP to 45 to 55 mmHg [6]. The lowest IOP that permits ocular autoregulation as indicated by blue-field entopic leukocyte speed in acutely induced ocular hypotension in healthy subjects is 6 mmHg [7].

AUTONOMIC DYSFUNCTION

Patients with autonomic failure can experience dimming of their vision as they assume an upright posture. These symptoms improve with treatment of their autonomic dysfunction. Some also will report ocular pain with wide fluctuations in blood pressure. Untreated patients have significant declines in systolic and diastolic blood pressures, IOPs, and mean ocular perfusion pressures compared with matched control subjects when changing from supine to standing positions [8].

A patient with unbuffered autonomic activity from baroreflex failure can have a strong positive correlation

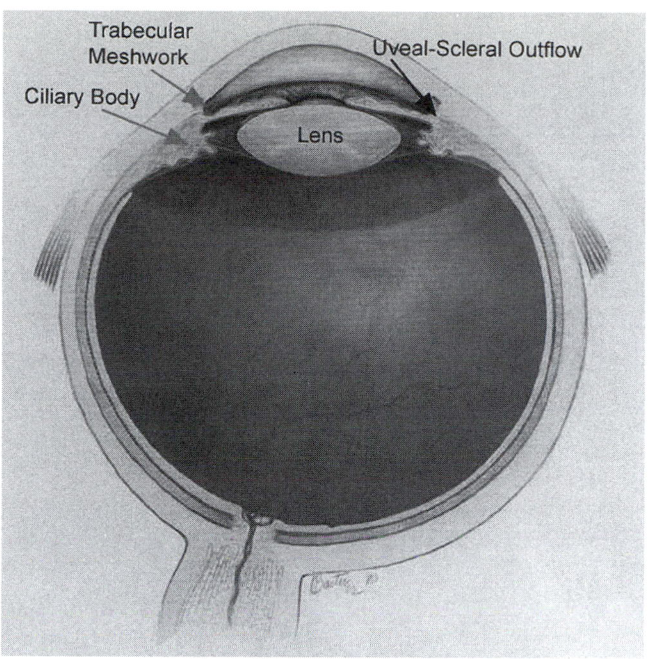

FIGURE 42.1 Ocular anatomy with aqueous inflow and outflow pathways indicated. (Courtesy National Eye Institute, National Institutes of Health, Bethesda, MD.)

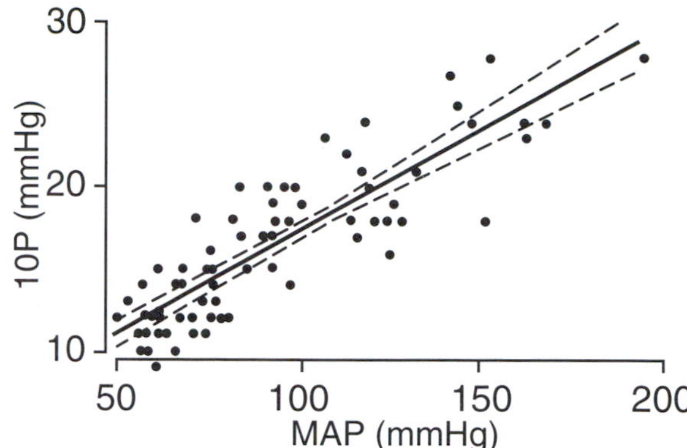

FIGURE 42.2 Correlation of mean arterial pressure (MAP) and intraocular pressure (IOP) in a patient with selective baroreflex failure. *Dotted lines*, 95% confidence interval. (Reprinted with permission from Elsevier: Joos, K. M., S. K. Kakaria, K. S. Lai, J. R. Shannon, and J. Jordan. 1998. Intraocular pressure and baroreflex failure. *Lancet* 351:1704).

between blood pressure and IOP fluctuations (Fig. 42.2) [9]. Values of IOP, mean arterial pressure, and mean ocular perfusion pressure are closest to corresponding control values in the standing position [8]. Through extrapolation, these values increase when position changes from standing to supine in untreated patients with baroreflex failure.

IOP also is associated with blood pressure readings in such forms of primary autonomic failure as multiple system atrophy and pure autonomic failure [8, 10]. A correlation between changes in mean arterial pressure and IOP occurs with variation of positions on a tilt table [10]. With physiologic positional changes in untreated patients, IOP, mean arterial pressures, and mean ocular perfusion pressures were closest to corresponding control values in the supine position [8]. These values decline to less than corresponding control values with a positional change from supine to standing in patients with peripheral or central autonomic dysfunction.

The autonomic system appears to have a significant role in stabilizing IOP and may indirectly act through blood pressure maintenance. Decreases in mean ocular perfusion pressure and the development of symptoms including dimming of vision, eye pain on standing, or both could suggest at least a temporarily overwhelmed ocular autoregulatory capacity.

References

1. Hayreh, S. S. 1997. Factors influencing blood flow in the optic nerve head. *J. Glaucoma* 6:412–425.
2. Shiose, Y. 1990. Intraocular pressure: New perspectives. *Surv. Ophthalmol.* 34:413–435.
3. Bulpitt, C. J., C. Hodes, and M. G. Everitt. 1975. Intraocular pressure and systemic blood pressure in the elderly. *Br. J. Ophthalmol.* 59: 717–720.
4. McLeod, S. D., S. K. West, H. A. Quigley, and J. L. Fozard. 1990. A longitudinal study of the relationship between intraocular and blood pressures. *Invest. Ophthalmol. Vis. Sci.* 31:2361–2366.
5. Leske, M. C., and M. J. Podgor. 1983. Intraocular pressure, cardiovascular risk variables, and visual field defects. *Am. J. Epidemiol.* 118:280–287.
6. Pillunat, L., D. R. Anderson, R. W. Knighton, K. M. Joos, and W. J. Feuer. 1997. Autoregulation of human optic nerve head circulation in response to increased intraocular pressure. *Exp. Eye Res.* 64:737–744.
7. Grunwald, J. E., S. H. Sinclair, and C. E. Riva. 1982. Autoregulation of the retinal circulation in response to decrease of intraocular pressure below normal. *Invest. Ophthalmol. Vis. Sci.* 23:124–127.
8. Singleton, C. D., D. Robertson, D. W. Byrne, and K. M. Joos. 2003. Effect of posture on blood and intraocular pressures in multiple system atrophy, pure autonomic failure, and baroreflex failure. *Circulation* 108:2349–2354.
9. Joos, K. M., S. K. Kakaria, K. S. Lai, J. R. Shannon, and J. Jordan. 1998. Intraocular pressure and baroreflex failure. *Lancet* 351:1704.
10. Dumskyj, M. J., C. J. Mathias, C. J. Dore, K. Bleasdale-Barr, and E. M. Kohner. 2002. Postural variation in intraocular pressure in primary chronic autonomic failure. *J. Neurol.* 249:712–718.

43 Angiotensin II/Autonomic Interactions

Debra I. Diz
Hypertension and Vascular Disease Center
Winston-Salem, North Carolina

David B. Averill
Hypertension and Vascular Disease Center
Winston-Salem, North Carolina

Anatomic studies indicate that Angiotensin (Ang) II receptors are abundant at all levels of the synaptic relays for both sympathetic and parasympathetic branches of the autonomic nervous system. Thus, activation of the renin-angiotensin system (RAS) may have profound consequences on regulation of various autonomic functions.

SYMPATHETIC NERVOUS SYSTEM

Angiotensin II Influence on the Sympathetic Nervous System

Ang II is noted for its facilitatory effects on the sympathetic nervous system (SNS). What is less frequently appreciated is the widespread distribution of Ang II receptors, which positions the peptide to influence function at each relay of the synaptic circuitry of the SNS. Ang II receptors are localized within central nervous system (CNS) sites involved in control of sympathetic outflow: hypothalamus, pons, dorsal medullary centers processing visceral afferent input, and the caudal and rostral ventrolateral medullary (CVLM and RVLM, respectively) centers that ultimately project to sympathetic preganglionic neurons (SPNs). The excitatory actions of Ang II on neurons within hypothalamic and pontine sites are pressor and tachycardic, largely activating descending pathways to increase sympathetic nerve activity in general and to the kidney in particular. Figure 43.1 is a schematic of medullary, spinal, and peripheral sites where Ang II receptors exist. At the level of the dorsal medulla, Ang II excites neurons of the nucleus tractus solitarii (NTS) and A_2 catecholamine cell group. It attenuates baroreceptor reflex actions that restrain sympathetic outflow to heart and vasculature in response to increases in blood pressure. Sympathetic activity to various peripheral organs is the result of the ability of RVLM neurons to integrate inputs from other CNS sites. A number of studies show that Ang II endogenous to the RVLM enhances sympathoexcitation produced by activation of paraventricular neurons of the hypothalamus or by elicitation of the somatosympathetic reflex. In addition, Ang II receptors are located on SPN, in sympathetic chain ganglia, and on sympathetic nerve terminals. At the ganglion, Ang II facilitates synaptic neurotransmission by direct excitation of ganglionic neurons. Complex effects of Ang II at nerve terminals include several important long- and short-term actions. Ang II increases the synthesis of tyrosine hydroxylase in sympathetic nerves, facilitates release of norepinephrine, and prevents reuptake. The adrenal medulla is another site where Ang II receptors exist in great abundance to facilitate catecholamine release.

Sympathetic Nervous System Influence on the Renin-Angiotensin System

The earlier focus on Ang II modulation of SNS activity should not overshadow the considerable influence of the SNS on the RAS. Increased renal sympathetic nerve activity (SNA) is a major stimulus for release of renin through β-adrenergic receptors on juxtaglomerular cells. Along with intrarenal baroreceptors, sodium status and Ang II receptor subtype 1 (AT_1)-mediated feedback is one of four major stimuli regulating renin release. Thus, the SNS and RAS have a reciprocal relation akin to a positive feedback loop. Disorders of this pathway, as seen in certain dysautonomias, may render suboptimal renin release in response to increases in SNS. The resulting postural hypotension with tachycardia reflects the importance of the interplay of these two systems to orthostatic competence.

PARASYMPATHETIC NERVOUS SYSTEM

Angiotensin II Influence on the Parasympathetic Nervous System

Although early studies on the effects of Ang II on the baroreflex yielded information on inhibition of vagal control of heart rate, the sites and mechanisms for these effects were not known. With the revelation in the mid-1980s that Ang II receptors were associated with central and peripheral components of vagal sensory and motor systems, a neuroanatomic substrate was provided for these actions. Subsequent studies clearly show that Ang II receptors are distributed at each synaptic relay within the parasympathetic

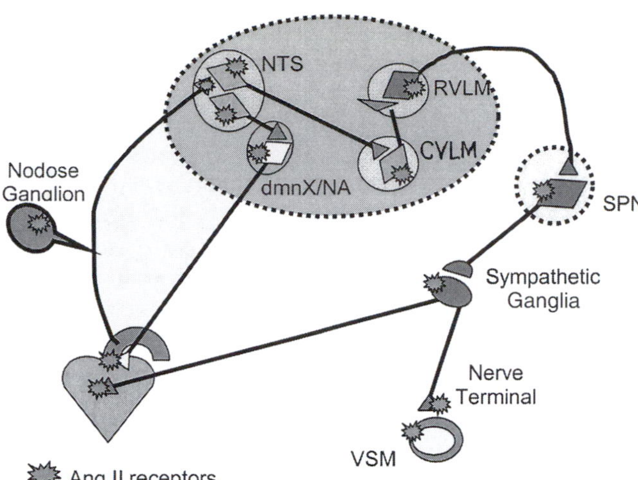

FIGURE 43.1 Neural pathways participating in baroreceptor reflex control of sympathetic and parasympathetic nervous systems. This schema emphasizes the multiple sites where angiotensin (Ang) II may exert actions on reflex control of the autonomic nervous system. Identification of these sites (indicated by the *burst icon*) is based on studies using receptor binding or functional assessment of actions of Ang II on sympathetic or parasympathetic nerve activity. CVLM, caudal ventrolateral medulla; DMN, dorsal motor nucleus of the vagus; NA, nucleus ambiguus; NTS, nucleus tractus solitarii; RVLM, rostral ventrolateral medulla; SPN, sympathetic preganglionic neurons of the intermediolateral cell column; VSM, vascular smooth muscle.

nervous system (PSNS). Ang II influences PSNS outflow through actions at sites in CNS, ganglia, and peripheral end organs (see Fig. 43.1), similar to what is seen for the SNS. Receptors for Ang II are present in the dorsal motor nucleus of the vagus (DMN) and nucleus ambiguus, sites of parasympathetic motor neurons, and in the NTS, site of the first CNS synapse of visceral afferent fibers in the vagus nerve. Ang II has excitatory actions on cells in the NTS and DMN; injection of the peptide at these sites produces depressor and bradycardic actions mediated largely through the cardiac vagus. In the NTS, the response is dependent on substance P. Ang II receptors are found on cell bodies in the nodose ganglion, where excitatory actions are consistent with direct effects on sensory afferent fibers. Potter showed that Ang II inhibited release of acetylcholine from cardiac vagal fibers, evidence consistent with effects on the efferent limb of the system and the presence of receptors in the peripheral vagus nerve.

PHYSIOLOGIC EXAMPLES OF REGULATION/INTERACTIONS

Baroreceptor Reflex

Ang II attenuates the gain or sensitivity of the baroreceptor reflex. Injection of Ang II into the NTS impairs vagally mediated reflex bradycardia demonstrating inhibition of baroreceptor reflex control of heart rate. Blockade of Ang II receptors in the dorsomedial medulla facilitates vagally mediated reflex bradycardia, which underscores the importance of Ang II in tonic modulation of the cardiac baroreflex. This effect occurs particularly by inhibiting the limb of the reflex arc mediating activation of the vagus to slow the heart and inhibition of the sympathetics to slow the heart and reduce tone to the vasculature. The overall effect to control sympathetic outflow is mixed with the most striking influence being to increase or to maintain renal nerve activity even in the face of reductions in other sympathetic nerve activities.

Chemoreceptor Reflex

The role of Ang II in responses to chemoreceptor stimulation is complex (see Reference 4 for review). There are distinct differences in effects depending on the site of action (central or peripheral) and whether the carotid body chemoreceptors or cardiopulmonary chemosensitive afferents are being studied. Facilitation of increases in sympathetic outflow by Ang II in the face of activation of the carotid chemoreceptors may occur at the carotid body itself or at the dorsal and ventral medullary centers serving as sites of integration and relay for the information. In contrast, increased brain Ang II in hypertensive animals is associated with an inhibitory influence on the response to activation of vagal cardiopulmonary sensory afferent fibers that respond to serotonergic stimuli (e.g., phenylbiguanide). This would be consistent with the inhibitory influence of the peptide on baroreceptor responses involving activation of the aortic depressor nerve, another component of the sensory vagus nerve.

Other Sensory Modalities

The presence of Ang II receptors in the motor and sensory vagal system is far more extensive than projections of cardiopulmonary afferent and efferent fibers. This indicates a more widespread role of the peptide in modulation of noncardiovascular aspects of vagal function than currently appreciated including gastric and respiratory function. The association of Ang II receptors at numerous sites in the spinal cord, dorsal root ganglia, and higher CNS areas responsible for integration of sensory neural input provides a potential role for the peptide in influencing pain, stress and anxiety, memory and learning, and temperature regulation (see Reference 4 for review). That each of these contributes to overall autonomic function suggests that important discoveries linking Ang II to a variety of sensorimotor processes await further research.

PATHOPHYSIOLOGY

Hypertension

Enhanced activity of the SNS contributes to the pathogenesis and maintenance of hypertension. Given the evidence presented earlier, it is not surprising that Ang II has been implicated as playing an important role in regulation of sympathetic outflow in hypertension. Experimental studies demonstrated that blockade of Ang II receptors on vasomotor neurons in the RVLM causes a drastic reduction in sympathetic nerve activity emanating from SPNs. With hypertension, the sympathoexcitatory effect of Ang II in the RVLM is even more pronounced, thereby driving enhanced activity of the SNS. In hypertension, Ang II has two actions to significantly alter baroreceptor reflex regulation of SNA. First, the peptide acts in the NTS to reduce the sensitivity of the baroreflex. Thus, for a given increase in arterial pressure, the baroreceptor reflex is less capable of appropriately reducing SNA or activating vagal activity. Second, although Ang II has long been recognized as being a potent vasoconstrictor, this peptide has an independent action in the CNS to shift baroreflex regulation of SNA to greater arterial pressures. This pressure-independent resetting of the baroreflex was demonstrated in rats in which the RAS was stimulated by a low-salt diet. More recently, pressure-independent resetting of the baroreflex to greater arterial pressure was demonstrated in transgenic hypertensive rats that overexpress Ang II in the CNS. Figure 43.2 depicts some of these effects of Ang II on baroreflex control of sympathetic outflow.

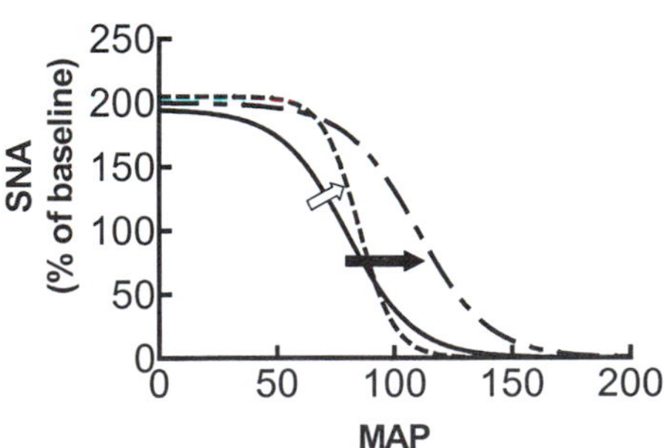

FIGURE 43.2 Influence of Angiotensin (Ang) II on baroreceptor reflex control of sympathetic nerve activity. Each curve illustrates the relation between increases and decreases in mean arterial pressure (MAP) and sympathetic nerve activity (SNA). During resting conditions, the prevailing levels of SNA and MAP are found at the midpoint of each curve. The baroreflex function curve for subjects and animals with normal blood pressures is depicted by the *solid curve*. Ang II–dependent hypertension is associated with a rightward shift of the baroreflex function curve (*solid arrow* and *interrupted line*). Blockade of Ang II receptors shifts the baroreflex curve to decrease pressures and increases the slope of the linear portion of the curve (*open arrow* and *dashed line*).

Congestive Heart Failure

β-Adrenergic blockade and inhibition of angiotensin-converting enzyme dramatically improve the management of patients with congestive heart failure (CHF). Conversely, patients with less heart rate variability and lower vagal tone have increased rates of mortality. These clinical findings underscore important interactions between activation of the RAS and enhanced sympathetic outflow/reduced vagal tone that characterizes CHF. It is particularly interesting that Ang II has dual but opposite actions in regulation of SNA. Studies from Zucker and colleagues show that Ang II increases sensitivity of the cardiac sympathetic afferent reflex, whereas other investigators have found that Ang II blunts arterial baroreflex sensitivity. Although these effects appear opposite, the net effect is to promote enhanced sympathetic outflow to the heart and kidney. Evidence indicates that Ang II acts at AT_1 receptors in the hypothalamus (paraventricular nucleus [PVN]) and the RVLM to modulate reflex regulation of SNA. For both reflexes (cardiac sympathetic afferent reflex and arterial baroreflex) Ang II may down-regulate nitric oxide (NO) synthase activity in the CNS such that reduced production of NO contributes to enhancement of cardiac sympathetic afferent reflex and blunting of arterial baroreflex. Although the PVN has been implicated in these actions of Ang II, further studies need to explore whether this modulation of NO exists at other brain sites implicated in Ang II-mediated regulation of SNA.

Consequences of Ang II–Mediated Enhancement of Sympathetic Nerve Activity to the Kidney

Both hypertension and CHF are typified by dysregulation of salt and water balance by the kidney. In both situations, Ang II may act directly in the kidney to promote salt and water retention. However, it is currently appreciated that increased SNA to the kidney also promotes sodium reabsorption. Thus, the aforementioned actions of Ang II in the CNS may be directed importantly to increase renal SNA, thereby reinforcing the direct renal actions of Ang II for retention of salt and water. Ang II also is associated with renal nerve activation in the face of ganglionic blockade, suggesting direct ganglionic effects to increase nerve activity.

Receptor Pharmacology

Ang II acts through at least two separate receptors: the AT_1 and AT_2 subtypes. The majority of actions of Ang II on the SNS and PSNS are mediated by AT_1 receptors. Within the CNS, however, AT_2 receptors may play a role in neuronal cell maturation and differentiation, growth, repair, and pain threshold. In the adrenal, both AT_2 and AT_1 receptors are responsible for the increase in catecholamine release. An important consideration in understanding the complexities of the interactions between the SNA and RAS are reports suggesting that Ang II alters α_2-receptor affinity. These studies suggest a decreased function of the major receptor involved in mitigating activation of the SNS at the level of the CNS.

Antihypertensive therapy with converting enzyme inhibitors or AT_1 receptor blockers removes the positive modulatory actions of Ang II on SNS activity. As indicated earlier in heart failure or hypertension, the improvements seen are largely because of attenuation of SNS overactivity mediated by actions at each level of the system. With the increasing use of AT_1 receptor blockers in treatment of hypertension, it should be noted that many of these compounds contain imidazole moieties. At greater doses, potential interactions with other biologically important receptors, such as the thromboxane A_2 receptor and imidazoline/guanidinium receptor sites, may occur to confound interpretation of results.

CONCLUSIONS

Ang II is well positioned for regulation of both SNS and PSNS, which emphasizes the importance and multiplicity of pathways by which Ang II contributes to cardiovascular homeostasis. The wider role of this peptide with respect to noncardiovascular actions includes potential influences on learning and cognitive function, pain and anxiety, vagally mediated insulin release, control of G-I function, and regulation of whole body metabolism. These latter aspects require further elucidation.

References

1. Averill, D. B., and D. I. Diz. 2001. Angiotensin peptides and baroreflex control of sympathetic outflow: Pathways and mechanisms of the medulla oblongata [Review]. *Brain Res. Bull.* 51:119–128.
2. Dampney, R. A., Y. Hirooka, P. D. Potts, and G. A. Head. 1996. Functions of angiotensin peptides in the rostral ventrolateral medulla [Review]. *Clin. Exp. Pharmacol. Physiol.* 3:S105–S111.
3. DiBona, G. F. 2001. Peripheral and central interactions between the renin-angiotensin system and the renal sympathetic nerves in control of renal function. *Ann. NY Acad. Sci.* 940:395–406.
4. Diz, D. I. 1999. Commentary: Angiotensin II receptors in central nervous system physiology. In *Drugs, enzymes and receptors of the renin angiotensin system: Celebrating a century of discovery*, ed. A. Husain and R. Graham. New York: Harwood Academic Publishers.
5. Diz, D. I., J. A. Jessup, B. M. Westwood, S. M. Bosch, S. Vinsant, P. E. Gallagher, and D. B. Averill. 2001. Angiotensin peptides as neurotransmitters/neuromodulators in the dorsomedial medulla [Review]. *Clin. Exp. Pharmacol. Physiol.* 29:473–482.
6. Jordan, J., J. Shannon, and D. Robertson. 1997. The physiological conundrum of hyperadrenergic orthostatic intolerance. *Chin. J. Physiol.* 40:1–8.
7. Langer, S. Z., and P. E. Hicks. 1984. Physiology of the sympathetic nerve ending [Review]. *Br. J. Anaesth.* 56:689–700.
8. Ma, X., F. M. Abboud, and M. W. Chapleau. 2001. A novel effect of angiotensin on renal sympathetic nerve activity. *J. Hypertens.* 19(3 Pt 2):609–618.
9. McKinley, M. J., A. L. Albiston, A. M. Allen, M. L. Mathai, C. N. May, R. M. McAllen, B. J. Oldfield, F. A. Mendelsohn, and S. Y. Chai. 2003. The brain renin-angiotensin system: Location and physiological roles. *Int. J. Biochem. Cell Biol.* 35:901–918.
10. The Heart Outcomes Prevention Evaluation Study Investigators. 2000. Effects of an angiotensin-converting-enzyme inhibitor, ramipril, on cardiovascular events in high-risk patients. *N. Engl. J. Med.* 342:145–153.
11. Zucker, I. H., W. Wang, R. U. Pliquett, J.-L. Liu, and K. P. Patel. 2001. The regulation of sympathetic outflow in heart failure: The roles of angiotensin II, nitric oxide, and exercise training [Review]. *Ann. NY Acad. Sci.* 940:431–433.

44 Autonomic Effects of Anesthesia

Thomas J. Ebert
Department of Anesthesiology
Medical College of Wisconsin
Milwaukee, Wisconsin

Anesthetic agents vary in their chemical structure and also vary in their ability to influence the autonomic nervous system (ANS). The anesthetic agents with the most significant effects on the ANS are the potent volatile anesthetic gases, which are derivatives of ether. They include halothane, isoflurane, sevoflurane, and desflurane. Liquid anesthetics also are used for intravenous (IV) induction of anesthesia (establish unconsciousness); the three most common liquid anesthetics are sodium thiopental, etomidate, and propofol. Propofol (2,6-di-isopropylphenol) is a sedative/hypnotic that can be used in low doses for sedation and in greater doses to induce anesthesia. Of these IV anesthetic agents, the one with the least influence on the ANS and baroreflex control of autonomic outflow is etomidate [1]. Etomidate is commonly used to initiate anesthesia in the compromised patient, including those with impaired autonomic control.

DIRECT EFFECTS OF ANESTHETICS ON SYMPATHETIC OUTFLOW

Intravenous Anesthetics (Sedative/Hypnotics)

One of the more popular techniques is to establish general anesthesia with an IV bolus of propofol followed by a maintenance infusion. This is commonly associated with substantial hypotension. Investigations using human sympathetic microneurography have clearly identified propofol to be a potent inhibitor of sympathetic efferent activity [1, 2]. The mechanism is probably central in origin, but also may involve depression of baroreflex function. For maintenance of anesthesia, propofol is commonly infused in combination with inhalation of the nonpotent anesthetic, nitrous oxide (typically 50–70% inspired concentration). This allows the use of less propofol and results in modest return of sympathetic outflow, baroreflex function, and blood pressure. Earlier work has indicated that nitrous oxide maintains or slightly increases sympathetic outflow when used in concentrations of 20 to 40% [3].

Another common anesthetic agent is the sedative/hypnotic and amnestic drug, midazolam. This is a benzodiazepine that has the ability to decrease sympathetic outflow, although not to the extent of propofol. It is not commonly associated with decreases in blood pressure, which suggests that the recorded decrease in sympathetic outflow may be regional and that other sympathetic beds might respond differently to this drug, such that blood pressure is maintained.

The potent anesthetic gases appear to have multiple effects on the ANS, and detailed dissection of these effects has been reported in animal studies (Fig. 44.1). These gases impair cardiac–vagal activity as suggested by a loss of respiratory sinus arrhythmia. The anesthetic gases (aside from halothane) are associated with dose-dependent decreases in blood pressure. This effect is most likely because of their ability to directly relax vascular smooth muscle rather than to inhibit sympathetic outflow. Direct recordings of human sympathetic outflow indicate that the commonly used anesthetic gases, isoflurane and sevoflurane, have little effect on basal sympathetic activity (Fig. 44.2) [4]. The outlier is desflurane. For unclear reasons, desflurane increases sympathetic outflow and norepinephrine levels with increasing concentrations.[1] The curious finding with desflurane is that the increase in sympathetic outflow does not sustain blood pressure (see Fig. 44.2). Desflurane also has the ability to cause substantial surges in sympathetic outflow when the inspired concentration is increased rapidly [5]. This is likely related to the pungency of this anesthetic and subsequent activation of airway irritant receptors when desflurane is used in high concentrations [6]. Halothane is the single volatile anesthetic still in limited clinical use that maintains sympathetic outflow and peripheral resistance. Blood pressure decreases from halothane have been attributed to direct myocardial depression.

[1] Anesthetic gases are typically given as a fraction of the total inspired gas concentration and range anywhere from 0.5 to 11% inspired concentrations. They are expressed as multiples of MAC (minimum alveolar concentration). This is the concentration of anesthetic gas at steady state that will prevent 50% of patients from moving to a surgical stimulus. One MAC of sevoflurane, isoflurane, and desflurane in a 45-year-old patient is 2%, 1.2%, and 6% expired concentration, respectively.

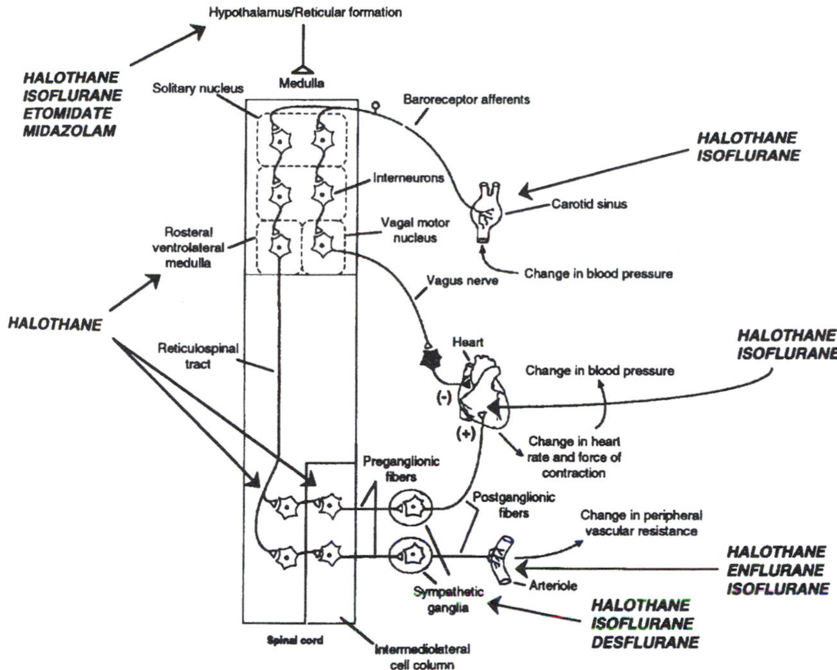

FIGURE 44.1 This schematic of the baroreflex pathway exemplifies neural mechanisms of cardiovascular control. Specific sites of anesthetic action are summarized. Volatile anesthetics can sensitize baroreceptors to increase afferent activity, but most efferent sites are depressed by anesthetic agents. Other agents such as barbiturates, propofol, narcotics, desflurane, and sevoflurane also are known to affect neural control of the vasculature at various levels. However, the actions of the agents at sites indicated in this figure have been specifically identified in different studies. (Reprinted with permission from Stekiel, T. A., W. J. Stekiel, and Z. J. Bosnjak. 1997. The peripheral vasculature. In *Anesthesia biologic foundations*, ed. T. L. Yaksh, C. Lynch, W. M. Zapol, M. Maze, J. F. Biebuyck, and L. J. Saidman, 1159. Philadelphia, Lippincott-Raven.)

HUMAN BAROREFLEX FUNCTION AND ANESTHETIC GASES

The maintenance of baroreflex control of the circulation would serve as an important counter-regulatory mechanism in the face of surgical blood loss. Unfortunately, the baroreflex is reasonably attenuated during general anesthesia.

Low-Pressure (Cardiopulmonary) Baroreflexes

Although little information exists on the function of this reflex during anesthesia, several studies performed with lower body negative pressure (LBNP) have provided some important insights. Cardiopulmonary baroreflex activation of sympathetic outflow and peripheral resistance can be triggered by graded applications of LBNP to reduce central venous pressure. In awake patients, blood pressure (BP) does not decrease during this preload reduction because peripheral resistance is increased (Fig. 44.3). However, during general anesthesia with clinically relevant doses of halothane, the reflex increase in sympathetic outflow, and therefore vascular resistance, is markedly attenuated during LBNP. Thus, BP is not well maintained, which predisposes patients to exaggerated effects of blood volume loss during anesthesia [7]. This is not true for all anesthetics. Sometimes combinations of greater doses of fentanyl with diazepam or midazolam are used to achieve a general anesthetic state. This combination of drugs clearly preserves reflex function during application of LBNP [8] (see Fig. 44.3).

High-Pressure Baroreflexes

Many anesthetics sensitize the baroreceptors themselves, such that afferent activity of these receptors has been found to increase. However, recordings from both preganglionic and postganglionic sites have indicated a decrease in efferent activity (see Fig. 44.1).

Intravenous Anesthetics

The primary IV anesthetic used for general anesthesia is propofol. It is clear that this substance impairs reflex control of sympathetic outflow [2]. Interestingly, reflex control of

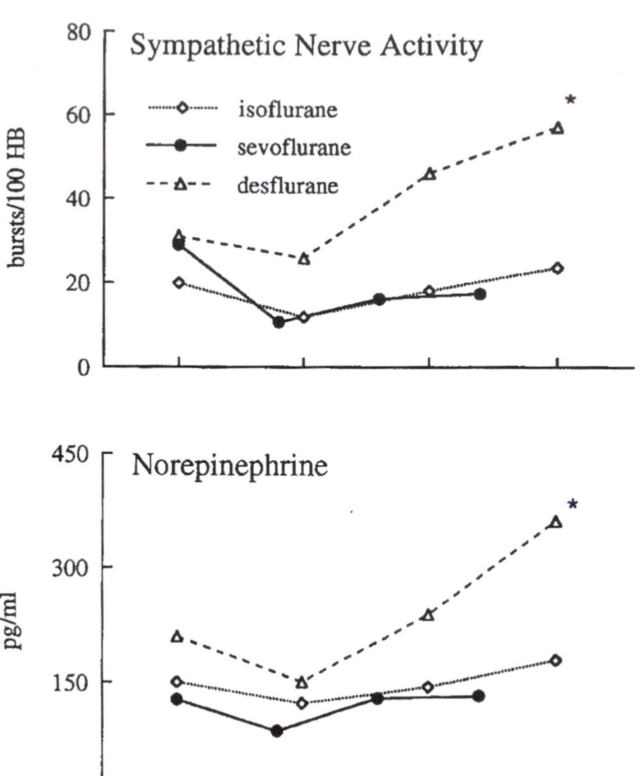

FIGURE 44.2 Sympathetic nerve activity and plasma norepinephrine concentration responses to steady-state periods of anesthesia with desflurane, isoflurane, or sevoflurane in healthy volunteers. During the administration of isoflurane and sevoflurane, there were no significant changes in basal levels of sympathetic nerve activity and circulating norepinephrine concentrations. However, at desflurane concentrations greater than 0.5 minimum alveolar anesthetic concentration, there were increases in sympathetic outflow leading to significant increases in plasma norepinephrine. Bursts/100HB, bursts per 100 heart beats. (Reprinted with permission from Ebert, T. J., C. P. Harkin, and M. Muzi. 1995. Cardiovascular responses to sevoflurane: A review. *Anesth. Analg.* 81:S11–S22.)

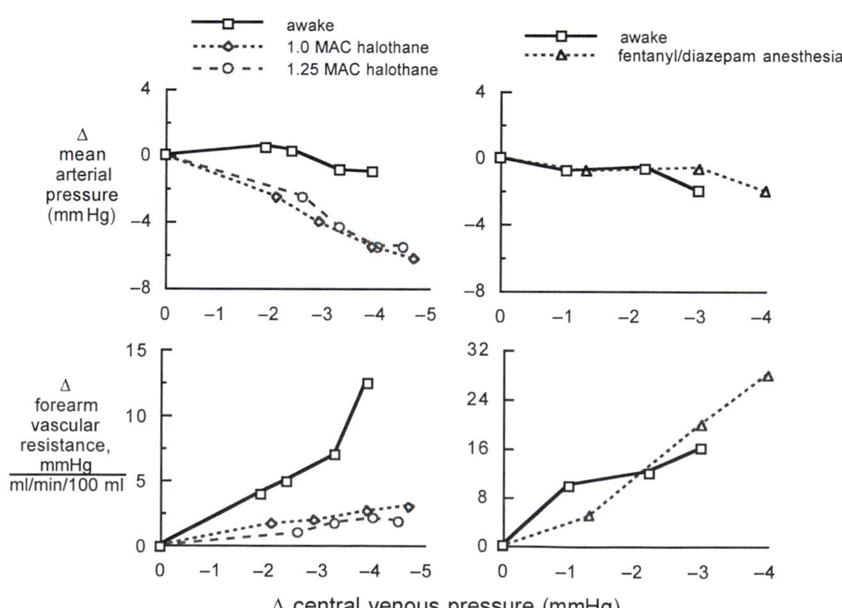

FIGURE 44.3 Low-pressure cardiopulmonary baroreflex control of peripheral resistance during two different approaches to general anesthesia. Lower body negative pressure (LBNP) was used to produce progressive reductions in central venous pressure triggering increases in peripheral resistance. Halothane anesthesia at each of two clinically relevant doses impaired the reflex response and blood pressure (BP) was compromised. In contrast, general anesthesia with a combination of fentanyl and diazepam preserved reflex vasoconstriction to LBNP, and therefore prevented BP from decreasing.

heart rate (a vagal mechanism) is well preserved with the use of propofol.

Inhaled Agents

The three most common clinical inhaled anesthetic gases appear to have similar effects on baroreflex function in humans (Fig. 44.4). At low concentrations, slightly less than clinically relevant concentrations, there is only a slight depression of the reflex control of sympathetic outflow and heart rate. However, at 1.0 and 1.5 MAC, these gases clearly depress baroreflex control of heart rate and sympathetic outflow. There do not appear to be differences among the three commonly used anesthetic gases [4].

In summary, most anesthetic gases and IV agents have relatively consistent effects to diminish autonomic control mechanisms in humans. This removes an important compensatory mechanism to maintain blood pressure in the face of blood volume decreases during surgical procedures. Despite this adverse situation, cardiovascular homeostasis, specifically blood pressure support for patients under anesthesia, typically is through direct acting pharmacologic agents and generous IV fluid supplementation to help maintain or increase intravascular volume. Other techniques used to achieve anesthesia include spinal and epidural regional anesthesia with drugs such as lidocaine or bupivacaine given into either the cerebrospinal fluid at the lumbar level or the epidural space. Commonly, sympathetic denervation below the mid-thoracic level is achieved through spinal or epidural anesthesia, resulting in vasodilation and decreases in blood pressure. Compensatory baroreflex control of upper extremity and cardiac function is maintained to help offset many of these unwanted peripheral vasodilating effects.

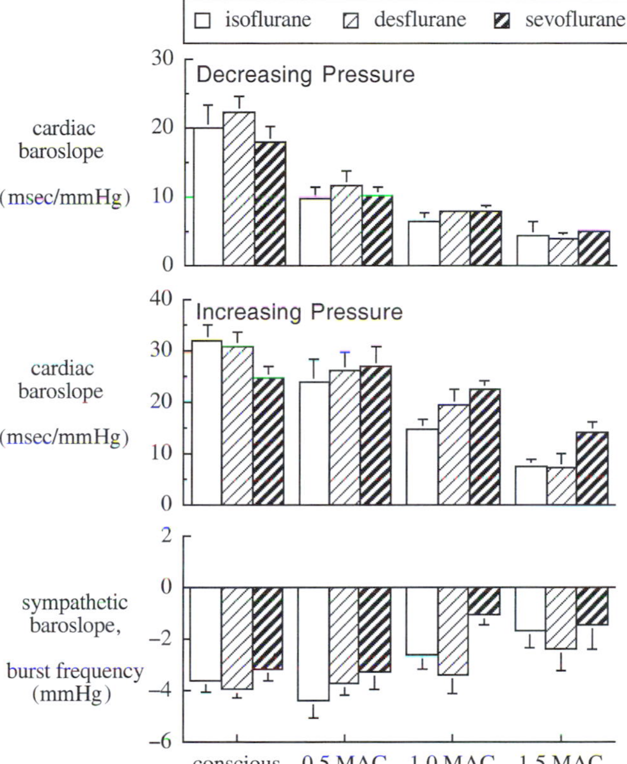

FIGURE 44.4 Summary data of the high-pressure, arterial baroreflex regulation of heart rate (R-R interval, cardiac baroslope) and sympathetic nerve activity (sympathetic baroslope) in response to pharmacologically induced blood pressure changes. In general, the reflex control of heart rate and of sympathetic outflow are decreased progressively with increasing clinically relevant concentrations of these three popular anesthetic gases. Choosing lower concentrations of these potent gases in combination with intravenous drugs such as fentanyl (an opioid) and benzodiazepines best preserves reflex control. (Reprinted with permission from Ebert T. J., C. P. Harkin, and M. Muzi. 1995. Cardiovascular responses to sevoflurane: A review. *Anesth. Analg.* 81:S11–S22.)

References

1. Ebert, T. J., M. Muzi, R. Berens, D. Goff, and J. P. Kampine. 1992. Sympathetic responses to induction of anesthesia in humans with propofol or etomidate. *Anesthesiology* 76:725–733.
2. Ebert, T. J., and M. Muzi. 1994. Propofol and autonomic reflex function in humans. *Anesth. Analg.* 78:369–375.
3. Ebert, T. J., and J. P. Kampine. 1989. Nitrous oxide augments sympathetic outflow: Direct evidence from human peroneal nerve recordings. *Anesth. Analg.* 69:444–449.
4. Ebert, T. J., C. P. Harkin, and M. Muzi. 1995. Cardiovascular responses to sevoflurane: A review. *Anesth. Analg.* 81:S11–S22.
5. Ebert, T. J., M. Muzi, and C. W. Lopatka. 1995. Neurocirculatory responses to sevoflurane in humans: A comparison to desflurane. *Anesthesiology* 83:88–95.
6. Muzi, M., T. J. Ebert, W. G. Hope, B. J. Robinson, and L. B. Bell. 1996. Site(s) mediating sympathetic activation with desflurane. *Anesthesiology* 85:737–747.
7. Ebert, T. J., K. J. Kotrly, E. J. Vucins, C. Z. Pattison, and J. P. Kampine. 1985. Halothane anesthesia attenuates cardiopulmonary baroreflex control of peripheral resistance in humans. *Anesthesiology* 63:668–674.
8. Ebert, T. J., K. J. Kotrly, K. E. Madsen, J. S. Bernstein, and J. P. Kampine. 1988. Fentanyl-diazepam anesthesia with or without N_2O does not attenuate cardiopulmonary baroreflex-mediated vasoconstrictor responses to controlled hypovolemia in humans. *Anesth. Analg.* 67:548–554.

45 Peripheral Dopamine Systems

Graeme Eisenhofer
Clinical Neurocardiology Section
National Institutes of Neurological Disorders and Stroke
National Institutes of Health
Bethesda, Maryland

David S. Goldstein
Clinical Neurocardiology Section
National Institutes of Neurological Disorders and Stroke
National Institutes of Health
Bethesda, Maryland

Dopamine is usually thought of as a neurotransmitter in the brain or as an intermediate in the production of norepinephrine and epinephrine in the periphery. It has been presumed that these sources account for the large amounts of dopamine and its metabolites excreted in urine. The contribution of the brain to circulating levels and urinary excretion of dopamine metabolites is now known to be minor. Also, in sympathetic nerves and the adrenal medulla, most dopamine is converted to norepinephrine. Therefore, other sources and functions of dopamine in the periphery have to be considered. Emerging evidence suggests the presence of a third peripheral catecholamine system, in which dopamine functions not as a neurotransmitter or circulating hormone, but as an autocrine or paracrine substance (Table 45.1).

DOPAMINE IN THE KIDNEYS

In the kidneys, dopamine is now well established as an autocrine/paracrine effector substance contributing to the regulation of sodium excretion. Unlike neuronal catecholamine systems, production of dopamine in the kidneys is largely independent of local synthesis of L-dihydroxyphenylalanine (L-dopa) by tyrosine hydroxylase. Thus, renal denervation does not affect urinary dopamine excretion. Instead, production of dopamine in the kidneys depends mainly on proximal tubular cell uptake of L-dopa from the circulation. The L-dopa is then converted to dopamine by aromatic amino acid decarboxylase, the activity of which is up-regulated by a high-salt diet and down-regulated by a low-salt diet.

It is not exactly clear how the dopamine produced in renal tubules is secreted to exert its natriuretic actions. The presence in kidneys of plasma membrane transporters that use dopamine as a substrate suggests one possible mechanism of secretion of the amine. Other possible points of regulation include the uptake of L-dopa through another transporter and intracellular metabolism of dopamine by catechol-O-methyltransferase and monoamine oxidase.

The presence of a renal dopamine paracrine/autocrine system explains the considerable amounts of free dopamine excreted in the urine, which exceeds amounts for the other catecholamines. Most dopamine in urine derives from renal uptake and decarboxylation of circulating L-dopa and reflects the function of the renal dopamine paracrine/autocrine system.

DOPAMINE IN THE GASTROINTESTINAL TRACT

Although the kidneys represent the major source of urinary free dopamine, this source does not account for the larger amounts of excreted dopamine metabolites, such as homovanillic acid and dopamine sulfate. Findings of large arterial to portal venous increases in plasma concentrations of dopamine and its metabolites imply that substantial amounts of dopamine are produced in the gastrointestinal tract. Mesenteric organs account for between 40 and 50% of the dopamine produced in the body that is not converted to norepinephrine or epinephrine.

The substantial production and metabolism of dopamine in the human gastrointestinal tract suggests that dopamine functions as an enteric neuromodulator or paracrine/autocrine substance. Dopamine and dopamine receptor agonists stimulate bicarbonate secretion and protect against ulcer formation, whereas dopamine antagonists augment secretion of gastric acid and promote ulcer development. Dopamine also appears to influence gastrointestinal motility, sodium transport, and gastric and intestinal submucosal blood flow. In the pancreas, dopamine may modulate secretion of digestive enzymes and bicarbonate.

Morphologic studies have demonstrated the presence of cells in the gastrointestinal tract that contain dopamine and express components of dopamine-signaling pathways, including catecholamine biosynthetic enzymes and specific dopamine receptors and transporters. In the stomach, tyrosine hydroxylase is expressed in epithelial cells, including acid-secreting parietal cells. In the small intestine, cells of the lamina propria, including immune cells, also express tyrosine hydroxylase. The enzyme is additionally found in pancreatic exocrine cells.

The high rates of dopamine production by mesenteric organs cannot be accounted for by local extraction and decarboxylation of circulating L-dopa. Thus, unlike in the

TABLE 45.1 Peripheral Catecholamine Systems

Catecholamine	System	Mechanism	Disorder
Norepinephrine (noradrenaline)	Sympathetic nervous system	Neurotransmitter	Hypertension Heart failure PAD/MSA/PD
Epinephrine (adrenaline)	Adrenomedullary hormonal system	Hormone	Distress
Dopamine	Dopa–dopamine system	Autocrine/paracrine substance	Hypertension? Peptic ulcer?

kidneys, where dopamine is produced mainly from circulating L-dopa, in the gastrointestinal tract, production of dopamine requires the presence of tyrosine hydroxylase or other sources of L-dopa.

DIET AND DOPAMINE SULFATE

Consumption of food increases plasma concentrations of L-dopa, dopamine, and dopamine metabolites, particularly dopamine sulfate, indicating that dietary constituents may also represent an important source of peripheral dopamine. Such a source does not, however, account for the substantial amounts of dopamine produced in peripheral tissues outside of the digestive tract, or of that produced in digestive tissues of fasting individuals. In particular, plasma concentrations of both L-dopa and dopamine sulfate remain high even after a 3-day fast.

The source and physiologic significance of dopamine sulfate, which is present in plasma at much greater concentrations than of free dopamine, have long posed a puzzle. Although liver, brain, and platelets have all been suggested sources, it is now clear that dopamine sulfate is mainly produced in the gastrointestinal tract from both dietary and locally synthesized dopamine. The substantial contribution of mesenteric organs to the production of the sulfate conjugates of dopamine and other catecholamines and their metabolites is consistent with findings that the gastrointestinal tract contains high concentrations of the sulfotransferase isoenzyme, SULT1A3. In humans, a single amino acid substitution confers on this isoenzyme a high affinity for metabolism of monoamines, particularly dopamine. Production of sulfate conjugates in the digestive tract could provide an enzymatic "gut–blood barrier," for detoxifying dietary biogenic amines and delimiting physiologic effects of locally produced dopamine.

PERSPECTIVES

Because of the different sources of dopamine in the periphery, sources that are distinct from those of the other catecholamines, one may speculate that abnormalities of peripheral dopamine systems will manifest clinically in ways that the concept of a unitary "sympathoadrenal system" would not predict. For example, dopamine deficiency in the digestive tract might contribute to gastric or duodenal ulcers; abnormalities in the enzymatic "gut–blood barrier" might increase toxicity from ingested monoamines; and interferences with the renal L-dopa–dopamine system might promote sodium-retaining states.

References

1. Goldstein, D. S., E. Mezey, T. Yamamoto, A. Åneman, P. Friberg, and G. Eisenhofer. 1995. Is there a third peripheral catecholaminergic system? Endogenous dopamine as an autocrine/paracrine substance derived from plasma DOPA and inactivated by conjugation. *Hypertens. Res.* 18:S93–S99.
2. Carey, R. M. 2001. Theodore Cooper Lecture. Renal dopamine system: Paracrine regulator of sodium homeostasis and blood pressure. *Hypertension* 38:297–302.
3. Soares-da-Silva, P, and M. A. Vieira-Coelho. 1998. Nonneuronal dopamine. *Adv. Pharmacol.* 42:866–869.
4. Eisenhofer, G., A. Aneman, P. Friberg, D. Hooper, L. Fandriks, H. Lonroth, B. Hunyady, and E. Mezey. 1997. Substantial production of dopamine in the human gastrointestinal tract. *J. Clin. Endocrinol. Metab.* 82:3864–3871.
5. Flemstrom, G., and B. Safsten. 1994. Role of dopamine and other stimuli of mucosal bicarbonate secretion in duodenal protection. *Dig. Dis. Sci.* 39:1839–1842.
6. Mezey, E., G. Eisenhofer, S. Hansson, G. Harta, B. J. Hoffman, K. Gallatz, M. Palkovits, and B. Hunyady. 1999. Non-neuronal dopamine in the gastrointestinal system. *Clin. Exp. Pharmacol. Physiol. Suppl.* 26:S14–S22.
7. Eisenhofer, G., M. W. Coughtrie, and D. S. Goldstein. 1999. Dopamine sulphate: An enigma resolved. *Clin. Exp. Pharmacol. Physiol. Suppl.* 26:S41–S53.

46 Dopamine Mechanisms in the Kidney

Robert M. Carey
Division of Endocrinology
University of Virginia Health Systems
Charlottesville, Virginia

RENAL DOPAMINE FORMATION AND EXCRETION

Dopamine (DA) biosynthesis in the kidney occurs in proximal tubule cells (PTC) as a result of uptake of filtered L-dihydroxyphenylalanine (L-dopa) by way of a sodium transporter in the apical (brush border) membrane. Once inside the PTC, L-dopa is rapidly decarboxylated to DA through aromatic amino acid decarboxylase, the activity of which is dependent on the sodium load to the tubule. DA is secreted by PTC either across the apical or basolateral membrane. The basolateral outward transporter also is dependent on sodium and pH.

The supply of L-dopa to the PTC is the major regulator of DA synthesis and secretion. *In vivo*, DA is preferentially secreted across the apical membrane into the tubule lumen, as the increase in urinary DA far exceeds its increment in the renal interstitial fluid [1]. In contrast to the usual pathway for DA biosynthesis in neurons, in the kidney DA is synthesized independently of nerve activity. Figure 46.1 depicts the scheme of DA formation and secretion in the PTC.

RENAL DOPAMINE RECEPTOR EXPRESSION

D_1-Like and D_2-like receptor families are expressed at postjunctional sites within the kidney. The D_1 receptor (D_{1A} in the rodent) and probably also the D_5 receptor (D_{1B} in the rodent) are localized in the smooth muscle cells of renal arterioles, juxtaglomerular cells, PTC, and cortical collecting duct (CCD) both by immunohistochemistry and by *in situ* amplification of mRNA [2, 3]. The D_3 receptor is localized in renal arterioles, glomeruli, PTC, medullary thick ascending limb cells, and the CCD by immunohistochemistry [4]. The D_4 receptor is localized specifically in the CCD. Renal DA receptor distribution is shown in Table 46.1.

DOPAMINERGIC REGULATION OF RENAL SODIUM EXCRETION

D_1-Like Receptors

The renal D_1-like receptor family plays a major role in the regulation of tubule sodium transport. The natriuretic action of DA is caused by inhibition of both proximal and distal tubule sodium reabsorption. The action of endogenous DA to inhibit tubule sodium transport is distinct from the renal vasodilator action of exogenous DA, which depends on increased plasma concentrations of DA [5].

A major cell-signaling process whereby renal DA induces natriuresis is inhibition of Na^+,K^+-ATPase along the entire nephron (PTC, thick ascending limb of Henle's loop, distal tubule, and CCD). This action is thought to be mediated by the D_1-like receptor family, although synergism between D_1- and D_2-like receptors in the inhibition of Na^+,K^+-ATPase has been demonstrated.

The signaling processes whereby DA inhibits Na^+,K^+-ATPase activity are nephron-specific [6]. Both protein kinase A (PKA) and protein kinase C (PKC) are involved in the PTC, whereas only PKA is required in the medullary thick ascending limb and CCD. PKA and PKC phosphorylate the catalytic subunit of the enzyme inhibiting its activity.

A primary component of the regulation of Na^+,K^+-ATPase by DA is the action to inhibit the Na^+/H^+ exchanger (NHE) and the Na^+/P_1 cotransporter in the apical membrane of the tubule cell. This action of DA inhibits transport of Na^+ into the cell, thus rendering intracellular Na^+ too low to stimulate Na^+,K^+-ATPase. The ability of DA to inhibit NHE activity is primarily because of activation of cyclic adenosine monophosphate (cAMP) and PKA, but also can occur through D_1-like receptors directly without involving cAMP and PKA. DA also can inhibit NHE activity by stimulation of P-450 eicosanoids such as 20-HETE.

Endogenous intrarenal DA is a major physiologic regulator of urinary sodium excretion *in vivo* [7]. About 50% of basal sodium excretion during normal sodium balance is controlled by DA. There is currently clear evidence that renal DA acts as a paracrine substance (cell-to-cell

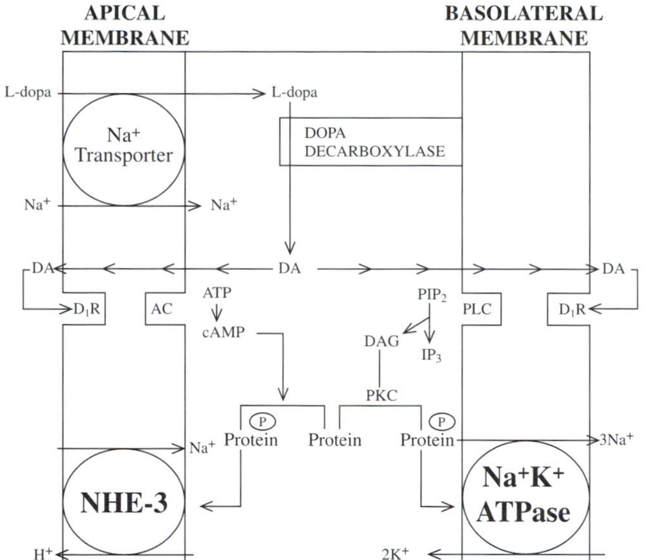

FIGURE 46.1 Schematic depiction of dopamine formation and cell-signaling mechanisms activating sodium transport across the proximal tubule cell. AC, adenylyl clyclase; DA, dopamine; DAG, diacylglycerol; D_1R, dopamine D_1 receptor; PLC, phospholipase C.

TABLE 46.1 Renal Dopamine Receptor Expression

	Receptor subtype				
Tissue Expression	D_1	D_2	D_3	D_4	D_5
Arterioles	+	−	+	−	+
Glomerulus	−	−	+	−	−
Proximal tubule	+	−	+	−	+
mTal	+	−	+	−	+
Distal tubule	+	−	+	−	+
Cortical collecting duct	+	−	+	+	+
Renal nerves	−	+	−	+	−
Juxtaglomerular cells	+	−	+?	−	+?

mediator) locally modulating renal sodium excretion by an action at the renal tubule independently of renal hemodynamic function [7]. This has been demonstrated both by pharmacologic blockade of the renal D_1-like receptor family and also by antisense oligonucleotide-induced inhibition of D_{1A} receptor protein expression [7, 8].

D_2-Like Receptors

Evidence suggests that the renal D_3 receptor may increase glomerular filtration rate through postglomerular (efferent) arteriolar constriction. Also, a D_2-like receptor, possibly D_4, in the basolateral membrane of CCD cells is probably responsible for a natriuretic action of DA in this tubule segment. However, relatively little is known about the D_2-like receptor family, compared with D_1-like receptors, in the control of sodium excretion.

TABLE 46.2 Effects of Renal Dopamine Receptor Stimulation

D_1-LIKE RECEPTORS (D_1 and D_5)
- Vasodilation of renal arterioles (requires circulating DA)
- Inhibition of proximal and distal tubule sodium reabsorption
- Stimulation of renin secretion
- Inhibition of angiotensin AT_1 receptor expression

D_2 RECEPTOR
- Inhibition of norepinephrine release from renal sympathetic neurons

D_3 RECEPTOR
- Inhibition of renin secretion
- Inhibition of angiotensin AT_1 receptor expression
- Possible increase in glomerular filtration
- Possible vasodilation of renal arterioles
- Possible inhibition of tubule sodium reabsorption (natriuresis)

D_4 RECEPTOR
- Possible inhibition of sodium reabsorption in the cortical collecting duct

PHYSIOLOGIC INTERACTIONS OF THE RENAL DOPAMINERGIC SYSTEM AND THE RENIN-ANGIOTENSIN SYSTEM

In addition to direct modulation of renal tubule sodium transport, DA stimulates renin release from renal juxtaglomerular cells through the D_1-like receptor family. The interaction of DA with the renin-angiotensin system (Fig. 46.2) is an area of continuing investigation. DA has been demonstrated to decrease PTC angiotensin AT_1 receptor expression through the D_{1A} receptor; therefore it appears that the net effect of DA is to increase intrarenal angiotensin II and to down-regulate its actions. Current evidence suggests that DA may promote natriuresis both by direct action at the renal tubule and indirectly by decreasing angiotensin II–stimulated sodium reabsorption [9]. The renal D_3 receptor is thought to inhibit renin secretion and may also inhibit AT_1 receptor expression.

Renal DA serves as one of several paracrine mediators of renal sodium excretion. During low sodium intake, sodium is retained to meet the body's requirement for sodium homeostasis. Under these conditions, the renin-angiotensin system is stimulated and DA biosynthesis is markedly curtailed, both leading to antinatriuresis during sodium loading; conversely, the renin-angiotensin system is suppressed and DA biosynthesis is activated, both leading to natriuresis. When DA synthesis is increased, DA stimulates renin secretion, which serves to increase the activity of the renin-angiotensin system, which was suppressed by sodium loading. Thus, the interaction between these two systems leads to a series of overlapping steps, which attempt to normalize each other to bring the control of sodium excretion into equilibrium.

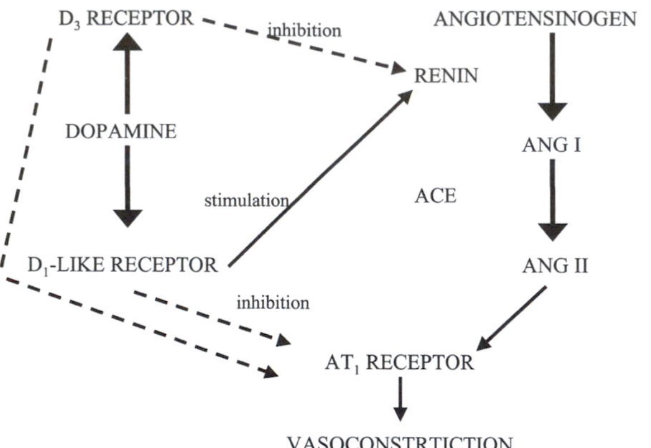

FIGURE 46.2 Schematic depiction of the interactions between the renal dopaminergic system and the renal renin-angiotensin system. ACE, angiotensin-converting enzyme; ANG I, angiotensin I; ANG II, angiotensin II.

RENAL DOPAMINE AND HYPERTENSION

Two fundamental defects in the renal DA system have been described in hypertension: (1) deficient DA production caused by decreased PTC uptake, decarboxylation of DOPA, or both; and (2) defective D_1-like receptor/G protein coupling, so that DA is ineffective in transmitting a signal to inhibit sodium excretion. The latter defect is confined to the PTC and evidence suggests that the defect is caused by hyperphosphorylation of the D_1 receptor by a mutation in G protein–coupled receptor kinase-4 [10]. Under these circumstances, the hyperphosphorylated D_1 receptor is internalized in the cytoplasm and is desensitized. More research needs to be done to determine whether this defect is responsible for states of salt sensitivity and sodium-dependent hypertension in humans.

Clearly, the role of DA receptors in hypertension has been substantial by studies in animals in which a specific DA receptor has been disrupted. Knockout of the D_1 receptor in mice leads to hypertension, but a mutation in the coding region of the receptor has not been found in human essential hypertension or in genetically hypertensive rats. Disruption of the D_2 receptor also induces hypertension, but the increase in blood pressure is related to noradrenergic discharge at the whole body level, and there is no sodium retention. Absence of the D_3 receptor generates a renin-dependent form of hypertension with an inability to excrete a sodium load. Although these studies show potentially interesting interactions, particularly between renin-angiotensin and dopaminergic systems, compensatory mechanisms may alter the resulting phenotype. Additional research needs to be done, especially with renal-specific knockout of the individual DA receptors and combinations of receptors of the DA and renin-angiotensin systems.

References

1. Wang, Z-Q., H. M. Siragy, R. A. Felder, and R. M. Carey. 1997. Intrarenal dopamine production and distribution in the rat: Physiological control of sodium excretion. *Hypertension* 29:228–234.
2. O'Connell, D. P., S. J. Botkin, S. P. Ramos, D. R. Sibley, M. A. Ariano, R. A. Felder, and R. M. Carey. 1995. Localization of dopamine D_{1A} receptor protein in the rat kidney. *Am. J. Physiol.* 268:F1185–F1197.
3. O'Connell, D. P., A. M. Aherne, E. Lane, R. A. Felder, and R. M. Carey. 1998. Detection of dopamine receptor D_{1A} subtype-specific mRNA in rat kidney by in situ amplification. *Am. J. Physiol.* 43:232–241.
4. O'Connell, D. P., C. J. Vaughan, A. M. Aherne, S. J. Botkin, Z.-Q. Wang, R. A. Felder, and R. M. Carey. 1998. Expression of the dopamine D_3 receptor protein in rat kidney. *Hypertension* 32:886–895.
5. Hughes, J., N. V. Ragsdale, R. A. Felder, R. L. Chevalier, B. King, and R. M. Carey. 1988. Diuresis and natriuresis during continuous dopamine-1 receptor stimulation. *Hypertension* 11(Suppl 1):I-169–I-174.
6. Aperia, A. C. 2000. Intrarenal dopamine: A key signal in the interactive regulation of sodium metabolism. *Ann. Rev. Physiol.* 62:621–647.
7. Siragy, H. M., R. A. Felder, N. L. Howell, R. L. Chevalier, M. J. Peach, and R. M. Carey. 1989. Evidence that intrarenal dopamine acts as a paracrine substance at the renal tubule. *Am. J. Physiol.* 257:F469–F477.
8. Wang, Z.-Q., R. A. Felder, and R. M. Carey. 1999. Selective inhibition of renal dopamine subtype D_{1A} receptor induces antinatriuresis in conscious rats. *Hypertension* 33:504–510.
9. Cheng, H.-F., B. N. Becker, and R. C. Harris. 1996. Dopamine decreases expression of type-1 angiotensin II receptors in renal proximal tubule. *J. Clin. Invest.* 97:2745–2752.
10. Felder, R. A., H. Sanada, J. Xu, P.-Y. Yu, Z. Wang, W. Wang, I. Yamaguchi, D. Hazen-Martin, L.-J. C. Wong, R. M. Carey, and P. A. Jose. 2002. G protein-coupled receptor kinase 4 gene variants in human essential hypertension. *Proc. Natl. Acad. Sci. USA* 97:3872–3877.

PART IV

STRESS

47 Exercise and the Autonomic Nervous System

Vernon S. Bishop
Department of Pharmacology
University of Texas Health Sciences Center
San Antonio, Texas

The autonomic nervous system plays a key role in the regulation of the cardiovascular response during exercise. The general concept is that at the onset of exercise, the central nervous system generates a cardiorespiratory pattern (central command) appropriate to the somatomotor signal. The central command then initiates a withdrawal of parasympathetic activity to the heart and an increase in ventilation rate, and it is also probably involved in the resetting of the arterial baroreflex toward greater pressures. Although little is known about the central neural connections involved in initiating the changes in parasympathetic and sympathetic outflow in the exercised state, it is known that central command and the arterial baroreflexes are critical to the sympathoexcitatory response at the onset of exercise (Fig. 47.1).

At the onset of exercise, it is generally accepted that heart rate (HR) is increased primarily by central command (decrease in vagal activity to the heart). As exercise continues or its level increases, further increases in HR may occur as a result of increases in sympathetic outflow to the heart. If the resulting increase in cardiac output is inadequate to increase the arterial pressure to the level required by the new operating point of the arterial baroreflex, then sympathetic outflow to the peripheral circulation will increase. The net effect of this increase in sympathetic outflow is to increase vascular resistance in regions not involved in the exercised response. Upward resetting of the operating point of the arterial baroreflex appears to be the major factor responsible for the sympathoexcitatory response to exercise (see Fig. 47.1). As a result of this upward resetting, an error signal is created between the actual arterial pressure and the pressure of the new operating point. To minimize the error, sympathetic outflow is increased. Notably, once the error signal is corrected and the system is operating on the new baroreflex curve, not only is the systemic pressure increased, but the level of sympathetic outflow relative to the pressure also is increased. This resetting of the operating point of the reflex provides an effective means of increasing sympathetic outflow and arterial pressures. In addition, to the sympathoexcitatory response resulting from the resetting of the arterial baroreflexes, reflexes initiated from muscle mechanosensitive and chemosensitive receptors, as well as from cardiac vagal afferents, contribute to the regulation of sympathetic activity to the peripheral circulation.

Mechanosensitive and chemosensitive receptors located in the muscle provide important afferent signals relative to the activity and perfusion of exercising muscles. In general, we assume that mechanical activation of the muscle receptor signals muscle activity and that the resulting afferent activity contributes to central command. Activation of the chemosensitive receptors by metabolites released during muscle contraction are probably involved when a mismatch between vascular resistance and cardiac output occurs. Increased activity from these receptors results in an increase in sympathetic activity to active and inactive muscles.

In most animal models and humans, there is a redistribution of cardiac output to the exercising muscle. Basically, this involves an increase in sympathetic outflow to the visceral organs, which results in an increase in vascular resistance in these regions. Conversely, the resistance to the exercising muscle is diminished. The increased resistance to the nonexercising regions is initially the result of the upward resetting of the arterial baroreflex. As the exercise continues, an additional increase in vascular resistance may occur because of activation of chemosensitive muscle afferents [1, 2].

In addition to the arterial baroreflexes and chemosensitive reflexes from the exercising muscle, cardiac vagal afferents also contribute to the redistribution of cardiac output during exercise. In rabbits, renal and mesenteric vascular resistances increase during running, whereas systemic resistance decreases. Blockade of cardiac vagal afferents by intrapericardial injections of procainamide results in further increases in renal and mesenteric vascular resistance. However, it does not significantly affect systemic vascular resistance (Fig. 47.2A). This observation suggests that cardiac afferents modulate the magnitude of the sympathetic-mediated vasoconstriction of the visceral organs. Furthermore, when the tonic influence of the cardiac vagal afferents is increased by exercise training, the role of the cardiac vagal afferents in modulating vascular resistance of the visceral organs also is increased. Note that in the exercised endurance-trained state, the increase in renal and mesenteric vascular resistance is substantially less than in

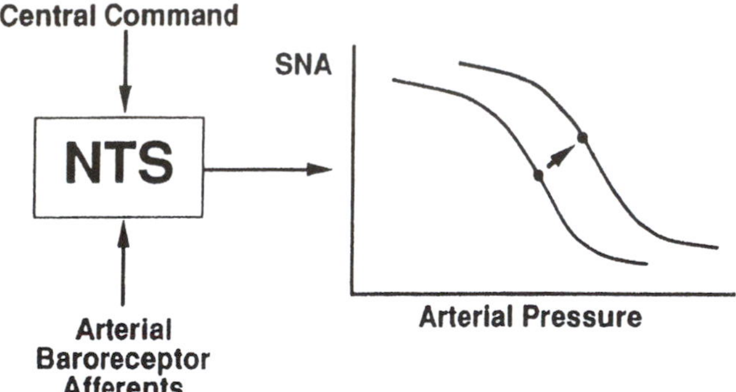

FIGURE 47.1 Schematic illustration of the role of central command and arterial baroreceptor afferents on the sympathetic component of the arterial baroreflex. Studies from DiCarlo and Bishop [3] indicate that central command and baroreceptor afferents are required for the upward resetting of the baroreflex. (Adapted from Rowell, L. B., and D. S. O'Leary. 1990. Reflex control of the circulation during exercise: Chemoreflexes and mechanoreflexes. *J. Appl. Physiol.* 69(2):407–418, with permission.)

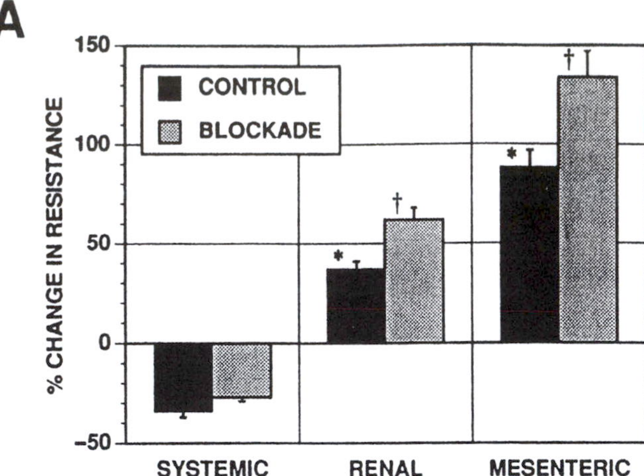

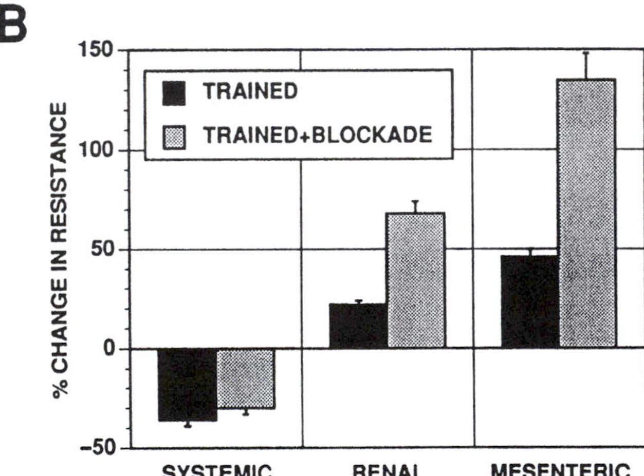

FIGURE 47.2 A, The change in systemic, renal, and mesenteric resistance during exercise with cardiac afferents intact (control) and when cardiac afferents are blocked with procainamide (blockade). **B**, Illustration of the influence of cardiac afferents on systemic, renal, and mesenteric resistance during exercise in rabbits after endurance exercise training. Trained: response to exercised in endurance-trained rabbits with cardiac afferents intact. Trained plus blockade: response of the endurance-trained rabbits with cardiac afferents blocked with procainamide.

the untrained state (see Fig. 47.2). However, in the exercise-trained rabbit, blockade of the cardiac vagal afferents causes a greater increase in renal and mesenteric vascular resistance than in the untrained exercising rabbit. These findings suggest that cardiac vagal afferents may be involved in determining the cardiovascular responses to a given workload [4, 5].

In conclusion, one must realize that the role of neural mechanisms in the exercise response varies depending on many factors, including the type of exercise, the number of muscle groups involved, the duration of the exercise, and the level of endurance training.

References

1. Rowell, L. B., and D. S. O'Leary. 1990. Reflex control of the circulation during exercise: Chemoreflexes and mechanoreflexes. *J. Appl. Physiol.* 69(2):407–418.
2. DiCarlo, S. E., and V. S. Bishop. 1990. Regional vascular resistance during exercise: Role of cardiac afferents and exercise training. *Am. J. Physiol.* 258(27):H842–H847.
3. DiCarlo, S. E., and V. S. Bishop. 1992. Onset of exercise shifts operating point of arterial baroreflex to higher pressures. *Am. J. Physiol.* 262(1 Pt 2):H303–H307.
4. DiCarlo, S. E., and V. S. Bishop. 1990. Exercise training enhances cardiac afferent inhibition of baroreflex function. *Am. J. Physiol.* 258(27):H212–H220.
5. DiCarlo, S. E., and V. S. Bishop. 1988. Exercise training attenuates baroreflex regulation of nerve activity in rabbits. *Am. J. Physiol.* 255(4):H974–H979.

48 Effects of High Altitude

Luciano Bernardi
Department of Internal Medicine
University of Pavia
Pavia, Italy

Ascent to high altitude reduces the inspired partial pressure of O_2, leading to hypobaric hypoxia. This requires a complex adaptive process (acclimatization), which, in its early phases, is largely influenced by the autonomic nervous system. This process is complex, and the integrated response depends on a number of factors, including the extent and duration of hypoxic exposure. Acute responses are modified by chronic adaptations that restore circulatory function toward normoxic levels, over periods that may range from a few days or weeks for the sea-level sojourner, to years for the high-altitude native. Tolerance to hypoxia varies greatly among individuals, and subjects with a particular susceptibility may develop inappropriate responses, leading to acute mountain sickness and even to life-threatening conditions, such as high-altitude cerebral and pulmonary edema (HAPE). Sympathetic overactivity seems to play an important role in HAPE.

EFFECTS OF ACUTE HYPOXIA

The main oxygen sensors involving the autonomic nervous system response are the peripheral chemoreceptors, which are located in the carotid body and in the arch of the aorta. The carotid sensors respond mainly to a decrease in arterial oxygen pressures (Pa_{O_2}); aortic sensors respond mainly to arterial oxygen content (Ca_{O_2}). Chemoreceptor afferents synapse in the primary cardiovascular control center of the rostral ventrolateral medulla. Stimulation of this center by hypoxia leads to hyperventilation and excitation of sympathetic and parasympathetic neurons. However, this response is modified by numerous secondary influences of hypoxia, such as hyperventilation and hypocapnia [1]. The hyperventilation, which is proportional to the decreases in Pa_{O_2}, stimulates lung stretch receptors (during inspiration), whose final response is an inhibition of vagal tone. In addition, hyperventilation induces hypocapnia, which attenuates the sympathetic activation associated with the peripheral chemoreflex, and also reduces the stimulus for the central chemoreflex [2]. Because of the increase in ventilation, the respiratory changes in stroke volume also are increased, and this contributes to increased baroreceptor loading and unloading during expiration and inspiration, respectively. The baroreflexes remain able to maintain adequate cardiovascular modulation during chemoreflex activation [3]. Thus, arterial baroreceptors, central chemoreceptors, and pulmonary stretch receptors all may modulate the sympathetic activation associated with peripheral chemoreflex excitation [1].

The purpose of this combined cardiovascular and autonomic response is to maintain systemic and regional oxygen despite the decrease in Pa_{O_2} [4]. This is achieved by an increase in cardiac output (proportional to the altitude), mainly because of an increase in heart rate; tachycardia results from increased sympathetic activity caused by chemoreceptor stimulation, and probably also from vagal withdrawal, as a consequence of hyperventilation (central pathways, feedback from pulmonary stretch receptors, and hypocapnia) [2].

Acute hypoxia provokes vasodilation in all vascular beds [5], except the lung (where hypoxic vasoconstriction in susceptible subjects often is exaggerated and may be a crucial factor leading to HAPE). Peripheral vasodilation, in addition to increases in heart rate and cardiac output, causes a remarkably effective redistribution of flow to vascular beds with the greatest metabolic demand, similar to physical exercise [6]. The increment in blood flow associated with hypoxia, at rest and during exercise, precisely matches the decrease in arterial oxygen content, keeping O_2 delivery to tissues constant. Endothelial and neurally derived NO may be involved in this integrated autonomic and cardiovascular response to hypoxia [1, 7].

Blood pressure depends on the balance between hypoxic vasodilation and the vasoconstrictor effect of sympathetic activation, and it changes little during acute hypoxia. When peripheral vasodilation is not effectively compensated by sympathetic activity, syncope may occur; this is more frequent after rapid ascent to high altitude. Hypoxia also causes cerebral vasodilation, which is counteracted partially by hypocapnia, so that pulsating headache is a common symptom on arrival at high altitude.

EFFECTS OF CHRONIC HYPOXIA

Over a period of days to weeks, reduction in plasma volume and later increase in red cell mass increase hemoglobin concentration and Cao_2 (also with contribution of hyperventilation). The increased Cao_2 reduces the hyperdynamic circulation and both cardiac output and peripheral blood flow returns toward normal. However, the still low Pao_2 maintain chemostimulation and, hence, sympathetic activation. This results in a progressive increase in vascular resistance and blood pressure, as the increase in CaO_2 reduces the vasodilatory effect of hypoxia. The arterial baroreflexes, although diminished, continue to function at high altitude despite the marked increase in chemoreflexes [3], suggesting a central resetting of the baroreflex with exposure to hypoxia [1].

Cardiac output is consistently depressed after acclimatization to high altitude, often to less than baseline sea-level values, because of a decrease in stroke volume (with preserved contractile function), in turn caused by a reduction in left ventricular end-diastolic volume, the latter because of a 20 to 30% reduction in plasma volume. Sympathetic activation and slower acting neurohormones, such as angiotensin, aldosterone, or vasopressin, may be important in sustaining the reduction in plasma volume in chronic hypoxia. This relative dehydration unloads low-pressure cardiopulmonary receptors and arterial baroreceptors (by reducing aortic dimensions and by decreasing pulsatile flow through arterial baroreceptors [1]).

Chronic sympathetic hyperactivity leads to downregulation of peripheral β receptors, with gradual diminution of the heart rate response to sympathetic activation [8]. After prolonged sojourn to high altitude, sympathetic activity diminishes and blood pressure normalizes. After years of acclimatization, lowlanders and high-altitude natives appear similar to sea-level natives [9].

Whereas this response is typically observed at altitudes varying from 3000 to 5000 m, at extreme altitudes, the acclimatization process cannot normalize Cao_2; as a result, peripheral vasodilation and reduction in peripheral resistance persist as in acute hypoxia.

AUTONOMIC NERVOUS SYSTEM AND HIGH-ALTITUDE ILLNESS

HAPE is associated with severe pulmonary hypertension (probably with uneven distribution, thus allowing pulmonary areas of hyperperfusion), pulmonary capillary leak, endothelial dysfunction, possibly a late inflammation, and alveolar edema.

Although the origin of HAPE is still debated, recent studies in the Italian/Swiss Alps on patients with HAPE susceptibility have confirmed the essential role of pulmonary hypertension. Such patients have a marked increase in sympathetic activity during acute exposure to hypoxia, even before the development of HAPE. Sympathetic activation may thus play at least a facilitatory role in HAPE, presumably by contributing to the development of pulmonary hypertension in susceptible individuals [10].

References

1. Levine, B. D. 2000. Mountain medicine and the autonomic nervous system. In *Handbook of clinical neurology, Vol 75. The autonomic nervous system,* ed. O. Appenzeller, 259–280, Amsterdam: Elsevier.
2. Somers, V. K., A. L. Mark, D. C. Zavala, and F. M. Abboud. 1989. Influence of ventilation and hypocapnia on sympathetic nerve responses to hypoxia in normal humans. *J. Appl. Physiol.* 67:2095–2100.
3. Bernardi, L., C. Passino, G. Spadacini, A. Calciati, R. Robergs, E. R. Greene, E. Martignoni, I. Anand, and O. Appenzeller. 1998. Cardiovascular autonomic modulation and activity of carotid baroreceptors at altitude. *Clin. Sci.* 95:565–573.
4. Wolfel, E. E. 1993. Sympatho-adrenal and cardiovascular adaptation to hypoxia. In *Hypoxia and molecular medicine,* ed. J. R. Sutton, C. S. Houston, and G. Coates, 62–80. Burlington, VT: Queen City.
5. Heistad, D. D., and F. M. Abboud. 1980. Dickinson W. Richards Lecture: Circulatory adjustments to hypoxia. *Circulation* 61:463–470.
6. Cerretelli, P., C. Marconi, O. Deriaz, and D. Giezendanner. 1984. After effects of chronic hypoxia on cardiac output and muscle blood flow at rest and exercise. *Eur. J. Appl. Physiol.* 53:92–96.
7. Thomas, G. D., and R. G. Victor. 1998. Nitric oxide mediates contraction-induced attenuation of sympathetic vasoconstriction in rat skeletal muscle. *J. Physiol. (Lond)* 506:817–826.
8. Voelkel, N. F., L. Hegstrand, J. T. Reeves, I. F. McMurtry, and P. B. Molinoff. 1981. Effects of hypoxia on density of beta-adrenergic receptors. *J. Appl. Physiol.* 50:363–366.
9. Passino, C., L. Bernardi, G. Spadacini, A. Calciati, R. Robergs, I. Anand, E. R. Greene, E. Martignoni, and O. Appenzeller. 1996. Autonomic regulation of heart rate and peripheral circulation: Comparison of high altitude and sea level residents. *Clin. Sci.* 91:81–83.
10. Duplain, H., L. Vollenweider, A. Delabays, P. Nicod, P. Bartsch, and U. Scherrer. 1999. Augmented sympathetic activation during short-term hypoxia and high-altitude exposure in subjects susceptible to high altitude pulmonary edema. *Circulation* 99:1713–1718.

49 Hypothermia

Bruce C. Paton
University of Colorado
Denver, Colorado

Hypothermia is defined as a core body temperature of less than 35°C. It may range from mild (32–35°C) to profound (<30°C). Several types of hypothermia exist.

Induced hypothermia protects organs in cardiac and transplantation surgery and preserves isolated tissues such as blood and skin. Profound cold (cryotherapy) is used to destroy tissues and preserve cells such as sperm. Accidental hypothermia occurs if there is unexpected heat loss exceeding heat production and maintenance. Incidental hypothermia develops in neurologic, metabolic, dermatologic, and other diseases that interfere with body temperature control such as hypothyroidism, diabetes, stroke, and brain tumors affecting the hypothalamus. Gram-negative sepsis is frequently associated with hypothermia.

ETIOLOGIC FACTORS

Heat is lost by four modes: conduction, convection, evaporation, and radiation. Pathophysiologic responses depend on speed of hypothermia development and duration. Immersion in very cold water induces hypothermia quickly with only minor changes in physiologic balance. Prolonged exposure to ambient hypothermia may cause severe changes in metabolism, electrolyte, and acid-base balance.

GENERAL RESPONSE TO HEAT LOSS

The hypothalamus controls responses on the basis of signals received from the periphery (skin) and the temperature of the blood. Shivering increases metabolism and vasoconstriction restricts further heat loss. Changes in skin temperature trigger shivering that can increase heat production fivefold, at the expense of increased oxygen consumption. Oxygen consumption decreases 7% per degree Celsius decrease in core temperature, and there is commensurate slowing or reduction of many physiologic functions.

SPECIFIC SYSTEMATIC CHANGES

Systematic changes include progressive diminishing of heart rate. Less than 30°C blood pressure may be difficult to measure by usual means because of stiff arteries and low blood pressure. Less than 29°C cardiac arrhythmias are likely, of which atrial fibrillation is the most common. Less than 27°C ventricular fibrillation or bradycardia may lead to asystole and death. Vasoconstriction shunts blood to core structures, maintains blood pressure, and reduces peripheral heat loss.

Respiratory rate decreases and ventilation becomes shallow, partly because of increasing stiffness of the chest wall muscles. Respiration may cease below 29°C, but occasionally continues to as low as 20°C. Tracheal and bronchial ciliary function stops; the cough reflex is suppressed and pneumonia is a common complication. Pulmonary edema is frequent in prolonged hypothermia.

Between 32 and 35°C, cognitive functions deteriorate with disorientation, confusion, and character changes; unconsciousness usually occurs at 25 to 28°C. Reflexes slow, then cease; pupils dilate and become fixed, simulating death. Diminished oxygen demand protects the central nervous system, permitting occasional prolonged submersion or cessation of blood flow without residual damage. The spinal cord is similarly protected from prolonged ischemia.

Gastrointestinal motility decreases, stress ulcers may occur, and pancreatitis is found after prolonged exposure to hypothermia. Serum sodium decreases, potassium increases, and glucose levels are variable with hypothermia. Metabolic acidosis is common if hypothermia is prolonged. The hematocrit and viscosity increase, the coagulation cascade slows without a specific abnormality, disseminated intravascular coagulation occurs occasionally, and thrombotic complications are common in fatal cases.

There is no correlation between thyroid-stimulating hormone and temperature: thyroid hormone levels are normal unless the patient is hypothyroid, and adrenal corticosteroids are usually normal, but may be reduced in prolonged exposure with adrenocortical exhaustion. Cortisol levels may increase during rewarming. Endogenous insulin levels remain normal. Both endogenous and exogenous insulin are ineffective if body temperature is less than 31°C. Thermoregulation is impaired with age. There is diminished perception of ambient temperature with lower body temperature, metabolic rate, and peripheral blood flow.

DIAGNOSIS

Core temperature (rectal, esophageal, tympanic, bladder) is essential for correct diagnosis. Hypothermia is possible in (1) healthy victims of exposure or drowning; (2) otherwise healthy persons intoxicated by drugs or alcohol; (3) individuals with predisposing diseases such as hypothyroidism, hypopituitarism, malnutrition, muscular dysfunction and inactivity, hypoglycemia, or ketoacidosis; and (4) elderly, without serious illness, who are exposed to mild cold.

Physical findings include slurred speech; impaired coordination; shivering; cold trunk; pale skin color (but color may be bright pink if there is vasodilation); diminished or absent reflexes; dilated and fixed pupils; slow respirations; slow heart rate, imperceptible pulses, blood pressure not measurable; and no bowel sounds. Sometimes patients initially appear dead.

Clinical management consists of assessing consciousness, cardiorespiratory function, temperature, associated diseases, and/or injuries, etiologic factors, and duration of hypothermia. Laboratory evaluation should include a complete biochemical blood screen including blood urea nitrogen, sugar, and electrolytes, and in severe cases, a coagulation screen, acid-base measurement. A chest x-ray also should be obtained. Severely affected patients should be treated in intensive care with full physiologic monitoring (temperature, arterial and venous pressures, fluid balance, cardiac output); endotracheal intubation may be necessary. The risk for inducing ventricular fibrillation is small if the patient is actively ventilated and oxygenated before intubation.

Treatment includes correction of physiologic abnormalities with rewarming. Rewarming methods are: (1) Passive: remove cold wet clothing, place in warm dry environment, allow spontaneous rewarming; (2) active-external: hot water tub, hot water bottles, hydraulic or warm air blankets; and (3) active-internal: hot food and drink, warmed intravenous fluids, warmed humidified air, lavage (gastric, thoracic, peritoneal, bladder), hemodialysis, and extracorporeal circulation. The method chosen should be appropriate to severity. The patient should be rewarmed as rapidly as possible with full physiologic control. Choose a method that permits access to the patient for resuscitation in case of need. Mortality (0–80%) depends on severity, duration, associated diseases, and injuries. Serum potassium greater than 10 mEq/liter or need for cardiopulmonary resuscitation may predict fatal outcome.

References

1. Danzl, D. F. 2001. Accidental hypothermia. In *Wilderness medicine,* 4th ed., ed. P. Auerbach, 135–177. St. Louis: Mosby.
2. Giesbrecht, G. G., and G. K. Bristow. 1997. Recent advances in hypothermia research. *Ann. NY Acad. Sci.* 813:676.
3. Gilbert, M., R. Busund, A. Skagseth, P. A. Nilsen, and J. P. Solbo. 2000. Resuscitation from accidental hypothermia of 13.7°C with circulatory arrest. *Lancet* 355:375.

50 Psychological Stress and the Autonomic Nervous System

Michael G. Ziegler
UCSD Medical Center
San Diego, California

Autonomic responses to psychological stress prepare the body for fight or flight. Cannon and Selye described stereotypic responses to stress that involved activation of sympathetic nerves and adrenocortical hormone release. Corticotropin-releasing factor (CRF) in the central nervous system activates autonomic and adrenocortical responses to stressors. CRF injected into the brain increases arousal and responsiveness to stressful stimuli. Conversely, CRF antagonists can reverse behavioral responses to many stressors. CRF alters the discharge of locus ceruleus neurons in the brainstem, and these effects are mimicked by some stressors. Locus ceruleus noradrenergic neurons project into the cerebral cortex. In the paraventricular nucleus of the hypothalamus, norepinephrine stimulates further CRF release. Other central nervous system pathways also mediate stress-induced activation of the sympathetic nervous system, but they generally have not been studied as thoroughly as the CRF pathways [1].

NORMAL PSYCHOLOGICAL STRESSES AND AUTONOMIC ACTIVITY

There is a 24-hour rhythm in the plasma levels of norepinephrine and epinephrine that tend to be lowest at 3 AM, and increase rapidly until a peak at 9 AM, similar to the cortisol rhythm. Sleep decreases sympathetic nerve activity. Arousals during sleep cause a rapid increase in muscle sympathetic nerve electrical activity, which decreases back to baseline when sleep resumes. Muscle sympathetic nerve activity nearly doubles when going from sleep to wake, and doubles yet again when going from recumbent to standing posture. Exercise, pain, and cold lead to even more dramatic increases in sympathetic nerve activity, which is detailed elsewhere in this textbook. These are normal responses to the stresses of day-to-day life. These autonomic responses to the stresses of daily life may help to explain why there is a preponderance of myocardial infarction and sudden death between 6:00 AM and 12 PM. The autonomic responses to stress might also help to explain early mortality during both unemployment and bereavement.

PATTERNS OF AUTONOMIC RESPONSE TO STRESS

The general response to both physical and psychological stress is activation of the sympathetic nervous system with inhibition of the parasympathetic nervous system. When stress becomes severe or uncontrolled, then adrenomedullary release of epinephrine ensues. As stress increases even further, then CRF not only activates the sympathetic nervous system but leads to the release of adrenocorticotropic hormone and adrenocortical steroids.

Sympathetic nervous stimulation to the muscles activates vasoconstriction and increases peripheral vascular resistance. Sympathetic nerves that supply the skin both vasoconstrict and supply sweat glands through sympathetic cholinergic innervation. Activation of this skin sympathetic pathway can precipitate a "cold sweat" or perspiration and flushing of the skin. During sleep, muscle sympathetic nervous activity and skin sympathetic nervous activity have similar firing intensity and frequency. However, during stress, muscle and skin sympathetic nerves activities diverge. When a doctor took patients' blood pressure, skin sympathetic nerve activity increased by 38%, whereas muscle sympathetic nerve activity decreased by 25%. This was accompanied by an apparent increase in sympathetic nerve activity to the heart as heart rate and blood pressure increased [2] (Table 50.1).

Some stimuli such as hypoglycemia elicit a fairly specific activation of adrenomedullary epinephrine release without a marked increase in sympathetic nerve activity. When medical residents climbed stairs, their plasma norepinephrine increased; however, when they presented a public speech, epinephrine levels showed an even greater increase. Psychological stress not only tends to increase epinephrine disproportionately, it also tends to increase sympathetic nerve activity to the heart, leading to increased cardiac output. As we age, norepinephrine release in response to the cold pressor test increases. Less epinephrine is released from the adrenal medullae in the elderly; however, epinephrine blood levels are similar because of diminished clearance of epinephrine from the circulation with advancing age.

TABLE 50.1 Sympathetic Nerve Responses to Stress

Organ	Response	Receptor
Cardiac atrium	Heart rate	β_1
Cardiac ventricle	Inotropism	β_1
Eye	Pupil dilation	α_1
Skin blood vessel	Constriction	α_1
Hand sweat glands	Sweat	Cholinergic
Blood vessels	Constriction	α_1
Salivary glands	Constriction, dry mouth	α_1, α_2
Gut	Decrease motility	α_1, α_2, β_2
Gut sphincters	Contraction	α_1
Kidney	Renin release	β_1
Bladder	Relaxation	β_2
Bladder sphincter	Contraction	α_1
Hair	Piloerection	α_1
Muscle cells	Glycogenolysis	β_2
Muscle cells	K^+ uptake	β_2
Muscle blood vessels	Dilation	β_2

GASTROINTESTINAL CONTROL

The thought of food can elicit salivation, gastric motility, and acid secretion. Stress inhibits gastrointestinal (GI) motility when it activates the sympathetic nervous system, primarily through release of norepinephrine at its synaptic interface with the enteric nervous system. Postganglionic projections from sympathetic nerves terminate in myenteric submucous ganglia of the enteric nervous system where they suppress motility and secretion. α-Adrenergic stimulation inhibits both GI secretion and GI blood flow. In animal models, cold water immersion is associated with an inhibition of gastric emptying. Although stress decreases gastric emptying and intestinal motility, it does not decrease colonic motility. Activation of the sympathetic nervous system cannot explain the symptoms of secretory diarrhea and abdominal discomfort associated with psychological stress. Current evidence suggests that degranulation of enteric mast cells by nerve input releases inflammatory mediators, and this is postulated to underlie the secretory diarrhea and abdominal discomfort associated with stress [3].

PSYCHOSOMATIC DISORDERS AND THE AUTONOMIC NERVOUS SYSTEM

Autonomic responses to stress frequently lead to medical care. Feelings of warmth and cold, palpitations, tachycardia, nausea, abdominal pain, diarrhea, and constipation can all be the consequence of autonomic stress responses. Twenty percent of patients with borderline hypertension in the doctor's office have entirely normal home blood pressures. Sympathetic nervous stimulation of the heart increases heart rate, cardiac output, and blood pressure in novel or stressful environments. This cardiovascular stress response increases myocardial oxygen consumption and can precipitate angina pectoris in patients with coronary artery disease.

A vasovagal response can be triggered by a stressful situation that makes a person want to run away even though social constraints prevent the person from leaving. When this happens, hypothalamic activation of medullary cardiovascular responses triggered by emotional stress can lead to venodilation and increased inotropic stimulation to the heart. This can stimulate ventricular mechanoreceptors and promote vasodilation, bradycardia, and fainting.

POSTTRAUMATIC STRESS DISORDER, PANIC, AND ANXIETY

Posttraumatic stress disorder (PTSD) occurs when intrusive thoughts elicit memories of an unusually stressful event. Nineteenth century descriptions of "soldier's heart" noted abnormal excitability of the cardiac nervous system in the absence of serious cardiac disease. PTSD often is accompanied by tachycardia, palpitations, and high blood pressure [4].

In panic disorder, a psychological stimulus elicits an autonomic response characterized by flushing, tachycardia, palpitations, hypertension, and GI symptoms. The autonomic response can sometimes be extinguished by repeated exposure to the stimulus under reassuring circumstances. In anxiety disorder, similar autonomic symptoms occur with no inciting stimulus. In all three of these psychological disorders baseline norepinephrine and epinephrine are normal, but there are increased plasma and urinary catecholamines when symptomatic reactions are triggered [5]. β-Adrenergic blocking drugs tend to diminish subjective symptoms of palpitations and tremor, and they often eliminate episodes of tachycardia.

Autonomic responses to psychological stress serve the useful function of preparing us for action by increasing muscle blood supply and slowing vegetative functions. However, inappropriate stress responses are the basis for many psychosomatic disorders. Familiarity with the patterns of autonomic response to psychological stress is essential to understanding human disease.

References

1. Koob, G. F. 1999. Corticotropin-releasing factor, norepinephrine, and stress. *Biol. Psychiatry* 46:1167–1180.
2. Grassi, G., C. Turri, S. Vailati, R. Dell'Oro, and G. Mancia. 1999. Muscle and skin sympathetic nerve traffic during the "white-coat" effect. *Circulation* 100:222–225.
3. Plourde, V. 1999. Stress-induced changes in the gastrointestinal motor system. *Can. J. Gastroenterol.* 13(A):26A–31A.
4. Lamprecht, F., and M. Sack. 2002. Posttraumatic stress disorder revisited. *Psychosom. Med.* 64:222–237.
5. Hoehn-Saric, R., and D. R. McLeod. 2000. Anxiety and arousal: Physiological changes and their perception. *J. Affect. Disord.* 61(3): 217–224.

51 Aging and the Autonomic Nervous System

Vera Novak
Division of Gerontology
Beth Israel Deaconess Medical Center
Harvard Medical School
Boston, Massachusetts

Lewis A. Lipsitz
Division of Gerontology
Beth Israel Deaconess Medical Center
Harvard Medical School
Boston, Massachusetts

Healthy aging is associated with several abnormalities in autonomic nervous system function that can impair adaptation to orthostatic stress in older people. Aging affects central and peripheral autonomic regulations and it is associated with loss of small nerve fibers. However, aging should be differentiated from symptoms of autonomic failure, because many mechanisms compensating for demands of daily living remain intact.

Orthostatic and postprandial hypotension are the two most prominent manifestations of age-associated autonomic nervous system impairment. Both are defined as a 20–mmHg or greater decline in systolic blood pressure on assumption of the upright posture, or within 1 hour of eating a meal, respectively [1, 2]. These are two distinct conditions that may or may not occur in the same patient. Orthostatic hypotension is observed in less than 7% of healthy normotensive elderly people and in as many as 30% of elder older than 75 years with multiple pathologic conditions. The epidemiology of postprandial hypotension is unknown, but it is particularly common in the nursing home population and in patients with unexplained falls and syncope. Orthostatic hypotension is an important symptom that may hallmark onset of generalized autonomic failure associated with diabetes, malignancy, amyloidosis, parkinsonism, and other syndromes. Medications used to treat comorbidities may contribute to orthostatic hypotension. Pathophysiologic mechanisms predisposing healthy elderly people to hypotension are summarized in Table 51.1.

The following sections address the effects of normal aging on autonomic function. These effects are most obvious in the cardiovascular system, where they have received the most rigorous investigation.

BAROREFLEX FUNCTION

Normal human aging is associated with impairment in baroreflex sensitivity. This is evident from the blunted cardioacceleration to stimuli that decreases blood pressure, such as standing up, nitroprusside infusions, and lower body negative pressure, as well as reduced bradycardic response to drugs such as phenylephrine, which increase blood pressure. Reduced baroreflex sensitivity also manifests as larger blood pressure reductions to straining during Valsalva maneuver and hypotensive stimuli such as standing up or eating a meal. The baroreflex may be impaired at any one of multiple sites along its arc, including carotid and cardiopulmonary pressure receptors, afferent pathways, brainstem (nucleus tractus solitarii) and higher regulatory centers, efferent sympathetic and parasympathetic neurons, postsynaptic cardiac β receptors, or defects in intracellular signal transduction pathways within the myocardium. Age-associated blood pressure increase contributes to baroreflex impairment.

SYMPATHETIC ACTIVITY

Studies of sympathetic nervous system activity in healthy human subjects demonstrated an age-related increase in resting plasma norepinephrine levels, muscle sympathetic nerve activity, and vascular resistance, as well as the plasma norepinephrine response to upright posture and exercise. The increase in plasma norepinephrine is primarily caused by an increase in norepinephrine spillover at sympathetic nerve endings and secondarily caused by a decrease of its clearance. Despite apparent increases in sympathetic tone with aging, cardiac and vascular responsiveness is diminished. Infusions of β-adrenergic agonists result in smaller increases in heart rate (HR), left ventricular ejection fraction, cardiac output, and vasodilation in older compared with younger men [3].

PARASYMPATHETIC ACTIVITY

Previous studies demonstrating age-related reductions in HR variability in response to respiration, cough, and the Valsalva maneuver suggest that aging is associated with impaired cardiac–vagal control. Elderly patients with orthostatic hypotension or syncope have even greater reduction in HR responses to cough and deep breathing than healthy

TABLE 51.1 Age-Related Physiologic Changes Predisposing to Hypotension

1. Decreased baroreflex sensitivity
   a. Diminished heart rate response to hypotensive stimuli
   b. "Impaired" adrenergic vascular responsiveness
2. Impaired defense to reduced intravascular volume
   a. Reduced secretion of renin, angiotensin, and aldosterone
   b. Increased atrial natriuretic peptide, supine and upright
   c. Decreased plasma vasopressin response to orthostasis
   d. Reduced thirst after water deprivation
3. Impaired early cardiac ventricular filling (diastolic dysfunction)

age-matched subjects without syncope. Loss of the respiratory sinus arrhythmia and attenuation of the HR response to vagal maneuvers suggest that impaired parasympathetic HR control can be associated with length-dependent autonomic neuropathy with aging. Reflex responses to respiratory maneuvers have to be evaluated under standardized conditions and compared with age-matched normative values to quantify the severity of cardiac–vagal impairment.

VARIABILITY OF CARDIOVASCULAR SIGNALS

The complexity of HR signal reflects interactions between the cardiovascular and autonomic nervous systems in response to environmental demands. HR spectral analysis is used to quantify the relative contributions of sympathetic and parasympathetic nervous systems to HR variability [4]. The HR power spectrum can be divided into low- and high-frequency components. Previous studies using β-blockade, atropine, or both demonstrated that the low-frequency oscillations (0.05–0.1 Hz) in blood pressure reflect sympathetic modulation of vasomotor tone and in HR reflect a combination of baroreflex-mediated sympathetic and parasympathetic influences. Spectral power at high-frequency portions of the HR power spectrum (0.15–0.5 Hz) is under parasympathetic control and represents the respiratory sinus arrhythmia. Spectral analysis techniques have confirmed that healthy aging is associated with reductions in baroreflex and parasympathetic modulation of HR, with a relatively greater loss of the high-frequency parasympathetic component. Reduced complexity of cardiovascular signals can hallmark cardiac disease, but also central or peripheral autonomic nervous system impairment.

NEUROTRANSMITTERS AND RECEPTORS

Plasma norepinephrine levels increase with advancing age, in large part because of increased spillover at adrenergic nerve terminals, and to a smaller extent because of decreased plasma clearance [5]. Likewise, any change in the level of a neurotransmitter must be interpreted with regard to changes in production and clearance. Other catecholamines, as well as serotonin and acetylcholine neurotransmitters, that influence autonomic nervous system functions have received much less attention in humans. In the brain, a decline in dopamine and norepinephrine is related to a loss of dopaminergic and noradrenergic neurons in the substantia nigra and locus ceruleus. The clinical implications of these changes are not fully understood. The enzymes choline acetyltransferase and acetylcholinesterase, which are responsible for synthesis and degradation of acetylcholine, respectively, decrease in the cerebral cortex with aging. Furthermore, muscarinic and nicotinic receptors have been reported to decrease in cortical structures. These findings provide indirect evidence for a decrease in central cholinergic neurotransmission with normal aging.

CARDIAC β-ADRENERGIC RECEPTORS

The age-related decrease in chronotropic response to sympathetic stimulation has been attributed to multiple molecular and biochemical changes in β receptor–coupling and postsynaptic signaling. The number of β receptors in cardiac myocytes is unchanged with advancing age, but the affinity of β receptors for agonists is reduced. Postsynaptic changes with aging include a decrease in the activity of Gs protein and the adenylate cyclase catalytic unit, and a decrease in cyclic adenosine monophosphate–dependent phosphokinase-induced protein phosphorylation. As a result of these changes, G protein–mediated signal transduction is impaired. The decrease in cardiac contractile response to sympathetic stimulation has been studied in rat ventricular myocytes, where it appears to be related to decreased influx of calcium ions through sarcolemmal calcium channels and a reduction in the amplitude of the cytosolic calcium transient after β-adrenergic stimulation. These changes are similar to those seen in receptor desensitization caused by prolonged exposure of myocardial tissue to β-adrenergic agonists. Thus, age-associated alterations in β-adrenergic response may be caused by desensitization of the adenylate cyclase system in response to chronic increases of plasma catecholamine levels.

VASCULAR REACTIVITY

Aging is associated with increased vascular stiffness and peripheral resistance. Vasoconstriction responses are preserved, and endothelium-dependent vasodilation is progressively impaired with aging. The vasorelaxation response of both arteries and veins to infusions of the β-adrenergic agonist isoproterenol is attenuated in elderly people. Hyperlipidemia and other cardiovascular risk factors further affect vasodilation response. Arterial adrenergic responses to norepinephrine infusion also appear to be reduced in healthy elderly subjects. However, this impairment is reversible by suppression of sympathetic nervous system activity with guanadrel. This remarkable observation suggests that the abnormality in α-adrenergic response also represents receptor desensitization caused by heightened sympathetic nervous system activity. It also indicates that some of the physiologic changes associated with aging may be reversible.

VOLUME REGULATION

Aging is associated with a progressive decline in plasma renin, angiotensin II, and aldosterone levels, and increases in atrial natriuretic peptide, all of which promote salt wasting by the kidney. In many healthy elderly individuals, there is also a defective plasma vasopressin response to upright posture. These physiologic changes predispose elderly people to volume contraction and hypotension [6]. Furthermore, healthy elderly individuals do not experience the same sense of thirst as younger subjects when they become hyperosmolar during water deprivation or hypertonic saline infusion. Consequently, dehydration may develop rapidly during conditions such as an acute illness, preparation for a medical procedure, diuretic therapy, or exposure to a warm climate when fluid losses are increased, access to oral fluids is limited, or both.

Conditions that reduce preload, such as upright posture, meal digestion, or volume contraction, may threaten cardiac output and predispose older people to hypotension.

CEREBRAL VASOREGULATION

Cerebral vasoregulation reflects the ability of the cerebral circulation to maintain stable perfusion pressure when blood pressure changes occur [7]. It is maintained by active vasodilation of cerebral microvasculature during hypotensive stimuli and by vasoconstriction during blood pressure increases. Cerebral vasomotor reserve can be evaluated from blood flow increment with CO_2 rebreathing (vasodilation) and reduction during hyperventilation (vasoconstriction). Vasomotor reserve is reduced with aging, and cardiovascular risk factors further contribute to this decline. Cerebral autoregulation is effective within the pressure range of 80 to 150 mmHg. Autoregulation range is narrowed with aging and the lower limits are shifted toward greater values with hypertension. Orthostatic hypotension can be associated with normal or impaired autoregulation [8]. With impaired autoregulation, cerebral blood flow follows decreasing blood pressure. Therefore, older people may be at risk for cerebral hypoperfusion, if blood pressure decreases to less than an autoregulated range during hypotension.

References

1. Lipsitz, L. A. 1989. Orthostatic hypotension in the elderly. *N. Engl. J. Med.* 321:952–957.
2. Lipsitz, L. A., R. P. Nyquist, J. Y. Wei, and J. W. Rowe. 1983. Postprandial reduction in blood pressure in the elderly. *N. Engl. J. Med.* 309:81–83.
3. Lakatta, E. G. 1993. Deficient neuroendocrine regulation of the cardiovascular system with advancing age in healthy humans. *Circulation* 87:631–636.
4. Lipsitz, L. A., J. Mietus, G. B. Moody, and A. L. Goldberger. 1990. Spectral characteristics of heart rate variability before and during postural tilt: Relations to aging and risk of syncope. *Circulation* 81:1803–1810.
5. Hogikyan, R. V., and M. A. Supiano. 1994. Arterial alpha-adrenergic responsiveness is decreased and sympathetic nervous system activity is increased in older humans. *Am. J. Physiol.* 266(5 Pt 1):E717–E724.
6. Davis, K. M., and K. L. Minaker. 1994. Disorders of fluid balance: Dehydration and hyponatremia. In *Principles of geriatric medicine and gerontology*, 3rd ed., ed. W. E. Hazzard, J. P. Blass, J. B. Halter, J. G. Ouslander, and M. E. Tinetti, 1183–1190. New York: McGraw-Hill.
7. Aslid, A. R. 1992. Cerebral hemodynamics. In *Transcranial Doppler*, ed. D. W. Newell and R. Aaslid, 49–55. New York: Raven Press.
8. Novak, V., P. Novak, J. M. Spies, and P. A. Low. 1998. Autoregulation of cerebral blood flow in orthostatic hypotension. *Stroke* 29:104–111.

52 Mind–Body Interactions

Daniel Tranel
Department of Neurology
University of Iowa
College of Medicine
Iowa City, Iowa

The electrodermal skin conductance response (SCR) is a remarkably powerful and informative psychophysiologic index. The SCR is considered to be part of the sympathetic division of the autonomic nervous system (ANS), although the neural mechanisms for the higher level control skin conductance are complex and not well understood [1]. Because SCRs are relatively easy to measure and provide reliable indexes of a wide variety of psychologic states and processes, SCRs have been arguably the most popular aspect of ANS activity used to study human cognition and emotion [2]. We have used SCRs in neurologic patients with brain damage, to study processes such as nonconscious memory, nonconscious learning, and emotional processing.

NONCONSCIOUS MEMORY

Nonconscious Face Recognition in Prosopagnosia

Individuals who sustain brain damage to modality-related association cortexes can manifest impairments of recognition of stimuli presented through that modality (*agnosia*). For example, bilateral damage to visual association cortexes, in the vicinity of the occipitotemporal region, causes the condition known as *prosopagnosia*, which is an inability to recognize familiar faces. When patients with prosopagnosia see faces of family members, friends, or even their own face, the patients have no sense that they know the people, and they cannot remember who the people are. Each face looks like a complete stranger.

Using SCRs, we discovered that patients with prosopagnosia, despite their profound inability to recognize familiar faces, could still discriminate those faces nonconsciously [3]. In these experiments, skin conductance was recorded while the patients viewed faces that they used to know (*targets*), mixed in random order with faces the patients had never seen before (*nontargets*). A summary of these experiments is presented in Figure 52.1. All of the six patients with prosopagnosia that we studied produced significantly larger amplitude SCRs to target faces, compared with nontargets. This occurred in two separate experiments, one in which target faces were family members, friends, and self, and another in which target faces were famous individuals (movie stars, politicians, and sports figures). These experiments showed that patients with prosopagnosia could generate nonconscious discrimination of familiar faces they could not otherwise recognize and for which even a remote sense of familiarity was lacking. The results suggest that some part of the physiologic process of face recognition remains intact in the patients, although the results of this process are not available at a conscious level. The neural structures that mediate this "recognition without awareness" may involve a dorsal pathway that goes through parietal–frontal and ventromedial prefrontal structures to activate ANS control nuclei, such as the amygdala and various brainstem nuclei.

Nonconscious Recognition in the Auditory Modality

The phenomenon of nonconscious recognition of familiar stimuli also has been revealed in the auditory modality. We studied a patient who, after damage to the right auditory association cortexes, developed a special form of auditory agnosia: specifically, an inability to recognize familiar music and singing voices (including his own; he was a professional opera singer). A paradigm akin to the one described earlier for prosopagnosia was used: we played a series of music pieces, or singing voices, and included a randomly ordered mix of items that should have been familiar (targets), and ones the patient had never heard before (nontargets). The patient produced discriminatory SCRs to the target stimuli in both experiments. This outcome suggests that, as was the case for the visual modality, there is a preserved route from sensory input to ANS effectors such as the amygdala, probably again through the ventromedial prefrontal cortex. It is intriguing that for both the visual and auditory modalities, the brain can preserve a type of ANS-based discrimination mechanism (which can be indexed through SCRs), even when conscious recognition processes have been precluded by brain damage.

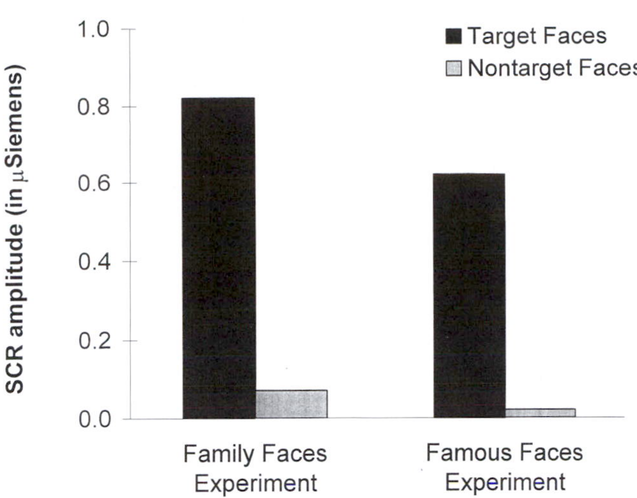

FIGURE 52.1 Nonconscious face recognition in prosopagnosia. Six patients with prosopagnosia produced large-amplitude skin conductance responses to pictures of family members and famous individuals, despite their inability to recognize those faces at conscious level.

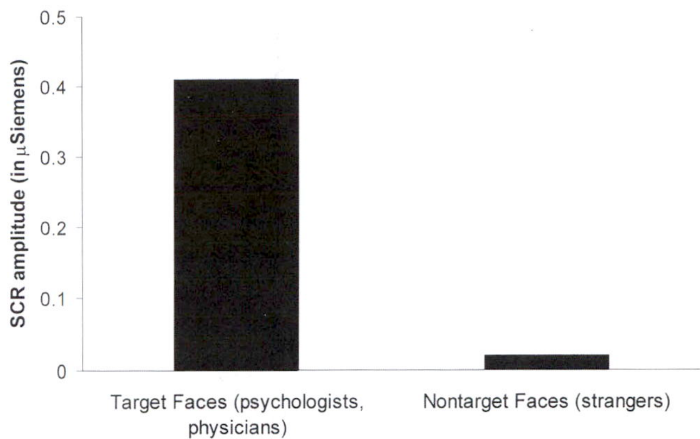

FIGURE 52.2 Nonconscious face learning in prosopagnosia. Five patients with prosopagnosia produced large-amplitude SCRs to pictures of individuals with whom they had extensive exposure after the onset of their brain damage, but not before (e.g., psychologists and physicians). This occurred despite that the patients had failed to learn the faces of these individuals at a conscious level.

NONCONSCIOUS LEARNING

Nonconscious Face Learning in Prosopagnosia

In the experiments reviewed earlier, SCRs were indexing knowledge that had been stored in the brain before the onset of brain damage. What about *learning*—that is, acquiring new information? To address this question, we studied five patients with prosopagnosia with the same type of experiment as described earlier, except that the target faces were persons the patients had encountered only *after* the onset of their brain injury. All five patients produced discriminatory SCRs to the target faces (Fig. 52.2), suggesting that despite the patients' inability to learn new faces consciously, some mechanism for acquiring new information about faces was preserved. We have speculated that this mechanism involves ANS-related structures, including ventromedial prefrontal cortex and amygdala.

Nonconscious Learning of Affective Valence

One of our patients, known as Boswell, experienced development of a profound amnesic syndrome after damage to the entire mesial temporal lobes, bilaterally. Boswell is incapable of learning any new declarative information, including facts, faces, and names. We conducted an experiment in which we exposed Boswell to three stimulus individuals: a "Good Guy," who always treated Boswell exceptionally well; a "Bad Guy," who always was stern and grumpy; and a "Neutral Guy," who was always neutral in

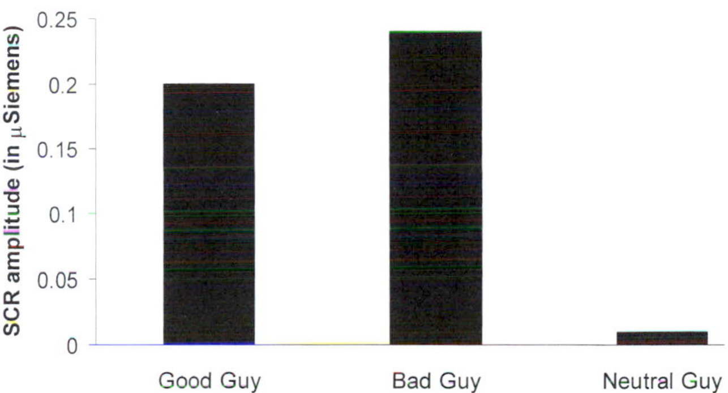

FIGURE 52.3 Covert learning of affective valence in patient Boswell. Boswell generated large-amplitude SCRs to the Good Guy and Bad Guy, but not to the Neutral Guy. This occurred despite his complete inability to learn the faces of those individuals at a conscious level.

demeanor. In one experiment, this exposure took place over the course of a week; in another, we carried out this manipulation over the course of several years [4]. Despite his profound amnesia, Boswell demonstrated nonconscious learning of the individuals. For example, when we showed him pairs of faces, one of which was one of the stimulus persons and one of which was a complete stranger, and asked him to "choose the one you would prefer to ask for a treat," Boswell reliably selected the Good Guy. He reliably selected *against* the Bad Guy, and his selection of the Neutral Guy was at chance. Moreover, Boswell generated discriminatory SCRs to both the Good Guy and the Bad Guy (Fig. 52.3). And all of this occurred despite that Boswell never produced a shred of evidence that he had learned any of the individuals at conscious level. We have proposed that the neostriatum, and the caudate nucleus in particular, may be part of the neural substrate that supports this nonconscious learning of affective valence.

Conditioning Without Awareness

Another remarkable example of learning without conscious influence comes from an experiment in which a patient with bilateral hippocampal damage, which caused severe amnesia for declarative knowledge, was shown to demonstrate intact emotional conditioning [5]. This patient went through an experiment in which he was exposed to a long series of differently colored slides, one of which (the conditioned stimulus [CS], a blue slide) was paired with an aversive unconditioned stimulus (UCS, a loud noise). The patient demonstrated normal conditioning: after several CS-UCS pairings, the patient began to produce reliable SCRs to the CS presented alone—that is, the blue slide evoked a conditioned emotional response from the patient. This occurred despite that the patient was incapable of factual learning—for example, mere minutes after the experiment, he could not remember which color of slide had been the CS, or even what had happened in the experiment. Given that the patient had intact amygdalae, this experiment supports a role for the amygdala in emotional conditioning, a result that is consistent with some recent functional imaging studies [6, 7].

EMOTION

In the situations reviewed earlier, SCRs were informative of brain processes that operate below the level of conscious awareness. We also have learned from the opposite scenario—that is, situations in which SCRs are *missing* despite conscious knowledge of the stimuli. Two such examples are presented in the following sections.

Impaired Skin Conductance Responses to Emotionally Charged Stimuli

Patients with damage to the ventromedial prefrontal sector of the brain develop striking changes in personality and emotional functioning. In the hallmark cases, the patients develop a sort of psychopathic personality style and seem to lose their ability to learn from their mistakes. We made a remarkable discovery in these patients: when presented with emotionally charged pictures that normally evoke large-amplitude SCRs (e.g., mutilation scenes and nudity), patients with ventromedial damage failed to produce such SCRs—their polygraph record was almost completely flat (Fig. 52.4) [8]. This occurred despite the fact that the patients were fully capable of producing normal SCRs under other circumstances, for example, in response to a sudden loud noise or light flash.

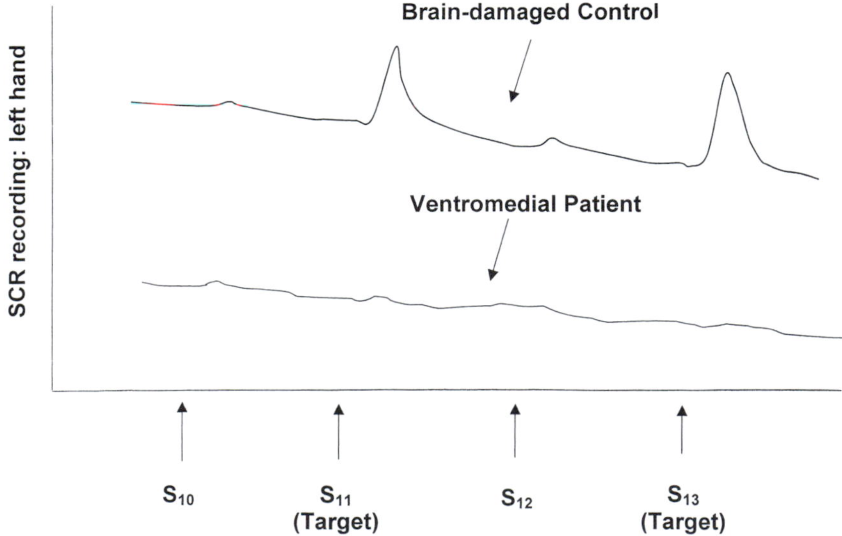

FIGURE 52.4 Impaired skin conductance responses (SCRs) to emotionally charged stimuli after ventromedial prefrontal damage. The polygraph record shows four stimulus presentations: stimuli S_{10} and S_{12} are nontargets (farm scenes), and stimuli S_{11} and S_{13} are targets (a nude and mutilation scene, respectively). A control patient with brain damage produced normal, large-amplitude SCRs to the target stimuli; the patient with ventromedial prefrontal damage did not.

Impaired Skin Conductance Responses to Familiar Faces

In another experiment with patients with ventromedial damage, we found that the patients failed to produce SCRs to well-known faces [9]. In fact, the pattern was exactly the opposite of the one we had obtained in patients with prosopagnosia: the ventromedial patients had completely normal conscious recognition of familiar faces, but they failed to produce discriminatory SCRs. As in the case of the emotionally charged pictures, the patients with ventromedial damage seemed to be oblivious to the emotional significance of the stimuli.

The Somatic Marker Hypothesis

The findings reviewed here, and other related observations, have led to the development of a framework that is termed the *somatic marker hypothesis* [10]. In summary, the theory posits that feelings and emotions give rise to "somatic markers," which serve as guideposts that help steer behavior in an advantageous direction. Deprived of these somatic markers, patients with ventromedial damage lose the ability to experience appropriate emotional responses to various stimuli and events. And we have proposed that the absence of these emotional responses—evidenced, for example, by the missing SCRs in the experiments described earlier—leads to defective planning and decision making; this, in turn, leads to the psychopathic-like behavior that is characteristic of patients with ventromedial damage.

References

1. Tranel, D., and H. Damasio. 1994. Neuroanatomical correlates of electrodermal skin conductance responses. *Psychophysiology* 31:427–438.
2. Dawson, M. E., A. M. Schell, and D. L. Filion. 2000. The electrodermal system. In *Handbook of psychophysiology*, ed. J. T. Cacioppo, L. G. Tassinary, and G. G. Berntson, 200–223. Cambridge, MA: Cambridge University Press.
3. Tranel, D., and A. R. Damasio. 1985. Knowledge without awareness: An autonomic index of facial recognition by prosopagnostics. *Science* 228:1453–1454.
4. Tranel, D., and A. R. Damasio. 1993. The covert learning of affective valence does not require structures in hippocampal system or amygdala. *J. Cogn. Neurosci.* 5:79–88.
5. Bechara, A., D. Tranel, H. Damasio, R. Adolphs, C. Rockland, and A. R. Damasio. 1995. Double dissociation of conditioning and declarative knowledge relative to the amygdala and hippocampus in humans. *Science* 269:1115–1118.
6. Morris, J. S., A. Öhman, and R. J. Dolan. 1998. Conscious and unconscious emotional learning in the human amygdala. *Nature* 393: 467–470.
7. Whalen, P. J., S. L. Rauch, N. L. Etcoff, S. C. McInerney, M. B. Lee, and M. A. Jenike. 1998. Masked presentations of emotional facial expressions modulate amygdala activity without explicit knowledge. *J. Neurosci.* 18:411–418.
8. Damasio, A. R., D. Tranel, and H. Damasio. 1990. Individuals with sociopathic behavior caused by frontal damage fail to respond autonomically to social stimuli. *Behav. Brain Res.* 41:81–94.
9. Tranel, D., H. Damasio, and A. R. Damasio. 1995. Double dissociation between overt and covert face recognition. *J. Cogn. Neurosci.* 7:425–432.
10. Damasio, A. R. 1994. *Descartes' error: Emotion, reason and the human brain.* New York: Grosset/Putnam.

P A R T V

NEUROPATHOLOGY

53 Oxidative Processes

Jing Zhang
Department of Pathology
Vanderbilt University
Nashville, Tennessee

Thomas J. Montine
Department of Pathology
University of Washington
Harborview Medical Center
Seattle, Washington

OXIDATIVE STRESS

Oxidative stress results from excess generation of free radicals and related reactive molecules. Free radicals are atoms or molecules with one or more unpaired electron(s) in the outer valence shell. A growing body of research indicates that free radical production under controlled conditions is a component of second messenger signaling in cells. However, excess or uncontrolled free radical production is detrimental to cells either by direct damage to macromolecules or liberation of toxic second messengers.

A number of sources of free radical generation exist in cells including cytochromes, oxygenases, and oxidases; however, the major source is thought to be mitochondrial oxidative phosphorylation, given that more than 90% of oxygen delivered to a cell is consumed by this organelle. In disease states, other sources of free radical generation may become pathophysiologically significant—that is, myeloperoxidase and inducible nitric oxide synthase in inflammatory conditions, advanced glycation end products in aging and diabetes, xanthine oxidase in ischemia/reperfusion injury, and possibly cyclooxygenases in some neurodegenerative diseases.

Although there are many types of free radicals, research in biologic systems has focused largely on reactive oxygen species (ROS) and reactive nitrogen species (RNS) [1]. During the sequential four electron reduction of molecular oxygen to water (Fig. 53.1, Reaction 1), two free radicals—superoxide anion (O_2^-) and hydroxyl radical (OH)—are produced along with hydrogen peroxide (H_2O_2); because H_2O_2 is not a radical, these three molecules are collectively referred to as ROS. Both O_2^- and H_2O_2 are signaling molecules under normal physiologic conditions. Conversely, OH is the most reactive and is capable of oxidizing lipids, carbohydrates, proteins, and nucleic acids at a rate limited by its own diffusion. OH is formed from O_2^- and H_2O_2 by the Haber–Weiss reaction (see Fig. 53.1, Reaction 2) or from H_2O_2 by Fenton chemistry (see Fig. 53.1, Reaction 3). Several metal ions may participate in the Fenton reaction including, Fe(II), Cu(I), Mn(II), Cr(V), and Ni(II).

Nitric oxide (NO), a free radical product of nitric oxide synthase–catalyzed oxidation of L-arginine to citrulline, initiates a cascade of RNS. NO has several physiologic functions including vasodilator and neuromodulator. NO also may directly inhibit some enzymes such as ribonucleotide reductase because it reacts efficiently with tyrosyl radical (rate constant $> 10^9 M^{-1} S^{-1}$). NO reacts with O_2^- to produce peroxynitrite ($ONOO^-$), a potent oxidant (Fig. 53.1, Reaction 4). In turn, reaction of $ONOO^-$ with ubiquitous CO_2 forms nitrosoperoxy carbonate that spontaneously cleaves to form a nitrating agent, nitrogen dioxide radical, and an oxidant, carbonate anion radical (see Fig. 53.1, Reaction 5). Finally, $ONOO^-$ may decompose to nitrous oxide and OH on protonation.

MECHANISMS TO LIMIT REACTIVE OXYGEN SPECIES AND REACTIVE NITROGEN SPECIES ACCUMULATION

A number of low molecular weight molecules and enzyme-catalyzed mechanisms have evolved to limit the accumulation of ROS and RNS in cells [1]. Low molecular weight antioxidants include glutathione, α-tocopherol, and ascorbate. Enzymes include superoxide dismutases (SODs), catalase, and peroxidases such as glutathione peroxidase (GPX). SODs are high-capacity enzymes located in the cytosol (Cu/Zn-SOD), mitochondria (Mn-SOD), or extracellular space (EC-SOD) that catalyze the conversion of O_2^- to H_2O_2. H_2O_2 is reduced to water by cytosolic GPX or peroxisomal catalase. Detoxification of $ONOO^-$ is obtained largely by preventing its formation, that is, metabolism of O_2^-. However, $ONOO^-$ can be reduced to nitrite (ONO^-) by GPX and selenoprotein P. As noted earlier, if not reduced to water by GPX or catalase, H_2O_2 is labile to Fenton chemistry and thereby generates OH. There are no known enzymes that detoxify OH. Moreover, glutathione, α-tocopherol, and ascorbate are not especially effective at detoxifying OH.

OXIDATIVE DAMAGE TO CELLULAR MACROMOLECULES

Lipid Peroxidation

Free radical–mediated damage to polyunsaturated fatty acids, termed lipid peroxidation, is a self-propagating

$$O_2 \longrightarrow O_2^{-} \longrightarrow H_2O_2 \longrightarrow {}^{\cdot}OH \longrightarrow H_2O \quad (1)$$

Molecular Oxygen — Superoxide Anion — Hydrogen Peroxide — Hydroxyl Radical — Water

$$O_2^{-} + H_2O_2 \longrightarrow O_2 + OH^{-} + {}^{\cdot}OH \quad (2)$$

$$H_2O_2 + Me^{+} \longrightarrow OH^{-} + {}^{\cdot}OH + Me^{++} \quad (3)$$

$$NO + O_2^{-} \longrightarrow ONOO^{-} \quad (4)$$

Nitric Oxide — Peroxynitrite

$$ONOO^{-} + CO_2 \longrightarrow ONOOCO_2^{-} \longrightarrow NO_2 + CO_3 \quad (5)$$

Nitrosoperoxy Carbonate — Nitrogen Dioxide — Carbonate Anion Radical

FIGURE 53.1 Some reactions that underlie oxidative stress, including reduction of molecular oxygen to water (1), Haber-Weiss reaction (2), Fenton reaction (3), peroxynitrite formation (4), and carbonate anion radical formation (5).

process that both damages cellular membranes and generates cytotoxic by-products [2]. Membrane damage derives from the generation of fragmented fatty acyl chains, lipid–lipid crosslinks, and lipid–protein crosslinks. In addition, lipid hydroperoxyl radicals can undergo endocyclization to produce novel fatty acid esters that may disrupt membranes. Bioactive secondary products are formed by fragmentation of lipid hydroperoxides to liberate a number of diffusible products, some of which are potent electrophiles. The most abundant diffusible products of lipid peroxidation are chemically reactive aldehydes such as acrolein, 4-hydroxy-2-hexenal, and 4-hydroxy-2-nonenal (HNE) (Fig. 53.2) [3]. In addition, enzymatic hydrolysis of the abnormal fatty acyl groups generated by lipid peroxidation also can liberate novel byproducts.

Some products of lipid peroxidation are thought to contribute significantly to its deleterious effects in tissue. Reactive aldehydes produced from lipid peroxidation react with a number of cellular nucleophiles, including protein, nucleic acids, and some lipids [3]. Indeed, many of the cytotoxic effects of lipid peroxidation can be reproduced directly by electrophilic lipid peroxidation products such as acrolein and HNE. These include depletion of glutathione, dysfunction of structural proteins, reduction in enzyme and transporter activities, and induction of cell death.

In addition to chemically reactive lipid peroxidation products, chemically stable products of lipid peroxidation also may contribute to disease through receptor-mediated signaling. For example, peroxidation and fragmentation of polyunsaturated fatty acyl groups in phosphatidylcholines can generate platelet-activating factor (PAF) analogues that stimulate the PAF receptor, thereby stimulating inflammatory responses [4]. In addition, one isomer of the isoprostanes, products of arachidonic acid peroxidation, has been shown to be a potent vasoconstrictor both peripherally and in the cerebrovasculature, likely through a receptor-mediated mechanism [5].

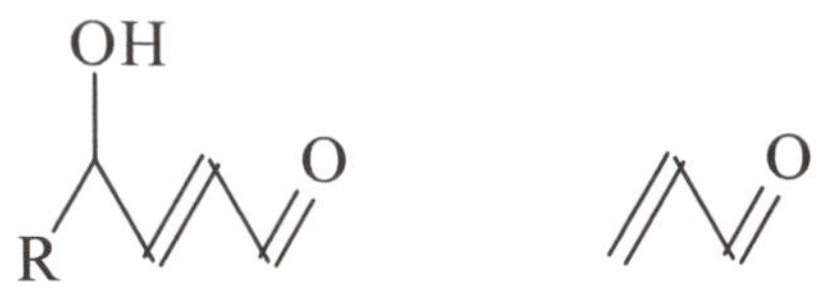

OH R O O

HNE: $R = C_5H_{11}$ Acrolein

HHE: $R = C_2H_5$

FIGURE 53.2 Some reactive alpha-beta unsaturated aldehydes generated during lipid peroxidation, including 4-hydroxy-2-nonenal (HNE), 4-hydroxy-2-hexenal (HHE), and acrolein.

Nucleic Acid

Unlike lipid peroxidation, oxidative damage to DNA is not self-propagating and is not thought to release cytotoxic effectors. However, if oxidative damage does cause a mutation, then DNA replication propagates the consequences of DNA oxidative damage to progeny. Oxidative damage to DNA can result in several structural changes to DNA such as single- and double-strand breaks, abasic sites, and a number of chemically modified nucleotides including thymine and cytosine glycols, 5-hydroxycytidine, 8-hydroxyguanine, and 8-hydroxyadenine [6]. In addition, many other products can be formed; for example, oxidative damage to cytosine alone generates more than 40 different species. One study of urinary concentrations of 8-hydroxyguanine and thymine glycol estimated that approximately 20,000 bases in DNA per cell per day are damaged by ROS. In addition to direct attack by ROS, reactive products of lipid peroxidation mentioned in the previous section also chemically modify DNA to form a variety of species.

Oxidative damage to DNA, either directly from ROS or by lipid peroxidation products, can lead to mutations; among the most common mutations are $C \rightarrow T$ substitutions, $G \rightarrow C$ transversions, and $G \rightarrow T$ transversions. However, it must be stressed that the common oxidative damage–induced mutations are not specific because they also are produced by errors by DNA polymerase copying of undamaged DNA. Thus, although there is substantial circumstantial evidence that oxidative damage–induced mutations can contribute to the initiation or progression of cancer, this lack of oxidative damage–specific mutations confounds definite demonstration of oxidative damage as a cause of malignancy.

Protein

Unlike lipid peroxidation, oxidative damage to protein is not self-propagating, and unlike oxidative damage to DNA, structural damage to protein from oxidative processes is not propagated to progeny. Nevertheless, oxidative damage to protein is thought to be the major effector of oxidative damage–mediated cellular dysfunction and death. As with DNA, protein may be directly modified by ROS and by products of lipid peroxidation. Given the ubiquitous distribution and much greater susceptibility of polyunsaturated fatty acids to free radical attack, it is proposed that lipid peroxidation products are the major source of protein modification from oxidative damage to cells.

CELLULAR REPAIR AND DETOXIFICATION MECHANISMS FOR OXIDATIVE DAMAGE

Glutathione-*S*-transferases

Glutathione-*S*-transferases (GSTs) are a nearly ubiquitous multigene enzyme superfamily that catalyze nucleophilic attack of glutathione on a broad group of electrophiles, including reactive compounds generated from lipid peroxidation. Typically, glutathionyl thioether formation results in a less toxic product, the exceptions being some aromatic compounds [7]. Organisms that have GST activity generally express multiple forms of the enzyme. Indeed, there are at least 21 human GST genes, of which 15 encode cytosolic GSTs; the main cytosolic classes are alpha, mu, and pi.

GSTs catalyze the committed step in the mercapturic acid pathway, a multistep mechanism to detoxify and excrete electrophiles. GSH-conjugates are transported out of the cell where they are cleaved sequentially by two ectoenzymes. The first, membrane-bound γ-glutamyltranspeptidase, cleaves the γ-glutamyl moiety. After this, a dipeptidase catalyzes removal of the glycine residue, leaving the cysteinyl thioether conjugate. The cysteinyl conjugate is then transported back into cells where it is *N*-acetylated by microsomal cysteine *S*-conjugate *N*-acetyltransferase. This *N*-acetylcysteine thioether, or mercapturic acid, conjugate is then exported from cells. Mercapturic acids conjugates formed in the kidney go directly into urine, whereas those synthesized in the liver may be transported into bile. Mercapturic acids synthesized in other tissues enter the bloodstream and are cleared by the kidney or liver.

Aldo-keto Oxidoreductases

Several cytotoxic products of lipid peroxidation, such as HNE and acrolein, are reactive carbonyls, similar to precursors of advanced glycosylation end products. Aldo-keto oxidoreductases oxidize or reduce carbonyl groups, thereby diminishing cytotoxicity from "carbonyl stress." This class includes a large number of enzymes involved in phase I metabolism. Examples of enzymes that reduce reactive carbonyls to alcohols are aldose reductase, aldehyde reductases, and members of the alcohol dehydrogenase family. Prominent among the enzymes that catalyze the oxidation of reactive carbonyls to carboxylic acids are the aldehyde dehydrogenases, for which there are multiple genes in humans.

DNA Repair

In broad terms, there are two pathways by which cells cope with DNA damage. If the damage is extensive, cells initiate cell death programs that result in apoptosis. Alternatively, in less extreme circumstances, cells use several different mechanisms to repair DNA damage. Overall, the fundamental processes of DNA repair are (1) recognition of the damage, (2) removal of the structurally altered base if appropriate, (3) new DNA synthesis, and (4) ligation [8]. The outcome is either true repair, disrepair, or nonrepair, the latter two having the potential to be propagated as mutations. The major mechanisms of DNA repair are base excision repair, nucleotide excision repair, double-strand break repair, mismatch repair, and O^6-methylguanine-DNA methyltransferase repair. Of these, base excision repair is thought to be especially important in repairing oxidative damage to DNA.

SUMMARY

ROS and RNS play critical roles in normal physiology and the pathophysiology of several diseases, including atherosclerosis, cancer, and neurodegeneration. Multiple modes for the production of ROS and RNS exist, and they can have diverse effects on cellular macromolecules. Numerous mechanisms have evolved by which cells defend themselves from these reactive species and their toxic consequences. Although complex, these offer multiple potentially therapeutic targets to intervene in the initiation and progression of these common diseases.

References

1. Gregus, Z., and C. D. Klaassen. 2001. Mechanisms of toxicity. In *Casarett and Doull's toxicology*, ed. C. D. Klaassen, 35–82. New York: McGraw-Hill.
2. Farber, J. L. 1995. Mechanisms of cell injury. In *Pathology of environmental and occupational disease*, ed. J. E. Craighead, 287–302. St. Louis: Mosby.
3. Esterbauer, H., R. J. Schaur, and H. Zollner. 1991 Chemistry and biochemistry of 4-hydroxynonenal, malondialdehyde and related aldehydes. *Free Radic. Biol. Med.* 11:81–128.
4. McIntyre, T. M., G. A. Zimmerman, and S. M. Prescott. 1999. Biologically active oxidized phospholipids. *J. Biol. Chem.* 274:25,189–25,192.
5. Morrow, J. D., and L. J. Roberts. 1997. The isoprostanes: Unique bioactive products of lipid peroxidation. *Prog. Lipid. Res.* 36:1–21.
6. Jackson, A. L., and L. A. Loeb. 2001. The contribution of endogenous sources of DNA damage to the multiple mutations in cancer. *Mutat. Res.* 477:7–21.
7. Parkinson, A. 2001. Biotransformation of xenobiotics. In *Casarett & Doull's toxicology*, ed. C. Klaassen, 133–224. New York: McGraw-Hill.
8. Preston, R. J., and G. R. Hoffmann. 2001. Genetic toxicology. In *Casarett and Doull's toxicology*, ed. C. D. Klaassen, 321–350. New York: McGraw-Hill.

54

α-Synuclein and Neurodegeneration

Michel Goedert
MRC Laboratory of Molecular Biology
Cambridge, United Kingdom

Parkinson's disease (PD) is the most common movement disorder. Neuropathologically, it is defined by nerve cell loss in the substantia nigra and the presence there of Lewy bodies and Lewy neurites. Nerve cell loss and Lewy body pathology also are found in a number of other brain regions, such as the dorsal motor nucleus of the vagus, the nucleus basalis of Meynert, and some autonomic ganglia. Lewy bodies and Lewy neurites also constitute the defining neuropathologic characteristics of dementia with Lewy bodies (DLB), a common late-life dementia that exists in a pure form or overlaps with the neuropathologic characteristics of Alzheimer's disease (AD). Unlike PD, DLB is characterized by large numbers of Lewy bodies in cortical brain areas.

Ultrastructurally, Lewy bodies and Lewy neurites consist of abnormal filamentous material. Despite that the Lewy body was first described in 1912, its biochemical composition remained unknown until 1997 [1].

Two developments have imparted a new direction to research on the etiology and pathogenesis of PD and DLB. First, the discovery that a missense mutation in the α-synuclein gene is a rare genetic cause of PD [2]. Second, the identification of the α-synuclein protein as the main component of Lewy bodies and Lewy neurites in PD, DLB, and several other diseases [3] (Fig. 54.1). Subsequently, the filamentous glial and neuronal inclusions of multiple system atrophy (MSA) also were found to be made of α-synuclein, revealing an unexpected molecular link with Lewy body diseases (Fig. 54.2). These findings have placed α-synuclein dysfunction at the center of several common neurodegenerative diseases (Table 54.1).

THE SYNUCLEIN FAMILY

Synucleins are proteins that are abundant in the brain; their physiologic functions are poorly understood. The synuclein family consists of three members—α-synuclein, β-synuclein and γ-synuclein—that range from 127 to 140 amino acids in length and are 55 to 62% identical in sequence, with a similar domain organization [1]. The amino-terminal half of each protein is taken up by imperfect 11 amino acid repeats that bear the consensus sequence KTKEGV. The repeats are followed by a hydrophobic intermediate region and a negatively charged carboxy-terminal domain. Synucleins are natively unfolded proteins with little ordered secondary structure that have only been identified in vertebrates. Of the three synucleins, only α-synuclein is associated with the filamentous inclusions of Lewy body diseases and MSA. Experimental studies have shown that α-synuclein can bind to lipid membranes through its amino-terminal repeats, indicating that it may be a lipid-binding protein. Mice that lack α-synuclein have been produced by homologous recombination [4, 5]. In the hippocampus of these mice, a marked reduction in the number of undocked synaptic vesicles was observed [5], suggesting that α-synuclein may influence the mobilization of synaptic vesicles in nerve terminals.

THE α-SYNUCLEIN DISEASES

Two missense mutations (A30P and A53T) in the 140-amino acid α-synuclein have been identified in familial cases of PD [1, 6]. Where examined, abundant Lewy bodies and Lewy neurites consisting of filamentous α-synuclein were present. Therefore, it is clear that the basis of this autosomal-dominant inherited form of PD resides in a toxic property conferred by the mutation in α-synuclein. A corollary of this thought is that a similar toxic property of wild-type α-synuclein may underlie the much more common forms of Lewy body diseases and MSA. The pathway leading from soluble to filamentous α-synuclein is probably central to Lewy body diseases and MSA (Fig. 54.3). It remains to be established whether the mere presence of filaments is sufficient to cause neurodegeneration or whether other toxic moieties, such as protofibrils, play a major role [7]. Filaments are space-occupying lesions that are likely to be detrimental to the long-term survival of nerve cells, especially when present in neurites (Table 54.1).

The α-synuclein filaments are unbranched, with a length of 200 to 600 nm and a width of 5 10 nm. Full-length α-synuclein is found in the filaments. Biochemically, the presence of inclusions correlates with the accumulation of

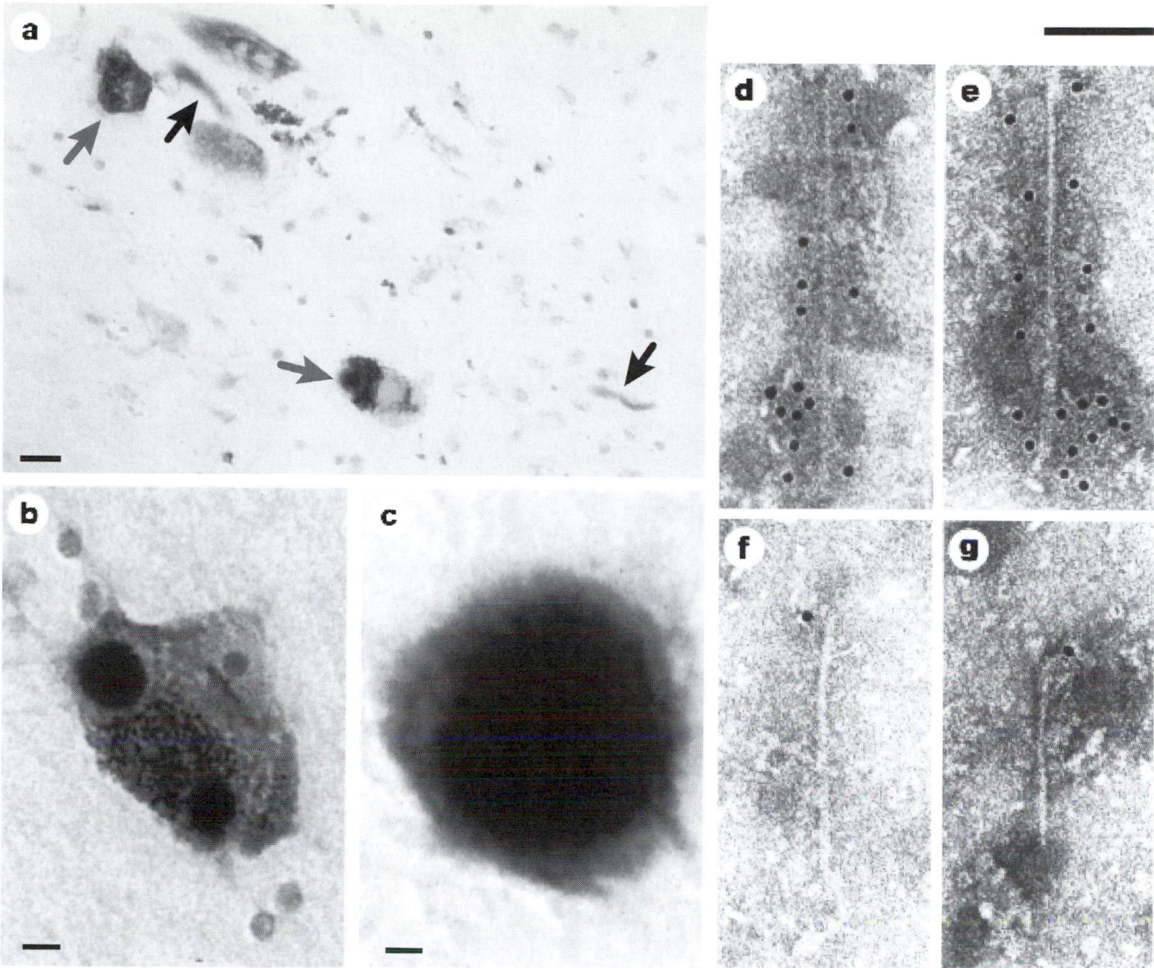

FIGURE 54.1 The α-synuclein pathology of Parkinson's disease. Lewy bodies and Lewy neurites in the substantia nigra and several other brain regions define Parkinson's disease at a neuropathologic level. These entities are shown here at the light (**A–C**) and electron microscopic (**D–G**) levels, labeled by α-synuclein antibodies. **A**, Two pigmented nerve cells, each containing an α-synuclein–positive Lewy body (*red arrows*). Lewy neurites (*black arrows*) also are immunopositive. Scale bar = 20 μm. **B**, Pigmented nerve cell with two α-synuclein–positive Lewy bodies. Scale bar = 8 μm. **C**, α-Synuclein–positive extracellular Lewy body. Scale bar = 4 μm. **D–G**, Isolated filaments from the substantia nigra of patients with Parkinson's disease are decorated with an antibody directed against the carboxyl-terminal (**D** and **E**) or the amino-terminal (**F** and **G**) region of α-synuclein. The gold particles conjugated to the second antibody appear as *black dots*. Note the uniform decoration in **D** and **E**, and the labeling of only one filament end in **F** and **G**. Scale bar (for **D–G**) = 100 nm. (See Color Insert)

TABLE 54.1 α-Synuclein Diseases

Lewy body diseases
Idiopathic Parkinson's disease
Dementia with Lewy bodies
Pure autonomic failure
Lewy body dysphagia
Incidental Lewy body disease
Inherited Lewy body diseases (mutations of the α-synuclein gene, PARK3 and PARK4)
Multiple system atrophy
Olivopontocerebellar atrophy
Striatonigral degeneration
Shy–Drager syndrome

insoluble α-synuclein. Phosphorylation, nitration, and ubiquitination are posttranslational modifications of filamentous α-synuclein. Phosphorylation at serine residue 129 and nitration appear to be common to all filaments. It remains to be seen whether they precede the assembly into filaments. By contrast, ubiquitination of α-synuclein is a late event that follows its assembly into filaments.

MODELS OF α-SYNUCLEINOPATHIES

In cell-free systems, α-synuclein assembles into filaments that share many of the morphologic and ultrastruc-

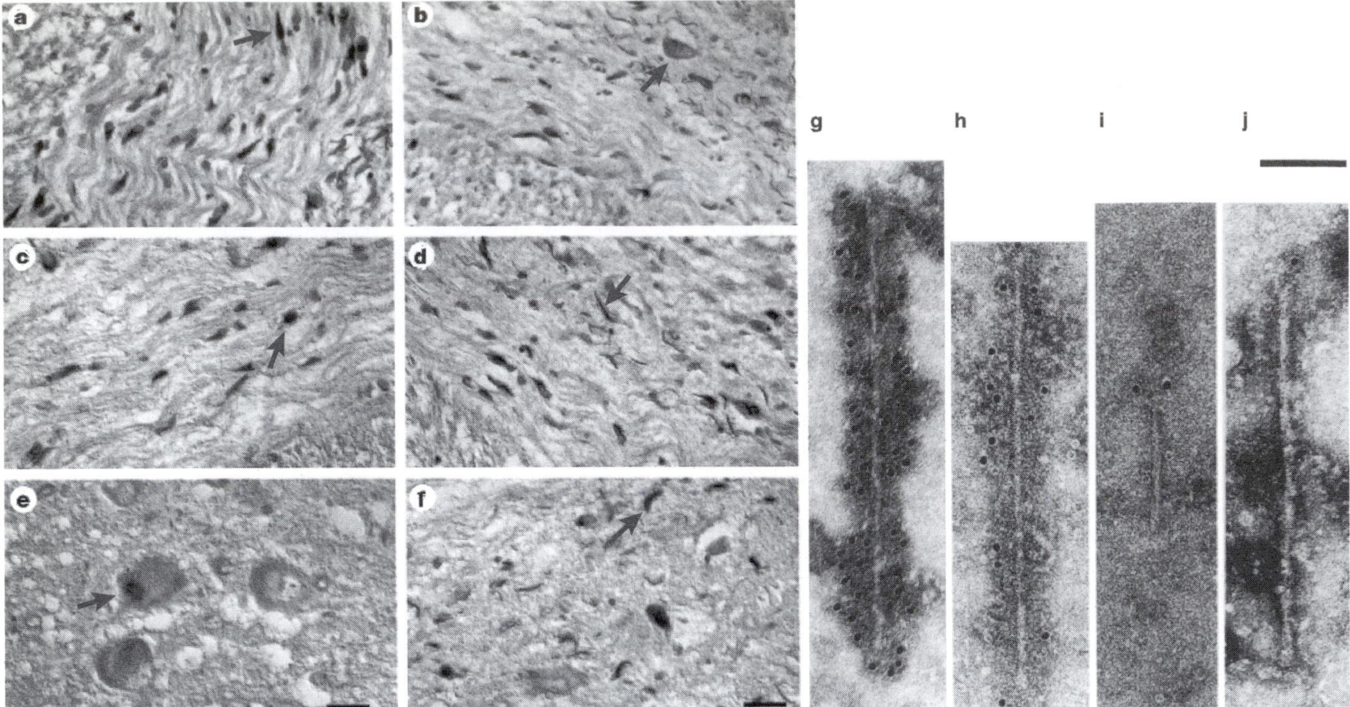

FIGURE 54.2 The α-synuclein pathology of multiple system atrophy. Glial cytoplasmic inclusions in several brain regions define multiple system atrophy at a neuropathologic level. Similar inclusions also are present in the nucleus of some glial cells, the cytoplasm and nucleus of some nerve cells, and in nerve cell processes. Here, these entities are shown at the light (**A–F**) and electron microscopic (**G–J**) levels, labeled by α-synuclein antibodies. **A–D**, α-Synuclein–immunoreactive oligodendrocytes and nerve cells in white matter of pons (**A**, **B**, and **D**) and cerebellum (**C**). **E** and **F**, α-Synuclein–immunoreactive oligodendrocytes and nerve cells in gray matter of pons (**E**) and frontal cortex (**F**). *Arrows* identify examples of each of the characteristic lesions stained for α-synuclein: cytoplasmic oligodendroglial inclusions (**A** and **F**), cytoplasmic nerve cell inclusions (**B**), nuclear oligodendroglial inclusion (**C**), neuropil threads (**D**), and nuclear nerve cell inclusion (**E**). Scale bars = 33 μm (**E**); 50 μm (**A–D**, **F**). **G–J**, Isolated filaments from the frontal cortex and cerebellum of patients with multiple system atrophy are decorated with an antibody directed against the carboxyl-terminal (**G** and **H**) or the amino-terminal (**I** and **J**) region of α-synuclein. The gold particles conjugated to the second antibody appear as *black dots*. Note the uniform decoration in **G** and **H**, and the labeling of only one filament end in **I** and **J**. A "twisted" filament is shown in **G**, whereas **H** shows a "straight" filament. Scale bar = 100 nm. (See Color Insert)

tural characteristics of filaments present in humans. The A53T mutation increases the rate of filament assembly, suggesting that this may be its primary effect. The mechanism of action of the A30P mutation in α-synuclein is less clear. An increase in the rate of oligomer formation and reduced lipid binding have been described. The assembly of α-synuclein is accompanied by the transition from random coil conformation to a β-pleated sheet. By electron diffraction, α-synuclein filaments show a conformation characteristic of amyloid fibers. Under the conditions of these experiments, β- and γ-synuclein failed to assemble into filaments and remained in a random coil conformation. However, when incubated with α-synuclein, they inhibited assembly into filaments.

Numerous laboratories are currently engaged in the production of animal models of α-synucleinopathies. Most work has involved the overexpression of wild-type or mutant human α-synuclein in nerve cells. To date, two studies, one in *Drosophila* and one in mouse, have described the formation of filamentous α-synuclein inclusions and nerve cell loss, confirming the direct link between dysfunction of α-synuclein and neurodegeneration [8, 9]. An intriguing model of α-synuclein pathology has been developed in the rat by the chronic intravenous infusion of the pesticide rotenone [10]. The rats developed a progressive degeneration of nigrostriatal neurons and filamentous, Lewy body–like inclusions that were immunoreactive for α-synuclein and ubiquitin. It would thus seem that oxidative stress can lead to the assembly of α-synuclein into filaments. During the last two decades, oxidative stress has received much attention as a pathogenic mechanism, because the metabolism of dopamine is a potential source of reactive oxygen species. Therefore, the rotenone model could have a direct bearing on the mechanisms by which Lewy bodies and Lewy neurites form in the substantia nigra in idiopathic PD.

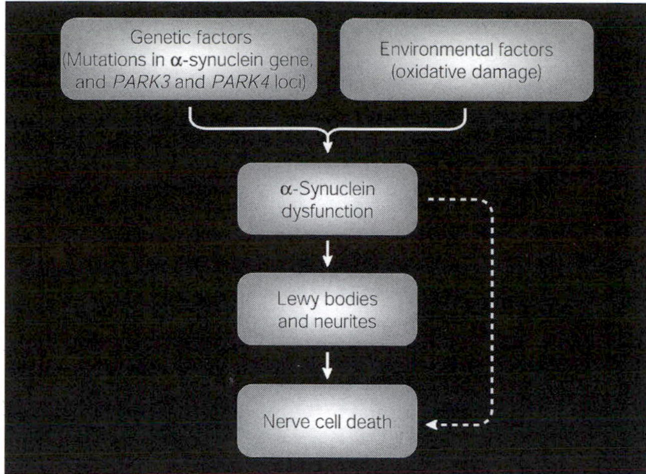

FIGURE 54.3 Model of disease pathway in Parkinson's disease. Genetic factors (mutations in the α-synuclein gene and mutations at the PARK3 and PARK4 loci) or environmental factors (oxidative damage, as exemplified by the experimental effects of rotenone) lead to a dysfunction of α-synuclein, which results in its ordered assembly into the filaments that characterize Lewy bodies and neurites. It is probable that the space-occupying Lewy body pathology contributes directly to nerve cell death. In addition, it is possible that conformationally altered, nonfilamentous α-synuclein is toxic to nerve cells.

References

1. Goedert, M. 2001. Alpha-synuclein and neurodegenerative diseases. *Nat. Rev. Neurosci.* 2:492–501.
2. Polymeropoulos, M. H., C. Lavedan, E. Leroy, S. E. Ide, A. Dehejia, A. Dutra, B. Pike, H. Root, J. Rubenstein, R. Boyer, E. S. Stenroos, S. Chandrasekharappa, A. Athanassiadou, T. Papapetropoulos, W. G. Johnson, A. M. Lazzarini, R. C. Duvoisin, G. Di Iorio, L. I., Golbe, and R. L. Nussbaum. 1997. Mutation in the α-synuclein gene identified in families with Parkinson's disease. *Science* 276:2045–2047.
3. Spillantini, M. G., M. L. Schmidt, V. M.-Y. Lee, J. Q. Trojanowski, R. Jakes, and M. Goedert. 1997. α-Synuclein in Lewy bodies. *Nature* 388:839–840.
4. Abeliovich, A., Y. Schmitz, I. Farinas, D. Choi-Lundberg, W. H. Ho, P. E. Castillo, N. Shinsky, J. M. Verdugo, M. Armanini, A. Ryan, M. Hynes, H. Phillips, D. Sulzer, and D. Rosenthal. 2000. Mice lacking α-synuclein display functional deficits in the nigrostriatal dopamine system. *Neuron* 25:239–252.
5. Cabin, D. E., K. Shimazu, D. Murphy, N. B. Cole, W. Gottschalk, K. L. McIllwain, B. Orrison, A. Chen, C. E. Ellis, R. Paylor, B. Lu, and R. L. Nussbaum. 2002. Synaptic vesicle depletion correlates with attenuated synaptic responses to prolonged repetitive stimulation in mice lacking α-synuclein. *J. Neurosci.* 22:8797–8807.
6. Krüger, R., W. Kuhn, T. Müller, D. Woitalla, S. Graeber, S. Kösel, H. Przuntek, J. T. Epplen, L. Schols, and O. Riess. 1998. Ala30Pro mutation in the gene encoding α-synuclein in Parkinson's disease. *Nat. Genet.* 18:106–108.
7. Conway, K. A., S. J. Lee, J. C. Rochet, T. T. Ding, R. E. Williamson, and P. T. Lansbury. 2000. Acceleration of oligomerization, not fibrillization, is a shared property of both α-synuclein mutations linked to early-onset Parkinson's disease: Implications for pathogenesis and therapy. *Proc. Natl. Acad. Sci. USA* 97:571–576.
8. Feany, M. B., and W. W. Bender. 2000. A *Drosophila* model of Parkinson's disease. *Nature* 404:394–398.
9. Giasson, B. I., J. E. Duda, S. M. Quinn, B. Zhang, J. Q. Trojanowski, and V. M.-Y. Lee. 2002. Neuronal α-synucleinopathy with severe movement disorder in mice expressing A53T human α-synuclein. *Neuron* 34:521–533.
10. Betarbet, R., T. B. Sherer, G. MacKenzie, M. Garcia-Osuna, A. V. Panov, and J. T. Greenamyre. 2000. Chronic systemic pesticide exposure reproduces features of Parkinson's disease. *Nat. Neurosci.* 3:1301–1306.

55 Experimental Autoimmune Autonomic Neuropathy

Steven Vernino
Department of Neurology
Mayo Clinic
Rochester, Minnesota

Autoimmune autonomic neuropathy is an acquired pandysautonomia often associated with autoantibodies against the acetylcholine receptor in autonomic ganglia. An animal model of this disorder, experimental autoimmune autonomic neuropathy (EAAN), can be induced in rabbits by immunization with the ganglionic acetylcholine receptor. Rabbits with EAAN manifest symptoms of autonomic failure similar to those seen in patients. Histologic and electrophysiologic studies of EAAN indicate that this autoimmune form of autonomic neuropathy is caused by an immune-mediated impairment in ganglionic synaptic transmission.

AUTOIMMUNE AUTONOMIC NEUROPATHY

Many cases of acute and subacute autonomic neuropathy likely result from neurologic autoimmunity. These include cases of Guillain–Barré syndrome with dysautonomia, paraneoplastic autonomic neuropathy, and idiopathic autoimmune autonomic neuropathy (AAN). Several clinical features of AAN, including the observation that some patients respond to intravenous immunoglobulin, suggest that this disorder is caused by pathogenic autoantibodies.

In myasthenia gravis (the prototypical antibody-mediated neurologic disorder), antibodies against the muscle acetylcholine receptor (AChR) impair transmission at the neuromuscular junction. In the autonomic nervous system, neuronal AChRs mediate fast synaptic transmission through both sympathetic and parasympathetic autonomic ganglia. The ganglionic neuronal AChR (nAChR) is a pentameric ion channel receptor that is structurally similar to the muscle nAChR and is typically composed of two α_3 subunits in combination with β_4 subunits [1]. Transgenic mice that are homozygous for null mutations in the α_3 gene lack ganglionic nAChRs and have profound autonomic dysfunction [2]. By analogy with myasthenia gravis, ganglionic AChR antibodies could impair transmission through autonomic ganglia and cause autonomic failure.

Indeed, many patients with AAN have serum autoantibodies specific for the neuronal ganglionic nAChR (see Chapter 87). Greater antibody levels are significantly correlated with more severe dysautonomia [3] and with a predominance of "cholinergic" symptoms (impaired bowel and bladder motility, impaired pupillary function and sicca symptoms) [4]. These observations strongly support the concept that AAN is an antibody-mediated disorder.

EXPERIMENTAL AUTOIMMUNE AUTONOMIC NEUROPATHY

Rigorous criteria for proving that a disorder is antibody-mediated have been advanced [5]. A critical step is demonstration that the specific autoantibodies reproduce the cardinal features of the disease in animals. Antibodies can be obtained from affected individuals and administered to the animal (passive transfer) or induced in the animal by immunization with the antigen of interest (active immunization). In the ideal setting (as with myasthenia gravis and experimental autoimmune myasthenia gravis), both passive transfer and active immunization reproduce the disease.

An active immunization model of ganglionic AChR autoimmunity has been reported. EAAN is produced by immunizing rabbits with a recombinant α_3 neuronal nAChR subunit fusion protein and adjuvant [6]. Within a few weeks of immunization, rabbits begin to produce ganglionic AChR antibodies and develop chronic severe generalized dysautonomia with prominent "cholinergic" failure.

EAAN recapitulates the clinical phenotype of human AAN. Rabbits producing high levels of ganglionic AChR antibody develop gastrointestinal dysmotility and fail to gain weight because of reduced food intake [6]. Gastroparesis and impaired intestinal motility are evident by fluoroscopy and by examination of the gut at autopsy. Severe parasympathetic dysfunction manifests as dilated and poorly responsive pupils (Fig. 55.1A), decreased lacrimation, reduced heart rate variability (especially at respiratory frequencies, see Fig. 55.1B), and dilated bladder [6, 7]. EAAN rabbits also have reduced levels of plasma catecholamines indicating reduced sympathetic tone. As in patients with AAN, the severity of autonomic disturbances is greater in rabbits with greater antibody levels. Individual measures of autonomic function in EAAN rabbits also correlate with antibody level [7].

In the animal model, the pathophysiology of autoimmune autonomic neuropathy can be elucidated. Neurons in autonomic ganglia from EAAN rabbits are intact but show a selective loss of surface ganglionic AChR [7]. Electrophysiologic studies of mesenteric ganglia isolated from EAAN rabbits demonstrate a failure of ganglionic synaptic transmission consistent with the loss of postsynaptic receptors (Fig. 55.2) [6].

This animal model serves to define human AAN as an antibody-mediated disorder. Studies of EAAN suggest that the autonomic deficits in AAN may be reversible (at least early in the disease course). An animal model also facilitates the preclinical development and testing of novel therapeutic strategies for autonomic failure.

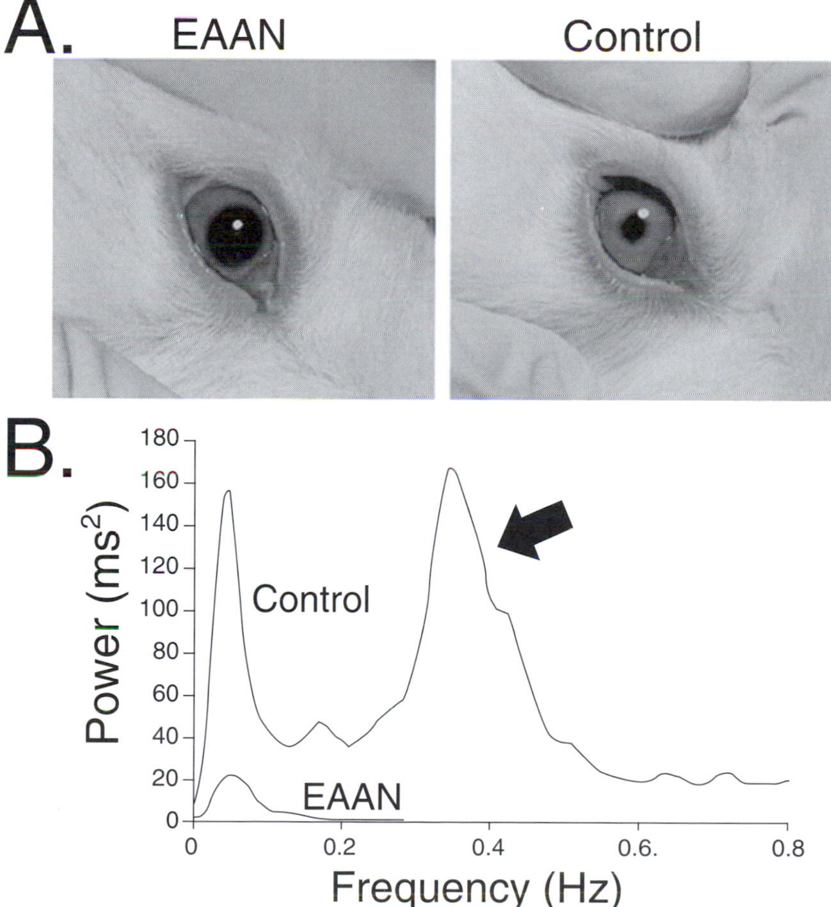

FIGURE 55.1 Parasympathetic failure in experimental autoimmune autonomic neuropathy (EAAN). **A**, Pupillary response to light. EAAN rabbits have dilated pupils with impaired pupillary light response. **B**, Power spectral analysis of heart rate variability in a control rabbit (top trace) reveals large high-frequency (*arrow*) and low-frequency peaks. In a rabbit with high antibody level (bottom trace), there is a complete loss of high-frequency variability (reflecting impairment of cardiovagal innervation) [6, 7].

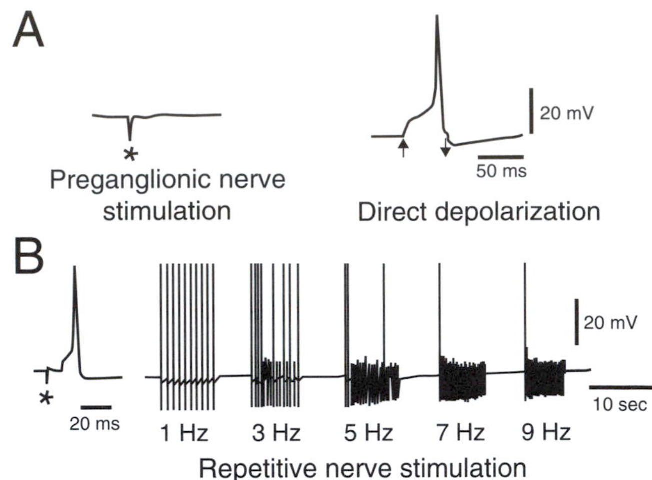

FIGURE 55.2 Ganglionic synaptic transmission failure in experimental autoimmune autonomic neuropathy (EAAN) [6]. Intracellular electrode recordings from neurons in an isolated inferior mesenteric ganglia preparation. Neurons in this ganglia provide extrinsic control of gut motility and receive cholinergic innervation from the spinal cord and gut. **A**, Supramaximal stimulus of lumbar colonic nerve (*asterisk*) fails to elicit a response in most neurons (70% showed no response), whereas direct depolarization of the neuron readily elicits an action potential. In contrast, preganglionic stimulation produced an action potential response in all neurons studied from ganglia of control rabbits (not shown). **B**, A minority of ganglionic neurons from EAAN rabbits respond to a single stimulation of the preganglionic lumbar colonic nerves. In these neurons, repetitive nerve stimulation at increasing stimulation frequency was applied. At low stimulation frequency (up to 1 Hz), each stimulus produces an action potential in the postsynaptic neuron. At greater stimulus frequencies, synaptic transmission begins to fail frequently. A similar failure of synaptic transmission with repetitive stimulation is seen at the neuromuscular junction in animals with experimental myasthenia gravis. Repetitive stimulation studies in control ganglia (not shown) showed no synaptic failure during repetitive stimulation up to 7 Hz. This finding indicates a reduced safety margin for synaptic transmission at the ganglionic synapse as the cause of EAAN.

References

1. Patrick, J., P. Seguela, S. Vernino, M. Amador, C. Luetje, and J. Dani. 1993. Functional diversity of neuronal nicotinic acetylcholine receptors. In *Progress in brain research*, ed. A. C. Cuello, 113–120. Amsterdam: Elsevier Science.
2. Xu, W., S. Gelber, A. Orr-Urtreger, D. Armstrong, R. A. Lewis, C. N. Ou, J. Patrick, L. Role, M. De Biasi, and A. L. Beaudet. 1999. Megacystis, mydriasis, and ion channel defect in mice lacking the alpha3 neuronal nicotinic acetylcholine receptor. *Proc. Natl. Acad. Sci. USA* 96:5746–5751.
3. Vernino, S., P. A. Low, R. D. Fealey, J. D. Stewart, G. Farrugia, and V. A. Lennon. 2000. Autoantibodies to ganglionic acetylcholine receptors in autoimmune autonomic neuropathies. *N. Engl. J. Med.* 343: 847–855.
4. Klein, C. M., S. Vernino, V. A. Lennon, P. Sandroni, R. D. Fealey, L. Benrud-Larson, D. Sletten, and P. A. Low. 2003. The spectrum of autoimmune autonomic neuropathies. *Ann. Neurol.* 53:752–758.
5. Drachman, D. B. 1990. How to recognize an antibody-mediated autoimmune disease: Criteria. In *Immunologic mechanisms in neurologic and psychiatric disease*, ed. B. H. Waksman, 183–186. New York: Raven Press.
6. Lennon, V. A., L. G. Ermilov, J. H. Szurszewski, and S. Vernino. 2003. Immunization with neuronal nicotinic acetylcholine receptor induces neurological autoimmune disease. *J. Clin. Invest.* 111:907–913.
7. Vernino, S., P. A. Low, and V. A. Lennon. 2003. Experimental autoimmune autonomic neuropathy. *J. Neurophysiol.* 90:2053–2059.

PART VI

EVALUATION OF AUTONOMIC FAILURE

56 Clinical Assessment of Autonomic Failure

David Robertson
Vanderbilt University Medical Center
Clinical Research Center
Nashville, Tennessee

There are more tests of the autonomic nervous system than of any other neurologic system. Many of these tests are readily applied at the bedside. Unfortunately, although these bedside autonomic tests are easy to perform, they may be difficult to interpret in an individual patient. Most physicians who routinely treat patients with autonomic disorders develop a small armamentarium of tests they feel comfortable with and rely on. For the neurologist, tests of peripheral sudomotor function may form the organizing nucleus of autonomic evaluation; for the cardiologist, it may be tests of blood pressure and heart rate; for the endocrinologist, it may be circulating catecholamines and renin; for the ophthalmologist, it may be pupillary tests; and for the pharmacologist, it may be drug tests for evidence of stimulated autonomic function or hypersensitivity. Despite such dramatically divergent diagnostic approaches, it is remarkable how much consensus is often achieved in terms of the actual diagnosis and therapy of an individual patient.

A carefully taken history is obviously the single most valuable diagnostic resource. A brief listing of important points in questioning patients is shown in Table 56.1. More detailed discussions of some of these may be found in the Low text. Key features for evaluation in the physical examination are shown in Table 56.2.

In this section, attention is given to highly informative autonomic tests. A listing of widely used tests is shown in Tables 56.3, 56.4, and 56.5. Because many of these tests provide redundant information, most of them are unnecessary outside of a research environment.

ORTHOSTATIC TEST

Orthostatic symptoms are usually the most debilitating aspect of autonomic dysfunction readily amenable to therapy, and for this reason the blood pressure and heart rate response to upright posture should be the starting point of any autonomic laboratory evaluation. In healthy human subjects, the cardiovascular effect of upright posture has been carefully defined. When assumption of the upright posture is active (standing), the vigorous contraction of large muscles leads to a transient muscle vasodilation and minor decrease in arterial pressure for which the reflexes are not immediately able to completely compensate, but this short-lived depressor phase is not usually seen with passive (tilt-table) upright posture. Immediately after 90-degree head-up tilt, about 500 ml blood moves into the veins of the legs and about 250 ml into the buttocks and pelvic area. There is a rapid, vagally mediated increase in heart rate followed by a sympathetically mediated further increase. As right ventricular stroke volume declines, there is depletion of blood from the pulmonary reservoir and central blood volume decreases. Stroke volume decreases, and cardiac output decreases about 20%. With this decline in cardiac output, blood pressure is maintained by vasoconstriction that reduces splanchnic, renal, and skeletal muscle blood flow in particular, but other circulations as well.

In the orthostatic test, mild autonomic impairment usually leads to a dramatic tachycardia with relatively little change in blood pressure (Table 56.6). In the presence of a still functioning baroreflex, the increased heart rate can compensate for the mild peripheral denervation, thus preventing significant decrement in blood pressure. With moderate autonomic neuropathy, the tachycardia may still be present, but may be unable to compensate completely and mild orthostatic hypotension may occur. As the neuropathy becomes more severe, the orthostatic decrease in blood pressure becomes greater and greater, and the ability of the efferent autonomic system to manifest a tachycardia is progressively attenuated. In the severe autonomic failure, the decrease in blood pressure may be more than 100 mmHg, and yet the heart rate may not increase at all.

Orthostatic tolerance is challenged by a number of factors. Important among these factors are food ingestion, high environmental temperature, hyperventilation, endogenous vasodilators, and many pharmacologic agents. If no abnormality in orthostatic blood pressure or heart rate is detected in the hour after ingestion of a large meal, autonomic neuropathy of sufficient severity to cause cardiovascular instability is effectively ruled out.

An important aspect of evaluation of responses to orthostasis is the rapid reduction in total blood volume that

TABLE 56.1 Key Features in the Autonomic History

- Orthostatic intolerance or hypotension
  - Dizziness or lightheadedness
  - Visual changes
  - Neck and shoulder discomfort
  - Weakness
  - Confusion
  - Slurred speech
  - Presyncope or syncope
  - Postprandial angina pectoris
  - Nausea
  - Palpitations
  - Tremulousness
  - Flushing sensation
  - Nocturia
  - Worsening by the following:
    - Bedrest
    - Food ingestion
    - Alcohol
    - Fever
    - Hot weather/environment
    - Hot bath
    - Environmental heat
    - Exercise
    - Hyperventilation
- Hypohidrosis
  - Dry skin
  - Dry socks and feet
  - Reduced skin wrinkling
  - Excessive sweating in intact regions
- Genitourinary dysautonomia
  - Impotence
  - Nocturia
  - Urinary retention
  - Urinary incontinence
  - Recurrent urinary tract infection
- Gastrointestinal dysautonomia
  - Constipation
  - Postprandial fullness
  - Anorexia
  - Diarrhea
  - Fecal urgency and incontinence
  - Weight loss
- Poorly characterized dysautonomia features
  - Early transient autonomic hyperfunction
  - Anemia
  - Ptosis
  - Supine nasal stuffiness
  - Supine hypertension and diuresis
  - Fatigue
- Nonautonomic features in multiple system atrophy
  - Problems with balance/movement
  - Loud respirations/snoring
  - Episodic gasping respirations
  - Sleep apnea
  - Brief crying spells
  - Emotional lability
  - Leg pain
  - Altered libido
  - Hypnagogic leg jerking
  - Hallucinations
  - Difficulty swallowing
  - Aspiration pneumonia
  - Drooling
  - Other cerebellar and extrapyramidal symptoms

TABLE 56.2 Key Features in the Autonomic Physical Examination

- Skin
  - Dryness
  - Dry socks and feet
  - Reduced hand wrinkling
  - Absent pilomotor reaction
  - Pallor
- Eyes
  - Impaired pupillary motor function
  - Dryness of eyes (redness and itching)
  - Ptosis
- Cardiovascular
  - Low standing blood pressure ± tachycardia
  - Unchanging pulse rate on standing
  - Increased supine blood pressure
  - Loss of respiratory arrhythmia
- Gastrointestinal
  - Reduced salivation
  - Stomach fullness
  - Reduced transit time
  - Impaired anal tone
- Genitourinary
  - Impaired morning erection
  - Retrograde ejaculation
  - Urgency
  - Sphincter weakness
  - Atonic bladder
- Other
  - Abnormal temperature regulation
  - Extrapyramidal signs (rigidity > tremor)
  - Cerebellar signs
  - Impaired ocular movements
  - Slurred speech
  - Laryngeal paralysis
  - Muscle wasting

TABLE 56.3 Tests of Baroreflex Function

Test	Afferent	Integration	Efferent	Response
Orthostasis	IX, X, CNS	Medulla	Autonomic	↑ HR
Deep breathing	X	Medulla	X	↑ HR (inspiration)
Valsalva maneuver	IX, X, CNS	Medulla	Autonomic	↑ HR then ↓ HR
Cuff occlusion	IX, X	Medulla	Autonomic	↓ BP, ↑ HR
Saline infusion	IX, X	Medulla	Autonomic	↑ BP, ↓ HR
Barocuff (suction)	IX	Medulla	X	↓ HR
Barocuff (pressure)	IX	Medulla	X	↑ HR
LBNP	IX, X	Medulla	Autonomic	↑ HR
Carotid massage	IX	Medulla	Autonomic	↓ HR, ↓ BP
Phenylephrine	IX, X	Medulla	Autonomic	↓ HR
Nitroprusside	IX, X	Medulla	Autonomic	↑ HR

BP, blood pressure; CNS, central nervous system; HR, heart rate; LBNP, lower body negative pressure; IX, glossopharyngeal; X, vagus.

TABLE 56.4 Tests of Neurotransmitter Receptor Responsiveness

Name	Administration	Receptor	Response
Agonists			
Phenylephrine	IV, eye	α_1	Pressor; pupillary dilation
Clonidine	Oral	α_2, I	Depressor (central); MSNA
Isoproterenol	IV	β_1	Increased HR
Isoproterenol	IV local	β_2	Depressor; vascular resistance
Acetylcholine	IV local	Muscarinic	Decreased vascular resistance
Methacholine	Eye	Muscarinic	Pupillary constriction
Nicotine	IV	Nicotinic	Increase HR
Antagonists			
Phentolamine	IV	α_1, α_2	Depressor
Yohimbine	IV	α_2	Increased BP, plasma NE
Propranolol	IV	β_1	Reduced HR
Propranolol	IV local	β_2	Increased vascular resistance
Atropine	IV	Muscarinic	Increased HR
Trimethaphan	IV	Nicotinic	Depressor; MSNA
Neurotransmitter-releasing agents			
Tyramine	IV	α, β	Increased BP; plasma NE
Hydroxyamphetamine	eye	α_1	Pupillary dilatation
Pheochromocytoma-provoking agents			
Histamine	IV	α_1, β	Increased BP; plasma NE
Glucagon	IV	α_1, β	Increased BP; plasma NE

BP, blood pressure; HR, heart rate; I, imidazoline; IV, intravenous; MSNA, muscle sympathetic nerve activity; NE, norepinephrine.

TABLE 56.5 Other Autonomic Tests

Test	Afferent	Integration	Efferent	Response
Cold pressor	Pain fibers	CNS	Sympathoadrenal	↑ BP
Handgrip	Muscle afferents	CNS	Autonomic	↑ BP, ↑ HR
Mental arithmetic	CNS	CNS	Sympathoadrenal	↑ BP
Startle	Auditory	CNS	Sympathoadrenal	↑ BP, ↑ HR
Face immersion	V	Medulla	Autonomic	↓ HR
Pupil cycle time	Optic nerve	Edinger–Westphal	III	Dilate/constrict
Venous response venoconstriction (inspiratory gasp)	Spinal nerve	Cord	Sympathetic	
Venoarterial reflex vasoconstriction	Noradrenergic axon	neuron	noradrenergic axon	
Reflex heating	Spinothalamic	Hypothalamus	Sympathetic	Vasodilatation
Thermoregulatory	Temperature receptors	Hypothalamus	Sympathetic	Sweating
QSART	Sympathetic cholinergic axon	Neuron	Sympathetic cholinergic axon	Sweating

BP, blood pressure; CNS, central nervous system; III, oculomotor nerve; QSART, quantitative sudomotor axon reflex test; V, trigeminal nerve.

TABLE 56.6 Hemodynamics of Autonomic Failure on Standing

	ΔBP	ΔHR
Normal	—	↑
Mild AF	—	↑↑↑
Moderate AF	↓↓	↑↑
Severe AF	↓↓↓	—

AF, autonomic failure; BP, blood pressure; HR, heart rate.

occurs. It is not unusual for a 12% decrease in total plasma volume to occur within 10 minutes of assumption of the upright posture as fluid goes from the vascular compartment into the extravascular space. This accounts for the delay in appearance of symptoms in patients with mild autonomic impairment for some minutes after the actual assumption of upright posture. Therefore, the long stand (30 minutes) test is a much more severe orthostatic stress than the short stand (5 minutes) test commonly used.

TILT-TABLE TESTING

Many investigators prefer the use of upright tilt to the orthostatic test in the evaluation of the variables. In general, analogous but not identical results are obtained. The use of upright tilt is described in detail in the Grubb text (7). Although there is no proof that upright tilt offers any diagnostic advantage over carefully obtained upright blood pressure data, many investigators use tilt because of its convenience, its capacity to calibrate the gravity stimulus, and its safety for the patient.

PHARMACOLOGIC TESTS

Information about prevailing sympathetic and parasympathetic activation and denervation hypersensitivity can be achieved by use of muscarinic and adrenergic agonists and antagonists. References 1 and 3 provide instructive examples of how biochemical and physiologic tests may be combined to make novel diagnostic discoveries.

References

1. Low, P. A., Ed. 1997. *Clinical autonomic disorders: Evaluation and management*, 2nd ed., 179–209, 383–403. Philadelphia: Lippincott.
2. Eckberg, D. L. 1980. Parasympathetic cardiovascular control in human disease: A critical review of methods and results. *Am. J. Physiol.* 239:H581–H593.
3. Eckberg, D. L. 2003. The human respiratory gate. *J. Physiol.* 548:339–352.
4. Robertson, D., M. R. Goldberg, A. S. Hollister, J. Onrot, R. Wiley, J. G. Thompson, and R. M. Robertson. 1986. Isolated failure of autonomic noradrenergic neurotransmission: Evidence for impaired beta-hydroxylation of dopamine. *N. Engl. J. Med.* 314:1494–1497.
5. Robertson, D. 1981. Assessment of autonomic function. In *Clinical diagnostic manual for the house officer*, ed. K. L. Baughman KL, 86–101. Baltimore, Williams & Wilkins.
6. Malik M, Ed. 1998. *Clinical guide to cardiac autonomic tests.* Dordrecht: Kluwer.
7. Grubb, B. P. 1998. *Syncope*. New York: Futura.
8. Julu, P. O., V. L. Cooper, S. Hansen, and R. Hainsworth. 2003. Cardiovascular regulation in the period preceding vasovagal syncope in conscious humans. *J. Physiol.* 549:299–311.
9. Goldstein, D. S. 2000. *The autonomic nervous system in health and disease.* New York: Dekker.

57 Evaluation of the Patient with Syncope

Horacio Kaufmann
Autonomic Nervous System Laboratory
Department of Neurology
Mount Sinai School of Medicine
New York, New York

Syncope (Greek, "synkcope": cessation, pause) is a transient loss of consciousness and postural tone with spontaneous recovery and no neurologic sequelae. Syncope is caused by a global reversible reduction of blood flow to the reticular activating system, the neuronal network in the brainstem responsible for supporting consciousness. Temporary loss of consciousness caused by noncardiovascular mechanisms such as seizure and metabolic and psychiatric disorders may stimulate syncope but can usually be distinguished from true syncope by clinical features.

Syncope is a common clinical problem. In the 26-year surveillance of the Framingham study, syncope occurred in 3% of men and in 3.5% of women [1]. Moreover, syncope accounts for up to 6% of hospital admissions.

MECHANISMS OF SYNCOPE

Three hemodynamic abnormalities may produce syncope (Table 57.1): (1) a decrease in systemic blood pressure, which usually occurs in the standing position (i.e., orthostatic hypotension) and is mainly caused by ineffective control of peripheral vascular resistance; (2) an acute decrease in cardiac output; and (3) an acute increase in cerebrovascular resistance.

Orthostatic Hypotension

In the standing position, arterial pressure at brain level is 15 to 20 mmHg less than arterial pressure at the level of the aortic arch. Local autoregulatory mechanisms maintain cerebral blood flow fairly constant despite changes in cerebral arterial pressure. However, if cerebral arterial pressure decreases to less than 40 mmHg, cerebral autoregulation does not prevent decreases in cerebral blood flow. Thus, if a person is standing and mean aortic pressure decreases to less than 70 mmHg, cerebral blood flow is likely to decrease sufficiently for syncope or presyncope to occur.

Orthostatic hypotension can be secondary to drugs, to chronic autonomic failure (which is discussed elsewhere in this book), and to neurally mediated syncope (i.e., vasovagal syncope).

Orthostatic hypotension caused by drugs is a common but often overlooked cause of syncope, particularly in the elderly in whom baroreflexes may be impaired. Another frequent reason for syncope in the elderly is postprandial hypotension. This is believed to be caused by impaired baroreflex-mediated vasoconstriction that fails to compensate for the splanchnic vasodilation induced by food [2].

The most frequent cause of syncope in apparently healthy subjects is neurally mediated syncope. Neurally mediated syncope (also referred to as vasovagal, vasodepressor, or reflex syncope) is an acute hemodynamic reaction produced by a sudden change in autonomic nervous system activity. In neurally mediated syncope, the normal pattern of autonomic outflow that maintains blood pressure in the standing position (increased sympathetic and decreased parasympathetic activity) is acutely reversed. Parasympathetic outflow to the sinus node increases producing bradycardia, whereas sympathetic outflow to blood vessels is reduced and there is profound vasodilation, which, interestingly, is heterogeneous. Vasodilation occurs in skeletal muscle and probably in the splanchnic vascular bed, but not in the skin. Bradycardia is not the cause of hypotension because ventricular pacemakers prevent it but they do not prevent syncope. Whether the reduction in sympathetic activity is the sole mechanism responsible for vasodilation is unknown. Increased levels of adrenaline and an increase in nitric oxide–mediated vasodilation may also be involved [3].

Neurally mediated syncope can be triggered centrally by stimuli such as pain or fear, presumably, by descending signals from cortical, limbic, or hypothalamic structures to autonomic control centers in the medulla. Neurally mediated syncope also can be triggered peripherally by stimulation of sensory receptors located in the arterial tree or viscera. These receptors respond to pressure or mechanical deformation and have afferent fibers in the vagus and glossopharyngeal nerves, and when discharged excessively may inhibit vasomotor centers in the medulla (Fig. 57.1). For example, neurally mediated syncopal syndromes occur after compression of carotid baroreceptors in the neck, after rapid emptying of a distended bladder or distention of the gastrointestinal tract and during glossopharyngeal or trigeminal neuralgia.

In addition, in susceptible individuals, neurally mediated syncope may occur with no obvious trigger while the subject is standing or walking. It had been postulated that in these cases the trigger of syncope was excessive stimulation of afferent nonmyelinated nerves from the ventricle (i.e., neurocardiogenic or "ventricular" syncope) [4]. However, neurally mediated syncope has been induced in patients with heart transplants, in whom the ventricle is likely to be denervated. Perhaps, sensory receptors in the patient with heart transplant are in the arterial tree rather than the ventricle.

Neurally mediated syncope needs to be distinguished from syncope in autonomic failure. In autonomic failure, orthostatic hypotension is persistent and caused by chronic inability to appropriately activate efferent sympathetic fibers. In contrast, hypotension in neurally mediated syncope is an acute, self-limited event caused by a paroxysmal transient disruption of baroreflex function (Fig. 57.2). Between syncopal episodes, patients with neurally mediated syncope have normal autonomic cardiovascular responses.

TABLE 57.1 Causes of Syncope

Orthostatic hypotension (reduction in vascular resistance of intravascular volume or both):
Drugs
Chronic baroreflex failure
Neurally mediated syncope
Decrease in cardiac output:
Cardiac arrhythmia
Obstructions to flow
Myocardial infarction
Increased cerebrovascular resistance:
Hyperventilation
Increased intracranial pressure

ACUTE DECREASE IN CARDIAC OUTPUT

A decrease in cardiac output resulting in syncope may be caused by cardiac arrhythmias, by obstruction to flow in aortic stenosis or pulmonary embolism, and as a result of acute myocardial infarction. Episodes of profound sinus bradycardia or sinus arrest caused by sinoatrial disease may present as recurrent syncope. Similarly, supraventricular tachyarrhythmias and the sinus pauses that follow, as well as rapid ventricular tachycardia that progresses to ventricular fibrillation before reverting spontaneously to normal, may be responsible for recurrent episodes of syncope or near syncope.

ACUTE INCREASE IN CEREBROVASCULAR RESISTANCE

Rarely, syncope may occur when blood flow to the reticular activating system is compromised by acute increases in cerebrovascular resistance or intracranial pressure. A reduction in carbon dioxide in blood induced by alveolar hyperventilation, as it occurs in panic attacks, may produce diffuse cerebral vasoconstriction severe enough to induce syncope, particularly if the person is standing. An increase in intracranial pressure induced by coughing or straining against a closed glottis may precipitate syncope in patients with craniocervical malformations.

Atherosclerotic disease involving the posterior cerebral circulation is an infrequent cause of syncope and is usually accompanied by other neurologic abnormalities. A rare cause of syncope is the subclavian steal syndrome. It is caused by occlusive disease of the subclavian artery, proximal to the origin of the vertebral artery usually on the left side. Syncope occurs during upper arm exercise because blood is shunted through the circle of Willis retrograde through the vertebral artery to the distal subclavian artery to the arm.

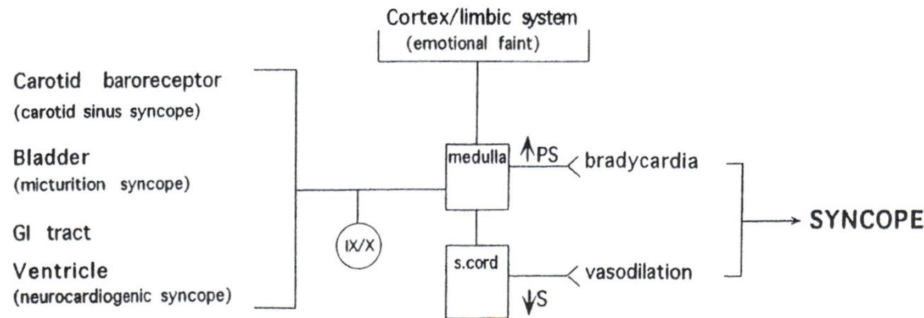

FIGURE 57.1 Afferent and efferent pathways in neurally mediated syncope.

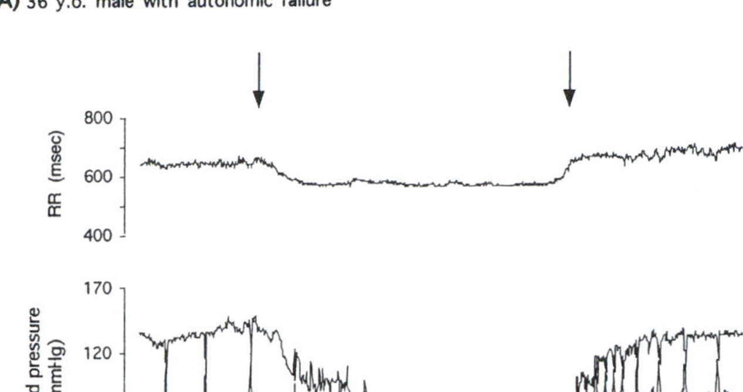

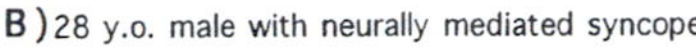

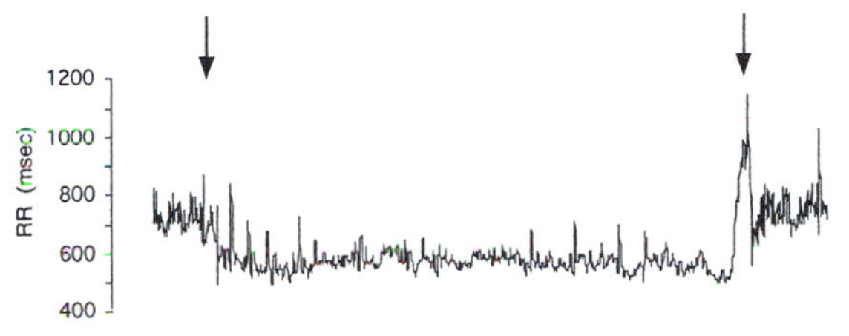

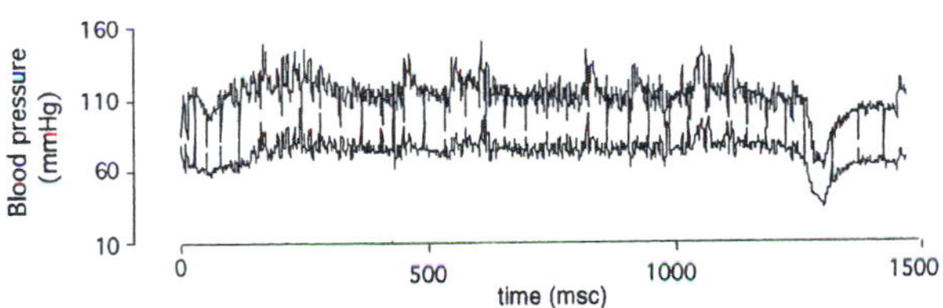

FIGURE 57.2 Continuous RR intervals and blood pressure (Finapres) recordings during passive head-up tilt in (**A**) subject with primary autonomic failure and (**B**) subject with neurally mediated syncope. *First arrow* indicates tilt up and *second arrow* tilt down after syncope occurred.

DIAGNOSIS

History, physical examination, and electrocardiography have a combined diagnostic yield of about 50%. A thorough history-taking may reveal the cause of syncope in a substantial number of cases [5]. Accounts of witnesses must be sought to rule out a seizure disorder. A few myoclonic jerks, tonic contractions of the limbs, or "rolling of the eyes" can occur in syncope, but frank tonic clonic convulsions suggest seizure. Urinary incontinence is rare in syncope, but it is frequent with seizures and postictal confusion is almost diagnostic of seizure activity.

A complete drug history is essential. The use of antihypertensives, neuroleptics, tricyclic antidepressants, and dopaminergic agonist is a frequent cause of orthostatic hypotension and syncope, particularly in the elderly.

When syncope is preceded by emotionally stressful or painful situations or by nausea, abdominal discomfort, pallor, diaphoresis, and blurred vision (all symptoms of autonomic activation), neurally mediated syncope should be suspected. When the victim falls, the horizontal position improves cerebral blood flow and consciousness is quickly regained, but hypotension and bradycardia may persist for several minutes; therefore, on attempting to stand, consciousness is frequently lost again. A characteristic setting is typical in several well known neurally mediated syncopal syndromes. For example, syncope after standing immobile, particularly in hot weather or after a period of bedrest; syncope occurring during micturition, coughing, or while playing a wind instrument such as the trumpet; and syncope with trigeminal or glossopharyngeal neuralgia are likely to be neurally mediated.

In marked contrast to the prodromal symptoms characteristic of neurally mediated syncope, syncope in patients with autonomic failure is never preceded by signs of autonomic activation.

Syncope during or after exercise suggests fixed or dynamic aortic stenosis. Syncope in aortic stenosis can be caused by obstruction to flow, arrhythmias, or reflex vasodilation. The latter resulting from increased ventricular mechanoreceptor discharge, a mechanism similar to that of neurally mediated syncope.

On physical examination, blood pressure and heart rate should be taken in the supine and upright position checking for orthostatic hypotension with or without a compensatory increase in heart rate. Special attention should be given to signs of cardiac valvular disease, autonomic failure, or other neurologic abnormalities commonly associated with autonomic failure, such as parkinsonism, cerebellar ataxia, or the presence of deafness as in Romano–Ward syndrome (congenital long QT syndrome). A bruit over the supraclavicular area and induction of symptoms by exercise of the arm are diagnostic of subclavian steal syndrome.

Because of its potential severity, the possibility of a cardiac arrhythmia causing syncope should always be considered first. A severe or potentially severe conduction defect such as third-degree atrioventricular block or the long QT syndrome are easily identified by 12-lead electrocardiography. In most cases, however, an arrhythmic cause of syncope is difficult to prove. Ambulatory electrocardiographic monitoring for 24 hours may be diagnostic, but the test is frequently inconclusive because arrhythmias that do not correlate with clinical symptoms are common. Portable and implantable loop electrocardiographic recorders that a patient can wear for weeks or months and that can be activated after a syncopal episode are currently available and have a diagnostic yield of 25 to 35% [5]. Invasive electrophysiologic studies, by introducing extra electrical stimuli into the heart, identify susceptibility to ventricular arrhythmias that can cause syncope. The procedure has shown some predictive value only in patients with structural heart disease. The use of signal-averaged electrocardiogram to identify late potentials in the terminal portion of the QRS complex (indicative of heterogeneous myocardial activation and a possible substrate of sustained ventricular tachyarrhythmias) has been reported to be useful.

TILT TESTING

In patients with syncope in whom a cardiac arrhythmia cannot be documented by electrocardiography, hemodynamic monitoring during passive tilt (i.e., tilt-table test) is the best available diagnostic procedure. Passive head-up tilt by preventing the pumping effect of skeletal muscle contraction exaggerates the reduction in venous return of the upright posture and triggers neurally mediated syncope in susceptible individuals.

During prolonged tilt, between 30 and 80% of patients with recurrent unexplained syncope experience neurally mediated syncope with symptoms similar to those they experience spontaneously. Their initial response to tilt is normal. However, after a variable period with well-maintained blood pressure and tachycardia, hypotension and sudden bradycardia develop. As shown in Figure 57.2, there is a differentiation between these patients and those with classic autonomic failure, because in patients with autonomic failure, blood pressure decreases progressively immediately after tilt and there is no bradycardia.

Although tilt-induced neurally mediated syncope appears to be identical to spontaneous syncope, the mechanism responsible for triggering this abnormal reflex response and the reason for individual susceptibility are still unknown.

The tilt-table test also is useful to assess the effect of drugs in orthostatic tolerance. Orthostatic hypotension caused by drugs may not be evident after a few minutes in the standing position, but may become apparent during prolonged tilt.

PROGNOSIS

The prognosis of syncope depends on the underlying cause. Among participants in the Framingham Heart Study, subjects with cardiac syncope were at increased risk for death from any cause and cardiovascular events, and those with syncope of unknown cause were at increased risk for death from any cause. There was no increased risk for cardiovascular morbidity or mortality associated with vasovagal syncope [6].

References

1. Savage, D. D., L. Corwin, D. L. McGee, W. B. Kannel, and P. A. Wolf. 1985. Epidemiologic features of isolated syncope: The Framingham Study. *Stroke* 16(4):626–629.
2. Lipsitz, L. A., R. P. Nyqvist, J. Y. Wei, and J. W. Rowe. 1983. Postprandial reduction in blood pressure in the elderly. *N. Engl. J. Med.* 309:81–83.
3. Kaufmann, H. 1997. Neurally mediated syncope and syncope due to autonomic failure: Differences and similarities. *J. Clin. Neurophysiol.* 14:183–196.
4. Abboud, F. M. 1989. Ventricular syncope. Is the heart a sensory organ? *N. Engl. J. Med.* 320(6):390–392.
5. Linzer, M., E. H. Yang, N. A. Estes III, P. Wang, V. R. Vorperian, and W. N. Kapoor. 1997. Diagnosing syncope. Part I. Value of history, physical examination, and electrocardiography: Clinical Efficacy Assessment Project of the American College of Physicians. *Ann. Intern. Med.* 126:989–996.
6. Soteriades, E. S., J. C. Evans, M. G. Larson, M. H. Chen, L. Chen, E. J. Benjamin, and D. Levy. 2002. Incidence and prognosis of syncope. *N. Engl. J. Med.* 347:878–885.

58 Evaluation of the Patient with Orthostatic Intolerance

Ronald Schondorf
Department of Neurology
Sir Mortimer B. Davis Jewish General Hospital
Montreal, Quebec, Canada

OVERVIEW

Autonomically mediated increases in heart rate and in systemic vascular resistance maintain normotension during any physiologic stress that diminishes central blood volume. Orthostatic intolerance (OI) is defined as the development of symptoms during standing that are relieved by recumbency. Typically these symptoms occur even in normal individuals once autonomic reflexes near the limit of compensation. There exists, however, a significant patient cohort who chronically or frequently have these symptoms to stressors that would have minimal or no effect on healthy subjects. These patients predictably experience disabling symptoms that are exacerbated by even the most basic activities of daily living (Table 58.1, parts A and B). The true prevalence of OI is unknown, although it has been estimated that as many as 500,000 individuals in the United States have OI [1]. Patients often have complaints dismissed because of the nonspecific nature of the symptoms reported and because **patients with OI do not have orthostatic hypotension**. Our understanding of chronic OI also is obscured by the large number of terms used to describe these patients (Table 58.2).

CLINICAL FEATURES

The age of presentation of OI is most commonly between 15 and 50 years, and women are five times as likely as men to be affected. The onset of symptoms is subacute and often a viral prodrome is noted [2]. The nonspecificity of symptoms may cause confusion between OI and panic disorder, but a history of a close relation between presence of orthostatic stressors and symptoms (see Table 58.1), as well as resolution of symptoms in the absence of these stressors, generally helps to clarify the diagnosis. Many patients with OI also will fulfill diagnostic criteria for chronic fatigue syndrome (CFS) [3, 4], and the presence of CFS should be documented. Other causes of OI such as prolonged bedrest, hypovolemia, dehydration, or medications must be eliminated. New-onset OI also must be differentiated from constitutional OI, in which patients have a history of mild OI since childhood. In some cases, a family history of OI is obtained. Physical examination should be directed to unmasking evidence of heightened sympathetic activity during orthostatic stress and evidence of excessive venous pooling (see Table 58.1, part C). There may also be evidence of impaired sudomotor function (reduced plantar sweating and compensatory hyperhidrosis) or small-fiber sensory neuropathy.

PATHOPHYSIOLOGY OF ORTHOSTATIC INTOLERANCE

The pathophysiology of OI is complex, and more than one etiologic factor for this condition is likely. The main putative mechanisms of OI are summarized in Table 58.3. A selective autonomic neuropathy that predominantly affects the lower extremities may explain the excessive venous pooling [5], and an impairment of renal sympathetic innervation may explain the decreases in plasma volume or red cell mass seen in OI. Conversely, the reduction in plasma volume in OI may be caused by an increase in sympathetic activity. Sympathetic overactivity and partial autonomic denervation have both been described in OI [6, 7]. Denervation supersensitivity has been suggested as a cause for cardiac ß-adrenergic hypersensitivity in OI, although direct testing failed to provide confirming evidence [8]. Other possible mechanisms for the increased tachycardia during infusion of ß-adrenergic agonists include reduced vagal cardioinhibitory activity (vagal braking effect) or a compensatory heart rate response to enhanced β-adrenergic vasodilation.

LABORATORY EVALUATION OF ORTHOSTATIC INTOLERANCE

The brief discussion of pathophysiology underscores the complexity of OI and highlights the limitations of "closed loop" measurements made in these patients. Objective documentation of OI is nonetheless required. Standard laboratory documentation requires provocation of symptoms of OI

TABLE 58.1 Clinical Evaluation of Orthostatic Intolerance

A: Symptoms of orthostatic intolerance
Lightheadedness
Dizziness
Exercise intolerance
Palpitations
Fatigue
Cognitive difficulties (fuzzy head)
Blurred vision
Tremulousness or anxiety
Nausea
Tight chest
Clamminess
B: Stressors contributing to symptoms of orthostatic intolerance
Rapid positional change
Standing (waiting in line)
Standing after prolonged recumbency
Exercise
Heat
Meals
Time of day
Medications
C: Signs of orthostatic intolerance
Tachycardia
Diastolic hypertension
Exaggerated blood pressure oscillations
Livedo reticularis
Cold extremities
Sudomotor dysfunction
Distal small-fiber neuropathy

TABLE 58.2 Terms for Orthostatic Intolerance

Mitral valve prolapse syndrome
Soldier's heart
Vasoregulatory asthenia
Neurocirculatory asthenia
Irritable heart
Orthostatic anemia
Hyperadrenergic orthostatic hypotension
Orthostatic tachycardia syndrome
Postural tachycardia syndrome
Sympathotonic orthostatic hypotension
Hyperdynamic β-adrenergic state
Idiopathic hypovolemia
Chronic orthostatic intolerance

TABLE 58.3 Putative Mechanisms of Orthostatic Intolerance

Length-dependent autonomic neuropathy
Hypovolemia
Impaired venous compliance
β-Adrenergic supersensitivity
α-Adrenergic hyposensitivity
Impaired baroreflex response
Impaired norepinephrine transporter
Centrally mediated increase in sympathetic activity
Paradoxic decrease in cerebral blood flow

in the absence of orthostatic hypotension within 5 minutes of active standing or head-up tilt. An increase in heart rate of 30 beats/min or more from baseline or a heart rate that exceeds 120 beats/min confirms the presence of OI (Fig. 58.1). Attention should be paid, however, to the chronotropic reserve following simple orthostatic stress. A heart rate increase from 50 to 80 beats/min cannot be equated with an increase from 100 to 130 beats/min, although in both cases an increase of 30 beats/min is observed. Other abnormal responses to orthostatic stress include diastolic hypertension, diminished pulse pressure, and large (0.1-Hz) fluctuations in blood pressure. The heart rate response to deep breathing is usually normal, indicating intact cardiovagal function. The heart rate response to the Valsalva maneuver is normal or exaggerated. Phase 2 blood pressure may be diminished, and phase 4 overshoot often is increased [2]. We recommend evaluation of sympathetic sudomotor function using a combination of quantitative sudomotor axon reflex test (QSART) and thermoregulatory sweat test to search for autonomic neuropathy. Routine biochemistry, complete blood count, thyroid function, serum cortisol, renin, aldosterone, and 24-hour urine collection for catecholamines and urinary sodium should be measured. Healthy subjects should have a sodium excretion greater than 150 mmol over 24 hours. A threefold increase in plasma norepinephrine from supine to standing may also help confirm the diagnosis of OI. Measurement of plasma volume, baroreflex sensitivity, the response to infusion of adrenergic agonists, and microneurographic of sympathetic nerve activity should not be done routinely (see "Pathophysiology of Orthostatic Intolerance").

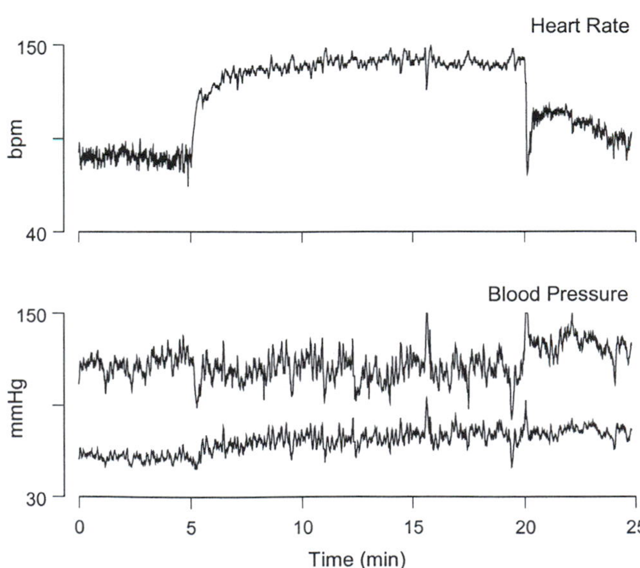

FIGURE 58.1 Hemodynamic profile of a patient with orthostatic intolerance during 15 minutes of head-up tilt (5–20 minutes). There is significant tachycardia without orthostatic hypotension. The head-up tilt reproduced the patient's typical symptoms of orthostatic intolerance.

SYMPTOMS OF ORTHOSTATIC INTOLERANCE

Even after sophisticated laboratory evaluation, our understanding of symptoms of OI remains incomplete. For example, lightheadedness and visual blurring may indicate cerebral hypoperfusion, but many patients have similar symptoms with normal cerebral blood flow [9]. Palpitations and tremulousness may be the result of sympathetic overactivity, although appropriate pharmacologic treatment often is ineffective in relieving OI. Other symptoms such as chest tightness and fatigue remain poorly understood. The hemodynamic abnormalities of OI may also be provoked in healthy individuals by combining simple stressors of orthostatic tolerance such as mild heat combined with head-up tilt. These healthy subjects do not experience the severe symptoms of OI that patients do. Patients with OI are undoubtedly severely disabled [10]. Increased recognition and standardized evaluation of OI will undoubtedly lead to improved treatment of this condition.

References

1. Robertson, D. 1999. The epidemic of orthostatic tachycardia and orthostatic intolerance. *Am. J. Med. Sci.* 317:75–77.
2. Low, P. A., R. Schondorf, V. Novak, P. Sandroni, T. L. Opfer-Gehrking, and P. Novak. 1997. Postural tachycardia syndrome (POTS). In *Clinical autonomic disorders*, ed. P. A. Low, 681–697. Philadelphia: Lippincott-Raven.
3. Fukuda, K., S. E. Straus, I. Hickie, M. C. Sharpe, J. G. Dobbins, and A. Komaroff. 1994. The chronic fatigue syndrome: A comprehensive approach to its definition and study. *Ann. Intern. Med.* 121:953–959.
4. Schondorf, R., and R. Freeman. 1999. The importance of orthostatic intolerance in the chronic fatigue syndrome. *Am. J. Med. Sci.* 317: 117–123.
5. Schondorf, R. and Low, P. A. 1993. Idiopathic postural orthostatic tachycardia syndrome: An attenuated form of acute pandysautonomia? *Neurology* 43:132–137.
6. Furlan, R., G. Jacob, M. Snell, D. Robertson, A. Porta, P. Harris, and R. Mosqueda-Garcia. 1998. Chronic orthostatic intolerance: A disorder with discordant cardiac and vascular sympathetic control. *Circulation* 98:2154–2159.
7. Jacob, G., F. Costa, J. R. Shannon, R. M. Robertson, M. Wathen, M. Stein, I. Biaggioni, A. Ertl, B. Black, and D. Robertson. 2000. The neuropathic postural tachycardia syndrome. *N. Engl. J. Med.* 343:1008–1014.
8. Jordan, J., J. R. Shannon, A. Diedrich, B. K. Black, and D. Robertson. 2002. Increased sympathetic activation in idiopathic orthostatic intolerance: Role of systemic adrenoreceptor sensitivity. *Hypertension* 39:173–178.
9. Schondorf, R., J. Benoit, and R. Stein. 2001. Cerebral autoregulation in orthostatic intolerance. *Ann. N Y Acad. Sci.* 940:514–526.
10. Benrud-Larson, L. M., M. S. Dewar, P. Sandroni, T. A. Rummans, J. A. Haythornthwaite, and P. A. Low. 2002. Quality of life in patients with postural tachycardia syndrome. *Mayo Clin. Proc.* 77:531–537.

59

Sympathetic Microneurography

B. Gunnar Wallin
The Sahlgren Academy at Göteborg University
Institute of Clinical Neuroscience
Sahlgren University Hospital
Göteborg, Sweden

Microneurography was developed in the mid-1960s for percutaneous recordings of action potentials in human peripheral nerves. The technique was intended for myelinated sensory fibers, but it was found to be useful also for recordings from unmyelinated postganglionic sympathetic axons [1]. Since then, many studies have been published on human sympathetic nerve traffic to skin and muscle, mostly in groups of sympathetic fibers (multiunit activity), but also in single axons. Large extremity nerves are commonly used, but recordings have been made from face and mouth nerves. The methodology has provided valuable new knowledge on autonomic physiology and pathophysiology, but it is not suitable for diagnostic assessment in individual patients. This chapter summarizes methodologic aspects of microneurography from biological and technical viewpoints. Detailed accounts have been published previously [2–4].

METHODOLOGY

Equipment

Commonly used equipment includes insulated monopolar tungsten microelectrodes with tip diameters of a few micrometers, but a concentric needle electrode has been described [5]. Electrodes are available commercially or may be produced in the laboratory. Impedances range from about 50 kΩ to several MΩ; single fiber recordings require electrodes with smaller uninsulated tips and higher impedance. Usually, the neurogram is amplified (gain 50–100 k) in two steps: first in a preamplifier/impedance converter positioned close to the recording site, and then in a main amplifier. To quantify multiunit activity, the raw neurogram is full wave rectified and passed through a leaky integrator with a time constant of 0.1 second. Audio monitoring, which facilitates the actual recording, is made after noise reduction. This is achieved by filters (e.g., bandwidth 500–2000 Hz) and a discriminator, which cuts out the central portion of the neurogram, transmitting only the positive and negative peaks of the signals to the audio amplifier (see Reference 4, for technical details).

Procedure

The nerve is located by the paraesthesia/muscle twitches evoked first by percutaneous electrical stimulation, and then by stimulation through the microelectrode after it has been inserted through the skin. Peripheral nerves contain many fascicles, and, in the distal part of the extremities, fascicles are connected either to a defined skin area or to a muscle. The fascicle and its innervation zone are identified by the type of peripheral stimuli that evoke afferent mechanoreceptive impulses: muscle stretch and light touch stimuli for muscle and skin fascicles, respectively. Sympathetic nerve fibers are not evenly distributed within the fascicle; they lie together with afferent C fibers in bundles inside Schwann cells (Fig. 59.1); therefore, repeated small needle adjustments may be necessary before a sympathetic recording site is found.

Sympathetic fibers discharge spontaneously in synchronized bursts, which occur irregularly in characteristic temporal patterns, which differ between skin and muscle nerve fascicles (see Fig. 59.1). Furthermore, the activity increases in a predictable way with certain maneuvers (Fig. 59.2). In **muscle nerve fascicles**, multiunit bursts presumably contain only vasoconstrictor impulses, which occur in the cardiac rhythm, preferentially during reductions of arterial blood pressure; their number increases with apneas or Valsalva maneuvers. In **skin fascicles**, sympathetic bursts may contain vasoconstrictor, vasodilator, and/or sudomotor impulses; cardiac rhythmicity is usually absent but any surprising sensory stimulus regularly evokes a single discharge.

Recordings from **single sympathetic fibers** are achieved by repeated minute electrode adjustments in a region of a fascicle in which multiunit sympathetic bursts are present [6]. To facilitate fiber identification in skin nerves, experiments are done while subjects are cooled or heated; this

Sympathetic nerve recording

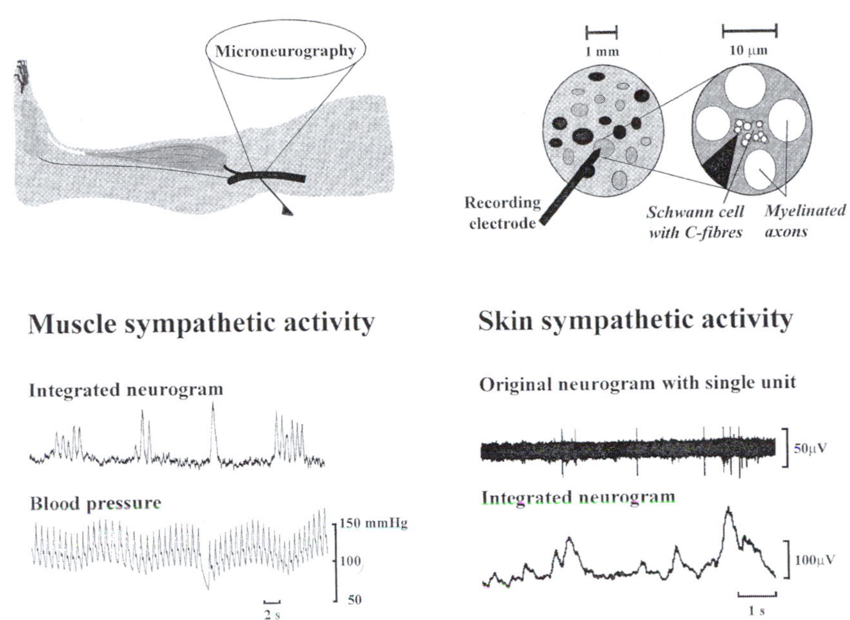

FIGURE 59.1 Schematic figure of microneurographic recording from the peroneal nerve at the fibular head (**top left**). The nerve contains skin and muscle fascicles, and, in both types of fascicles, sympathetic fibers are located in bundles inside Schwann cells and surrounded by myelinated axons (**top right**). **Bottom left**, Spontaneous variations of muscle sympathetic activity (integrated neurogram) and blood pressure. Note cardiac rhythmicity and the inverse relation between neurogram and blood pressure levels. **Bottom right**, Spontaneous skin sympathetic activity in original and integrated neurograms. Note that the single unit can be identified only in the original neurogram (bandpass, 0.3–5 kHz).

biases sympathetic traffic toward vasoconstriction and sweating, respectively. Sites with adequate signal-to-noise ratio for multiunit activity are obtained in ~90% of attempts; the corresponding figure for single-unit activity recordings is much less.

Analysis

Multiunit Activity

In a given electrode site, the strength of multiunit activity in the mean voltage neurogram can be quantified as the number of bursts multiplied by mean burst area (= total activity). In muscle nerves, burst duration is relatively constant; therefore, burst amplitude can be substituted for burst area. Measurement of total activity is suitable for quantifying **changes of activity** induced by maneuvers.

The strength of **resting sympathetic activity**, conversely, can only be quantified in terms of the number of bursts; burst amplitude cannot be compared among electrode sites because it depends on the proximity of the electrode tip to the active fibers, which varies among sites. Because muscle sympathetic activity always displays cardiac rhythmicity, the strength of activity is expressed both as number of bursts/100 heartbeats (burst incidence) and bursts/min (burst frequency). Burst detection often is made visually, but computer-assisted analysis is valuable because it is faster, reduces observer bias, and gives accurate measures of burst area (see Reference 7 for additional references).

Single-Unit Activity

Single-unit analysis requires (1) fiber identification and (2) evidence that all impulses derive from the same fiber. Fiber identification is difficult in skin nerves, which contain several different types of sympathetic fibers. Therefore, to aid the identification, a thermally induced bias of the activity during recordings and spike-triggered averaging of effector responses should be used whenever possible.

To ensure that all impulses derive from one fiber, spike amplitude is important. However, because signal-to-noise ratio often is low, considerable spike amplitude variability may be induced by the noise. Therefore, only triggering on spikes exceeding a certain amplitude level is inadequate; spikes may be missed or, alternatively, spikes from other axons may be included. For this reason, computer-assisted inspection of wave form and amplitude, com-

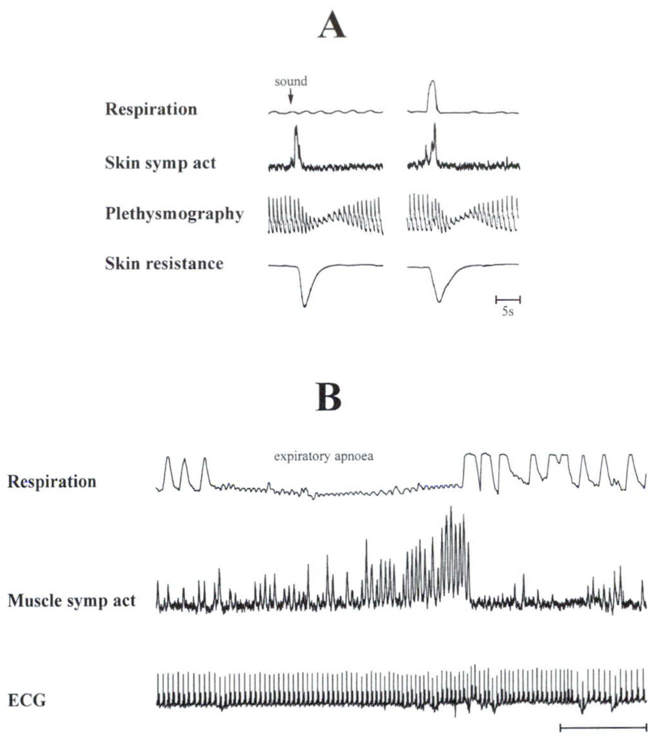

FIGURE 59.2 Simple maneuvers aiding the identification of skin and muscle sympathetic activity. In skin nerve fascicles (**A**), a single sympathetic discharge is regularly evoked by a deep breath (**right**) or any type of arousal stimulus—for example, a sudden sound (**left**). Note that the sympathetic burst is followed by transient signs of vasoconstriction (reduced pulse amplitudes in the plethysmogram) and sweating (reduction of skin resistance), indicating that vasoconstrictor and sudomotor fibers are activated in parallel. In muscle nerve fascicles (**B**), the activity increases markedly toward the end of an expiratory apnea.

bined with spike superimposition, is necessary before a population of spikes can be attributed to a single axon (Fig. 59.3).

Firing in single muscle sympathetic fibers displays cardiac rhythmicity; therefore, it is useful to quantitate not only firing frequency, but also the number of cardiac intervals with unit activity and the number of spikes/cardiac interval.

POTENTIAL DIFFICULTIES

Mixed Sites

Usually, the character of the sympathetic activity agrees with the classification of a fascicle on the basis of afferent mechanoreceptor responses to sensory stimuli. However, mixed sympathetic activity may be encountered in a fascicle that appeared "pure" based on afferent testing. To avoid such mistakes, careful testing of the sympathetic responsiveness is needed before accepting a recording site as "pure."

Changes of Electrode Site

Movements of the electrode tip during a recording (e.g., in association with a maneuver) are usually easy to detect. A slow change of site without obvious artifacts may, however, lead to problems. If signs of such changes are present (e.g., a drifting baseline level or slowly increasing burst amplitudes in the mean voltage neurogram), burst amplitude/area cannot be used in the quantitative analysis.

Acknowledgment

The author thanks Göran Pegenius for excellent technical assistance. Work was supported by Swedish Medical Research Council Grant no. 12170.

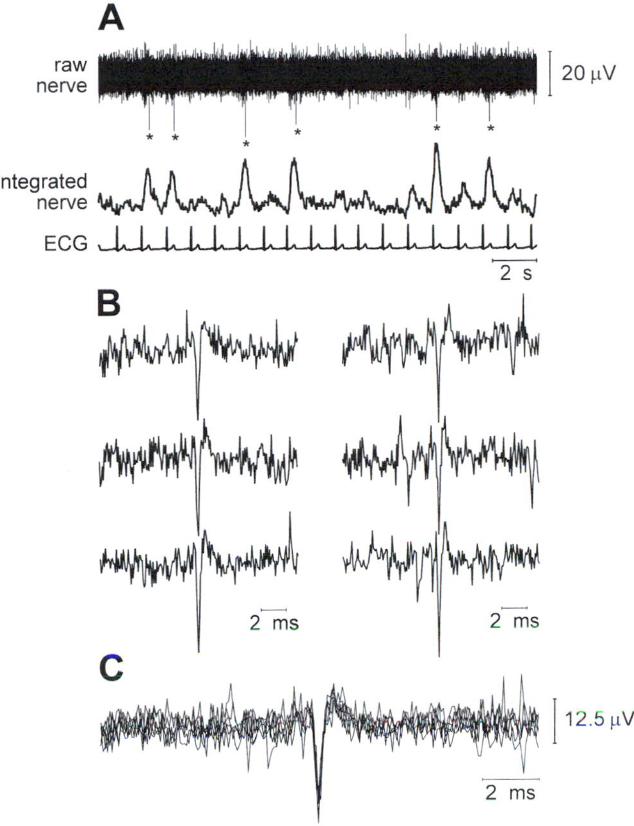

FIGURE 59.3 Recording from a single sympathetic vasoconstrictor fiber in a muscle nerve fascicle. **A**, In association with six multiunit bursts (see integrated neurogram), the fiber discharges a single impulse (*). Variations in spike amplitude in raw neurogram are a consequence of low signal-to-noise ratio. Reproduced with permission from Macefield, G. V., B. G. Wallin, and A. B. Vallbo 1994. The discharge behaviour or single vasoconstrictor motoneurones in human muscle nerves. *J. Physiol. (Lond.)* 481:799–809.

References

1. Hagbarth, K.-E., and Å. Vallbo. 1968. Pulse and respiratory grouping of sympathetic impulses in human muscle nerves. *Acta. Physiol. Scand.* 74:96–108.
2. Vallbo, Å. B., K.-E. Hagbarth, H. E. Torebjörk, and B. G. Wallin. 1979. Somatosensory, proprioceptive and sympathetic activity in human peripheral nerves. *Physiol. Rev.* 59:919–957.
3. Eckberg, D. L., and P. Sleight. 1992. *Human baroreflexes in health and disease.* New York: Oxford University Press.
4. Gandevia, S. C., and J. P. Hales. 1997. The methodology and scope of human microneurography. *J. Neurosci. Methods* 74:123–136.
5. Hallin, R. G., and G. Wu. 1998. Protocol for microneurography with concentric needle electrodes. *Brain Res. Protocols* 2:120–132.
6. Macefield, V. G., M. Elam, and B. G. Wallin. 2002. Firing properties of single postganglionic sympathetic neurones. *Auton. Neurosci.* 95:146–159.
7. Hamner, J. W., and J. A. Taylor. 2001. Automated quantification of sympathetic beat-by-beat activity, independent of signal quality. *J. Appl. Physiol.* 91:1199–1206.
8. Macefield, G. V., B. G. Wallin, and Å. B. Vallbo. 1994. The discharge behaviour of single vasoconstrictor motoneurones in human muscle nerves. *J. Physiol. (Lond.)* 481:799–809.

60 Assessment of the Autonomic Control of the Cardiovascular System by Frequency Domain Approach

Raffaello Furlan
Internal Medicine II
Ospedale L. Sacco
University of Milan
Milan, Italy

Alberto Malliani
Internal Medicine II
Ospedale L. Sacco
University of Milan
Milan, Italy

The neural control of heart rate is mainly regulated at the level of the sinoatrial node by the interaction of sympathetic and vagal efferent discharge. In most conditions, an increase of cardiac sympathetic activity is accompanied by a simultaneous inhibition of the vagal modulation to the heart and vice versa, hence the concept of sympathovagal balance [1]. It has been demonstrated that the state of sympathovagal balance can be broadly assessed by quantifying RR interval variability.

Similarly, arterial pressure spontaneously oscillates in part as a consequence of the sympathetic regulatory activity. The various types of blood pressure oscillations are represented in Figure 60.1. The second-order oscillations are produced mechanically by the respiratory activity. The third-order fluctuations, with a period of about 10 seconds, are related to vasomotion and are modulated by sympathetic activity; thus, they increase during conditions associated with a sympathetic excitation such as on standing. Therefore, the study of circulatory rhythms by spectrum analysis techniques may furnish a valuable insight into the autonomic regulation of the cardiovascular system in health and disease.

METHODOLOGY

Power spectrum analysis on the basis of Fast Fourier Transform [2] or autoregressive modeling [3] provides the center frequency of rhythmic fluctuations (see Fig. 60.1), their time relation (phase), and amplitude both in absolute and in normalized values [4]. Absolute values are computed as the integral of each oscillatory component (see Fig. 60.1, *hatched area*). Normalization procedure is obtained by dividing the absolute power of each oscillatory component by total variance (minus the power of the frequency components <0.03 Hz) and then multiplying by 100. Normalization overcomes the problems due to the marked changes in RR variance when comparing different subjects and experimental conditions [5]. The low-frequency/high-frequency component of RR variability (LF_{RR}/HF_{RR}) ratio, which is independent of units of measure, assesses the sympathovagal instantaneous relation (balance) [5].

FUNCTIONAL SIGNIFICANCE OF CARDIOVASCULAR RHYTHMS

Two major oscillatory components are observed in healthy subjects in recumbent position [5]. One is the high-frequency (HF $\approx$ 0.25 Hz) component. If extracted from RR variability (HF_{RR}), it is an accepted index of the vagal modulation of the sinoatrial node activity [2]. Indeed, HF_{RR} is reduced after muscarinic blockade [6] and is enhanced during the reflex increase of cardiac vagal activity obtained by phenylephrine administration. The HF component of systolic arterial pressure variability reflects the mechanical influence of respiratory activity. The other oscillatory component is indicated as low frequency (LF $\approx$ 0.10 Hz). In the case of systolic arterial pressure variability, LF_{SAP} is a marker of the sympathetic modulation of vasomotor activity [5] because it is increased in animals during baroreflex unloading induced by nitroglycerine and in humans during tilt test, moderate physical exercise, and mental stress. The LF_{RR}, when expressed in normalized units (n.u.), reflects primarily the sympathetic efferent modulation of the sinoatrial node [7]. Indeed, in conscious dogs, reflex increase of sympathetic activity by nitroglycerin administration enhanced LF_{RR} n.u., whereas the same stimulus after chronic bilateral stellectomy, which selectively abolishes cardiac sympathetic innervation, could not elicit any LF_{RR}. In humans, conditions characterized by an increased sympathetic activity such as gravitational, mental and mild physical stresses, baroreflex unloading induced by nitroprusside administration, and lower body negative pressure were associated with a remarkable increase of the normalized power of LF_{RR}. Chronic β-blocker consumption reduced LF_{RR} in n.u. [5]. The same oscillatory component was undetectable in subjects with pure autonomic failure, a condition characterized by the degeneration of sympathetic efferent neurons.

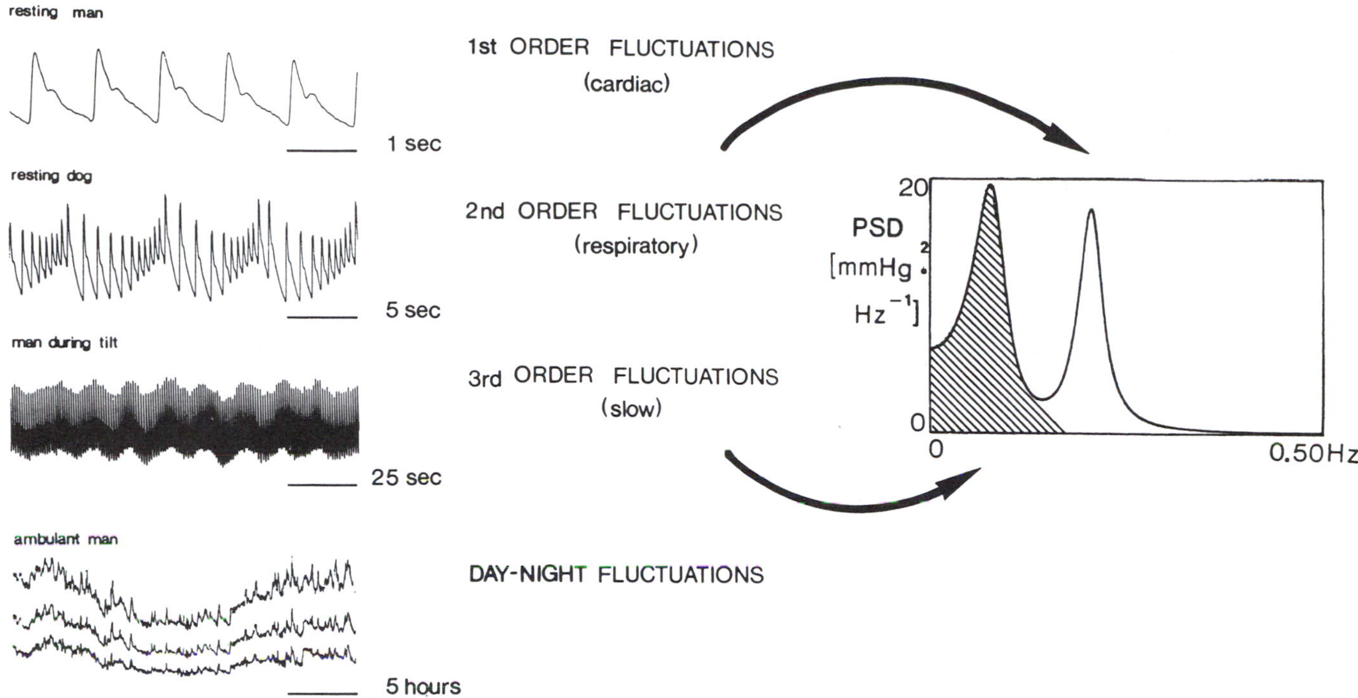

FIGURE 60.1 Examples of arterial pressure spontaneous fluctuations. Notice differences in both the amplitude and the period of the rhythmic oscillations. First-order fluctuations, generated by cardiac activity, are characterized by the interbeat period, and their amplitude is represented by the differential pressure. A period of 24 hours is the feature of day–night oscillations of systemic pressure. Second-and third-order fluctuations define the so-called short-term variability mostly related to neural influences.

RELATION BETWEEN CARDIOVASCULAR AND NEURAL RHYTHMS

Rhythmic discharge activity is a general property of the nervous system [1]. A 0.1-Hz rhythmicity linked with low-frequency fluctuations of RR interval and arterial pressure variability was found to characterize sympathetic neurons located in areas within the central nervous system involved in cardiovascular regulation. Interestingly, these fluctuations remain after baroreflex afferent inputs were removed by a stabilizer device connected to the arterial system of the animal, suggesting that baroreceptor activity is not necessary to the genesis of such fluctuations that, instead, may result from a central oscillator. Rhythmic LF and HF periodicities characterize the discharge activity of postganglionic sympathetic fibers of humans (muscle sympathetic nerve activity [MSNA]). In humans, the sympathetic activation induced by a gravitational stimulus was accompanied by a marked increase of the 0.1-Hz oscillatory component of MSNA, resembling the changes observed in the same oscillatory component of RR and systolic arterial pressure variability [8]. In addition, the linear coupling between LF fluctuations of MSNA and heart rate and MSNA and systolic arterial pressure was increased during the tilt maneuver, suggesting the onset of a common oscillatory pattern involving the different variables on the basis of prevailing 0.1-Hz fluctuations [8].

PHYSIOLOGY AND PATHOPHYSIOLOGY

In a study performed on habitual day workers based on spectral analysis of heart rate and arterial pressure variability over 24 hours, LF_{RR} in n.u. and LF_{SAP} were reduced during sleeping hours, increased with awakening in the early morning, and high during the work period. In habitual shift workers, LF_{RR} and the LF/HF ratio showed 24-hour oscillations with different time of maximum and minimum in accordance with the working and sleeping periods, respectively [9]. Lower values of LF_{RR} and LF/HF suggestive of a reduced cardiac sympathetic modulation were present when the job task was performed at night compared with the values observed when the work was performed during morning and evening [9]. The reduced values of the indexes of cardiac sympathetic modulation during night work might be related to the presence of sleepiness or reduced alertness that, in turn, could facilitate errors and accidents.

In a study based on time-variant spectrum analysis of RR variability, which enabled the monitoring of beat-by-beat changes of LF_{RR} and HF_{RR}, the two spectral components were relatively stable during a 15-minute tilt maneuver in healthy subjects. Conversely, in subjects with sudden syncope, the progression of tilt was characterized by wide fluctuations of LF_{RR} and HF_{RR}, suggestive of a marked instability of the cardiac autonomic control up to the onset of syncope [10].

References

1. Malliani, A. 2000. *Principles of cardiovascular neural regulation in health and disease*, 65–107. Boston: Kluwer Academic Publishers.
2. Akselrod, S., D. Gordon, F. A. Ubel, D. C. Shannon, A. C. Barger, and R. J. Cohen. 1981. Power spectrum analysis of heart rate fluctuation: A quantitative probe of beat-to-beat cardiovascular control. *Science* 213:220–222.
3. Baselli, G., S. Cerutti, S. Civardi, D. Liberati, F. Lombardi, A. Malliani, and M. Pagani. 1986. Spectral and cross-spectral analysis of heart rate and arterial blood pressure variability signals. *Comput. Biomed. Res.* 19:520–534.
4. Task Force of the European Society of Cardiology and the North American Society of Pacing and Electrophysiology. 1996. Heart rate variability: Standards of measurements, physiological interpretation, and clinical use. *Circulation* 93:1043–1065.
5. Pagani, M., F. Lombardi, S. Guzzetti, O. Rimoldi, R. Furlan, P. Pizzinelli, G. Sandrone, G. Malfatto, S. Dell'Orto, E. Piccaluga, M. Turiel, G. Baselli, S. Cerutti, and A. Malliani. 1986. Power spectral analysis of heart rate and arterial pressure variabilities as a marker of sympatho-vagal interaction in man and conscious dog. *Circ. Res.* 59:178–193.
6. Pomeranz, B., R. J. B. Macaulay, M. A. Caudill, I. Kutz, D. Adam, D. Gordon, K. B. Kilborn, A. C. Barger, D. C. Shannon, R. J. Cohen, and H. Benson. 1985. Assessment of autonomic function in humans by heart rate spectral analysis. *Am. J. Physiol.* 248:H151–H153.
7. Malliani, A., M. Pagani, F. Lombardi, and S. Cerutti. 1991. Cardiovascular neural regulation explored in the frequency domain. *Circulation* 84:482–492.
8. Furlan, R., A. Porta, F. Costa, J. Tank, L. Baker, R. Schiavi, D. Robertson, A. Malliani, and R. Mosqueda-Garcia. 2000. Oscillatory patterns in sympathetic neural discharge and cardiovascular variables during orthostatic stimulus. *Circulation* 101:886–892.
9. Furlan, R., F. Barbic, S. Piazza, M. Tinelli, P. Seghizzi, and A. Malliani. 2000. Modifications of cardiac autonomic profile associated with a shift schedule of work. *Circulation* 102:1912–1916.
10. Furlan, R., S. Piazza, S. Dell'Orto, F. Barbic, A. Bianchi, L. Mainardi, S. Cerutti, M. Pagani, and A. Malliani. 1998. Cardiac autonomic patterns preceding occasional vasovagal reactions in healthy humans. *Circulation* 98:1756–1761.

61

Assessment of Sudomotor Function

Phillip A. Low
Department of Neurology
Mayo Clinic
Rochester, Minnesota

Ronald Schondorf
Department of Neurology
Sir Mortimer B. Davis Jewish General Hospital
Montreal, Quebec, Canada

TESTS OF SUDOMOTOR FUNCTION

In the clinical neurophysiology laboratory, a number of tests of sudomotor function have been adapted or developed for clinical use. The most widely used tests are the TST (thermoregulatory sweat test), QSART (quantitative sudomotor axon reflex test), PASP (peripheral autonomic surface potential), and SIT (sweat imprint test). This chapter, therefore, focuses on these four tests; a comparison of the tests is shown in Table 61.1.

QUANTITATIVE SUDOMOTOR AXON REFLEX TEST

The physiologic basis of the QSART is summarized in Figure 61.1 [1]. The neural pathway consists of an axon "reflex" mediated by the postganglionic sympathetic sudomotor axon. The axon terminal is activated by acetylcholine (ACh). The impulse travels antidromically, reaches a branch point, and then travels orthodromically to release ACh from nerve terminal. ACh traverses the neuroglandular junction and binds to M_3 muscarinic receptors [2] on eccrine sweat glands to evoke the sweat response. Acetylcholinesterase in subcutaneous tissue cleaves ACh to acetate and choline, resulting in its inactivation and cessation of the sweat response.

The QSART specifically evaluates the functional status of postganglionic sympathetic axons. Current is applied through the anode of a constant current generator [2] within one compartment of a multicompartmental sweat cell, and the sweat response is recorded from a second compartment with a sudorometer (Fig. 61.2). To obtain an adequate sampling of postganglionic sudomotor function, the multicompartmental sweat cells are attached to four standard sites on the upper and lower extremity. This distribution permits the detection of dysfunction that can be localized to one specific peripheral nerve territory or of a length-dependent autonomic neuropathy.

There is an age effect on the axon reflex–mediated sweat response, which declined with age in the lower extremity [2]. There was no change with age in the forearm. In both sexes, the slope relating the decrease in sweat volume with age was steeper in the lower extremity compared with the upper extremity, suggesting a length-dependent mechanism of autonomic failure.

Complete or partial damage of sympathetic fibers is inferred from the resting sweat activity, latency to onset and morphology of the response, and by integrated sweat volume. An absent response indicates a lesion of the postganglionic axon, providing iontophoresis is successful and eccrine sweat glands are present. Milder axonal damage may be associated with persistent sweating or with a "hung-up" response. Many length-dependent neuropathies manifest a progressive reduction in sweat volumes occurring in a proximodistal distribution, maximal distally. The QSART also provides objective documentation of progression of neuropathies as sudomotor failure advances to more proximal sites. In most preganglionic or central disorders, the QSART is unimpaired, although with increasing duration of the preganglionic lesion, the QSART may be reduced. This suggests a transsynaptic defect or sweat gland atrophy.

SKIN IMPRINT RECORDINGS

The number and sizes of sweat droplets from sweat gland can be imprinted in rapidly setting silastic material [3]. Sweating can be evoked by directly stimulating muscarinic receptors of sweat gland (iontophoresis of pilocarpine) or indirectly through the axon reflex using nicotine or ACh [4]. Using this method it was demonstrated that sweat gland density was the same in men and women, but the greater sweat volume in men was caused by the larger volume secreted per sweat gland.

SKIN POTENTIAL RECORDINGS

The sympathetic skin response (SSR) is a polysynaptic reflex that requires integrity of hypothalamic, brainstem and spinal circuits, and postganglionic sympathetic sudomotor axons [5]. The SSR is generated in deep layers of the skin by sympathetically mediated activation of sweat glands. The

TABLE 61.1 Comparison of Quantitative Sudomotor Axon Reflex Test, Silastic Imprint, and Skin Potential Recordings

Test	QSART	TST	Silastic imprint	Skin potential
Principle	Sympathetic axon reflex	Central warming	Direct sweat gland muscarinic response	Somatosympathetic response
Stimulus	Acetylcholine	↑ Ambient temperature	Pilocarpine	Various reflex stimulation
Neural pathway				
Afferent	Sympathetic C	Mainly central	Nil	Groups II and III
Efferent	Sympathetic C	Sympathetic sudomotor	Nil	Sympathetic B and C
Effector	Eccrine sweat gland	Sweat gland	Sweat gland	Sweat gland secretion
Response characteristics				
Latency	Long (1–2 min)	V long (>30 min)	? brief	Brief (seconds)
Turn on	Rapid	Gradual (minutes)	Rapid	Rapid
Turn off	Relatively fast (2–3 min)	Slow (minutes)	Very slow (>2 hours)	Fast (seconds)
Neuropathy	Sensitive	Very Sensitive	Sensitive	Somewhat insensitive
Detection				
Advantages	Sensitive, reproducible, accurate, quantitative	Sensitive, reproducible	Sensitive, reproducible, accurate, quantitative	Standard electromyograph equipment
Disadvantages	Time-consuming, special equipment, rare problem with thick skin	Time-consuming, special equipment, qualitative	Time-consuming, special equipment	Variable (habituation), inaccurate, many factors affect the response
Dynamic recording	Yes	Semi	No	Yes
Histogram	No	No	Yes	No

QSART, quantitative sudomotor axon reflex test; TST, thermoregulatory sweat test.

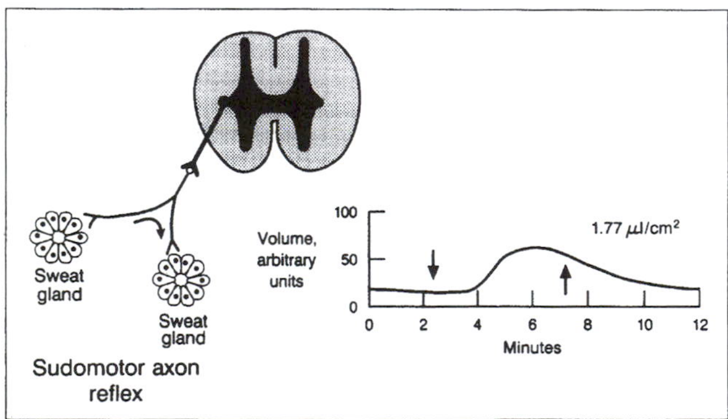

FIGURE 61.1 Quantitative sudomotor axon reflex test (QSART). Stimulus of nerve terminals by acetylcholine iontophoresis results in activation of postganglionic sympathetic sudomotor fibers, acetylcholine release, and activation of a new population of sweat glands.

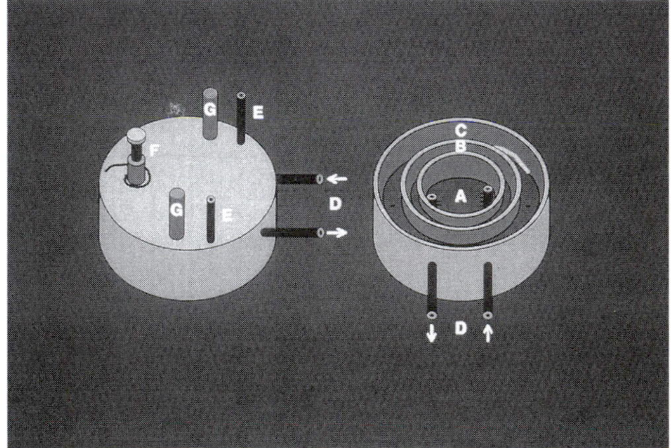

FIGURE 61.2 Multicompartmental sweat cell. Stimulus (acetylcholine) is iontophoresed through **C** and recorded in **A**. **A** and **C** are separated by air gap (**B**). Acetylcholine is administered through cannula **E** and current is applied through anode **F**. A stream of humidified nitrogen is run in through **D** to evaporate sweat. The capsule is held in place with straps applied to posts **G**.

morphology of the SSR potential is determined by the interaction between these sweat glands and the surrounding epidermal tissue. At normal ambient temperatures, SSR is recorded from the glabrous skin of the palms and soles. This activity is referenced to the adjacent hairy skin whose sweat glands are not typically active under these conditions. In routine clinical practice, the SSR is recorded after stimulation of median or posterior tibial nerve afferents at an intensity at three least times sensory threshold. In cases of peripheral neuropathy where afferent input may be insufficient to evoke an SSR, the response to acoustic stimuli or to an inspiratory gasp also should be recorded.

Although the SSR is easy to perform using standard electromyograph equipment, its clinical use in the evaluation of sympathetic sudomotor function is questionable. The criteria for what constitutes an abnormal SSR are controversial. Many only use lack of an SSR to define an abnormal result, but SSRs may not be obtained from the lower extremities in 50% of healthy subjects older than 60 years. There is often little correlation between severity of autonomic dysfunction and presence or absence of SSR. The SSR specifically tests sudomotor fibers that do not participate in thermoregulation, and hence the correlation between presence or absence of SSR and other modalities of measurement of sudomotor function is poor.

THERMOREGULATORY SWEAT TEST

The TST is a sensitive qualitative test of sudomotor function, providing important information on the pattern and degree of sweat loss. A color indicator (quinizarin powder [6]) is applied onto dry skin. The environmental temperature is increased until an adequate core temperature increase is attained and the presence of sweating causes a change in the indicator from brown to a violet color. Thermal stimulation using heat cradles or sweat cabinets can be used.

The test can be rendered semiquantitative by estimating the percent of anterior surface anhidrosis [7]. This percentage has proven to be a useful parameter in differentiating autonomic disorders. For example, multiple system atrophy (MSA) is usually associated with anhidrosis greater than 40%, and Parkinson's disease with and without orthostatic hypotension is usually associated with anhidrosis less than 40%. It also has been helpful in monitoring the status (improvement or worsening) of dysautonomias.

There are some characteristic patterns of anhidrosis in the peripheral neuropathies (Table 61.2) [7], including the following:

1. Distal anhidrosis is seen in distal small fiber neuropathy and length-dependent axonal neuropathy.
2. Global anhidrosis is generally seen in the generalized autonomic disorders such as MSA, pure autonomic failure, or the autonomic neuropathies.
3. Regional anhidrosis is another pattern; an example is the anhidrosis of chronic idiopathic anhidrosis, a form of restricted autonomic neuropathy.

The disadvantages of TST are its inability to distinguish between postganglionic, preganglionic, and central lesions; discomfort; the qualitative nature of the information obtained; and staining of clothing. There are many factors that affect the sweat response. These include sex, race, acclimation, and drugs, especially anticholinergic medications.

INTEGRATED EVALUATION OF SWEATING

By combining the different tests of autonomic function, it is possible to generate unique information. The TST and QSART can be combined to define the site of the lesion. A preganglionic lesion results in loss of sweating on TST with preserved sweating on QSART. TST and QSART can be combined to provide information on the distribution of anhidrosis (percentage of anhidrosis), whereas QSART can define the volume of sweat loss. Sweat imprint yields information on the diameter distribution of sweat droplets. Combined with QSART, it is possible to determine the volume per sweat droplet.

TABLE 61.2 Some Causes and Patterns of Anhidrosis and Hypohidrosis

Pattern	Examples	Site and mechanism
Distal	DSFN; many neuropathies	Postganglionic denervation
Global	Panautonomic neuropathy; multiple system atrophy	Preganglionic or postganglionic lesions
Segmental	Chronic idiopathic anhidrosis	Postganglionic ± preganglionic denervation
Dermatomal	Diabetic radiculopathy Ulnar neuropathy	Radicular postganglionic denervation Nerve trunk involvement
Hemianhidrosis	Cerebral infarction	Central lesion of sympathetic outflow Spinal cord tumor

DSFN, distal small fiber neuropathy.

References

1. Low, P. A., P. E. Caskey, R. R. Tuck, R. D. Fealey, and P. J. Dyck. 1983. Quantitative sudomotor axon reflex test in normal and neuropathic subjects. *Ann. Neurol.* 14:573–580.
2. Low, P. A. 1997. Laboratory evaluation of autonomic function. In *Clinical autonomic disorders: Evaluation and management*, ed. P. A. Low, 179–208. Philadelphia: Lippincott-Raven.
3. Kennedy, W. R., M. Sakuta, D. Sutherland, and F. C. Goetz. 1984. Quantitation of the sweating deficit in diabetes mellitus. *Ann. Neurol.* 15:482–488.
4. Low, P. A., T. L. Opfer-Gehrking, and M. Kihara. 1992. In vivo studies on receptor pharmacology of the human eccrine sweat gland. *Clin. Auton. Res.* 2:29–34.
5. Schondorf, R. 1993. The role of sympathetic skin responses in the assessment of autonomic function. In *Clinical autonomic disorders: Evaluation and management*, ed. P. A. Low, 231–241. Boston: Little, Brown and Company.
6. Low, P. A., J. C. Walsh, C. Y. Huang, and J. G. McLeod. 1975. The sympathetic nervous system in diabetic neuropathy: A clinical and pathological study. *Brain* 98:341–356.
7. Fealey, R. D. 1997. Thermoregulatory sweat test. In *Clinical autonomic disorders: Evaluation and management*, ed. P. A. Low, 245–257. Philadelphia: Lippincott-Raven.

62 Biochemical Assessment of Sympathoadrenal Activity

Joseph L. Izzo, Jr.
Department of Medicine
SUNY-Buffalo
Buffalo, New York

Stanley F. Fernandez
Department of Pharmacology and Toxicology
SUNY-Buffalo
Buffalo, New York

To respond to the many acute stressors presented by everyday life, the sympathoadrenal system (SAS) can be activated in an extremely pleiotropic pattern that results in varying contributions of adrenal and regional neuronal catecholamine release. At the same time, catecholamines are metabolized by a redundant series of degradative enzymes that differ in their relative activities within different tissues. Thus, the patterns of responses of catecholamines and metabolites found in biologic fluids are affected by the nature of the stimulus, the characteristics of the accompanying physiologic response, and potentially by disease states. Because of this complex pattern, it logically follows that no single measurement of a catecholamine or its metabolites can provide a full assessment of SAS activity at any given time. Rather, full assessment of SAS activation requires the integration of information from several diverse analytic approaches that are generally more complementary than redundant. This chapter discusses the major biochemical techniques for assessment of SAS activity that have been developed during the about last 40 years, largely in order of historical appearance.

CATECHOLAMINE METABOLISM

Knowledge of the usual patterns of intraneuronal and extraneuronal metabolism is the first requirement in assessing the strengths and limitations of each potential marker of SAS activity (Fig. 62.1).

URINARY EXCRETION OF CATECHOLAMINES AND METABOLITES

Urinary Vanillylmandelic Acid Excretion

Vanillylmandelic acid is the major end product of combined oxidation and transmethylation of norepinephrine (NE) and epinephrine. As such, it is completely insensitive to physiologic variations in regional sympathetic output, and because of the 24-hour collection, has limited value in any physiologic assessment of SAS activity. There is still occasional use of 24-hour urinary VMA excretion in the diagnosis of pheochromocytoma (≥7 mg/day by the Pisano assay is consistent with pheochromocytoma), but plasma and urinary metanephrines are substantially more specific and sensitive than urinary VMA, which retains little if any clinical usefulness.

Urinary-Free Catecholamines

Total or fractionated urinary catecholamines are used occasionally in the determination of 24-hour sympathetic nervous activity and are still quite commonly used in the diagnosis of pheochromocytoma. Under usual conditions, the bulk of urinary NE is derived from circulatory rather than renal sources. Normal total urinary catecholamine values are usually 100 mcg or less per day.

Urinary Metanephrines

Metanephrines, the primary O-methylated metabolites of catecholamines, have limited usefulness in the physiologic assessment of sympathetic tone. Metanephrines exist in both free and sulfate-conjugated forms. Pheochromocytoma cells release mostly free metanephrines, whereas sulfoconjugated metanephrines are produced principally in the gastrointestinal tract. Metanephrines have become the primary screening test for pheochromocytoma; total 24-hour metanephrine excretion less than 150 mcg/day is usually considered normal in most laboratories.

Urinary Methoxyhydroxyphenyl Glycol

Methoxyhydroxyphenyl glycol (MHPG) is produced in two steps: (1) oxidative metabolism in neural tissue, and (2) O-methylation by the liver or kidney. MHPG also can be sulfoconjugated or further metabolized to VMA. Urinary MHPG excretion was originally thought to represent central nervous system (CNS) sympathetic output, but MHPG is now known to be principally derived from peripheral sympathetic neuronal NE metabolism.

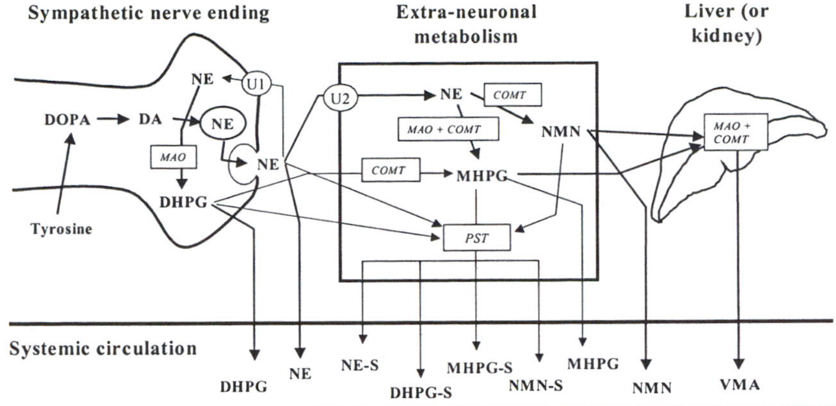

FIGURE 62.1 Metabolism of catecholamines. Norepinephrine (NE) is produced in postganglionic neurons and the adrenal medulla, through the actions of dopamine β-hydroxylase, the enzyme that incorporates dopamine into granules and converts it to NE. In the adrenal, and to a much lesser extent in certain brain regions and cardiac chromaffin cells, the presence of the enzyme phenylethanolamine-*N*-methyltransferase (PNMT) confers the ability to produce epinephrine from NE. The principal mechanism for the clearance of catecholamines from synaptic clefts is neuronal reuptake (U1). Enzymatic degradation of catecholamines within neurons occurs largely through monoamine oxidase (MAO), which produces dihydroxyphenyl glycol (DHPG), a marker of neuronal NE turnover. The other major pathway for inactivation of NE, epinephrine, or DHPG requires uptake by nonneuronal cells (U2) followed by o-methylation through catechol-O-methyl transferase (COMT) to form normetanephrine, metanephrine, or methoxyhydroxyphenyl glycol (MHPG), respectively. Sulfoconjugates (-S) of a variety of catecholamines and metabolites arise through the actions of phenyl sulfotransferase (PST) in platelets and in a variety of nonneural tissues. Vanillylmandelic acid (VMA) is the product of both MAO and COMT actions. DA, dopamine.

PLASMA CATECHOLAMINES AND METABOLITES

Plasma Norepinephrine

Plasma NE remains the most durable and widely used biochemical index to assess physiologic and pathologic increases in sympathetic activity. The NE in plasma is derived both from adrenal and peripheral neuronal sources, but under usual circumstances, the latter predominates. In general, venous plasma NE concentrations are about 30% greater than corresponding arterial values, indicating net release of catecholamines from peripheral sympathetic nerves. Variation in plasma NE caused by alterations in clearance and metabolism have not proven to be a major problem in using plasma NE within or between individuals. Forearm venous plasma NE is closely related to the corresponding muscle sympathetic activity. In addition to the assessment of SAS activity, plasma catecholamines are still useful in the diagnosis of pheochromocytoma. One caveat to their use is that the normal range reported by most commercial laboratories is derived from young volunteers, not appropriately controlled "at risk" patients. Increased plasma NE occurs with age, obesity, hypertension, cardiac decompensation, and other conditions in which false-positives can exist. There are few false-negatives, however, and a plasma NE less than 1000 pg/ml is highly unusual in pheochromocytoma.

Despite repeated attacks by some investigators on the basis of poor sensitivity, plasma NE remains a reliable and highly specific index of peripheral nerve traffic. The sensitivity of venous plasma NE to detect small changes in sympathetic activity is clearly less than that of direct nerve traffic studies, but the latter technique simply cannot be applied to large clinical studies. The technical inability to perform adequate microneurography studies in as many as half of all subjects, the need to maintain subjects in an uncomfortable motionless position for relatively long periods, and the expense of the procedure are some of the problems that justify the continued use of plasma catecholamines in clinical studies. There are also major barriers to microneurography caused by the difficulties of comparing data between or within individuals on different study days. Other investigators have proposed that potential differences in NE clearance within and between individuals necessitates a kinetic approach. It is further stated that because unequal sympathetic innervation across different organs causes differential NE release rates from these organs, assessment of whole body SAS activity requires use of arterial rather than venous NE. Yet, further analysis reveals that this stance also can be problematic, not only because of the varying responses that may occur during different stimuli, but because the lung also metabolizes catecholamines. As a reasonable compromise, it may be appropriate to measure arteriovenous differences across the organ of interest. If regional blood flow is measured and the Fick equation is used, a highly specific regional NE release rate can be obtained. For the most part, however, standard venous plasma NE values are reasonable indexes of organ-specific catecholamine production and are at least the equivalent of turnover studies in a variety of conditions.

Plasma Epinephrine

In contrast to NE, epinephrine in plasma simply reflects adrenal output. In general, venous values are slightly lower than corresponding arterial values because of peripheral uptake. Thus, there is a slight advantage to the measurement of arterial rather than venous epinephrine, but the difficulty of arterial sampling probably justifies use of venous values in many studies.

Plasma Dopamine

Free plasma dopamine normally circulates in very low concentrations (<50 pg/ml, which is often the limit of assay sensitivity); approximately 20 times as much dopamine circulates in the sulfoconjugated form compared with free dopamine. Plasma dopamine has no direct relation to other indexes of SAS activity and is not a diagnostic test in any well-accepted clinical syndromes. Why commercial laboratories continue to report plasma dopamine values as part of a "fractionated catecholamine" profile remains unclear.

Plasma Dihydroxyphenyl Glycol

Dihydroxyphenyl glycol (DHPG), the principal neuronal metabolite of NE, can be quantitated in plasma and has been shown to correlate closely with plasma NE and with neuronal NE turnover in humans. Catalyzed by monoamine oxidases (MAOs), it is formed from oxidative deamination of NE. Despite the presence of MAO in both neural and extraneural sites, a primarily neuronal source of circulating DHPG is suggested from experiments showing minimal conversion of infused NE to DHPG and minimal DHPG production by NE-secreting pheochromocytomas. In nerve terminals, DHPG formed from NE is derived from reuptake of NE through $Uptake_1$ or from NE that leaked out from storage vesicles. Granular leakage may be the predominant mechanism for DHPG formation because $Uptake_1$ inhibitors have minimal effects on plasma DHPG levels, whereas inhibition of granular transport mechanisms decreases DHPG.

Plasma Metanephrines

Evidence suggests that free plasma normetanephrine and metanephrine concentrations are the most sensitive (99%) and specific (89%) test for detection of hereditary and sporadic pheochromocytoma. This test is not yet in widespread clinical use, but its popularity appears to be increasing.

Sulfoconjugates

In contrast to dopamine, sulfoconjugated NE and epinephrine circulate in concentrations only about threefold greater than their respective free catecholamines. Acute changes in plasma catecholamines do not necessarily affect sulfoconjugate concentrations. Some investigators have postulated that tissue sulfatases can liberate free catecholamines from their respective sulfoconjugates, but the biologic and clinical significance of this possibility remain unclear.

OTHER PROTEINS AND PEPTIDES IN PLASMA

Dopamine β-Hydroxylase

Dopamine β-hydroxylase (DBH) is the enzyme responsible for the uptake and conversion of dopamine into NE in neuronal storage granules. DBH is a membrane-associated protein in granules that is released in limited quantities during the process of neuronal NE release; therefore, plasma DBH is a marker of SAS activity. DBH is much less sensitive to change than plasma NE or its metabolites, however, and it is not a reliable diagnostic tool in pheochromocytoma.

Chromogranin A

Chromogranin A (CGA) is the major intravesicular storage protein that acts to shield NE from oxidation. Like DBH, CGA is released during degranulation; but unlike DBH, CGA can be used in the diagnosis of pheochromocytome. Both DBH and CGA are quite stable in plasma and can be considered to be additional surrogates for increased SAS activity that may be preferable to catecholamines or metabolites in conditions in which sample preservation is difficult.

Neuropeptide Y

Neuropeptide Y (NPY) is stored in catecholamine-containing granules and also is released with NE during postganglionic sympathetic nerve stimulation. Although its role as cotransmitter is well established, the plasma NPY level as an independent indicator of SAS activity is not universally accepted. If SAS activation is intense, plasma NPY responses parallel those of NE, but during milder degrees of SAS stimulation, such as orthostatic stress or handgrip, circulating NPY changes often are undetectable. Plasma NPY also exhibits different kinetics from NE, with a slower rate of appearance after SAS activation, in part because of a slower diffusion rate from tissues. Its circulating level is further prolonged by its longer plasma half-life.

TISSUE CATECHOLAMINE CONCENTRATIONS

Tissue Catecholamines

Catecholamine turnover in neural and peripheral tissues can be relatively reliably assessed by the measurement of total tissue content, which is usually expressed in concentration per milligram of tissue. Peripheral tissue catecholamine content is generally inversely proportional to the sympathetic nerve traffic in that tissue because as catecholamine release increases, tissue stores are depleted. Tissue concentrations have been used most widely in the brain and heart, both in animal and human experiments.

Platelet Catecholamine

Platelet catecholamine content also has been used as a global integrated index of sympathetic function and in the diagnosis of pheochromocytoma. In platelets, nonspecific uptake ($Uptake_2$) causes platelet catecholamine content to increase in parallel with systemic sympathoadrenal activity.

CEREBROSPINAL FLUID CATECHOLAMINES AND METABOLITES

Free catecholamines and glycolic metabolites have been quantitated in cerebrospinal fluid (CSF) and exist in concentrations similar to those observed in plasma. The glycolic metabolites move rapidly from the CNS to the periphery, but the greater volume of peripheral NE-containing synapses is reflected in the large contribution of peripheral sympathetic nerves to plasma DHPG concentration. Nevertheless, in most experiments, it is unnecessary to collect CSF to quantitate SAS activity.

KINETIC (TURNOVER) STUDIES

General Methodology

Modified clearance techniques have been used to estimate SAS activity. These studies are based on the assumption that the rate of appearance of NE in the plasma is a more reliable index of SAS activity than the plasma NE concentration, which can be theoretically affected by different rates of removal from plasma. The approach uses relatively standard formulas for the kinetic turnover of a given substance. First, the plasma clearance rate is determined using a steady-state infusion by the following formula:

$$\underset{(\mathrm{Cx,\ ml/min})}{\text{Clearance of X}} = \frac{\text{infusion rate of X (mg/min)}}{\text{steady-state plasma concentration X(mg/ml)}}$$

If the infused substance is identical to a native substance, it is also necessary to account for the basal plasma X concentration (subtracting this value from the plateau concentration of X achieved during the steady-state infusion). From the plateau plasma X value (corrected if necessary) and the corresponding Cx, the basal plasma appearance rate of X can be calculated:

$$\text{Appearance of X (mg/min)} = [\text{basal plasma X (mg/ml)}] \times [\text{Cx (ml/min)}]$$

When these formulas have been applied to the infusion of exogenous NE, the NE appearance rate has been called the "NE spillover rate." Because about 80% of neuronally released NE is removed from the synapses by reuptake mechanisms, about 20% of the NE that is release is part of the "spillover." As long as the activities of the uptake mechanisms remain constant, the NE spillover rate (or plasma appearance rate) is a reasonable index of neuronal NE release and sympathetic nervous activity. As discussed earlier, the basic rationale for the use of turnover studies is the largely hypothetic concern that interindividual or interorgan variations in catecholamine metabolism limit the reliability of free plasma catecholamines as indexes of whole body or organ-specific SAS activity. In some cases, however, turnover studies may increase the likelihood of artifact by virtue of the complex assumptions and calculations involved.

Radiotracer Infusions

Objections have been made to the use of unlabeled NE infusions, largely on the theoretic grounds that the vasoactive properties of infused catecholamines could alter their own clearances. As a result, Esler [4] and others developed a tracer technique using tiny amounts of labeled catecholamines to quantitate the NE spillover rate according to the following formula:

$$\text{Regional NE spillover} = [(\mathrm{Cv} - \mathrm{Ca}) + \mathrm{Ca} * \mathrm{E}] * \mathrm{PF}$$

where C = concentration, a = arterial, v = venous, E = extraction, and PF = plasma flow. Central to the validity of this technique is the assumption that true steady-state, radiolabeled, NE concentrations are achieved across all cellular compartments, an assertion that has not been fully proven.

Kinetic techniques have confirmed that different organ beds can respond differently to systemic SAS stimulation, and that plasma catecholamines are not always sensitive enough to detect differences among organ beds or between populations. For example, the kidney may experience sympathetic activation during periods of reduced cardiac filling, whereas muscle beds are unaffected. Similarly, using spillover methodology, hypertensives have been found to release more NE than normotensives in response to mental stress, whereas parallel studies of plasma NE demonstrated no significant difference between the two conditions. There remain, however, significant limitations to the use of kinetic techniques. Perhaps the biggest drawback is the reluctance of many institutional review boards to approve the use of infused tritiated radiotracers for research purposes. Other major drawbacks include the great expense of the studies and the practice of infusing radiotracer through a fluoroscopically placed central venous catheter. This technique, therefore, is highly limited in use.

ANALYTIC METHODS FOR CATECHOLAMINES

The analysis of catecholamines and metabolites is always relatively expensive and can be artifactual if samples are not fastidiously collected and preserved before laboratory analysis.

Sample Preservation

Catecholamines and metanephrines are highly labile, whereas the glycolic metabolites are somewhat more stable. Plasma samples should be collected with antioxidant and iced immediately before plasma separation. Plasma should generally be stored at very low temperatures (<–70°C) before analysis. Urine samples for metanephrines or VMA should be collected with acid present to prevent spontaneous oxidation.

Analytic Techniques

Several methods are currently available for analysis of catecholamines and metabolites. Several of the techniques allow quantitation of several catecholamines or metabolites simultaneously, including glycolic metabolites. High-pressure liquid chromatography (HPLC) with electrochemical detection is the preferred method for catecholamine studies in urine and tissue, especially when the amount available for analysis is at least 50 pg per sample. Plasma NE concentrations can be reliably measured, but resting plasma epinephrine values (often <25 pg/ml) usually challenge HPLC sensitivity limits. Technical difficulties with the HPLC assay include the problems of consistency of catecholamine extraction and instability of the electrochemical detection system. Because of these difficulties, laboratories that remain consistently productive use more than one HPLC system for catecholamine analysis.

Radioenzymatic methods most commonly use catechol-O-methyl transferase to quantitatively incorporate a tritiated methyl group onto NE or epinephrine (to form normetanephrine or metanephrine, respectively) before chromatographic separation, oxidation, and extraction for scintillation counting. In a similar approach, NE can be measured by quantitating the amount of tritiated methylation caused by exposure of the sample to phenylethanolamine *N*-methyltransferase, which converts NE to epinephrine. Radioenzymatic methods for catecholamines are extremely sensitive (usually to 1 pg per sample) and are capable of detecting fentomolar quantities reliably. Unfortunately, they are the most labor intensive and are therefore extremely expensive. Radioenzymatic determinations are most clearly justified for the reliable quantitation of plasma epinephrine, analysis of samples with low catecholamine content, and repeated blood sampling in small animals.

Immunoassays are recent additions in quantifying plasma and urinary catecholamines. There are two methods in this category using the same basic principle: radioimmunoassay (RIA) and enzyme-linked immunoassay (ELISA). Immunoassays generally involve the use of capture antibodies that recognize the catecholamine of interest. This assay generally requires that the samples are chemically derivatized before incubation with capture antibodies. In the ELISA system, a second antibody conjugated with an enzyme is added to recognize another portion of the catecholamine. The amount of bound enzyme is proportional to the amount of catecholamine. Current commercially available RIAs are reported to have sensitivities of as low as 10 pg/ml, well within the physiologic range and consistent with HPLC data. Immunoassays offer the distinct advantage of lower cost and more readily accessible equipment but still require further validation.

References

1. Landsberg, L., and J. B. Young. 1992. Catecholamines and the adrenal medulla. In *Williams' textbook of endocrinology*, 8th ed., ed. J. D. Wilson and D. W. Foster, 637–640. Philadelphia: WB Saunders.
2. Goldstein, D. S., and I. J. Kopin. 1990. The autonomic nervous system and catecholamines in normal blood pressure control and in hypertension. In *Hypertension: Pathophysiology, diagnosis, and management*, ed. J. H. Laragh and B. Brenner, 711–732. New York: Raven Press.
3. Wallin, B. G., G. Sundlof, B. M. Eriksson, P. Dominiak, H. Grobecker, and L. E. Lindblad. 1981. Plasma noradrenaline correlates to muscle sympathetic nerve activity in man. *Acta. Physiol. Scand.* 111:69–73.
4. Esler, M. 1993. Clinical application of noradrenaline spillover methodology: Delineation of regional human sympathetic nervous responses. *Pharmacol. Toxicol.* 73:243–253.
5. Goldstein, D. S., G. Eisenhofer, M. Garty, C. J. Folio, R. Stull, J. E. Brush, Jr., F. L. Sax, H. R. Keiser, and I. J. Kopin. 1989. Implications of plasma levels of catechols in the evaluation of sympathoadrenomedullary function. *Am. J. Hypertens.* 2:133S–139S.
6. Lenders, J. W., K. Pacak, M. M. Walther, W. M. Linehan, M. Mannelli, P. Friberg, H. R. Keiser, D. S. Goldstein, and G. Eisenhofer. 2002. Biochemical diagnosis of pheochromocytoma: Which test is best? *JAMA* 287:1427–1434.

P A R T VII

CARDIOVASCULAR DISORDERS

63 Hypertension and Sympathetic Nervous System Activity

David A. Calhoun
Vascular Biology and Hypertension Program
University of Alabama Birmingham
Birmingham, Alabama

Suzanne Oparil
Vascular Biology and Hypertension Program
University of Alabama Birmingham
Birmingham, Alabama

Sympathetic nervous system activity is increased in both the developmental and chronic stages of primary hypertension. Animal and human studies demonstrate that sustained sympathetic stimulation of the kidney promotes sodium and fluid retention; stimulation of the heart increases cardiac output; and chronic stimulation of the vasculature induces smooth muscle cell hypertrophy and hyperplasia, resulting in sustained increases in peripheral resistance. These observations indicate that sympathetic activation plays a key role in both initiating and maintaining chronic increase of blood pressure.

RENAL SYMPATHETIC STIMULATION IN EXPERIMENTAL AND HUMAN HYPERTENSION

In animal models of hypertension, direct renal nerve stimulation induces renal tubular sodium and water reabsorption and decreases urinary water and sodium excretion, resulting in increased blood pressure secondary to increased intravascular volume. Direct assessments of renal sympathetic innervation have consistently demonstrated heightened sympathetic activation in rat models of primary hypertension. Denervation of the kidney, either surgically or pharmacologically, eliminates or blunts salt and water retention and prevents or reverses the development of hypertension in these models.

Renal sympathetic stimulation also is increased in human subjects with primary hypertension. Investigators in Australia have demonstrated that plasma norepinephrine spillover from the kidneys, an index of sympathetic activity, is increased in human patients with hypertension compared with normotensive control subjects. Renal arterial administration of phentolamine, an α-adrenoreceptor antagonist, reduces renal blood flow to a greater degree in hypertensive than normotensive subjects, which is consistent with increased greater renal sympathetic stimulation in hypertension.

In humans with renal failure, peripheral sympathetic activity is increased compared with normotensive control subjects. In a study using microneurography, resting muscle sympathetic nerve activity (MSNA) was more than doubled in patients with hypertension receiving hemodialysis compared with age-matched healthy normotensive individuals with normal renal function. Interestingly, MSNA is normal in patients receiving hemodialysis who have undergone bilateral nephrectomy, suggesting that sympathetic overactivity in patients with renal failure is caused by a neurogenic signal originating in the failing kidneys (Fig. 63.1).

CARDIAC SYMPATHETIC STIMULATION IN HUMAN HYPERTENSION

Multiple population-based studies have demonstrated a positive correlation between heart rate and future development of hypertension. For example, the multicenter longitudinal Coronary Artery Risk Development in Young Adults (CARDIA) study followed 4762 black and white men and women, initially aged 18 to 30 years, over a 10-year period. In this cohort, heart rate was an independent predictor of subsequent diastolic blood pressure in white men and women and black men. Overall, the mean increase in diastolic blood pressure was 1.3 mmHg per 10 heartbeats per minute. Because heart rate is, in large part, under sympathetic control, these results support the concept that chronic sympathetic overactivity induces hypertension. Because diastolic pressure relates more closely to vascular resistance and is less affected by cardiac function, the CARDIA investigators suggest that increased sympathetic tone, as evidenced by heart rate increase, may cause smooth muscle cell proliferation, resulting in reduced compliance of the peripheral vasculature and, consequently, increased diastolic blood pressure.

Consistent with population-based observations relating increased heart rate to the development of hypertension, norepinephrine spillover studies indicate that sympathetic cardiac stimulation is greater in young patients with hypertension compared with similarly aged normotensive control subjects. Together, these results suggest that increased

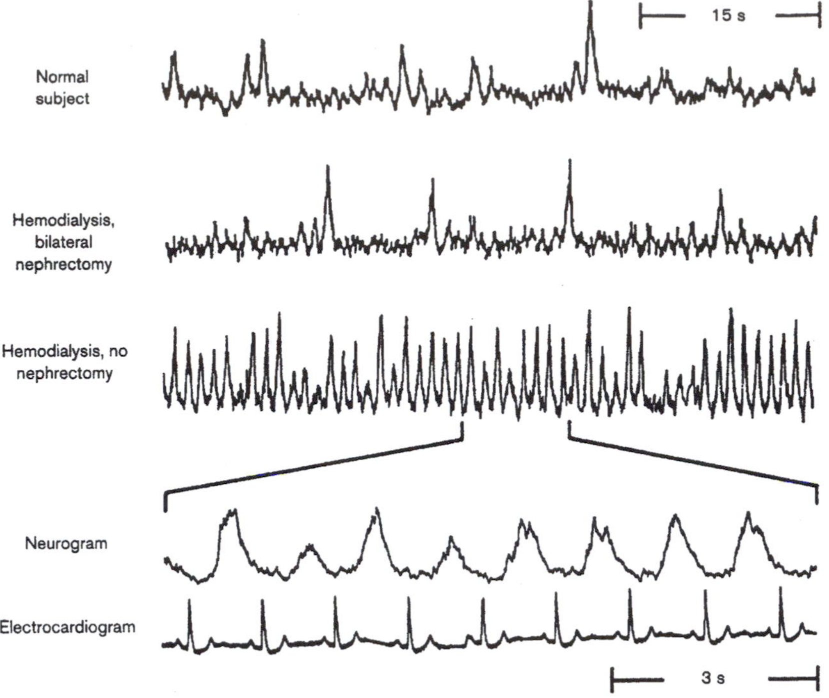

FIGURE 63.1 Recordings of sympathetic nerve discharge to the leg muscles in a healthy subject and in two patients receiving hemodialysis, one with and one without bilateral nephrectomy. The top three panels are representative segments of the neurograms from three subjects, and the bottom two panels display the neurogram and simultaneous electrocardiogram from the third subject on an expanded time scale. On these mean-voltage displays of muscle sympathetic nerve activity, each peak represents a spontaneous burst of sympathetic nerve discharge. The rate of sympathetic nerve discharge was much greater in the patient undergoing hemodialysis who had not had a nephrectomy than in the patient undergoing hemodialysis who had had a bilateral nephrectomy, with the rate in the latter being indistinguishable from that in the healthy subject. (Reproduced from Converse, R. L. Jr., T. N. Jacobsen, R. D. Toto, C. M. Jost, F. Cosentino, F. Fouad-Tarazi, and R. G. Victor. 1992. Sympathetic overactivity in patients with chronic renal failure. *N. Engl. J. Med.* 327:1912–1918, with permission.)

cardiac sympathetic stimulation correlates and likely contributes to the development of hypertension.

SYMPATHETIC NERVOUS SYSTEM ACTIVITY AND VASCULAR REMODELING

Vascular smooth muscle cell proliferation/hypertrophy is a consequence of the complex interaction of intravascular pressure, systemic and local hormones, genetic predispositions, and environmental factors. Animal and human studies demonstrate that sustained increases in sympathetic activation directly induce vascular remodeling. In cell culture and in whole animal models, norepinephrine promotes the synthesis and release of a variety of trophic substances, including transforming growth factor-β, insulin-like growth factor, and fibroblast growth factors. Inhibition of sympathetic stimulation, by sympathectomy, pharmacologic blockade, or both, prevents or diminishes cardiac and vascular hypertrophy in rat models of hypertension. Lastly, animal models demonstrate that local sympathetic denervation prevents hypertrophy and remodeling of cerebral arterioles.

Human studies likewise demonstrate vascular trophic effects of chronic sympathetic stimulation. In a large population-based study, circulating norepinephrine levels correlated positively with left ventricular mass. Italian investigators demonstrated that increased plasma norepinephrine levels are associated with reduced radial artery compliance, which is consistent with increased vascular hypertrophy.

PLASMA NOREPINEPHRINE LEVELS

Many studies report greater circulating levels of norepinephrine in patients with hypertension than in normotensive control subjects. A review of 64 studies found that 52 (81%) reported greater norepinephrine levels in patients with hypertension compared with normotensive subjects; but in only 25 (39%) of the 64 original studies were the greater norepinephrine levels statistically significant. Most studies that evaluated younger subjects (<40 years of age) found that norepinephrine levels were significantly greater in hypertensive versus normotensive subjects. Although plasma norepinephrine levels provide imprecise indexes of sympathetic nervous system activity, these studies provide indirect evidence that sympathetic activity is increased in human hypertension.

REGIONAL NOREPINEPHRINE SPILLOVER

The norepinephrine spillover technique is used to assess the tissue clearance of norepinephrine by determining the degree of dilution of a small amount of intravenously infused radiolabeled norepinephrine. The norepinephrine spillover rate is thought to reflect norepinephrine release from the sympathoeffector terminal and, thereby, sympathetic activity. In addition to the increased renal and cardiac norepinephrine spillover noted earlier, application of this technique has demonstrated that whole body norepinephrine spillover is increased in young patients with hypertension compared with normotensive control subjects, suggesting that heightened sympathetic activity contributes to the development of hypertension.

MICRONEUROGRAPHY

In the 1960s, Swedish neurophysiologists developed the technique of microneurography to directly record sympathetic activity from peripheral nerves in humans. Microneurography has been used to compare MSNA in patients with hypertension and normotensive subjects. The largest current study compared resting MSNA recorded from the tibial nerve in 63 Japanese subjects with hypertension (48 male and 15 female subjects) to 43 Japanese normotensive subjects (32 male and 11 female subjects). The Japanese investigators found that resting MSNA values were significantly greater in the subjects with hypertension compared with the normotensive subjects (31 vs 21 bursts/min; $P < 0.01$). MSNA was found to increase with age, but even when corrected for this factor, MSNA remain increased in the subjects with hypertension. Investigators at the University of Milan confirmed that MSNA is increased in patients with established hypertension. In this study, resting MSNA was found to be progressively greater in patients with mild, moderate, and serve hypertension (Fig. 63.2).

Resting MSNA also has been found to be greater in the developmental stages of hypertension than in normotensive control subjects. Investigators at the University of Iowa found that MSNA was significantly greater in 12 young male patients with "borderline" or intermittent hypertension compared with 15 age-matched normotensive control subjects regardless of high or low dietary NaCl ingestion. In a similar comparison, Canadian investigators found resting MSNA to be significantly greater in young patients with hypertension than in normotensive control subjects.

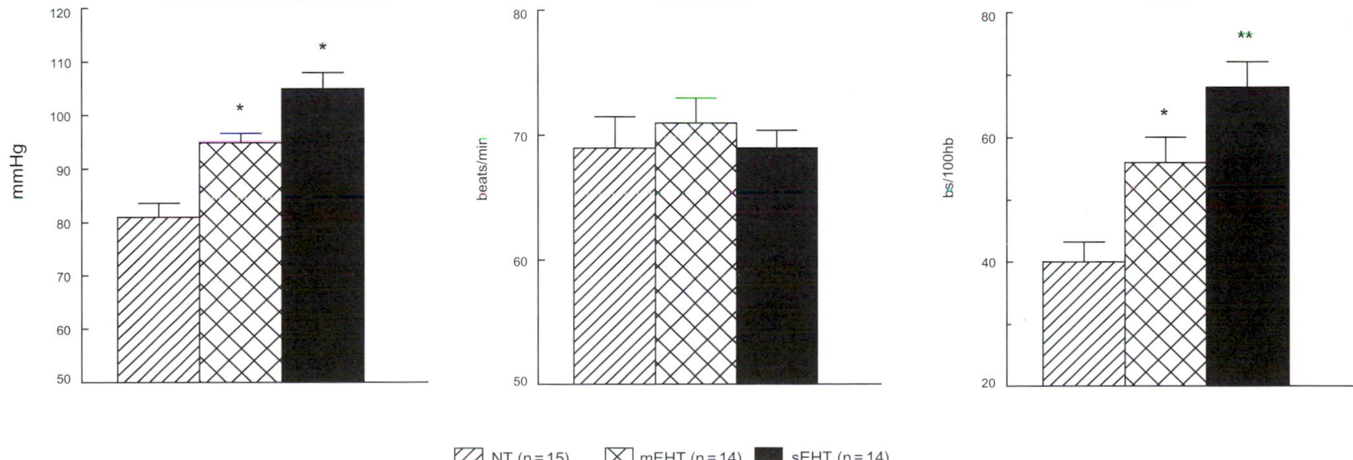

FIGURE 63.2 Values demonstrating relation between increasing blood pressure and increasing peripheral sympathetic activity. Mean arterial pressure (MAP), heart rate (HR) and muscle sympathetic nerve activity (MSNA) in normotensive (NT), mild primary hypertensive (mEHT), and more severe essential hypertensive (sEHT) subjects. Data are shown as mean ± SEM. *$P < 0.05$ vs NT; **$P < 0.01$ vs NT and mEHT. (Modified from Grassi, G., B. M. Cattaneo, G. Seravalle, A. Lanfranchi, and G. Mancia. 1998. Baroreflex control of sympathetic nerve activity in essential and secondary hypertension. *Hypertension* 31:68–72, with permission.)

SYMPATHETIC AND VASCULAR REACTIVITY

Patients with hypertension manifest greater vasoconstrictor response to infused norepinephrine than normotensive control subjects. In normotensive subjects, increased levels of circulating norepinephrine generally induce down-regulation of noradrenergic receptors. In patients with hypertension, however, such down-regulation appears not to occur, resulting in enhanced sensitivity to norepinephrine. The combination of enhanced sensitivity to and increased circulating levels of norepinephrine likely contributes significantly to sympathetic nervous system activity-related hypertension. Increased sensitivity to norepinephrine also has been observed in normotensive offspring of parents with hypertension compared with control subjects without a family history of hypertension, suggesting that the phenomenon may be genetic in origin and not simply a consequence of increased blood pressure.

Exposure to stress is well known to increase sympathetic output. A vicious circle is hypothesized to link stress and increases in sympathetic activity to the development of hypertension. According to this hypothesis, repeated stress-induced vasoconstriction causes vascular hypertrophy, which promotes even more vigorous vasoconstrictive responses to stress, leading to progressive increases in peripheral vascular resistance and blood pressure. Stress-induced hypertension has been observed in the laboratory setting. Stress may explain, in part, the greater incidence of hypertension in lower socioeconomic groups, because individuals in such groups must endure greater stress levels associated with day-to-day living.

Studies of sympathetic reactivity suggest that young subjects with a genetic predisposition to development of hypertension—that is, a positive family history of hypertension—manifest greater vasoconstrictive responses to laboratory stressors, such as mental stress, cold pressor testing, or physical exercise. In some studies, this greater vascular reactivity has been shown to correlate with a greater likelihood of hypertension development.

The results of stress testing are most consistent in young black individuals. The majority of studies report that young black individuals with normotension or mild hypertension manifest greater stress-induced vascular reactivity than age-matched white individuals, particularly in response to cold pressor testing. A study from this laboratory used microneurography to record MSNA responses in young normotensive black and white subjects and found that the greater pressor response to cold pressor testing observed in black individuals was attributable to greater increases in peripheral sympathetic nervous system activity (Fig. 63.3). It is hypothesized that greater stress-induced increases in sympathetic activity, in combination with the greater socioeconomic stress that black individuals often endure, likely contribute to the significantly greater incidence of hypertension in black compared with white individuals in the United States.

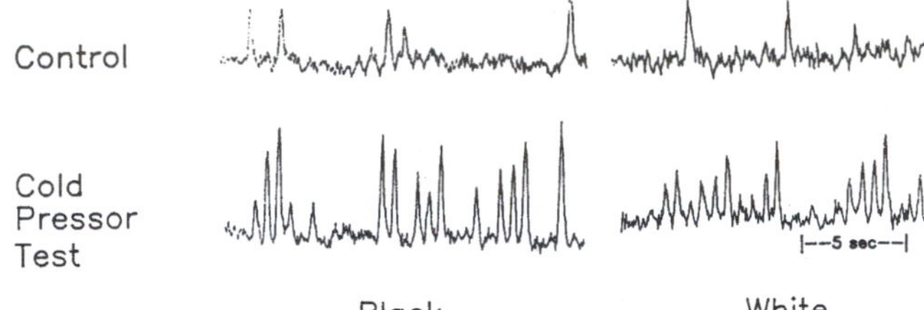

FIGURE 63.3 Tracings show muscle sympathetic nerve activity as recorded by microneurography (each spike represents an efferent burst) in a black normotensive subject and a white normotensive subject at rest (control) and during cold pressor test. Sympathetic nerve activity increased in both subjects during cold stress, but the magnitude of the increase was greater in the black subject. (Reproduced from Calhoun, D. A., M. L. Mutinga, A. S. Collins, S. Wyss, and S. Oparil. 1993. Normotensive blacks have heightened sympathetic response to cold pressor test. *Hypertension* 22:801–805, with permission.)

References

1. Converse, R. L. Jr., T. N. Jacobsen, R. D. Toto, C. M. Jost, F. Cosentino, F. Fouad-Tarazi, and R. G. Victor. 1992. Sympathetic overactivity in patients with chronic renal failure. *N. Engl. J. Med.* 327:1912–1918.
2. Grassi, G., B. M. Cattaneo, G. Seravalle, A. Lanfranchi, and G. Mancia. 1998. Baroreflex control of sympathetic nerve activity in essential and secondary hypertension. *Hypertension* 31:68–72.
3. Calhoun, D. A., M. L. Mutinga, A. S. Collins, S. Wyss, and S. Oparil. 1993. Normotensive blacks have heightened sympathetic response to cold pressor test. *Hypertension* 22:801–805.
4. Esler, M. 2000. The sympathetic system and hypertension. *Am. J. Hypertens.* 3:99S–105S.
5. Brook, R. D., and S. Julius. 2001. Autonomic imbalance, hypertension, and cardiovascular risk. *Am. J. Hypertens.* 13:112S–122S.
6. Kim, J.-R., C. I. Kiefe, K. Liu, O. D. Williams, D. R. Jacobs, and A. Oberman. 1999. Heart rate and subsequent blood pressure in young adults: The CARDIA Study. *Hypertension* 33:640–646.
7. Grassi, G. 1998. Role of the sympathetic nervous system in human hypertension. *J. Hypertens.* 16:1979–1987.
8. Palatini, P. 2001. Sympathetic overactivity in hypertension: A risk factor for cardiovascular disease. *Curr. Hypertens. Rep.* 3(Suppl. 1): S3–S9.
9. Jennings, G. L. 1998. Noradrenaline spillover and microneurography measurements in patients with primary hypertension. *J. Hypertens.* 16(Suppl. 3):S35–S38.
10. Calhoun, D. A., and M. L. Mutinga. 1997. Race, family history of hypertension, and sympathetic response to cold pressor testing. *Blood Press.* 6:209–213.

64 The Autonomic Nervous System and Sudden Cardiac Death

Dan M. Roden
Division of Clinical Pharmacology
Vanderbilt University
Nashville, Tennessee

In 1998, the last year for which figures are available, sudden cardiac death (SCD) killed an estimated 420,000 individuals in the United States [1]. This represented 64% of all cardiac deaths, up from 56% in 1989. In half of the patients, SCD is the first manifestation of heart disease. In the other half, the typical patient is a man in his 50 to 69 years old known to have heart disease, but who was in stable condition at the time of the fatal event. When heart rhythm is serendipitously recorded during sudden death, fast ventricular tachycardia (VT) or ventricular fibrillation (VF) is found as the primary precipitant in more than 80% of cases. The most common underlying heart disease is remote myocardial infarction; in one data set, the average time between index infarct and SCD was more than 6.5 years [2]. The other heart diseases associated with SCD include the cardiomyopathies and a group of increasingly frequently recognized familial arrhythmia syndromes, notably the long QT syndrome (LQTS) and hypertrophic cardiomyopathy. Although the latter are uncommon, study of underlying mechanisms has shed great light on mechanisms in the more usual patients.

CLINICAL LINKS BETWEEN AUTONOMIC DYSFUNCTION AND SUDDEN CARDIAC DEATH

Evidence from large clinical studies point to a prominent role for autonomic activation in SCD. In the late 1970s, landmark clinical trials established that β-blocker therapy in patients surviving acute myocardial infarction was highly effective in reducing overall mortality and SCD [3], and this has now become the standard of care. More recently, markers of activation of the autonomic nervous system (such as increased plasma norepinephrine) have been shown to be sensitive markers of mortality in patients with heart failure from all causes, and judicious use of β-blockers has been shown to reduce mortality in this setting as well [4]. Markers of autonomic dysfunction in patients with heart disease include reduced heart rate variability and blunted baroreflex sensitivity; both of these have been used to identify subsets of patients at high risk for SCD after acute myocardial infarction.

Some have termed LQTS as a "Rosetta stone" allowing translation of how autonomic function interacts with an arrhythmia-prone myocardium [5]. Elegant clinical and molecular genetic studies have established that mutations in at least seven different genes can cause congenital LQTS, characterized by QT prolongation on the surface electrocardiogram and arrhythmias [6]. This genetic heterogeneity, in turn, confers considerable phenotypic heterogeneity in this disease, and it is probably more appropriate to refer to the "long QT syndromes." The three commonest forms of LQTSs arise as a result of mutations in the genes encoding pore-forming subunits for potassium currents termed I_{Ks} (LQT1) and I_{Kr} (LQT2), and for the cardiac sodium current (LQT3). LQT1 and LQT2 together account for 80 to 90% of cases. In surveys of nongenotyped patients, adrenergic activation (e.g., awaking from sleep, exercise, or emotional stress) is a common precipitant for syncope and sudden death in LQTS. More recent studies in genotyped subjects have shown that these are characteristics of the LQT1 (and to a lesser extent the LQT2) forms of the disease, whereas the small minority with LQT3 generally have "events" at rest and die during sleep. These clinical findings, in turn, have driven research into basic mechanisms, as described in the following section.

BASIC MECHANISMS

A fundamental characteristic of diseased myocardium is the phenomenon of "electrophysiologic remodeling" in which the repertoire of ion channel (and other) genes expressed in individual myocytes change as a result of disease. Although such changes can be adaptive (e.g., to long-standing hypertension), they are frequently maladaptive. That is, they increase electrophysiologic heterogeneities with the result that the risk of reentrant excitation that underlies VT or VF is enhanced. These heterogeneities can occur at multiple levels, such as among action potential durations, cell-to-cell coupling, or activation of intracellular signaling pathways, including those controlling intracellular calcium. This formulation likely underlies arrhythmias in the LQTS and other monogenic arrhythmia syndromes, as well as in more common diseases such as coronary disease and cardiomyopathies. In animals, even small myocardial infarctions in the basal regions can result in denervation of more apically located myocytes with the resultant denervation hypersensitivity increasing arrhythmia risk.

A contemporary view of the way in which autonomic dysfunction modulates cardiac electrophysiology holds that receptor stimulation results directly or indirectly in changes in the function of individual molecules, usually the ion channels that underlie individual cardiac ion currents. An example of indirect changes is increased intracellular calcium, which can then activate enzymes, change patterns of gene expression, or activate protein kinases with direct channel phosphorylation.

Perhaps the most well-recognized acute autonomic effect on cardiac electrophysiology is increased heart rate and contractility with acute β-stimulation. Such changes presumably involve direct protein kinase A–mediated phosphorylation of channel proteins or modulating proteins, and in some cases, residues that are phosphorylated to mediate these electrophysiologic changes have been identified. Adrenergic stimulation results in prominent increases in inward current through L-type calcium channels caused by the phenomenon of "mode switching" in which the probability of open time of phosphorylated calcium channels is much increased. All things being equal, therefore, action potential durations (and thus QT intervals) would be increased by adrenergic stimulation. However, this is not the case under physiologic circumstances, thus indicating that other mechanisms are brought into play under these conditions. These mechanisms likely include increased activity of the electrogenic Na,K-ATPase (as a consequence of rate), as well as an increase in the magnitude of I_{Ks}. This formulation, then, leads directly to the prediction that mutations disrupting function of the genes underlying I_{Ks} will result in action potential prolongation that is especially marked under conditions of adrenergic stimulation. Indeed, this is the exactly the phenotype of patients with the LQT1 form of LQTS. In fact, in whole heart preparations, I_{Ks} block alone does not result in an arrhythmogenic substrate until β agonists are added, with a resultant marked increase in heterogeneity of action potential durations and reentrant excitation. Interestingly, an opposite phenomenon has been reported in animal models of LQT3, a form of the disease not linked to adrenergic stimuli. In this setting, considerable action potential heterogeneity is present at baseline, and adrenergic stimulation actually reverses these arrhythmogenic changes; whether, therefore, patients with the more uncommon LQT3 form of the disease should avoid β-blockers has not been settled.

The way in which kinase activation modulates channel function has received considerable attention. It is now apparent that, as with other target proteins, channels likely exist in macromolecular signaling complexes in association with kinases and specific anchoring proteins. Thus, it is close proximity (and in some cases the physical association) of the anchoring protein and the ion channel that is the final mediator of channel phosphorylation [7].

CONCLUSION

The problem of sudden death remains a huge public health issue. It is clear that there is a prominent autonomic influence on risk, and that β-blockers reduce risk whereas conventional antiarrhythmics targeting ion channels do not. Studies in human subjects and in cellular and animal models are currently elucidating molecular and genetic mechanisms modulating that risk. Ultimately, the development of improved therapies, possibly by modulating specifically targeted intracellular signaling pathways, may result in reduced risk for this devastating health issue.

References

1. Zheng, Z. J., J. B. Croft, W. H. Giles, and G. A. Mensah. 2001. Sudden cardiac death in the United States, 1989 to 1998. *Circulation* 104: 2158–2163.
2. de Vreede-Swagemakers, J. M., A. M. Gorgels, W. I. Dubois-Arbouw, and J. W. van Ree, M. J. Daemen, L. G. Houben, and H. J. Wellens. 1997. Out-of-hospital cardiac arrest in the 1990s: A population-based study in the Maastricht area on incidence, characteristics and survival. *J. Am. Coll. Cardiol.* 30:1500–1505.
3. Beta-Blocker Heart Attack Trial Research Group. 1982. A randomized trial of propranolol in patients with acute myocardial infarction. I. Mortality results. *JAMA* 247:1707–1714.
4. Bristow, M. R. 2000. Beta-adrenergic receptor blockade in chronic heart failure. *Circulation* 101:558–569.
5. Zipes, D. P. 1991. The long QT syndrome: A Rosetta stone for sympathetic related ventricular tachyarrhythmias. *Circulation* 84:1414–1419.
6. Roden, D. M., and P. M. Spooner. 1999. Inherited long QT syndromes: A paradigm for understanding arrhythmogenesis. *J. Cardiovasc. Electrophysiol.* 10:1664–1683.
7. Marx, S. O., J. Kurokawa, S. Reiken, H. Motoike, J. D'Armiento, A. R. Marks, and R. S. Kass. 2002. Requirement of a macromolecular signaling complex for beta adrenergic receptor modulation of the KCNQ1-KCNE1 potassium channel. *Science* 295:496–499.

65 Congestive Heart Failure

Mazhar H. Khan
Pennsylvania State University College of Medicine
Milton S. Hershey Medical College
Hershey, Pennsylvania

Lawrence I. Sinoway
Pennsylvania State University College of Medicine
Milton S. Hershey Medical College
Hershey, Pennsylvania

Congestive heart failure (CHF) is a complex syndrome resulting from an insult to the myocardium. Regardless of the etiology (ischemic, valvular, idiopathic, and others), the pathophysiology of the disease and the evoked compensatory mechanisms are similar. Of these compensatory responses, the autonomic nervous system adaptations are particularly important in discussions of CHF disease pathogenesis and progression. The sympathetic nervous system (SNS) component of the autonomic nervous system has been studied extensively in patients with CHF. Moreover, modern therapy for heart failure has been revolutionized by the use of agents that block some of the effects of the SNS.

SYMPATHETIC NERVOUS SYSTEM

In CHF, the increased plasma levels of norepinephrine (NE) and the increased urinary excretion of catecholamines indicate heightened activation of the SNS [1]. This activation of SNS occurs early in the course of the disease as shown in the Studies of Left Ventricular Dysfunction (SOLVD) trial [2]. SOLVD has demonstrated that NE is significantly greater in asymptomatic patients with impaired left ventricular (LV) function (ejection fraction <35%) than in control subjects. The magnitude of SNS activation is closely linked with prognosis in CHF. Individuals with high levels of SNS activation, as estimated by plasma NE values, have the worst prognosis [3].

REGULATION OF SYMPATHETIC NERVOUS SYSTEM ACTIVITY IN CONGESTIVE HEART FAILURE

The mechanisms that cause exaggerated SNS activity in patients with CHF remain unclear. Data from animal and human subjects with heart failure suggest that baroreceptor restraint of SNS drive is reduced [4, 5]. Altered baroreceptor function may be caused by a resetting of the reflex pathways, by altered Na,K-ATPase activity in the baroreceptor cell itself, or by both. In patients with CHF, intravenous administration of digitalis restores the sensitivity of baroreceptors as reflected by decreased muscle sympathetic nerve activity (MSNA) and forearm vascular resistance, implying that the increased activity of Na,K-ATPase may be responsible for altered baroreceptor sensitivity [6]. Interestingly, in CHF, sympathetic drive directed to skeletal muscle is enhanced, whereas sympathetic activity to skin is not increased [7].

Muscle afferents may also play an important role in regulation of SNS activity in patients with CHF [8, 9]. It is likely that muscle afferent activity contributes to heightened sympathetic tone during exercise but not to high resting SNS activity.

IMPLICATION OF SYMPATHETIC NERVOUS SYSTEM ACTIVATION IN CONGESTIVE HEART FAILURE

In acute heart failure, heightened sympathetic activation serves to counteract the effects of decreased cardiac output. Specifically, increased sympathetic drive will increase heart rate, myocardial contractility, peripheral vasoconstriction, and venous return. These compensatory responses serve to preserve blood pressure and to maintain perfusion to vital organs (i.e., heart and brain). However, in chronic heart failure, these compensatory responses have numerous deleterious effects that perpetuate the syndrome of CHF. These deleterious effects include decreased muscle perfusion and an impaired ability to maintain systemic sodium and water balance. These factors, in turn, contribute to the classic signs and symptoms of CHF: fatigue, shortness of breath, and peripheral edema.

At rest, the sympathetic vasoconstrictor tone regulates the blood flow to skeletal muscle. With exercise, despite an increase in SNS activity, vasodilation occurs, in part, because of local metabolite production resulting in augmentation of blood flow to the active muscle. Altered control of the peripheral circulation contributes to the reduced exercise capacity in patients with CHF. Zelis and colleagues [10] demonstrated that blood flow to exercising muscle was reduced in CHF. Musch and Terrell [11] demonstrated that the magnitude of muscle blood flow reduction was related to the amount of LV dysfunction and the degree of flow reduction was greatest in muscles having the largest percentage of oxidative muscle fibers. Shoemaker and colleagues [12] demonstrated that reduced flow with exercise in CHF is caused by increased sympathetic vasoconstriction. This increase in SNS activity with exercise is caused by heightened engagement of the muscle reflex.

Activation of the SNS in CHF is also a strong stimulus for the renin-angiotensin system (RAS). Activation of RAS causes salt and water retention and further vasoconstriction, leading to an increase in preload and afterload.

Augmented SNS activity is also largely responsible for the greater catecholamine exposure of cardiac myocytes in CHF. This leads to direct toxic effects of the catecholamine, as well as contributing to myocyte apoptosis. There is evidence suggesting that increased levels of NE associated with SNS activation along with other neuroendocrine factors play an important role in LV remodeling.

Finally, in patients with CHF, activation of SNS leads to sinus tachycardia, enhanced activity of ectopic atrial and ventricular foci, and increased transmural dispersion of refractoriness. These factors create a highly arrhythmogenic milieu and can produce chronic incapacitating, as well as acute and lethal, rhythm disturbances.

IMPLICATIONS FOR THERAPY

The current antiadrenergic treatment of CHF is based on the hypothesis that blockade of SNS will have positive effects on the course of this disease. Increased concentrations of NE cause down-regulation of β_1-adrenergic receptors. Blockage of these receptors with adrenergic antagonists ameliorates the negative effects of this down-regulation. Increased concentrations of catecholamines in CHF can be countered by administration of β-blockers that have been shown to improve cell function, increase ejection fraction, reduce end-diastolic pressures, enhance diastolic relaxation, improve myocardial energetics, and reduce the predilection to arrhythmias. Recent clinical trials have convincingly demonstrated the survival benefit of β-blockers added to the standard treatment for CHF (CIBIS II, MERIT). Survival benefit has been demonstrated even in patients with New York Heart Association Class IV heart failure (COPERNICUS trial). It has been hypothesized that attenuation of central sympathetic outflow using a centrally acting agent may be even more beneficial in the syndrome of CHF. A 2-month administration of clonidine reduces MSNA by 26% and plasma NE by 47% [13]. However, it must be emphasized that these beneficial laboratory findings do not translate into increased patient survival (MOXCON, MOXSE). Thus, it appears that some degree of sympathoexcitation and peripheral vasoconstriction are important in the physiologic response to heart failure.

References

1. Chidsey, C. A., D. C. Harrison, and E. Braunwald. 1962. Augmentation of the plasma nor-epinephrine response to exercise in patients with congestive heart failure. *N. Engl. J. Med.* 267:650–654.
2. The SOLVD Investigators. 1991. Effect of enalapril on survival in patients with reduced left ventricular ejection fractions and congestive heart failure. *N. Engl. J. Med.* 325:293–302.
3. Cohn, J. N., T. B. Levine, M. T. Olivari, V. Garberg, D. Lura, G. S. Francis, A. B. Simon, and T. Rector. 1984. Plasma norepinephrine as a guide to prognosis in patients with chronic congestive heart failure. *N. Engl. J. Med.* 311:819–823.
4. Rea, R. F., and W. J. Berg. 1990. Abnormal baroreflex mechanisms in congestive heart failure: Recent insights. *Circulation* 81:2026–2027.
5. Wang, W., J.-S. Chen, and I. H. Zucker. 1991. Carotid sinus baroreceptor reflex in dogs with experimental heart failure. *Circ. Res.* 68:1294–1301.
6. Ferguson, D. W., F. M. Abboud, and A. L. Mark. 1984. Selective impairment of baroreflex-mediated vasoconstrictor responses in patients with ventricular dysfunction. *Circulation* 69:451–460.
7. Middlekauff, H. R., M. A. Hamilton, L. W. Stevenson, and A. L. Mark. 1994. Independent control of skin and muscle sympathetic nerve activity in patients with heart failure. *Circulation* 90:1794–1798.
8. Silber, D. H., G. Sutliff, Q. X. Yang, M. B. Smith, L. I. Sinoway, and U. A. Leuenberger. 1998. Altered mechanisms of sympathetic activation during rhythmic forearm exercise in heart failure. *J. Appl. Physiol.* 84:1551–1559.
9. Middlekauff, H. R., E. U. Nitzsche, C. K. Hoh, M. A. Hamilton, G. C. Fonarow, A. Hage, and J. D. Moriguchi. 2001. Exaggerated muscle mechanoreflex control of reflex renal vasoconstriction in heart failure. *J. Appl. Physiol.* 90:1714–1719.
10. Zelis, R., J. Longhurst, R. J. Capone, and D. T. Mason. 1974. A comparison of regional blood flow and oxygen utilization during dynamic forearm exercise in normal subjects and patients with congestive heart failure. *Circulation* 50:137–143.
11. Musch, T. I., and J. A. Terrell. 1992. Skeletal muscle blood flow abnormalities in rats with a chronic myocardial infarction: Rest and exercise. *Am. J. Appl. Physiol. Heart Circ. Physiol.* 262:H411–H419.
12. Shoemaker, J. K., H. L. Naylor, C. S. Hogeman, and L. Sinoway. 1999. Blood flow dynamics in heart failure. *Circulation* 99:3002–3008.
13. Grassi, G., C. Turri, G. Seravalle, G. Bertinieri, A. Pierini, and G. Mancia. 2001. Effects of chronic clonidine administration on sympathetic nerve traffic and baroreflex function in heart failure. *Hypertension* 38:286–291.

66

Neurally Mediated Syncope

Satish R. Raj
Autonomic Dysfunction Unit
Division of Clinical Pharmacology
Vanderbilt University
Nashville, Tennessee

Rose Marie Robertson
Division of Cardiology
Vanderbilt University
Nashville, Tennessee

Syncope is a sudden, transient loss of consciousness with spontaneous recovery that is associated with a loss of postural tone. It is common, with conservative estimates that 3% of the general population has experienced at least one syncopal spell, with a greater proportion of groups such as the elderly affected [1]. Syncope is responsible for more than 1% of hospital admissions [1]. Syncope can have many possible causes, ranging from benign to life-threatening conditions. The common underlying mechanism of syncope is a transient decrease in cerebral perfusion. Neurally mediated syncope (NMS, or reflex fainting) is the most common cause of syncope, especially in those patients without evidence of structural heart disease. NMS most commonly occurs after prolonged sitting or standing, although it can also occur with exercise (initiation or peak exercise) or with emotional/psychological triggers (e.g., phlebotomy).

PATHOPHYSIOLOGY OF NEURALLY MEDIATED SYNCOPE

The pathophysiology of NMS is not completely understood [2]. The most common explanation for NMS is known as the "Ventricular Hypothesis" (Fig. 66.1). This hypothesis argues that the initiating event is a pooling of blood in the legs (from prolonged sitting or standing) with a resultant reduction in venous return (preload) to the heart. The resultant decrease in blood pressure leads to a baroreceptor-mediated increase in sympathetic tone. This increased sympathetic tone leads to an increased chronotropic and inotropic effect. The vigorous contraction, in the setting of an underfilled ventricle, is thought to stimulate unmyelinated nerve fibers ("ventricular afferents") in the left ventricle. This is thought to trigger a reflex loss of sympathetic tone and an associated vagotonia (with resultant hypotension, bradycardia, or both). In addition, there is a release of epinephrine from the adrenal gland that may also potentiate the hypotension.

This hypothesis seems to provide a plausible explanation for the "postural prodrome" to many of the episodes of NMS. It also provides a rationale for the use of the tilt-table test, which is currently commonly used to aid in the diagnosis of NMS. However, this hypothesis does not provide the complete truth. It fails to explain the mode of NMS in those patients with an emotional or psychological trigger, and it fails to account for episodes of NMS among denervated patients after cardiac transplantation. Even among patients with postural NMS, there are some experimental observations that do not fit with this hypothesis.

DIAGNOSIS OF NEURALLY MEDIATED SYNCOPE

The history and physical examination are at the heart of the diagnosis of NMS. A clinical diagnosis can be made with these alone in most cases. Much of the effort is focused on excluding more malignant causes of syncope. The history should focus on the circumstances surrounding the syncope, the associated symptoms before and after the event, and any collateral history from witnesses. The medical history may contain evidence of structural heart disease and coexisting medical conditions, which both point away from NMS. Medications may provoke syncope, and a family history of sudden death may point to an arrhythmic cause. Historical features of NMS have been found to include female sex, younger age, associated diaphoresis, nausea or palpitation, and postsyncopal fatigue [1]. A long duration of spells (from the first lifetime spell) also suggests NMS. Some historical features have been incorporated into a point score that can be used to distinguish between NMS and seizures (Table 66.1) [3].

The physical examination should focus on ruling out structural heart disease and focal neurologic lesions. The most useful examination maneuver is the carotid sinus massage. The current technique involves performing up to 10 seconds of massage to the carotid sinus (per side) in both the supine and upright posture, with a positive result requiring a decrease in blood pressure or heart rate with an associated reproduction in presenting symptoms [1]. This procedure is associated with a low rate of neurologic complications.

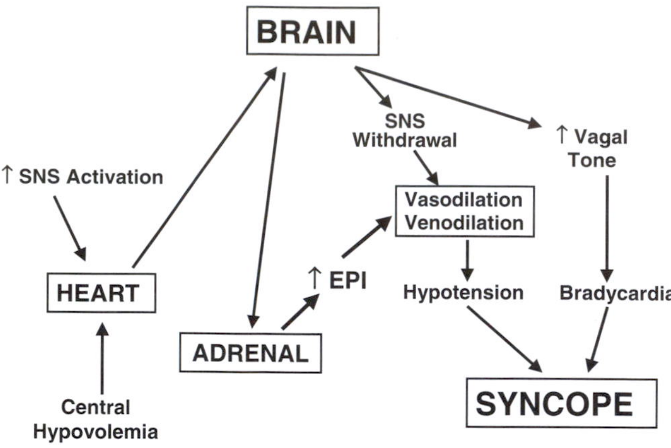

FIGURE 66.1 The "Ventricular Hypothesis of Neurally Mediated Syncope" is shown here. SNS = sympathetic nervous system.

TABLE 66.1 Diagnostic Questions to Determine Whether Loss of Consciousness Is Due to Seizures or Syncope

Question	Points (*If Yes*)
At times do you wake with a cut tongue after your spells?	2
At times do you have a sense of deja vu or jamais vu before your spells?	1
At times is emotional stress associated with losing consciousness?	1
Has anyone ever noted your head turning during a spell?	1
Has anyone ever noted that you are unresponsive, have unusual posturing or have jerking limbs during your spells or have no memory of your spells afterwards? *(Score as yes for any positive response)*	1
Has anyone ever noted that you are confused after a spell?	1
Have you ever had lightheaded spells?	−2
At times do you sweat before your spells?	−2
Is prolonged sitting or standing associated with your spells?	−2

The patient has seizures if the point score is ≥1, and syncope if the point score is <1. Reprinted with permission from Sheldon, R., M. S. Rose, D. Ritchie, et al. 2002. Historical criteria that distinguish syncope from seizures. *J. Am. Coll. Cardiol.* 40:142–148.

TILT-TABLE TESTING

Tilt-table testing has been widely used since the late 1980s. These tests subject patients to head-up tilt at angles of 60 to 80 degrees, and all aim to induce either syncope or intense presyncope, with a reproduction of presenting symptoms. Passive tilt tests simply use upright tilt for up to 45 minutes to induce vasovagal syncope (sensitivity ~40%, specificity ~90%) [1]. Provocative tilt tests use a simultaneous combination of orthostatic stress and drugs such as isoproterenol, nitroglycerin, or adenosine to provoke syncope with a slightly greater sensitivity, but reduced specificity. There is little agreement about the best protocol. Many physicians are more comfortable treating patients if a diagnosis can be established with a tilt-table test. Studies with implantable loop recorders have called the value of tilt testing into question. The International Study on Syncope of Uncertain Etiology (ISSUE) investigators have reported that in the absence of significant structural heart disease, patients with tilt-positive syncope and tilt-negative syncope have similar patterns of recurrence (34% in each group during a follow-up of 3–15 months), with electrocardiographic recording consistent with NMS [4]. Despite these data, tilt-table testing is still recommended for the evaluation of recurrent NMS [5]. Tilt tests are contraindicated in patients with severe aortic or mitral stenosis or critical coronary or cerebral artery stenosis.

NATURAL HISTORY OF NEURALLY MEDIATED SYNCOPE

Most people with NMS faint only once, but for some patients it can be a recurring and troublesome disorder. Most patients do well after assessment, with only a 25 to 30% likelihood of syncope recurrence after tilt testing in patients who receive neither drugs nor a device [6]. The cause for this apparently great reduction in syncope frequency may be spontaneous remission, reassurance, or advice about the pathophysiology of syncope, and postural maneuvers to prevent syncope. However, patients with a history of syncopal spells are more likely to faint in follow-up [7]. The time to the first recurrence of syncope after tilt testing is a simple and individualized measure of eventual syncope frequency, because those patients who faint early after a tilt test tend to continue to faint often [8].

Neurally Mediated Syncope Treatment

Most patients should simply be reassured about the usual benign course of NMS and should be instructed to avoid those situations that precipitate fainting. The use of support stockings or increased salt intake may be helpful. They should be taught to recognize an impending faint and urged to lie down (or sit down if lying down is not possible) quickly. However, these prevention methods will not be enough for some patients, and other treatment options may be necessary.

Some drugs may be helpful [1]. Although salt replenishment and fludrocortisone have not been rigorously studied, they are both commonly used because of their low side effect profile and probable efficacy. Although a common therapy, there is only poor evidence for the effectiveness of β-blockers. A large, international, multicenter, double-blind, randomized, placebo-controlled trial is currently underway to assess the effectiveness of oral metoprolol in NMS [9]. The α_1 agonist midodrine has been found to decrease the rate of recurrent syncope among patients who frequently faint [10], whereas another α_1 agonist, etilefrine, was not found to be useful [11]. The selective serotonin reuptake inhibitor paroxetine also has been shown to be useful in one well-designed study [12].

Orthostatic (tilt) training has been suggested as an effective nonpharmacologic therapy for patients with recurrent NMS [13]. This treatment involves having the patients lean upright against a wall for 30 to 40 minutes, 1 to 2 times per day. Although the initial results from this therapy are quite promising, this therapy has not yet been subjected to a proper trial.

Permanent dual-chamber pacemakers have been shown to be associated with a significant reduction in recurrent syncope among highly symptomatic patients with NMS in several unblinded randomized trials [14]. However, this therapy is expensive and invasive (requiring a small surgical procedure). A recent double blind placebo controlled trial found that the benefits of dual-chamber pacing are much more modest than was originally thought [15]. Currently, permanent pacemaker implantation cannot be recommended as a "first-line" therapy for NMS.

References

1. Raj, S. R., and A. R. Sheldon. 2002. Syncope: Investigation and treatment. *Curr. Cardiol. Rep.* 4:363–370.
2. Mosqueda-Garcia, R., R. Furlan, J. Tank, and R. Fernandez-Violante. 2000. The elusive pathophysiology of neurally mediated syncope. *Circulation* 102:2898–2906.
3. Sheldon, R., M. S. Rose, D. Ritchie, S. J. Connolly, M. L. Koshman, M. A. Lee, M. Frenneaux, M. Fisher, and W. Murphy. 2002. Historical criteria that distinguish syncope from seizures. *J. Am. Coll. Cardiol.* 40:142–148.
4. Moya, A., M. Brignole, C. Menozzi, R. Garcia-Civera, S. Tognarini, L. Mont, G. Botto, F. Giada, and D. Cornacchia. 2001. Mechanism of syncope in patients with isolated syncope and in patients with tilt-positive syncope. *Circulation* 104:1261–1267.
5. Benditt, D. G., D. W. Ferguson, B. P. Grubb, W. N. Kapoor, J. Kugler, B. B. Lerman, J. D. Maloney, A. Raviele, B. Ross, R. Sutton, M. J. Wolk, and D. L. Wood. 1996. Tilt table testing for assessing syncope. American College of Cardiology. *J. Am. Coll. Cardiol.* 28: 263–275.
6. Sheldon, R. S. 1997. Outcome of patients with neurally mediated syncope following tilt table testing. *Cardiologia* 42:795–802.
7. Sheldon, R., S. Rose, P. Flanagan, M. L. Koshman, and S. Killam. 1996. Risk factors for syncope recurrence after a positive tilt-table test in patients with syncope. *Circulation* 93:973–981.
8. Malik, P., M. L. Koshman, and R. Sheldon. 1997. Timing of first recurrence of syncope predicts syncopal frequency after a positive tilt table test result. *J. Am. Coll. Cardiol.* 29:1284–1289.
9. Sheldon, R. S., S. R. Raj, S. Rose, and S. J. Connolly. 2001. Beta-blockers in syncope: The jury is still out. *J. Am. Coll. Cardiol.* 38:2135–2136.
10. Perez-Lugones, A., R. Schweikert, S. Pavia, J. Sra, M. Akhtar, F. Jaeger, G. F. Tomassoni, W. Saliba, F. M. Leonelli, D. Bash, S. Beheiry, J. Shewchik, P. J. Tchou, and A. Natale. 2001. Usefulness of midodrine in patients with severely symptomatic neurocardiogenic syncope: A randomized control study. *J. Cardiovasc. Electrophysiol.* 12:935–938.
11. Raviele, A., M. Brignole, R. Sutton, P. Alboni, P. Giani, C. Menozzi, and A. Moya. 1999. Effect of etilefrine in preventing syncopal recurrence in patients with vasovagal syncope: A double-blind, randomized, placebo-controlled trial. The Vasovagal Syncope International Study. *Circulation* 99:1452–1457.
12. Di Girolamo, E., C. Di Iorio, P. Sabatini, L. Leonzio, C. Barbone, and A. Barsotti. 1999. Effects of paroxetine hydrochloride, a selective serotonin reuptake inhibitor, on refractory vasovagal syncope: A randomized, double-blind, placebo-controlled study. *J. Am. Coll. Cardiol.* 33:1227–1230.
13. Ector, H., T. Reybrouck, H. Heidbuchel, M. Gewillig, and F. Van de Werf. 1998. Tilt training: A new treatment for recurrent neurocardiogenic syncope and severe orthostatic intolerance. *Pacing Clin. Electrophysiol.* 21:193–196.
14. Raj, S. R., and R. S. Sheldon. 2002. Permanent cardiac pacing to prevent vasovagal syncope. *Curr. Opin. Cardiol.* 17:90–95.
15. Connolly, S. J., R. Sheldon, K. E. Thorpe, R. S. Roberts, K. A. Ellenbogen, B. L. Wilkoff, C. Morillo, and M. Gent. 2003. Pacemaker therapy for prevention of syncope in patients with recurrent severe vasovagal syncope: Second Vasovagal Pacemaker Study (VPS II): A randomized trial. *JAMA* 289:2224–2229.

67

Syncope in the Athlete

Victor A. Convertino
U.S. Army Institute of Surgical Research
Fort Sam Houston
Houston, Texas

Over the last half-century, anecdotal reports have described common experiences of dizziness, nausea, and symptoms of syncope in endurance-trained athletes. From these observations emerged the hypothesis that aerobically fit athletes were predisposed to orthostatic hypotension and intolerance. Although numerous investigations reported in the literature have failed to support a relation between aerobic fitness and orthostatic intolerance [1, 2], a few studies have provided evidence that individuals who habitually participate in endurance exercise training have demonstrated some degree of symptomatic orthostatism [1, 3, 4].

The mechanisms underlying syncope in athletes are unclear. Early cross-sectional investigations demonstrated that lower orthostatic tolerance was associated with greater venous compliance in the legs of athletes compared with nonathlete subjects [1, 2]. However, more recent cross-sectional and longitudinal studies have failed to demonstrate differences in leg compliance between trained and untrained states. High cardiac vagal tone or depressed carotid and aortic baroreceptor reflex responsiveness have been implicated as possible mechanisms that may limit the ability of athletes to increase heart rate during orthostatism [4]. However, cross-sectional and longitudinal data have demonstrated little difference in carotid–cardiac baroreflex responsiveness associated with exercise training [1, 2]. Furthermore, expanded blood volume, which is associated with endurance exercise training, is known to reduce heart rate and vasoconstrictive baroreflex responses to baroreceptor stimulation [5]. Because endurance athletes are hypervolemic, their reduced heart rate and vasoconstrictive responses may therefore represent a greater reserve for tachycardia and vascular resistance compared with nonathletes. It is important to emphasize that blood pressure is the product of heart rate × stroke volume × peripheral resistance. Athletes who have large stroke volumes secondary to eccentric hypertrophy and a large end-diastolic volume may require smaller baroreflex-mediated tachycardia and vasoconstriction in response to arterial hypotension to affect an appropriate corrective increase in cardiac output than does a nonathlete with a smaller stroke volume. This concept is supported by the observation that the lower tachycardia observed in athletes during an orthostatic challenge is compensated for by greater stroke volume, thus maintaining cardiac output at or above levels of nonathletes [1, 2]. Therefore, it is difficult to contend that syncope in athletes can be attributed to deficiencies in blood volume, compliance of the lower extremities, or baroreflex control of cardiac and vascular responses.

With the lack of evidence supporting the role of attenuated baroreflex function in athletes to explain their predisposition to syncope, an alternative hypothesis has emerged describing evidence that athletes have structural changes in the cardiovascular system that, although beneficial during exercise, can lead to an excessively large decrease in stroke volume during orthostatism. This hypothesis is based on the evidence that endurance-trained athletes demonstrate a greater effective left ventricular compliance and distensibility than nonathletes, and a steeper slope of the Frank–Starling relation between left ventricular filling pressure and stroke volume [3]. Thus, greater reduction in stroke volume for the same reduction in filling pressure may represent the most likely mechanism predisposing the athlete to syncope.

It should be emphasized that syncope in athletes occurs in few high-endurance–trained individuals. Because there is an important genetic component to being an elite athlete, it is not unreasonable to speculate that a steeper Frank–Starling curve may be an innate characteristic of some athletes, thus predisposing them to syncope. It is important that the predisposition to syncope in a few elite athletes not detract from the health benefits to be gained by sedentary individuals who undertake aerobic exercise programs. The phenomenon of syncope in the elite athlete most likely represents a mechanical change in the cardiovascular system that benefits the athlete during exercise and should not be interpreted as a clinical abnormality.

References

1. Convertino, V. A. 1987. Aerobic fitness, endurance training and orthostatic intolerance. *Exerc. Sports Sci. Rev.* 15:223–259.
2. Convertino, V. A. 1993. Endurance exercise training: Conditions of enhanced hemodynamic responses and tolerance to LBNP. *Med. Sci. Sports Exerc.* 25:705–712.

3. Levine, B. D. 1993. Regulation of central blood volume and cardiac filling in endurance athletes: The Frank–Starling mechanism as a determinant of orthostatic tolerance. *Med. Sci. Sports Exerc.* 25:727–732.
4. Raven, P. B., and J. A. Pawelczyk. 1993. Chronic endurance exercise training: A condition of inadequate blood pressure regulation and reduced tolerance to LBNP. *Med. Sci. Sports Exerc.* 25:713–721.
5. Mack, G. W., V. A. Convertino, and E. R. Nadel. 1993. Effect of exercise training on cardiopulmonary baroreflex control of forearm vascular resistance in humans. *Med. Sci. Sports Exerc.* 25:722–726.

P A R T VIII

CATECHOLAMINE DISORDERS

68

The Autonomic Storm

Alejandro A. Rabinstein
Department of Neurology
Mayo Clinic
Rochester, Minnesota

Eelco F. M. Wijdicks
Department of Neurology
Mayo Clinic
Rochester, Minnesota

Episodes of acute autonomic disturbances may occur after central nervous system catastrophic injury and are often misinterpreted. This is due, in part, to the confusing and scant literature on this topic and the lack of a systematic nomenclature [1]. Episodic hypersympathetic states have been variably named paroxysmal sympathetic storms [2], autonomic storms [3], diencephalic seizures [4], diencephalic epilepsy [5], autonomic dysfunction syndrome [6], or simply dysautonomia [1]. This chapter focuses on the diagnosis and management of paroxysmal autonomic derangements that occur after severe brain injury.

DEFINITION

Autonomic storms are acute disorders of sympathetic function that result in alterations of body temperature, blood pressure, heart rate, respiratory rate, sweating, and muscle tone. For the purpose of this chapter, use of the term *autonomic storm* is limited to patients with acute central nervous system disease.

CAUSES AND PATHOPHYSIOLOGY

Autonomic storms are most common after severe head trauma with diffuse axonal injury [1] and in postresuscitation encephalopathy caused by an anoxic–ischemic insult [7]. However, they can occur in patients with other forms of acute intracranial lesions, such as intracerebral hemorrhage [8], and in patients with brain or brainstem tumors [5] or hydrocephalus [9]. Immediately after an intracranial catastrophe, there is a massive catecholamine surge that may produce seizures, neurogenic pulmonary edema, and myocardial injury. Sympathetic outflow diminishes over time, and manifestations of autonomic dysfunction tend to disappear within a few days in most patients. However, some individuals go on to develop recurrent paroxysms of sympathetic overactivity (autonomic storms) during the acute hospitalization and later recovery phase.

The pathophysiology of autonomic storms remains unclear. Proposed mechanisms include heightened activity of diencephalic or brainstem sympathoexcitatory regions either caused by direct activation or by disinhibition (release phenomenon) secondary to loss of cortical and subcortical control [2, 4]. Resetting of baroreflex mechanisms could explain the coexistence of hypertension and tachycardia, whereas a combination of increased adrenomedullary catecholamines and neural sympathetic traffic could account for the increase in pulse pressure during the episodes [2]. Activation of somatosympathetic reflexes from muscle mechanoreceptors or chemoreceptors during episodes of hypertonia or fluctuations in intraventricular pressure could trigger the paroxysmal symptoms [2, 4, 6, 9]. Although epileptic discharges may cause a similar syndrome [5], they appear to be uncommon in patients with autonomic storms after severe head injury [2, 4, 6].

INCIDENCE

Autonomic storms may be much more common than suggested by the surprisingly scarce literature on this disorder. It is not infrequent to find patients with diffuse axonal injury showing features of dysautonomia both in intensive care and rehabilitation units. However, the lack of well-defined diagnostic criteria hampers the definition of true cases of autonomic storm. Currently, there is only one systematic review of consecutive patients ($n = 35$) with severe head trauma and paroxysmal dysautonomia available in the literature [1], and no prospective data have been published on this subject. Hence, currently, the real incidence of autonomic storms after traumatic brain injury and other forms of acute intracranial disease is unknown.

CLINICAL MANIFESTATIONS

The clinical features of autonomic storms include fever (often >39°C), tachycardia, hypertension (often with widening of the pulse pressure), tachypnea, hyperhidrosis, and extensor posturing. Pupillary dilation, intense flushing, and severe dystonia may also be present. Intracranial pressure may increase during the episodes; autonomic dysfunction usually precedes the increase in intracranial pressure [4, 6], except in patients whose episodes seem triggered by acute hydrocephalus [6].

The paroxysms usually begin 5 to 7 days after the injury, but may start earlier. The episodes follow a regular pattern, occurring on average 1 to 3 times per day; each episode may last between 2 and 10 hours. The changes in vital signs observed during a typical autonomic storm are illustrated in Figure 68.1. Over time, the episodes tend to become less frequent but more prolonged and severe before subsiding months after the inciting event [2, 4, 6].

DIFFERENTIAL DIAGNOSIS AND DIAGNOSTIC EVALUATION

The diagnosis of autonomic storm is based on the recognition of the regular pattern of dysautonomic spells in a patient with acute intracranial disease. It must be distinguished from other syndromes that also present with features of autonomic instability, such as neuroleptic malignant syndrome (see Chapter 82), malignant hyperthermia (see Chapter 49), and lethal catatonia. Lethal catatonia is most often seen in patients with psychiatric disorders, but also can occur after viral encephalitis. It begins subacutely with insomnia, anorexia, agitation, and rigidity with intermittent posturing. Labile blood pressure, tachycardia, fever, and diaphoresis become prominent, and extreme exhaustion and dehydration ensue. Outcome is fatal unless patients are timely treated with electroconvulsive therapy [10].

Cushing response, typically seen in patients with acute distortion of the lower brainstem, should not be confused with autonomic storm, because in these cases hypertension is associated with bradycardia, as opposed to tachycardia, and irregular breathing [3].

In all patients with suspected autonomic storm, sepsis should be excluded by serial blood cultures and encephalitis should be excluded by cerebrospinal fluid examination. However, the search for an infection should be efficient and must not preclude prompt recognition and treatment of autonomic storms. Epileptiform activity also should be ruled out by electroencephalography. The possibility of underlying spinal cord injury must be considered because autonomic dysreflexia can occur in patients with transections above the fifth or sixth thoracic level (see Chapter 81). Thus, magnetic resonance imaging of the cervical and upper thoracic spine should be obtained. Finally, all patients with autonomic storms need computed tomography or magnetic resonance scans of the brain to exclude the presence of hydrocephalus. Table 68.1 summarizes the differential diagnosis and diagnostic evaluation of autonomic storm.

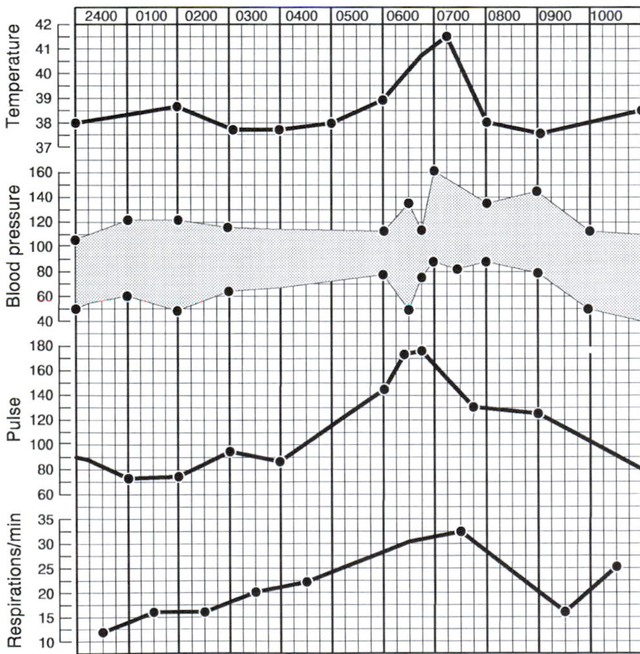

FIGURE 68.1 Changes in vital signs in a patient with typical autonomic storm after severe head trauma with diffuse axonal injury. Body temperature is measured in Celsius degrees, blood pressure in mmHg, and pulse in beats/minute. (Reproduced from Boeve, B. E., E. F. M. Wijdicks, E. E. Benarroch, and K. D. Schmidt. 1998. Paroxysmal sympathetic storms ("diencephalic seizures") after severe diffuse axonal head injury. *Mayo Clin. Proc.* 73:148–152, with permission.)

TREATMENT

Morphine sulfate (10 mg every 4 hours), bromocriptine (1.25–2.5 mg three times a day), and nonselective β-blockers such as labetalol (100–200 mg twice a day) or propranolol (20–60 mg four times a day) have been successfully used to treat autonomic storms [2, 4, 6, 11]. These agents may be used alone or in combination, especially during the acute phase. In our experience, morphine sulfate seems to be most effective. Once dysautonomic manifestations have been under control for several weeks, the medications may be tapered while carefully watching for symptom recurrence. Often, it is necessary to continue treatment for several months. The mechanisms by which opioids, dopamine agonists, and β-blockers improve dysautonomia remain speculative. Antiepileptic drugs are typically not helpful in true cases of autonomic storm but should be tried if questions about a possible epileptic nature of the spells persist. Systematic studies of different treatment regimens are needed to optimize outcome in patients with autonomic storm.

PROGNOSIS

Autonomic storms have been associated with poor functional outcome after severe traumatic brain injury [1].

TABLE 68.1 Differential Diagnosis and Diagnostic Evaluation of Autonomic Storm

Diagnosis	Diagnostic clue/evaluation/action
Neuroleptic malignant syndrome	History of neuroleptic use Remove antidopaminergic drugs Creatinine kinase*
Malignant hyperthermia	History of triggering event/drug Remove potential triggers Creatinine kinase* Muscle biopsy
Lethal catatonia	Subacute onset with agitation Creatinine kinase*
Cushing response	Bradycardia Irregular breathing pattern Brain MRI with upper brainstem distortion
Spinal cord injury	MRI of cervical and upper thoracic spine
Sepsis	Serial blood cultures Lactic acid Chest radiographs
Encephalitis	Cerebrospinal fluid examination
Seizures	Electroencephalography
Hydrocephalus†	CT or MRI scan of brain

*Serum creatinine kinase levels may fluctuate with the spells in patients with autonomic storm, whereas they remain persistently high in patients with unrelenting severe muscle rigidity such as seen in these three syndromes. However, the value of this potential differentiating clue has not been formally evaluated.

†Hydrocephalus could actually trigger true episodes of autonomic storm.

CT, computed tomography; MRI, magnetic resonance imaging.

Disabling dystonia and spasticity are the most common sequelae and may render patients almost unable to communicate [1]. Although these symptoms may simply be a reflection of the severity of the initial brain injury, the impact of secondary brain insult during dysautonomic episodes—from hyperthermia, extreme increase in energy expenditure, and increase in intracranial pressure—on neurologic outcome deserves further investigation. Permanent cardiac and skeletal muscle fiber damage also is possible because of the effects of massive catecholamine release.

References

1. Baguley, I. J., J. L. Nicholls, K. L. Felmingham, J. Crooks, J. A. Gurka, and L. D. Wade. 1999. Dysautonomia after traumatic brain injury: A forgotten syndrome? *J. Neurol. Neurosurg. Psychiatry* 67:39–43.
2. Boeve, B. E., E. F. M. Wijdicks, E. E. Benarroch, and K. D. Schmidt. 1998. Paroxysmal sympathetic storms ("diencephalic seizures") after severe diffuse axonal head injury. *Mayo Clin. Proc.* 73:148–152.
3. Ropper, A. H. 1997. Management of the autonomic storm. In *Clinical autonomic disorders*, 2nd ed., ed. P. A. Low, 791–801. Philadelphia: Lippincott-Raven.
4. Bullard, D. E. 1987. Diencephalic seizures: Responsiveness to bromocriptine and morphine. *Ann. Neurol.* 21:609–611.
5. Penfield, W., and H. Jasper. 1954. *Epilepsy and the functional anatomy of the human brain*. Boston: Little Brown.
6. Rossitch, Jr. E., and D. E. Bullard. 1988. The autonomic dysfunction syndrome: Aetiology and treatment. *Br. J. Neurosurg.* 2:471–478.
7. Wijdicks, E. F. M. 2002. *Neurologic complications of critical illness*, 2nd ed. New York: Oxford University Press.
8. Tong, C., M. W. Konig, P. R. Roberts, S. B. Tatter, and X. H. Li. 2000. Autonomic dysfunction secondary to intracerebral hemorrhage. *Anesth. Analg.* 91:1450–1451.
9. Talman, W. T., G. Florek, and D. E. Bullard. 1988. A hyperthermic syndrome in two subjects with acute hydrocephalus. *Arch. Neurol.* 45:1037–1040.
10. Mann, S. C., S. N. Caroff, H. R. Bleier, W. K. R. Weltz, M. A. Kliwg, and M. Hayashida. 1986. Lethal catatonia. *Am. J. Psychiatry*. 143:1374–1381.
11. Do, D., V. L. Sheen, and E. Bromfield. 2000. Treatment of paroxysmal sympathetic storm with labetalol. *J. Neurol. Neurosurg. Psychiatry* 69:832–833.

69 Pheochromocytoma

William M. Manger
New York University Medical Center
National Hypertension Association
New York, New York

Ray W. Gifford, Jr.
Cleveland Clinic Foundation
Cleveland, Ohio

Graeme Eisenhofer
Clinical Neurocardiology Section
National Institutes of Neurological Disorders and Stroke
National Institutes of Health
Bethesda, Maryland

Pheochromocytoma, a rare catecholamine-secreting tumor of neuroectodermal chromaffin cells, occurs in 0.01 to 0.05% of patients with sustained systolic and diastolic hypertension. Fifty percent of tumors cause sustained hypertension, often fluctuating and sometimes accompanied by orthostatic hypotension; 45% cause only paroxysmal hypertension and ~5% of patients remain normotensive, especially those with familial tumors.

Eighty-five percent of pheochromocytomas occur in the adrenal medulla; about 15% arise in extraadrenal sites (paragangliomas)—for example, organ of Zuckerkandl, urinary bladder (<1%), paraganglia chromaffin cells associated with sympathetic nerves elsewhere in the abdomen, pelvis, chest (<2%), neck (<0.1%), and rarely at the base of the skull. Extraadrenal and multiple pheochromocytomas are more frequent in children (30% and 35%, respectively) than adults (15% and 18%, respectively).

About 20% of pheochromocytomas are familial with an autosomal dominant mode of inheritance and may be associated with multiple endocrine neoplasms (MENs), von Hippel–Lindau disease (VHL), carotid body or multiple paragangliomas, and neurofibromatosis type-1. These familial pheochromocytomas are caused by genetic mutations, for example, RET protooncogene on chromosome 10 for MEN type 2a and 2b syndromes, on chromosome 3p for VHL, on chromosome 11q for carotid body and multiple paragangliomas, and on chromosome 17q for neurofibromatosis. Coexistence of pheochromocytoma with medullary thyroid carcinoma (MTC) or C cell hyperplasia and sometimes with parathyroid neoplasm or hyperplasia constitutes MEN type-2a. Coexistence of pheochromocytoma with MTC, mucosal neuromas, thickened corneal nerves, alimentary tract ganglioneuromatosis, and sometimes a marfanoid habitus constitutes MEN type-2b. Hyperparathyroidism occurs in ~50% of patients with MEN type-2a, but rarely in type-2b. MTC almost always precedes pheochromocytoma in MEN syndromes. von Recklinghausen's peripheral neurofibromatosis coexists in 5% of patients with pheochromocytoma; 1% of individuals with neurofibromatosis have a pheochromocytoma.

Embryologically related diseases arising from neural crest maldevelopment (e.g., pheochromocytoma, neuroblastoma, neurofibromatosis, MTC, carcinoid, and MEN) have been designated neurocristopathies. Some of these tumors are capable of amine and amine precursor uptake and decarboxylation (the APUD system) and may secrete catecholamines and a variety of peptides.

Pheochromocytomas coexist in ~14% of patients with VHL disease, which is characterized by central nervous system hemangioblastoma and retinal angioma; renal and pancreatic cysts, renal carcinoma, and cystadenoma of the epididymis may coexist. Familial paraganglioma and familial pheochromocytoma appear associated with genetic mutations in mitochondrial succinate dehydrogenase enzymes.

Pheochromocytomas average 3 to 5 cm in diameter but may be microscopic or weigh up to 4 kg. Average weight is ~70 g. Cells contain secretory granules that release catecholamines by diffusion, exocytosis, or both (along with dopamine β-hydroxylase, neuropeptide Y, and chromogranins); catecholamines exert cardiovascular and metabolic effects by stimulating α- and β-adrenergic receptors. Prolonged exposure to excess catecholamines can decrease receptor responsiveness (desensitization). Other peptides may be secreted and contribute to unusual clinical manifestations.

About 10% of adrenal pheochromocytomas and up to 40% of extraadrenal tumors are malignant (evidenced by metastases or invasion of adjacent structures), but histopathology cannot differentiate benign from malignant tumors.

Pheochromocytoma may be cured by surgical resection in ~90% of patients, but, if unrecognized, it almost invariably causes lethal cerebrovascular or cardiovascular complications from excess circulating catecholamines (e.g., stroke, myocardial infarction, arrhythmias, catecholamine cardiomyopathy, ischemic enterocolitis, shock, and multisystem organ failure).

Hypercatecholaminemia may cause manifestations suggesting many conditions, some with increased excretion of catecholamines and metabolites (Table 69.1). However,

TABLE 69.1 Differential Diagnosis of Pheochromocytoma

All hypertensive patients (sustained and paroxysmal) when diagnosis is unknown
Anxiety, panic attacks, psychoneurosis, tension states
Hyperthyroidism
Hyperdynamic β-adrenergic circulatory state
Menopause
Vasodilating headache (migraine and cluster headaches)
Coronary insufficiency
Renal parenchymal or renal arterial disease with hypertension
Focal arterial insufficiency of the brain; cerebral vasculitis
Intracranial lesions (with or without increased intracranial pressure)
Autonomic hyperreflexia
Diencephalic seizure; Page syndrome; dopamine surges
Preeclampsia (or eclampsia with convulsions)
Hypertensive crises associated with monoamine oxidase inhibitors
Hypoglycemia
Neuroblastoma; ganglioneuroblastoma; ganglioneuroma
Acute infectious disease; *acute abdomen* (cardiovascular catastrophe)
Unexplained shock
Neurofibromatosis (with hypertension)
Rare causes of paroxysmal hypertension (*adrenal medullary hyperplasia; acute porphyria; clonidine withdrawal; baroreflex failure; pseudopheochromocytoma;* factitious-induced by certain illegal, prescription, and nonprescription drugs); *fatal familial insomnia*

From Manger, W. M., and R. W. Gifford, Jr. 1996. *Clinical and experimental pheochromocytoma*, 2nd ed. Cambridge, MA: Blackwell Science.
Conditions in italics may increase the excretion of catecholamines, metabolites, or both.

TABLE 69.2 The Most Common Symptoms and Signs in Patients (Almost All Adults) with Pheochromocytoma Associated with Paroxysmal or Persistent Hypertension

	Paroxysmal (% of 37 patients)	Persistent (% of 39 patients)
Symptoms		
Headaches (severe)	92	72
Excessive sweating (generalized)	65	69
Palpitations with or without tachycardia	73	51
Anxiety, nervousness, fear of impending death, or panic	60	28
Tremulousness	51	26
Pain in chest, abdomen (usually epigastric), lumbar regions, lower abdomen or groin	48	28
Nausea with or without vomiting	43	26
Weakness, fatigue, prostration	38	15
Weight loss (severe)	14	15
Dyspnea	11	18
Warmth or heat intolerance	13	15
(Noteworthy are painless hematuria, urinary frequency, nocturia, and tenesmus in pheochromocytoma of the urinary bladder).		
Signs		
Hypertension with or without wide fluctuations (rarely paroxysmal hypotension or hypertension alternating with hypotension or hypertension absent)		
Hypertension induced by physical maneuver such as exercise, postural change, or palpation and massage of flank or mass elsewhere		
Orthostatic hypotension with or without postural tachycardia		
Paradoxic blood pressure response to certain antihypertensive drugs; marked pressor response with induction of anesthesia		
Inappropriate and severe sweating		
Tachycardia or reflex bradycardia, very forceful heartbeat and arrhythmia		
Pallor of face and upper part of body (rarely flushing)		
Anxious, frightened, troubled appearance		
Leanness or underweight		
Hypertensive retinopathy		

Modified from Manger, W. M., and R. W. Gifford, Jr. 1996. *Clinical and experimental pheochromocytoma*, 2nd ed. Cambridge, MA: Blackwell Science.

manifestations of "attacks" suggesting hypercatecholaminemia without hypertension are highly atypical. Symptomatic hypertensive attacks caused by pheochromocytoma usually occur 1 or more times a week and last less than 1 hour in ~75% of cases, but they may occur at any frequency. They may be precipitated by deep abdominal palpation, postural changes, exertion, anxiety, trauma, pain, ingestion of foods or beverages containing tyramine (certain cheeses, beer, and wine), use of certain drugs (β-blockers, phenothiazines, metoclopramide, monoamine oxidase inhibitors, tricyclic antidepressants, adrenocorticotropic hormone, and chemotherapy), intubation, anesthesia induction, operative manipulation, and micturition or bladder distension (with a bladder pheochromocytoma). Rarely, patients with predominantly epinephrine-secreting tumors have hypertension alternating with hypotension.

The most common symptoms and signs in patients with pheochromocytoma are listed in Table 69.2. Severe headaches (sometimes accompanied by nausea and vomiting) and/or generalized sweating and/or palpitations with tachycardia (rarely reflex bradycardia) occur in up to 95% of persons with functional pheochromocytomas. Anxiety, fear of death, and pallor (rarely flushing) are frequent during paroxysmal hypertension. Severe constipation or pseudo-obstruction may occur in patients with sustained hypertension because catecholamines inhibit peristalsis. Secretion of vasoactive intestinal peptide, serotonin, or calcitonin by some pheochromocytomas may cause diarrhea.

Retinopathy can occur with sustained hypertension. Fine tremors and slight fever (rarely hyperpyrexia) may occur. Polydipsia, polyuria, and convulsions may occur in children.

Transient arrhythmias, electrocardiogram (ECG) changes, or sudden heart failure may occur, and catecholamine cardiomyopathy, hypertension, and coronary atherosclerosis can cause persistent ECG changes.

Hypercatecholaminemia may cause hyperglycemia, increased triglycerides, and hyperreninemia. Endocrine abnormalities are sometimes caused by pheochromocytoma and coexisting conditions—for example, MEN type-2a or type-

2b or Cushing's syndrome. Rarely, pheochromocytomas or coexisting hemangioblastoma secrete erythropoietin and cause polycythemia.

Pheochromocytoma should be considered in all patients with unexplained paroxysmal or sustained hypertension associated with symptoms suggesting hypercatecholaminemia; when increased blood pressure is refractory to or sometimes aggravated by antihypertensive therapy; with a personal history of a previously resected or a family history of pheochromocytoma; or with discovery of an adrenal incidentaloma. Asymptomatic patients with unexplained hypertension and ECG abnormalities that may be caused by hypercatecholaminemia, with imaging evidence suggesting pheochromocytoma, or with diseases sometimes coexisting with pheochromocytoma should be screened. Also, first-degree relatives of patients with familial pheochromocytoma should be screened biochemically and genetically for evidence of pheochromocytoma and familial disease.

Plasma-free (unconjugated) metanephrine, normetanephrine, and catecholamines, and 24-hour urinary catecholamines, metanephrine, and normetanephrine (determined by high-pressure liquid chromatography) are almost always increased with sustained hypertension or during paroxysmal hypertension caused by pheochromocytoma. Total metanephrine determined by spectrophotometry and vanillylmandelic acid (VMA) measurements are less reliable. Even in the absence of hypertension, plasma-free metanephrine and normetanephrine will detect sporadic or familial pheochromocytoma with a sensitivity of 99% and 98%, respectively; however, measurement of urinary metanephrine and normetanephrine are almost as sensitive as their plasma measurements for detecting pheochromocytoma.

Because no biochemical test is totally specific, repeating a combination of tests may help in establishing or excluding presence of a pheochromocytoma. Physiologic stress and stress occurring with various diseases (e.g., heart or renal failure), hypotension, hypoglycemia, acidosis, some medications (e.g., acetaminophen, buspirone, tricyclic antidepressants, phenoxybenzamine, labetalol, sympathomimetics, and some vasodilators), and coffee may increase plasma or urinary concentrations of catecholamines and their metabolites or interfere with biochemical analyses.

Some patients with neurogenic or essential hypertension have increased plasma catecholamines and manifestations, which suggests pheochromocytoma. The clonidine suppression test permits differentiation of these conditions by suppressing plasma norepinephrine concentrations in patients without tumors but not in those with tumors (β-blockers, diuretics, and tricyclic antidepressants can interfere with this test). A glucagon provocative test combined with catecholamine quantitation may rarely be needed to establish presence of a pheochromocytoma.

Imaging localization of pheochromocytomas is indicated after establishing the diagnosis biochemically. Computerized tomography identified 95% of adrenal pheochromocytoma 1 cm or larger and 90% of extraadrenal tumors greater than 2 cm, but intravenous (IV) and oral contrast are necessary. Magnetic resonance imaging (MRI) is more sensitive than computed tomography for detecting pheochromocytoma and also is more specific, because high-signal intensity of T_2-weighted images on MRI may be fairly characteristic; it is noninvasive and is ideal for imaging children and pregnant patients, because no radiation is involved.

The radiopharmaceutical agents ^{131}I or ^{123}I metaiodobenzylguanidine (MIBG) concentrate in about 80% and 90%, respectively, of pheochromocytomas; MIBG is highly specific and may help to detect metastases and very small tumors. MIBG uptake may occur in neuroblastomas, MTC, carcinoids, and small cell lung carcinomas; uptake may be inhibited by some antihypertensives, antidepressants, sympathomimetics, and tranquilizers. Sometimes a combination of imaging studies can be especially helpful in detecting pheochromocytomas and confirming the diagnosis.

Optimal treatment of pheochromocytoma requires expertise. Preoperative adrenergic blockade with phenoxybenzamine or prazosin usually prevents clinical manifestations and reverses any hypovolemia and promotes a smooth anesthetic induction and a fairly stable blood pressure during surgery. Calcium channel blockers also can control pheochromocytic hypertension.

β-Blockade is used to prevent or to treat supraventricular arrhythmias and tachycardia. Ventricular arrhythmias are treated with IV lidocaine. β-Blockers should never be given without first creating α-blockade because β-blockade alone can cause marked hypertension.

Malignant hypertension, acute cardiovascular complications or acceleration of severity, and/or frequency of hypertensive crises may require immediate medical or surgical therapy, or both. Hypertensive crises are best controlled by IV phentolamine, nitroprusside, or nitroglycerin. If immediate surgery is necessary, hypovolemia is corrected with IV fluid, blood, or both. Morphine and phenothiazine should be avoided because they may precipitate hypertensive crises or shock.

With improvement of imaging techniques and with increasing experience with laparoscopic removal of adrenal and some extraadrenal pheochromocytomas, open surgical removal is indicated sometimes if tumors are multiple, greater than 6 cm in diameter, or difficult to remove laparoscopically.

Pheochromocytoma of the chest, neck, and urinary bladder require special surgical procedures. Pheochromocytoma or MEN (with MTC or C cell hyperplasia and/or hyperparathyroidism) may cause hypercalcitonemia, hypercalcemia, or both. Therefore, patients with these biochemical increases should be reevaluated after pheochromocytoma removal, because return of these increases to normal levels eliminates MEN as the cause.

Chemotherapy and radiation therapy may be helpful in treating aggressive malignant tumors and metastases. α- And β-adrenergic blockers may control symptomatology and blood pressure for many years. Metyrosine can markedly inhibit catecholamine synthesis and reduce symptomatology.

References

1. Bravo, E. L. 1994. Evolving concepts in the pathophysiology, diagnosis and treatment of pheochromocytoma. *Endocr Rev* 15:356–368.
2. Eisenhofer, G., T.-T. Huynh, M. Hiroi, and K. Pacak. 2001. Understanding catecholamine metabolism as a guide to the biochemical diagnosis of pheochromocytoma. *Rev. Endocr. Metab. Disord.* 2:297–311.
3. Lenders, J. W. M., K. Pacak, M. M. Walther, W. M. Linehan, M. Mannelli, P. Friberg, H. R. Keiser, D. S. Goldstein, and G. Eisenhofer. 2002. Biochemical diagnosis of pheochromocytoma: Which test is best? *JAMA* 287:1427–1434.
4. Pacak, K., W. M. Linehan, G. Eisenhofer, M. M. Walther, and D. S. Goldstein. 2001. Recent advances in genetics, diagnosis, localization and treatment of pheochromocytoma. *Ann. Intern. Med.* 134:315–329.
5. Manger, W. M., and R. W. Gifford, Jr. 1995. Pheochromocytoma: A clinical over view. In *Hypertension: Pathophysiology, diagnosis and management*, 2nd ed., ed. J. H. Laragh, and B. M. Brenner, 2225–2244. New York: Raven Press.
6. Manger, W. M., and R. W. Gifford, Jr. 1996. *Clinical and experimental pheochromocytoma*, 2nd ed. Cambridge, MA: Blackwell Science.
7. Manger, W. M., and R. W. Gifford, Jr. 2002. Pheochromocytoma: Diagnosis and treatment. *J. Clin. Hypertens*. 4:62–72.

70 Chemodectoma and the Familial Paraganglioma Syndrome

Terry Ketch
Autonomic Dysfunction Center
Vanderbilt University
Nashville, Tennessee

James L. Netterville
Division of Otolaryngology
Vanderbilt University
Nashville, Tennessee

The carotid body is one of the paraganglia located along the course of the vagus nerve in the head, neck, and chest. It functions as a chemoreceptor to stimulate respiration. Located on the medial surface of the carotid bifurcation, it is approximately 2 × 5 mm (Fig. 70.1). The carotid body is composed of clusters of epithelium-like cells in a richly vascular connective tissue stroma. Two cell types make up the cell nests. Chief cells (type 1, epithelioid cells) are the larger polygonal cells. They have an epithelioid appearance and contain neurosecretory granules. Sustentacular cells (type II, supporting cells) are smaller, irregularly shaped cells situated between the sinusoids and the type I cells. They are devoid of neurosecretory granules. These cell clusters are encased in a network of myelinated nerve fibers mixed with a rich vascular plexus.

Although there are no known tumors that arise from the carotid sinus, neoplastic growth of the carotid body can occur either as an isolated tumor or as part of the familial paraganglioma syndrome. Because of the chemoreceptor function of the carotid body, these tumors were first called chemodectomas or carotid body tumors (CBTs), but *carotid paraganglioma* is the most accurate histologic terminology for these lesions. Paragangliomas that develop from the paraganglia adjacent to the vagus nerve and the jugular bulb are usually described in the literature as glomus vagale and glomus jugulare, respectively.

Fewer than 1000 CBT cases were reported before 1980, indicating the rarity of these tumors. About 5% of these patients presented with bilateral CBTs. *Bilateral* or multiple paragangliomas, including those arising from the carotid, jugular, vagal, and tympanic regions, are most commonly seen in patients with familial paraganglioma syndrome.

The inheritance pattern of familial paraganglioma syndrome appears to be autosomal dominant modified by genomic imprinting. In genomic imprinting, the imprintable gene is transmitted in a Mendelian manner, but the expression of the gene is determined by the sex of the transmitting parent. In the case of paragangliomas, the gene does not result in the development of tumors when maternally inherited. Thus, male and female children of a male parent positive for the genetic defect have a 50% chance of manifesting paragangliomas. Children of a female parent positive for the abnormal trait will not experience development of paragangliomas, but they may pass the abnormal gene to their children. Because of potential complications from an undiagnosed tumor, recognition of potential expression of this gene in family members is of utmost importance. The paraganglioma gene (*PGL1*) has been mapped to 11q22.3–q23. Furthermore, analysis of families carrying the *PGL1* gene has revealed germ-line mutations in the *SDHD* gene on chromosome 11q23.

Paragangliomas, which grow by local extension, exhibit intimate anatomic association with the carotid artery, jugular vein, sympathetic chain, and lower cranial nerves (IX–XII). This accounts for both the symptoms and signs of patients, including dysphagia, dysphonia, aspiration, tinnitus, hearing loss, pain, chronic cough, and shoulder weakness. However, most patients with an isolated CBT present with an asymptomatic mass either in the high cervical region or in the lateral pharyngeal wall. On physical examination, if the tumor is larger than 2 cm, a mass is palpable just inferior to the angle of the mandible. The mass has moderate lateral mobility and limitations in vertical mobility because of its attachment to the carotid artery.

There are multiple imaging modalities used in the diagnosis of cervical paragangliomas. With clinical suspicion of a cervical or parapharyngeal space paraganglioma, magnetic resonance imaging (MRI) is the most informative and valuable imaging modality, allowing for greater soft-tissue resolution and imaging in multiple planes. Thus, for evaluation of suspected CBTs, we initially evaluate the patient with MRI with and without contrast. The lone advantage of computed tomography scanning is as an adjunct to the MRI, allowing for evaluation of bony involvement at the skull base. With clinical suspicion of a CBT, fine-needle aspiration is not indicated because of unnecessary costs and potential complications.

Unlike pheochromocytomas, less than 5% of paragangliomas secrete catecholamines. Jugular and vagal tumors have a greater rate of catecholamine excretion than CBT. Despite this, however, it is still prudent to evaluate patients with a 24-hour urine for fractionated catecholamines to

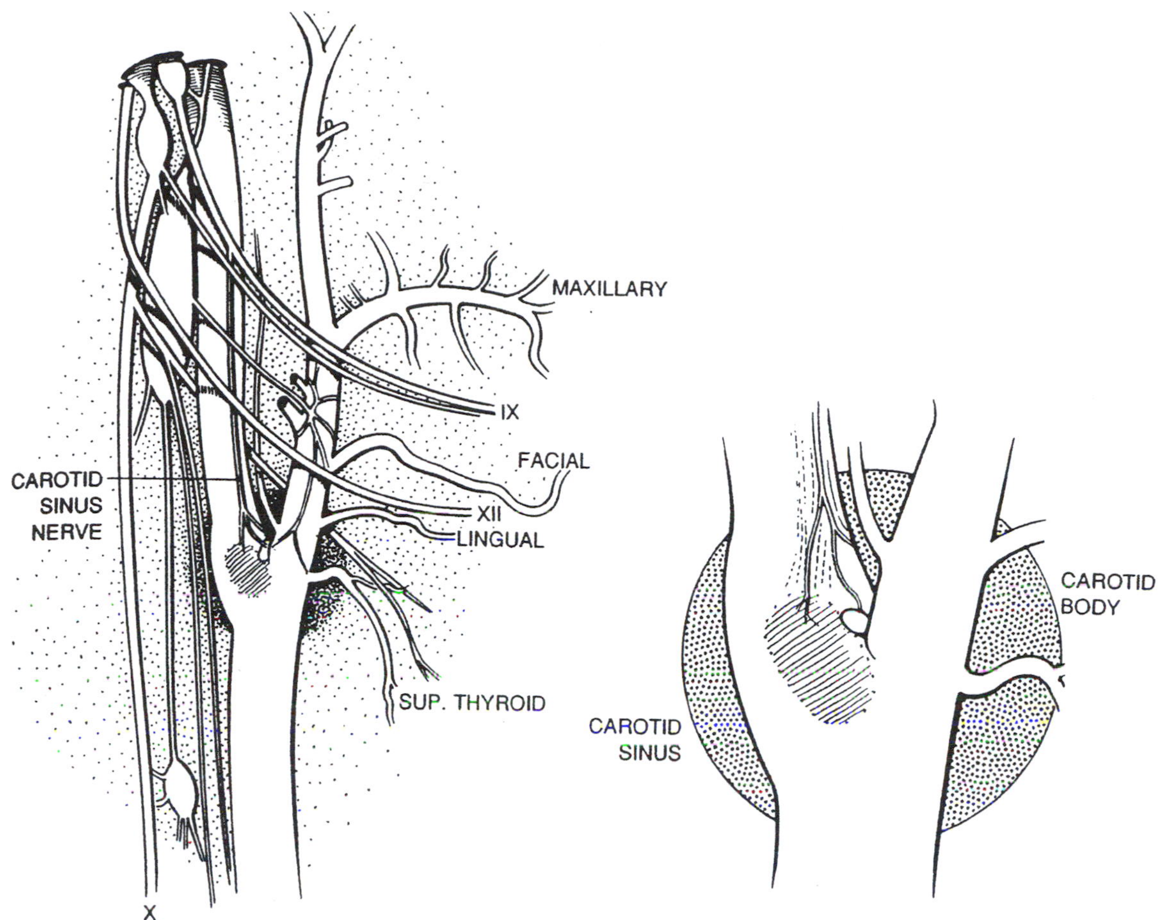

FIGURE 70.1 The carotid body lies on the medial surface of the carotid bifurcation adjacent to the carotid sinus in the lateral wall of the carotid bifurcation. The afferent signals travel up the carotid sinus nerve (nerve of Hering) to join with the glossopharyngeal nerve.

determine if catecholamine excretion is increased. At a minimum, patients with accompanying flushing, hypertension, palpitations, and headaches should undergo a 24-hour urine collection for catecholamine determination. To complicate matters, such increases of catecholamines may also occur as part of tumor-induced baroreflex failure.

Most CBTs grow from 1 to 2 mm per year. Some tumors, however, appear to advance at an even slower rate with minimal change over a several year period. Rarely, paragangliomas progress at a much faster rate. Because of this slow rate of enlargement, it is reasonable to initially observe some tumors to establish the rate of progression before deciding on a treatment course.

Surgical excision continues to be the mainstay of treatment for CBT, particularly for unilateral isolated CBT. This decision becomes more complicated in patients with bilateral CBT or patients with multiple bilateral paragangliomas. Tumors less than 4.0 cm have minimal neural involvement and can usually be separated from the carotid with minimal damage to the artery. Complication rates increase as the tumors enlarge to more than 5 cm. Preoperative embolization may decrease blood loss and facilitate surgical removal of these tumors, but its role has not been fully established.

Cranial nerve loss is the most common complication with surgical excision. In various series, the rate of loss ranges from 10 to 50%. The most commonly injured nerve is the superior laryngeal nerve, which provides sensory feedback from the superior half of the larynx and motor function to the cricothyroid muscle. Because of its location deep to the carotid bifurcation, it is usually enveloped within the vascular capsule on the medial surface of the tumor. Loss of the superior laryngeal nerve results in moderate dysphagia with mild aspiration caused by loss of sensory function and a decrease in the vocal range with the loss of motor function. Although the vocal range rarely returns to normal, compensation for the dysphagia occurs within several weeks to months after injury. Infrequently, the vagus and or the hypoglossal nerves must be resected with the tumor secondary to tumor involvement. More commonly, these nerves are injured because of retraction as they are separated away from the tumor. The hemilaryngeal and hemiglossal paralysis, which develops with retraction injury to these nerves, causes voice weakness, dysarthria, and significant aspiration. Other nerves that are occasionally injured during surgical resection include the glossopharyngeal, spinal accessory, and the sympathetic trunk.

First bite syndrome can occur after resection of CBTs. This is manifest by pain in the region of the parotid gland, which occurs with the first few bites of each meal. This pain results from the loss of the postganglionic sympathetic innervation to the parotid gland. These postganglionic fibers lie within the periadventitial tissue of the external carotid artery. This loss results in a denervation supersensitivity of the sympathetic receptors on the myoepithelial muscle cells within the parotid. It is hypothesized that crossover stimulation occurs during parasympathetic stimulation of the gland resulting in spasm of the myoepithelial cells. The pain decreases over time, but most patients alter their diets to stay away from strong sialogogues.

Baroreceptor dysfunction is usually mild and transient after unilateral CBT resection if there is normal innervation to the contralateral carotid sinus, although cases of baroreflex failure after unilateral resection have been reported. With bilateral CBT resection, most patients manifest baroreflex failure to some degree, thus requiring medical intervention. With baroreflex failure, the ability to maintain blood pressure and heart rate with a normal narrow range is impaired. This results in wide swings in pressure and heart rate in response to certain stimuli. An in-depth discussion of baroreflex failure is presented in Chapter 71.

Radiation therapy has had a limited role in the treatment of CBT. Although the series are small, it appears that radiation therapy can control tumor growth in a significant percentage of patients treated. Averaging several series, 25% of the tumors completely regressed, 25% of the tumors underwent a partial regression, and the final 50% either stayed the same size with no further growth or continued to advance in size.

Observation is a reasonable form of treatment in selected individuals. Because of the slow growth rate, these tumors can be observed to establish their rate of progression before final treatment planning. A few patients have been observed in some series for over a decade with minimal or no progression in the size of their tumors. We routinely observe tumors in patients older than 65 years, or in individuals whose life expectancy is decreased because of some other disease process. During this period of observation the size of the tumor is monitored to be sure that rapid growth does not unexpectedly occur.

References

1. Baysal, B. E., R. E. Ferrell, J. E. Willett-Brozick, E. C. Lawrence, D. Myssiorek, A. Osch, A. van der Mey, P. E. Taschner, W. S. Rubinstein, E. N. Myers, C. W. Richard, III, C. J. Cornelisse, P. Devilee, and B. Devlin. 2000. Mutations in SDHD, a mitochrondrial complex II gene, in hereditary paraganglioma. *Science* 287:848–851.
2. Sniezek, J. C., A. N. Sabari, and J. L. Netterville. 2001. Paranglioma surgery: Complications and treatment. *Otolaryngol. Clin. North. Am.* 34:993–1006.

71 Baroreflex Failure

Jens Jordan
Franz-Vohard-Klinik
Humboldt University
Berlin, Germany

Baroreflexes have a pivotal role in blood pressure regulation. Changes in blood pressure elicit changes in stretch of carotid and aortic baroreceptors. The altered stretch of carotid and aortic baroreceptors is conveyed to medullary brainstem nuclei through the glossopharyngeal and vagus nerves, respectively. In the brainstem, information from baroreceptors is integrated with input from other afferents and cortical input. Efferent parasympathetic and sympathetic activity are adjusted to compensate for the change in systemic blood pressure. Thus, the baroreflexes attenuate excessive swings in blood pressure. This effect serves to maintain blood flow to the organs, especially the brain. Moreover, the vasculature is protected from large, potentially deleterious, fluctuations in blood pressure.

Bilateral damage to structures of the afferent baroreflex arc results in baroreflex failure. Any afferent arc structure including baroreceptors, the afferent neurons transmitting the information from baroreceptors, or afferent brainstem nuclei may be involved. In contrast, damage to the efferent part of the baroreflex causes autonomic failure (Table 71.1). Whether the afferent baroreflex input must be completely lost to develop baroreflex failure is not known. In most patients with baroreflex failure, the lesion of the afferent arc of the baroreflex seems to be associated with damage to efferent neurons in the vagus nerve. The damage results in partial or complete parasympathetic denervation of the heart ("nonselective baroreflex failure," Fig. 71.1). In a minority of patients, efferent parasympathetic neurons are intact ("selective baroreflex failure," see Fig. 71.1).

There is a large body of literature on baroreflex function, both in different animal species and in humans. However, the number of patients with baroreflex failure reported in the literature is relatively small. The small number of reported cases may suggest that baroreflex failure is a rare condition. Perhaps the probability to experience bilateral damage to afferent baroreflex structures is low. An alternative explanation is that many cases of baroreflex failure go undetected.

CAUSES OF BAROREFLEX FAILURE

In most patients, the mechanism that led to bilateral interruption in afferent baroreflex input is suggested by the history. A common cause of baroreflex failure is extensive neck surgery and radiation therapy for cancers of the neck, which may damage baroreceptors, afferent baroreflex neurons, or both. In some patients, the bilateral loss results from repeated trauma to the neck. For example, surgical resection of the glossopharyngeal nerve resulted in baroreflex failure in a patient who had previously sustained injury to the contralateral glossopharyngeal and vagus nerves. Another patient reported in the literature experienced baroreflex failure after repeated surgery to the cervical spine and an auto accident. Baroreflex failure also has been described in patients with the familial paraganglioma syndrome. Bilateral damage to the nuclei of the solitary tract, the most important relay station for afferent autonomic input, is a rare cause of baroreflex failure. In a number of patients with typical signs and symptoms of baroreflex failure, no cause could be documented.

CLINICAL PRESENTATION

Most patients who are ultimately diagnosed with baroreflex failure are sent to tertiary care centers for the evaluation of volatile arterial hypertension. The hypertension can be sustained or episodic. Even with sustained hypertension, blood pressure is highly variable (Fig. 71.2). During hypertensive episodes, blood pressure recordings may be in the range of 170 to 280/110 to 135 mmHg. Hypertensive episodes are usually accompanied by tachycardia, a so-called tracking of blood pressure and heart rate. Patients may experience sensations of warmth or flushing, palpitations, headache, and diaphoresis. The hypertensive episodes are triggered by factors such as psychological stress, physical exercise, and pain. A minority of patients present with episodes of hypotension and bradycardia. Spontaneous hypotension and bradycardia is a feature of selective baroreflex failure. Hypotensive episodes can be observed when

Selective Baroreflex Failure

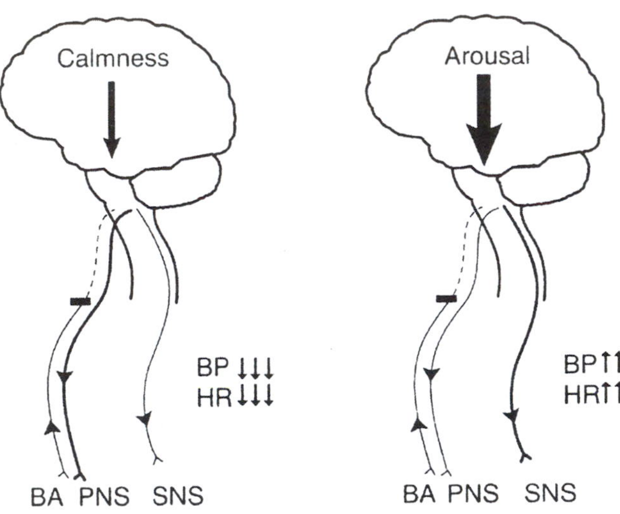

Nonselective Baroreflex Failure

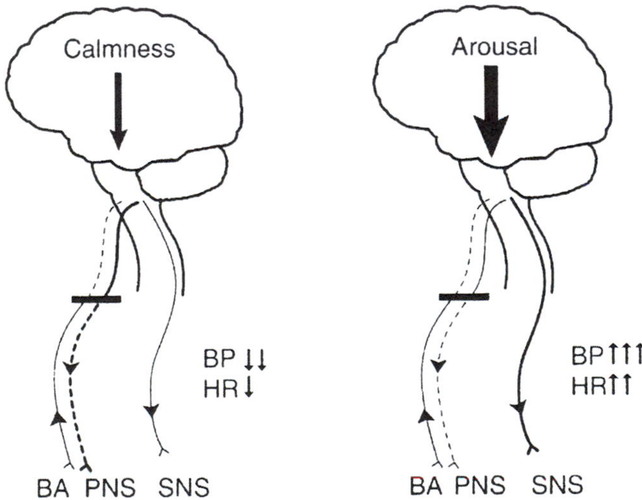

FIGURE 71.1 Selective baroreflex failure (**top**) contrasted to nonselective baroreflex failure (**bottom**). Baroreflex afferents (BA) are damaged in patients with selective and nonselective baroreflex failure. Efferent sympathetic (SNS) and parasympathetic nerves (PNS) are intact in selective baroreflex failure. In nonselective baroreflex failure, efferent parasympathetic nerves are at least in part damaged. BP, blood pressure; HR, heart rate. (From Jordan, J., J. R. Shannon, B. K. Black, F. Costa, A. C. Ertl, R. Furlan, I. Biaggioni, and D. Robertson. 1997. Malignant vagotonia due to selective baroreflex failure. *Hypertension* 30:1072–1077.)

patients are resting and cortical input is diminished. With profound hypotension, patients may experience presyncopal symptoms. Frank syncope seems to be uncommon. Severe orthostatic hypotension is not a typical symptom of baroreflex failure. Indeed, some patients feature a marked increase in blood pressure with standing, namely, orthostatic *hyper-*

TABLE 71.1 Distinction of Baroreflex Failure and Autonomic Failure

	Baroreflex failure	Autonomic failure
Labile hypertension	+++	+/–
Orthostatic hypotension	+/–	+++
Orthostatic hypertension	++	–
Supine hypertension	+/–	++
Postprandial hypotension	+/–	–
Episodic tachycardia	–	++
Bradycardic episodes	++*	+/–
Hypersensitivity to vasoactive drugs	+++	+++

* Bradycardia associated with hypotension is a typical feature of malignant vagotonia caused by selective baroreflex failure.

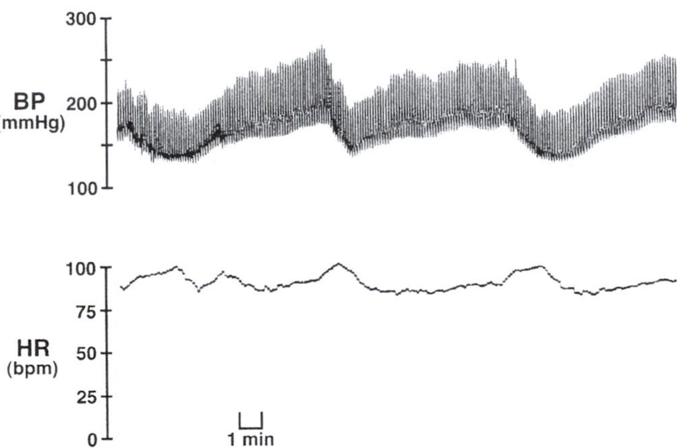

FIGURE 71.2 Continuous blood pressure (BP) and heart rate (HR) recordings at rest in a patient with baroreflex failure. There are large spontaneous oscillations of HR and BP that parallel each other. The decreases of BP are very brisk. (From Jordan, J., J. R. Shannon, B. K. Black, F. Costa, A. C. Ertl, R. Furlan, I. Biaggioni, and D. Robertson. 1997. Malignant vagotonia due to selective baroreflex failure. *Hypertension* 30:1072–1077.)

tension. Orthostatic hypotension may be observed in patients with baroreflex failure who are volume depleted or are treated with sympatholytic drugs. One possible explanation for the absence of severe orthostatic hypotension in most patients is sparing of cardiopulmonary stretch receptors. An alternative explanation is that other signals, such as visual and vestibular cues, are sufficient to increase sympathetic activity with assumption of the upright posture. The baroreflex buffers the effect of vasoactive medications. Therefore, patients with baroreflex failure may experience severe hypotension after ingestion of standard doses of antihypertensive medications (e.g., vasodilators, diuretics, and sympatholytic drugs). Medications that increase vascular tone can lead to dramatic increases in blood pressure. Clinical observations suggest that patients with baroreflex failure also feature emotional lability, particular during hypertensive episodes. However, this issue has not been systematically addressed.

The onset of baroreflex failure can be abrupt or more gradual. An abrupt onset of symptoms typically occurs in patients with baroreflex failure caused by neck surgery. A more gradual onset of baroreflex failure has been observed in some patients who had undergone radiation therapy of the neck. The degree of hypertension seems to be different during the acute and the chronic phase of the disease. After acute interruption of afferent baroreflex input, blood pressure is particularly high ("Entzügelungshochdruck"). Apneic spells can be seen during the first 24 hours when carotid body input to the central nervous system is lost. In the more chronic phase, the average blood pressure tends to decrease. Yet, blood pressure remains highly variable. A similar time effect has been observed in animal models of baroreflex failure.

DIAGNOSING BAROREFLEX FAILURE

Baroreflex failure should be suspected in patients with volatile arterial hypertension. However, in the majority of patients, volatile arterial hypertension is not caused by baroreflex failure. Alternative causes of volatile hypertension, such as renovascular hypertension, should be considered first. In patients in whom labile hypertension develops immediately after neck surgery, arriving at the correct diagnosis may be straightforward. Patients in whom the loss of afferent baroreflex function develops more gradually over time as a consequence of radiation therapy or a neuropathy may be difficult to diagnose. Pheochromocytoma can sometimes mimic baroreflex failure. Hypertensive episodes, tachycardia, flushing, and impaired baroreflex function have been described in both conditions. Therefore, the differential diagnosis pheochromocytoma should be considered and ruled out by appropriate testing. Other entities from which baroreflex failure needs to be distinguished are panic attack, generalized anxiety disorder, hyperthyroidism, alcohol withdrawal, and drug abuse (e.g., amphetamines and cocaine). Hyperadrenergic orthostatic intolerance may also present with volatility of blood pressure, but severe hypertension is uncommon. One patient reported in the literature who featured typical signs of baroreflex failure was later shown to have Munchausen syndrome. Baroreflex failure is a rare cause of hypotension and bradycardia.

Patients with baroreflex failure exhibit a normal or exaggerated pressor response to psychological (e.g., mental arithmetic test) and physiologic stimuli (e.g., cold pressor or handgrip testing). The pressor effect can be markedly prolonged in these patients. Baroreflex testing should be considered in patients with typical signs and symptoms of baroreflex failure. In patients with an atypical clinical presentation or a gradual onset of symptoms, more common entities should be ruled out before baroreflex testing is considered. The diagnostic abnormality in patients with baroreflex failure is the absence of a bradycardic response to pressor agents or a tachycardic response to vasodilators (Fig. 71.3). In healthy subjects, the heart rate will decrease 7 to 21 beats per minute (bpm) in response to a phenylephrine dose that increases systolic blood pressure 20 mmHg and the heart rate will increase 9 to 28 bpm in response to a nitroprusside dose that decreases blood pressure by 20 mmHg. In contrast, the heart rate in patients with baroreflex failure did not alter by more than 4 bpm with either maneuver. The loss of baroreflex blood pressure buffering in these patients is associated with about a 10- to 20-fold hypersensitivity to vasoactive medications (see Fig. 71.3). Therefore, baroreflex testing should be conducted starting with low doses of phenylephrine (e.g., 12.5 μg) and nitroprusside (e.g., 0.1 μg/kg). The doses should be increased to obtain a change in systolic blood pressure of at least 20 to 25 mmHg. Baroreflex heart rate control can be assessed noninvasively using cross-spectral analysis or the so-called sequence method. These methods have not been evaluated in patients with baroreflex failure and cannot be recommended as a diagnostic test in this setting. Theoretically, one would like to assess baroreflex regulation of heart rate and sympathetic nerve traffic, which are both impaired in baroreflex failure. However, recording of sympathetic activity is not feasible in the clinical setting. Abnormal baroreflex tests alone are not sufficient to diagnose baroreflex failure. Absence of heart rate changes during baroreflex testing also can be observed in patients with autonomic failure.

Biochemical assessment of patients with baroreflex failure demonstrates surges of sympathetic activity associ-

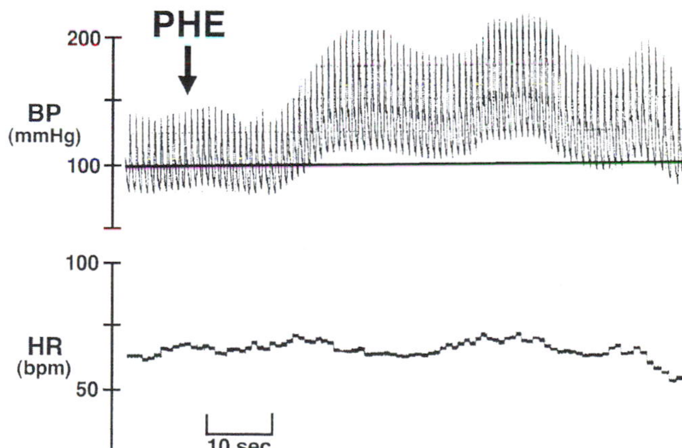

FIGURE 71.3 Blood pressure (BP) increase after a 25-mg bolus dose of phenylephrine (PHE) in a patient with baroreflex failure. Systolic blood pressure increased more than 40 mmHg. The same phenylephrine dose increases systolic blood pressure approximately 6 mmHg in healthy subjects. There was no baroreflex-mediated decrease in heart rate (HR). (From Jordan, J., J. R. Shannon, B. K. Black, F. Costa, A. C. Ertl, R. Furlan, I. Biaggioni, and D. Robertson. 1997. Malignant vagotonia due to selective baroreflex failure. *Hypertension* 30:1072–1077.)

ated with hypertensive episodes. Venous plasma norepinephrine concentrations as high as 2660 pg/ml have been reported. Conversely, levels drawn during normotensive periods may be within the normal range. Clonidine profoundly reduces blood pressure and plasma norepinephrine concentrations in patients with baroreflex failure. Determination of the norepinephrine response to clonidine can be useful to differentiate baroreflex failure from pheochromocytoma.

TREATMENT

Treating patients with baroreflex failure is a challenge. The first step in the treatment of baroreflex failure is the education of the patient, family members, and referring physicians. It is particularly important to convey the information that many medications that do not elicit changes in blood pressure may have a dramatic effect on patients with baroreflex failure. Medications that may change sympathetic activity or vascular tone, including a variety of over-the-counter drugs, must be used with great caution.

One of the main goals in treating patients with baroreflex failure is to prevent extreme hypertension (Table 71.2). The pharmacologic treatment of choice for the hypertension is clonidine. Clonidine can be given orally or applied as a skin patch. Clonidine decreases sympathetic activity in the central nervous system and in the periphery. Moreover, clonidine causes mild sedation. These effects attenuate pressure surges. α-Methyl-dopa also can be used in these patients but there are some concerns regarding possible hepatotoxicity. Some patients with baroreflex failure do not tolerate clonidine or α-methyl-dopa (e.g., exacerbation of depression). In these patients, peripherally acting sympatholytic agents, such as guanethidine and guanadrel, may be used. Because the hypertension in patients with baroreflex failure often is driven by cortical input, which is unopposed by the baroreflex, benzodiazepines elicit a reduction in blood pressure. Chronic treatment with relatively large doses of benzodiazepines can be used in selected patients. All the antihypertensive medications have to be taken very regularly even when blood pressure is relatively low. Discontinuation of the medication elicits a particularly severe rebound phenomenon in these patients.

TABLE 71.2 Treatment of Baroreflex Failure

Blood pressure reduction	Clonidine
	α-Methyl-dopa
	Guanethidine
	Guanadrel
	Diazepam
Blood pressure increase	Fludrocortisone
	Dietary salt
Prevention of bradycardia/asystole	Cardiac pacemaker

Some patients, particularly patients with selective baroreflex failure, experience hypotensive episodes. Sometimes, the hypotension is acutely exacerbated by the antihypertensive treatment. However, in the long term, prevention of hypertension may attenuate pressure-induced volume loss through the kidney. Thus, effective control of the hypertension may improve hypotension. We encourage patients who experience hypotension and are receiving chronic antihypertensive treatment to increase their dietary salt intake. In selected patients, pharmacologic treatment of the hypotension is required. Because of its long duration of action, fludrocortisone is a good choice for the treatment of hypotension in these patients. Other pressor agents should be used with great caution. Pacemakers generally are not indicated in persons with syncope. However, in a few patients with malignant vagotonia, hypotensive episodes may be accompanied by life-threatening bradycardia and asystole. Implantation of a cardiac pacemaker may be required in selected patients.

References

1. Aksamit, T. R., J. S. Floras, R. G. Victor, and P. E. Aylward. 1987. Paroxysmal hypertension due to sinoaortic baroreceptor denervation in humans. *Hypertension* 9:309–314.
2. Biaggioni, I., W. O. Whetsell, J. Jobe, and J. H. Nadeau. 1994. Baroreflex failure in a patient with central nervous system lesions involving the nucleus tractus solitarii. *Hypertension* 23:491–495.
3. Fagius, J., B. G. Wallin, G. Sundlof, C. Nerhed, and S. Englesson. 1985. Sympathetic outflow in man after anaesthesia of the glossopharyngeal and vagus nerves. *Brain* 108:423–438.
4. Ford, F. R. 1956. Fatal hypertensive crisis following denervation of the carotid sinus for the relief of repeated attacks of syncope. *Johns Hopkins Med. J.* 100:14–16.
5. Jordan, J., J. R. Shannon, B. K. Black, F. Costa, A. C. Ertl, R. Furlan, I. Biaggioni, and D. Robertson. 1997. Malignant vagotonia due to selective baroreflex failure. *Hypertension* 30:1072–1077.
6. Ketch, T., I. Biaggioni, R. Robertson, and D. Robertson. 2002. Four faces of baroreflex failure: Hypertensive crisis, volatile hypertension, orthostatic tachycardia, and malignant vagotonia. *Circulation* 105:2518–2523.
7. Kuchel, O., J. R. Cusson, P. Larochelle, N. T. Buu, and J. Genest. 1987. Posture- and emotion-induced severe hypertensive paroxysms with baroreceptor dysfunction. *J. Hypertens.* 5:277–283.
8. Lampen, H., P. Kezdi, E. Koppermann, and L. Kaufmann. 1949. Experimenteller Entzügelungshochdruck bei arterieller Hypertonie. *Zeitschrift für Kreislaufforschung*. 38:577–592.
9. Phillips, A. M., D. L. Jardine, P. J. Parkin, T. Hughes, and H. Ikram. 2000. Brain stem stroke causing baroreflex failure and paroxysmal hypertension. *Stroke* 31:1997–2001.
10. Robertson, D., A. S. Hollister, I. Biaggioni, J. L. Netterville, R. Mosqueda-Garcia, and R. M. Robertson. 1993. The diagnosis and treatment of baroreflex failure. *N. Engl. J. Med.* 329:1449–1455.
11. Tellioglu, T., J. A. Oates, and I. Biaggioni. 2000. Munchausen's syndrome presenting as baroreflex failure. *N. Engl. J. Med.* 343:581.

72 Deficiencies of Tetrahydrobiopterin, Tyrosine Hydroxylase, and Aromatic L-Amino Acid Decarboxylase

Keith Hyland
Department of Neurochemistry
Kimberly H. Courtwright and Joseph W. Summers Institute of Metabolic Diseases
Baylor University Medical Center
Dallas, Texas

Lauren A. Arnold
Department of Neurochemistry
Kimberly H. Courtwright and Joseph W. Summers Institute of Metabolic Diseases
Baylor University Medical Center
Dallas, Texas

BIOCHEMISTRY

Tetrahydrobiopterin (BH_4) is the cofactor for tyrosine hydroxylase (TH) and tryptophan hydroxylase (TRYPH), the rate-limiting enzymes required for the synthesis of the catecholamines (dopamine, norepinephrine, and epinephrine) and serotonin (5-HT). BH_4 is formed from guanosine triphosphate (GTP) in a multistep pathway and defects in its biosynthesis have been described at the level of GTP cyclohydrolase, 6-pyruvoyltetrahydropterin synthase (6-PTPS), and sepiapterin reductase (SR). In addition, deficiency of dihydropteridine reductase (DHPR) leads to the inability to regenerate BH_4 after its oxidation in the hydroxylase reactions (Fig. 72.1). All the defects affecting BH_4 metabolism are inherited in an autosomal recessive fashion, except GTP cyclohydrolase deficiency. In this disorder there is also an autosomal dominant form.

The various defects of BH_4 metabolism that occur within the central nervous system (CNS) lead to a deficiency of 5-HT and the catecholamines. There are, however, peripheral forms of 6-PTPS deficiency in which central neurotransmitter metabolism is normal [1]. BH_4 also is the cofactor for phenylalanine hydroxylase (PH); hence, defects in BH_4 metabolism generally lead to hyperphenylalaninemia. Dominantly inherited GTP cyclohydrolase deficiency and SR deficiency, however, only cause a lack of BH_4 within the CNS; therefore phenylalanine metabolism is unaffected. Another enzyme, pterin-4α-carbinolamine dehydratase, is involved in the hydroxylation of phenylalanine; deficiency again leads to hyperphenylalaninemia, but effects on central 5-HT and catecholamine metabolism are minimal, if present at all [1].

L-Dopa and 5-hydroxytryptophan (5-HTP), the products of the TH and TRYPH reactions, are decarboxylated by vitamin B_6, requiring aromatic L-amino acid decarboxylase (AADC) to form the respective neurotransmitters (see Fig. 72.1). Deficiency of TH leads to decreased concentrations of catecholamines [1], whereas a defect at the level of AADC leads to deficiencies of both 5-HT and the catecholamines [2]. A defect of TRYPH has not been described.

PRESENTATION AND NEUROLOGIC SYMPTOMS

The neurologic symptoms of the central BH_4 defects (except dominantly inherited GTP cyclohydrolase deficiency) and AADC deficiency are very similar and reflect a combined lack of both 5-HT and the catecholamine neurotransmitters. Patients present between 2 and 8 months of age with a fairly well-characterized syndrome. Symptoms include hypersalivation, temperature instability, pinpoint pupils, ptosis of the eyelids, oculogyric crises, hypokinesis, distal chorea, truncal hypotonia, swallowing difficulties, drowsiness, and irritability [3]. Autonomic features are variable with symptoms including ptosis, miosis, a reverse Argyll Robertson pupil, chronic or paroxysmal nasal congestion, paroxysmal sweating, temperature instability, gastrointestinal reflux, and constipation. In the first described cases of AADC deficiency, postural decrease in blood pressure was not present at 9 months but was noted at 1 year of age [2]. Some patients with DHPR deficiency develop long tract signs associated with multifocal perivascular calcification located mainly in the basal ganglia and, to a lesser degree, in areas of white and gray matter [4]. These changes are thought to occur as a result of an insidious folate deficiency that has been postulated to arise as a result of inhibition of folate metabolism by the unusual forms of biopterin that accumulate in this disease. The neurologic signs associated with peripheral forms of 6-PTPS deficiency and pterin-4α-carbinolamine dehydratase deficiency are minimal and disappear after correction of the hyperphenylalaninemia. A peripheral form of 6-PTPS deficiency progressing to give a central phenotype has been reported; thus, all patients should be reevaluated in terms of their central neurotransmitter status at a later age.

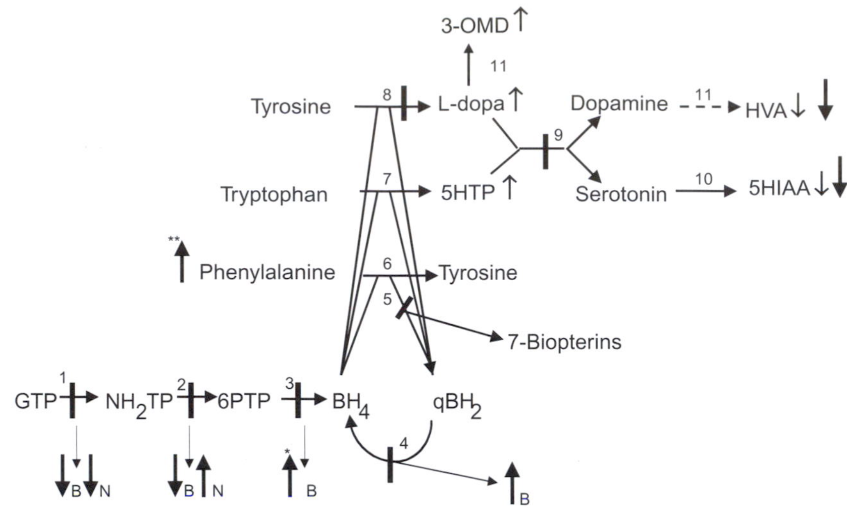

FIGURE 72.1 Biosynthesis of serotonin and dopamine, showing sites of metabolic block and abnormal metabolite profiles. 1 = GTP cyclohydrolase; 2 = 6-pyruvoyltetrahydropterin synthase; 3 = sepiapterin reductase; 4 = dihydropteridine reductase; 5 = pterin-4α-carbinolamine dehydratase; 6 = phenylalanine hydroxylase; 7 = tryptophan hydroxylase; 8 = tyrosine hydroxylase; 9 = aromatic L-amino acid decarboxylase; 10 = monoamine oxidase; 11 = catechol-*O*-methyltransferase. B, biopterin; N, neopterin; ↑ and ↓ represent changes seen in aromatic L-amino acid decarboxylase deficiency. **↑** and **↓** represent changes seen in the central forms of tetrahydrobiopterin deficiency. **I** shows the position of a metabolic block. *Change only seen in the central nervous system. **Excluding dominantly inherited GTP cyclohydrolase deficiency. 3-OMD, 3-*O*-methyldopa; 5-HIAA, 5-hydroxyindoleacetic acid; 5-HTP, 5-hydroxytryptophan; 6-PTP, 6-pyruvoyltetrahydropterin; BH_4, tetrahydrobiopterin; GTP, guanosine triphosphate; HVA, homovanillic acid; NH_2TP, dihydroneopterin triphosphate; qBH_2, quinonoid dihydrobiopterin.

Dominantly inherited GTP cyclohydrolase deficiency, otherwise known as Segawa's disease or dopa-responsive dystonia, does not present as in the other defects of BH_4 metabolism. Normal presentation is the appearance of a dystonic gait disorder at around 4 to 6 years of age; however, the age of presentation and the spectrum of clinical manifestations is broad. Occasionally, onset has been with arm dystonia, retrocollis, torticollis, poor coordination, or slowness in dressing before the development of leg signs. There may also be hyperreflexia and apparent extensor plantar responses, as well as other clinical features suggesting spasticity. The symptoms often, but not always, show a marked diurnal variation [5].

Clinical presentation in TH deficiency also is varied, ranging from exercise-induced dystonia, to progressive gait disturbance and tremor in childhood, to a severe infantile parkinsonism [6–8]. The patients reported to date appear to have a paucity of autonomic features, suggesting a compensatory peripheral mechanism.

DIAGNOSIS

Tetrahydrobiopterin Deficiencies

Defective BH_4 metabolism should be considered in all cases of hyperphenylalaninemia and in any child who presents with the neurologic syndrome described earlier. Methods for diagnosis rely initially on the appearance of characteristic high-pressure liquid chromatography profiles of neopterins and biopterins in urine [1]. The changes expected in each condition are marked on Figure 72.1.

A BH_4 loading test also can help to distinguish between BH_4 defects in which there is hyperphenylalaninemia and primary PH deficiency. Administering 2 to 20 mg/kg orally leads to a decrease in plasma phenylalanine in deficiencies of GTP cyclohydrolase, pterin-4α-carbinolamine dehydratase, and 6-PTPS; however, some cases of DHPR deficiency do not respond, and BH_4-responsive PH deficiency has been reported.

Further tests are required in suspected cases of dominantly inherited GTP cyclohydrolase deficiency, 6-PTPS, SR, and DHPR deficiency. The biopterin, neopterin profiles are similar in both DHPR and PH deficiency; therefore, it is necessary to measure DHPR activity in blood spots or erythrocytes. Pterin analysis also cannot distinguish between the peripheral and central forms of 6-PTPS deficiency; here it is necessary to measure cerebrospinal fluid (CSF) levels of 5-hydroxyindole acetic acid (5-HIAA) and homovanillic acid (HVA), the major catabolites of 5-HT and dopamine. These are normal in the peripheral condition, but they are reduced in the central forms of the disease [1]. Hyperphenylalaninemia does not develop in patients with dominantly inherited GTP cyclohydrolase deficiency and SR deficiency; diagnosis in these cases is again dependent on CSF analyses. Neurotransmitter metabolite levels are low and there are also characteristic abnormal pterin patterns (see Fig. 72.1) [1].

Tyrosine Hydroxylase Deficiency

The deficiencies of TH and AADC do not lead to abnormal profiles using traditional screening methods (blood spot screening, organic acid or amino acid analyses, etc.), and biopterin and neopterin levels also are normal. Recognition requires the clinician to consider an abnormality in biogenic amine metabolism in a child with clinical signs similar to those described earlier. Diagnosis of TH deficiency requires the analysis of catecholamine metabolites in CSF, where concentrations of HVA and 3-methoxy-4-hydroxyphenylglycol are low [1]. Confirmation of the diagnosis relies on mutation analysis because there is no easily available peripheral tissue that can be used for enzyme analysis.

Aromatic L-Amino Acid Decarboxylase Deficiency

The pattern of biogenic amine metabolites in AADC deficiency is very characteristic. There is marked increase of L-dopa, 5-HTP, and 3-*O*-methyldopa in CSF, plasma, and urine. HVA and 5-HIAA concentrations are greatly reduced in CSF, as are the levels of 5-HT, catecholamines, and their catabolites in blood and urine. Positive diagnosis is accomplished by analysis of AADC activity in plasma [2].

TREATMENT

BH_4 Deficiencies

Hyperphenylalaninemia may be corrected using a low phenylalanine diet or, in deficiencies of GTP cyclohydrolase, 6-PTPS and pterin 4α-carbinolamine, by administration of oral BH_4 (0.5–40 mg/day). BH_4 is usually ineffective in DHPR deficiency. Central neurotransmitter deficiency is corrected by oral administration of the precursors, L-dopa (2–20 mg/kg per day) and 5-HTP (0.8–12 mg/kg per day), in conjunction with carbidopa (0.3–4.0 mg/kg per day). Initial doses should be low, with clinical monitoring of the therapeutic effect. Adverse symptoms because of overtreatment are sometimes similar to the disease symptoms; therefore, monitoring by measuring CSF levels of HVA and 5-HIAA is crucial. Folinic acid (3 mg/day) should be administered in DHPR deficiency, with CSF 5-methyltetrahydrofolate levels measured at the same time as the neurotransmitter metabolites to ensure the adequacy of the dose.

Tyrosine Hydroxylase Deficiency

Treatment of TH deficiency aims to correct the abnormal catecholamine levels. Treatment with low-dose L-dopa/carbidopa (3 mg/kg and 0.75 mg/kg, respectively), three times daily has been extremely effective in some cases. In others, very slow institution of small doses of L-dopa/carbidopa, along with selegiline (monoamine oxidase B inhibitor) and an anticholinergic agent such as trihexyphenidyl, has been much more beneficial than L-dopa/carbidopa alone.

Aromatic L-Amino Acid Decarboxylase Deficiency

Treatment in the index cases of the disease consisted of bromocriptine (dopamine agonist, 2.5 mg twice daily), tranylcypromine (nonselective monoamine oxidase inhibitor, 4 mg twice daily), and pyridoxine (100 mg twice daily) in combination. Therapy led to a marked clinical and biochemical improvement [2]. Pergolide has since been shown to be an effective alternate to bromocriptine in some cases. As AADC is a B_6-requiring enzyme, high-dose pyridoxine monotherapy should be tried in all future cases.

References

1. Blau, N., B. Thony, R. G. H. Cotton, and K. Hyland. 2001. Disorders of tetrahydrobiopterin and related biogenic amines. In *The metabolic and molecular basis of inherited disease,* 8th ed., ed. C. R. Scriver, A. L. Beaudet, W. S. Sly, D. Valle, B. Childs, and D. Vogelstein, 1725–1776. New York: McGraw-Hill.
2. Hyland, K., R. A. H. Surtees, C. Rodeck, and P. T. Clayton. 1992. Aromatic L-amino acid decarboxylase deficiency: Clinical features, diagnosis and treatment of a new inborn error of neurotransmitter amine synthesis. *Neurology* 42:1980–1988.
3. Hyland, K. 1993. Abnormalities of biogenic amine metabolism. *J. Inherit. Metab. Dis.* 16:676–690.
4. Smith, I., K. Hyland, B. Kendall, and R. Leeming, R. 1985. Clinical role of pteridine therapy in tetrahydrobiopterin deficiency. *J. Inherit. Metab. Dis.* 8(Suppl. 1):39–45.
5. Nygaard, T. G., B. J. Snow, S. Fahn, and D. B. Calne. 1993. Dopa-responsive dystonia: Clinical characteristics and definitions. In *Hereditary progressive dystonia with marked diurnal fluctuation,* ed. M. Segawa, 3–13. Lancaster, UK: Parthenon.
6. De Lonlay, P., M. C. Nassogne, A. H. van Gennip, A. C. van Cruchten, T. Billatte de Villemeur, M. Cretz, C. Stoll, J. M. Launay, G. C. Steenberger-Spante, L. P. van den Heuvel, R. A. Wevers, J. M. Saudubray, and N. G. Abeling. 2000. Tyrosine hydroxylase deficiency unresponsive to L-dopa treatment with unusual clinical and biochemical presentation. *J. Inherit. Metab. Dis.* 23:819–825.
7. de Rijk-van Andel, J. F., F. J. Gabreels, B. Geurtz, G. C. Steenbergen-Spanjers, L. P. van den Heuvel, J. A. Smeitink, and R. A. Wevers. 2000. L-Dopa-responsive infantile hypokinetic rigid parkinsonism due to tyrosine hydroxylase deficiency. *Neurology* 55:1926–1928.
8. Ludecke, B., P. M. Knappskog, P. T. Clayton, R. A. Surtees, J. D. Clelland, S. J. Heales, M. P. Brand, K. Bartholome, and T. Flatmark. 1996. Recessively inherited L-DOPA-responsive parkinsonism in infancy caused by a point mutation (L205P) in the tyrosine hydroxylase gene. *Hum. Mol. Genet.* 5:1023–1028.

73 Dopamine β-Hydroxylase Deficiency

Anton H. van den Meiracker
Department of Internal Medicine
Erasmus Medical Center
Rotterdam, The Netherlands

Frans Boomsma
Department of Internal Medicine
Erasmus Medical Center
Rotterdam, The Netherlands

Jaap Deinum
Department of Internal Medicine
Erasmus Medical Center
Rotterdam, The Netherlands

The syndrome of dopamine β-hydroxylase (DBH) deficiency is characterized by sympathetic noradrenergic denervation and adrenomedullary failure, but intact vagal and sympathetic cholinergic function. It is a rare congenital form of severe orthostatic hypotension, caused by complete absence of DBH, the enzyme involved in the conversion of dopamine to norepinephrine, thus resulting in absence of both norepinephrine and epinephrine.

The first two reported patients with DBH deficiency were described in 1986 and 1987 by Robertson and colleagues [1] and Man in't Veld and co-workers [2]. A total of seven patients currently have been reported: two in the United States, two in the Netherlands, two in England (siblings), and one in Australia.

CLINICAL PRESENTATION

Despite congenital sympathetic noradrenergic failure, presence of orthostatic hypotension was not documented before the age of 20 years in 6 of the 7 patients with DBH deficiency, and at age 14 in one patient. During childhood, impaired exercise tolerance, fatigue, and episodes of fainting and syncope, usually worsening after exercise, were frequently present. All patients were born after an uneventful pregnancy, although one was four weeks premature. Orthostatic hypotension worsened in late adolescence and early adulthood. As is typical of autonomic failure, symptoms are more severe in the morning hours, during hot weather, after alcohol, but, interestingly, not after food ingestion. Physical and mental development and sexual maturation are normal with DBH deficiency. Sexual function is normal in female patients; however, in male patients, ejaculation is retrograde or unachievable.

Physical examination in DBH deficiency reveals a low normal supine blood pressure and a low supine heart rate caused by unopposed cardiac vagal innervation. In the upright position, systolic blood pressure always decreases to less than 80 mmHg; but, contrary to most other types of autonomic failure, the compensatory increase in heart rate because of vagal inhibition is preserved. Pupils may be small, but they respond to light and accommodation. Sweating is normal. Of the reported seven patients with DBH deficiency, blepharoptosis is present in five, whereas hyperextensible joints and sluggish deep tendon reflexes have been reported in three, and mild weakness of facial muscles and hypotonic skeletal musculature in two patients.

DIAGNOSIS

A 5- to 10-fold increased plasma dopamine concentration (i.e., values as high as plasma norepinephrine concentration in healthy subjects), together with undetectable concentrations of plasma norepinephrine and epinephrine, is pathognomonic for DBH deficiency. These findings are reflected in low or absent urinary norepinephrine, epinephrine, and their metabolites, whereas dopamine and its degradation products homovanillic acid and 3-methoxytyramine are increased. In cerebrospinal fluid norepinephrine and epinephrine also are undetectable and dopamine is markedly increased. Although DBH, measured either as enzymatic activity or immunologically, is absent, its measurement is not suitable as a key diagnostic criterion in DBH deficiency, because extremely low DBH values, genetically determined, are present in 3 to 4% of the population. The markedly increased plasma dopamine concentration in DBH deficiency is explained by induction of tyrosine hydroxylase, the rate-limiting enzyme in the formation of norepinephrine. Most likely, loss of the inhibitory feedback of norepinephrine in sympathetic nerves accounts for this induction and explains why the concentration of L-dopa, the precursor of dopamine, also is increased. Interestingly, the increased plasma dopamine concentration in DBH deficiency responds to various physiologic and pharmacologic stimuli, as does norepinephrine in healthy subjects. Thus, in response to upright posture a twofold to threefold increase in dopamine occurs. Likewise, in response to insulin-induced hypoglycemia, infusion of tyramine (which liberates neurotransmitters from sympathetic nerve terminals), and ganglionic stimulation with edrophonium, plasma dopamine increases several times, whereas plasma norepinephrine and epinephrine remain

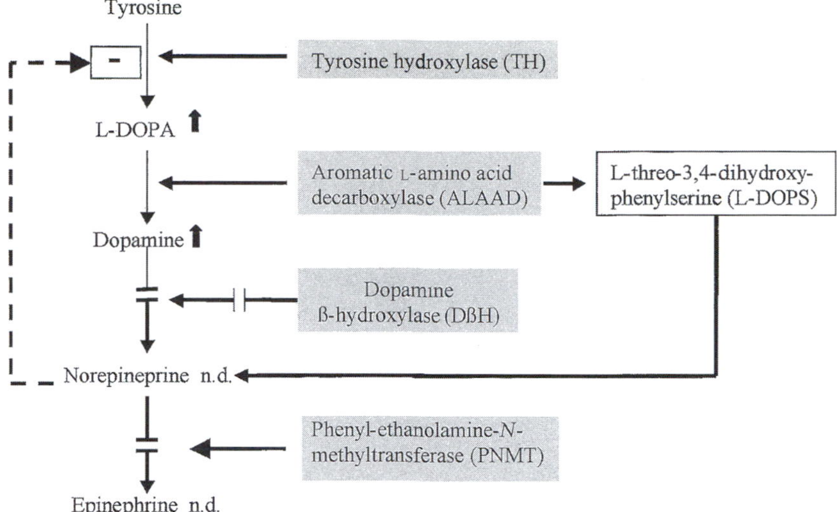

FIGURE 73.1 Biochemical consequences of dopamine β-hydroxylase (DBH) deficiency and conversion of L-threo-3,4-dihydroxyphenylserine (L-DOPS) to norepinephrine. Because of deficiency of DBH, norepinephrine and epinephrine are not formed in DBH deficiency. Loss of negative feedback of norepinephrine leads to induction of tyrosine hydroxylase, so that L-dopa and dopamine are increased. L-DOPS is converted to norepinephrine by aromatic L-amino acid decarboxylase (ALAAD), thereby bypassing DBH. n.d., not detectable; ↑, elevated.

undetectable. Conversely, a decrease in dopamine occurs in response to clonidine, a centrally acting sympatholytic agent. Microneurography, norepinephrine kinetics, and spectral analysis in one patient with DBH deficiency showed high resting nerve firing rate (2x normal) with appropriate increase during tilt, very low total-body norepinephrine spillover, and absence of low-frequency heart rate variability at rest with preservation of the respiratory-related high-frequency peak. All these observations imply that sympathetic nerves and reflex arcs are intact in DBH deficiency, but dopamine instead of norepinephrine is stored and released in sympathetic nerves. Analogous to other forms of autonomic failure, there is increased sensitivity to the hemodynamic effects of α- and β-adrenoceptor agonists in DBH deficiency, but because of complete (nor)adrenergic failure "denervation supersensitivity" is more extreme. Conversely, because of absent noradrenergic and adrenomedullary function, heart rate does not decrease in response to β-blockers and blood pressure does not decrease in response to α-blockers. As expected, heart rate increases normally in response to atropine, because parasympathetic innervation is intact.

DIFFERENTIAL DIAGNOSIS

DBH deficiency is easily differentiated from other types of autonomic insufficiency on clinical grounds (congenital orthostatic hypotension, intact cholinergic innervation) and biochemical grounds (markedly increased plasma dopamine and undetectable plasma norepinephrine and epinephrine levels). In another form of congenital orthostatic hypotension, familial dysautonomia (Riley–Day syndrome), there is combined sympathetic–parasympathetic insufficiency, as well as other neurologic abnormalities.

GENETICS

Mutations in the DBH gene causative for the lack of functioning enzyme have been reported. The two reported U.S. patients are heterozygous for an IVS1 + 2 T > C splice mutation; interestingly, this same mutation was independently found to be present in the two Dutch patients (homozygous in one). In the three heterozygous patients, four different other missense mutations have been found.

THERAPY

The treatment of choice in DBH deficiency is L-threo-3,4-dihydroxyphenylserine (DOPS), an unnatural amino acid devoid of direct pressor activity. DOPS is converted in one step into norepinephrine by aromatic L-amino acid decarboxylase (present in most tissues and in sympathetic nerves), thereby bypassing DBH. Administration of DOPS in a dose of 250 to 500 mg, twice daily, produces a moderate increase in blood pressure and a sustained dramatic relief of orthostatic symptoms, although postural hypotension is not completely cured. Plasma norepinephrine becomes detectable and plasma dopamine moderately decreases during administration of DOPS. In response to standing and tyramine infusion, plasma norepinephrine concentration increases further, indicating storage of norepinephrine in sympathetic nerves. Because in response to tyramine and standing increase in the plasma level of DOPS occurs as well, it may be that *de novo* formation of norepinephrine from DOPS takes place in the sympathetic nerves. Alternatively, norepinephrine may be formed extraneuronally and taken up by the sympathetic nerves.

In conclusion, DBH deficiency is a rare congenital cause of autonomic failure. Diagnosing DBH deficiency and differentiating it from other causes of autonomic failure is important, because with DOPS treatment almost complete relief of orthostatic symptoms is easily achievable.

References

1. Robertson, D., M. R. Goldberg, J. Ornot, A. S. Hollister, R. Wiley, J. G. Thompson, and R. M. Robertson. 1986. Isolated failure of autonomic noradrenergic neurotransmission. *N. Engl. J. Med.* 314:1494–1497.
2. Man in't Veld, A. J., F. Boomsma, P. Moleman, and M. A. D. H. Schalekamp. 1987. Congenital dopamine-beta-hydroxylase deficiency. *Lancet* i:183–188.
3. Man in't Veld, A. J., F. Boomsma, J. Lenders, A. H. van den Meiracker, C. Julien, J. Tulen, P. Moleman, T. Thien, S. Lamberts, and M. A. D. H. Schalekamp. 1988. Patients with dopamine beta-hydroxylase deficiency: A lesson in catecholamine physiology. *Am. J. Hypertens.* 1:231–238.
4. Mathias, C. J., R. B. Bannister, P. Cortelli, K. Heslop, J. M. Polack, S. Raimbach, R. Springall, and L. Watson. 1990. Clinical, autonomic and therapeutic observations in two siblings with postural hypotension and sympathetic failure due to the inability to synthesize noradrenaline from dopamine because of a deficiency of dopamine beta-hydroxylase. *Q. J. Med.* 278:617–633.
5. Biaggioni, I., D. S. Goldstein, T. Adkinson, and D. Robertson. 1990. Dopamine beta-hydroxylase deficiency in humans. *Neurology* 40: 370–373.
6. Robertson, D., V. Haile, S. E. Perry, R. M. Robertson, J. A. Phillips III, and I. Biaggioni. 1991. Dopamine beta-hydroxylase deficiency. *Hypertension* 18:1–8.
7. Thompson, J. M., C. J. O'Callaghan, B. A. Kingwell, G. W. Lambert, G. L. Jennings, and M. D. Esler. 1995. Total norepinephrine spillover, muscle sympathetic nerve activity and heart-rate spectral analysis in a patient with dopamine-beta-hydroxylase deficiency. *J. Auton. Nerv. System* 55:198–206.
8. Kim, C.-H., C. P. Zabetian, J. F. Cubells, S. Cho, I. Biaggioni, B. M. Cohen, D. Robertson, and K.-S. Kim. 2002. Mutations in the dopamine beta-hydroxylase gene are associated with human norepinephrine deficiency. *Am. J. Med. Gen.* 108:140–147.

74

Menkes Disease

Stephen G. Kaler
National Institute for Child Health and Human Development
National Institutes of Health
Bethesda, Maryland

Menkes disease is an inborn disorder of copper metabolism with multisystem ramifications. It is caused by defects in an X-chromosomal gene that encodes an intracellular copper-transporting adenosine phosphatase (ATPase). This gene product is localized to the *trans-Golgi* network and normally governs incorporation of copper into secreted copper enzymes, including dopamine β-hydroxylase (DBH). Clinical autonomic abnormalities in Menkes disease (and its allelic variants) reflect partial deficiency of this enzyme. Levels of plasma and cerebrospinal fluid (CSF) catechols influenced by DBH activity are distinctively abnormal and provide a highly sensitive and specific diagnostic marker for this disorder. In fact, plasma catechol analysis is arguably the best diagnostic test for at-risk newborns during the first month of life because other biochemical parameters are unreliable in this period and molecular analysis is less rapid. Early identification of affected infants is a fundamental requirement for successful medical intervention, underscoring the assay's importance.

EPIDEMIOLOGY

Menkes disease is a rare condition with incidence estimates ranging from 1/100,000 live births to 1/250,000 [1]. On the basis of recent annual birth rates in the United States (≈3.5 million), an estimated 15 to 30 affected babies are expected to be born in the United States each year. One third of these are predicted to be nonfamilial cases, representing new mutations [2]. The clinical and biochemical features important for the diagnosis of Menkes disease are summarized in Table 74.1.

CLINICAL PHENOTYPE

As an X-linked recessive condition, Menkes disease typically occurs in male infants who present at 2 to 3 months with loss of previously obtained developmental milestones and the onset of hypotonia, failure to thrive, and seizures. Characteristic physical changes of the hair and facies (Fig. 74.1), in conjunction with typical neurologic findings, often suggest the diagnosis. The presenting signs and symptoms of 127 patients reported in the medical literature up to 1985 have been compiled [3]. In the natural history of classical Menkes disease, death usually occurs by 3 years of age.

BIOCHEMICAL PHENOTYPE

The biochemical phenotype in Menkes disease and its variants involves the following: (1) low levels of copper in plasma, liver, and brain because of impaired intestinal absorption; (2) reduced activities of numerous copper-dependent enzymes; and (3) paradoxic accumulation of copper in certain tissues (i.e., duodenum, kidney, spleen, pancreas, skeletal muscle, and placenta). The copper-retention phenotype also is evident in cultured fibroblasts in which reduced egress of radiolabeled copper is demonstrable in pulse-chase experiments [4].

AUTONOMIC MANIFESTATIONS

Clinical Signs of Dysautonomia in Menkes Disease

Clinical features of Menkes patients attributable to DBH deficiency include temperature instability, hypoglycemia, and eyelid ptosis, autonomic abnormalities that may result from selective loss of sympathetic adrenergic function. Similar clinical problems have been described in patients with Riley–Day dysautonomia in which DBH deficiency has been documented, in patients with congenital absence of DBH [1], or both. In patients with milder variants of Menkes disease (e.g., occipital horn syndrome), in which overall neurologic functioning is greater, orthostatic hypotension and chronic diarrhea are common complaints.

Neurochemical Abnormalities

Partial deficiency of DBH is responsible for a distinctively abnormal plasma and CSF neurochemical pattern in patients with Menkes disease [5–9]. In our experience, the ratio of a proximal compound in the catecholamine biosynthetic pathway (Fig. 74.2), dihydroxyphenylalanine, to a distal metabolite dihydroxyphenyl glycol, provides a better index of DBH deficiency in patients with Menkes disease than norepinephrine (NE) levels alone. Plasma and especially CSF levels of NE, the direct product of DBH, are relatively well maintained in some patients with Menkes disease, presumably because of compensatory mechanisms. Peptidyl glycine α-amidating monooxygenase (PAM) is a copper enzyme related to DBH, which is required for removal of the carboxyl-terminal glycine residue characteristic of numerous neuroendocrine peptide precursors [1]. Failure to amidate these precursors can result in 100- to 1000-fold diminution of bioactivity compared with the mature, amidated forms. PAM deficiency may have important and wide-ranging physiologic effects that contribute to the Menkes phenotype.

Molecular Diagnosis

Rapid and robust molecular diagnosis of Menkes disease has become available [10], although this approach typically is still not as fast as neurochemical analysis.

TABLE 74.1 Diagnosis of Classical Menkes Disease

Clinical Characteristics	
Age/Sex	Birth to 1 year/male
History	Neonatal hypothermia, hypoglycemia
	Loss of early developmental milestones
	Poor weight gain
	Seizures
Physical examination	Profound hypotonia
	Abnormal hair
	Loose skin
	Pectus excavatum
Laboratory findings	
Local hospital or clinic	Serum copper <70 µg/liter*
	Serum ceruloplasmin <200 mg/liter*
	Pili torti on microscopic examination of hair
Specialized testing	Copper egress in cultures fibroblasts
	Plasma catecholamine analysis†
	Placental copper level†
	Mutation analysis†

*Unreliable in newborns during first several weeks of life.
†Rapid diagnostic test in newborns.

Treatment

Early diagnosis and institution of subcutaneous copper injections has been successful in about 20% of our cohort of infants treated within the first 2 weeks of life (n = 18). The type and severity of the underlying mutation appears to be an important factor in response to early treatment.

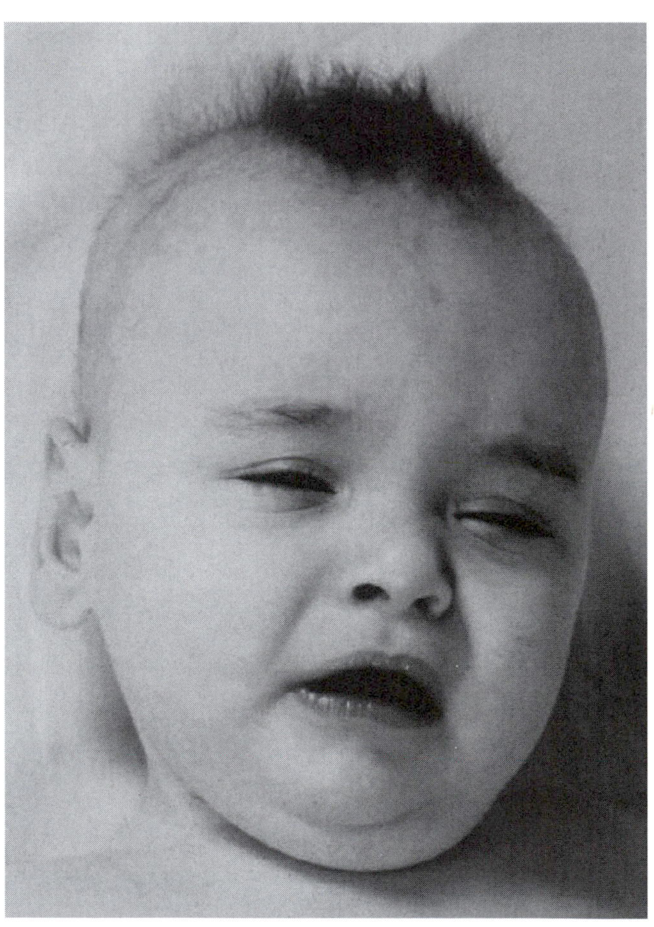

FIGURE 74.1 Menkes disease in an eight-month-old male infant. Note the abnormal hair, eyelid ptosis, and jowly facial appearance.

DBH

Dihydoxyphenylalanine (DOPA) ⇒ Dopamine (DA) ⇒⇒⇒ Norepinephrine (NE)

Dopamine (DA) ⇓ Dihydroxyphenylacetate (DOPAC)

Norepinephrine (NE) ⇓ Dihydroxyphenylglycol (DHPG)

FIGURE 74.2 Conversion of dopamine to norepinephrine by the copper-dependent enzyme dopamine β-hydroxylase (DBH) is a critical step.

References

1. Kaler, S. G. 1994. Menkes disease. In *Advances in pediatrics, Vol. 41*, ed. L. A. Barnes, 263–304. St. Louis: Mosby.
2. Haldane, J. B. S. 1935. The rate of spontaneous mutation of a human gene. *J. Genet.* 31:317–326.
3. Baerlocher, K., and D. Nadal. 1988. Das Menkes-syndrom. *Ergeb. Inn. Med. Kinderheilkd.* 57:77–144.
4. Kaler, S. G., L. K. Gallo, V. K. Proud, A. K. Percy, Y. Mark, N. A. Segal, D. S. Goldstein, C. S. Homes, and W. A. Gahl. 1994. Occipital horn syndrome and a mild Menkes phenotype associated with splice site mutations at the MNK locus. *Nat. Genet.* 8:195–202.
5. Rohmer, A., J. P. Krug, M. Mennesson, P. Mandel, G. Mack, and R. Zawislak. 1982. Maladie de Menkes: Etude de deux enzymes cupro-dependants. *Pediatrie* 32:447–456.
6. Grover, W. D., R. I. Henkin, M. Schwartz, N. Brodsky, E. Hobdell, and J. M. Stolk. 1982. A defect in catecholamine metabolism in kinky hair disease. *Ann. Neurol.* 12:263–266.
7. Hoeldtke, R. D., S. T. Cavanaugh, J. D. Hughes, K. Mattis-Graves, E. Hobdell, and W. D. Grover. 1988. Catecholamine metabolism in kinky hair disease. *Pediatr. Neurol.* 4:23–26.
8. Kaler, S. G., D. S. Goldstein, C. Holmes, J. A. Salerno, and W. A. Gahl. 1993. Plasma and cerebrospinal fluid neurochemical pattern in Menkes disease. *Ann. Neurol.* 33:171–175.
9. Kaler, S. G., C. S. Holmes, and D. S. Goldstein. 2002. Perfect sensitivity and specificity of plasma catechol analyses for neonatal diagnosis of Menkes disease. *Pediatr Res* 51(Pt 2):225A.
10. Liu, P. C., P. E. McAndrew, and S. G. Kaler. 2002. Rapid and robust screening of the Menkes disease/occipital horn syndrome gene. *Genet. Test.* 6:255–260.

75 Norepinephrine Transporter Dysfunction

Maureen K. Hahn
Center for Molecular Neuroscience
and Department of Pharmacology
Vanderbilt University Medical Center
Nashville, Tennessee

ROLE OF THE NOREPINEPHRINE TRANSPORTER

Norepinephrine (NE) is the major neurotransmitter in postganglionic sympathetic synapses and also is released at synaptic terminals of brainstem neurons that control cardiovascular function. A presynaptically localized NE transporter (NET) retrieves released NE to limit the spread and duration of synaptic excitability and allows repackaging of NE into synaptic vesicles [1]. The uptake mechanism is particularly important in the heart [2] where NET binding sites and activity show compromise in heart disease [3]. NET also is present at NE synapses in the brain, mediating functions of cognition, learning and memory, and emotions and stress responding. The importance of NET to the regulation of NE signaling and its implication in disease processes suggest that genetic variability that directs NET expression and activity contributes to individual differences in vulnerability to disease.

THE HUMAN NOREPINEPHRINE TRANSPORTER GENE

Organization of the human NET (hNET) gene suggests a susceptibility to the influence of polymorphic sequences (Fig. 75.1) [4]. hNET is a single-copy gene; thus, opportunity for compensation by other gene products in response to hNET genetic variation is limited. This is supported by studies of transgenic mice in which disruption of NET modifies behavioral and biochemical measures [5]. Furthermore, alternative splicing of exon 16 in hNET yields two protein variants that confer differing levels of transport activity in heterologous cells [6, 7]. Although evidence of *in vivo* expression of variants has yet to be demonstrated, polymorphisms that direct a favored use of one splice pattern over others pose a potential influence on hNET function.

HUMAN NOREPINEPHRINE TRANSPORTER SINGLE-NUCLEOTIDE POLYMORPHISMS

The examination of hNET genetic variation is in its infancy, with limited evidence for association of polymorphisms with disease. Single-nucleotide polymorphisms (SNPs) are the most common type of genetic variability, the most likely to contribute to disease susceptibility differences among individuals; thus, the information assembled for hNET comes mainly in the form of SNPs (Fig. 75.2) [4]. Several nonsynonymous SNPs (polymorphisms that result in the substitution of a single amino acid) were observed at frequencies of less than 0.02 and were not associated with bipolar disorder, schizophrenia, or Tourette syndrome. G155A, a synonymous polymorphism in exon 10, present at the relatively high frequency of 0.35 for the A allele, lacked association with major depression and suicidal ideation. Our laboratory has examined a group of nonsynonymous SNPs identified in a study of blood pressure variance for their effects on hNET expression and transport in transfected cells (see Fig. 75.2). This revealed both loss-of-function and gain-of-function hNET alleles that now must be explored in the context of individual patient phenotypes [8].

A457P AND ORTHOSTATIC INTOLERANCE

To increase the probability of uncovering hNET SNPs, our laboratory has focused on autonomic disturbances in which hNET dysfunction has been described. Orthostatic intolerance (OI) is a disorder characterized by an increase in standing heart rate of at least 30 beats per minute that is not accompanied by hypotension [9]. In some patients, a hyperadrenergic state characterized by increased plasma NE exists that may be caused by increased sympathetic outflow. Another way of achieving the same end-point would be dysfunction of hNET, thus preventing uptake of NE and prolonging sympathetic nervous system response. Indeed, treatment of healthy individuals with reboxetine, a selective NET blocker, recapitulates many of the salient characteristics of OI, including increased upright heart rate with a lack of a pressor response [10]. A proband with OI was identified who demonstrated features of hNET deficiency, including standing-induced increased NE spillover and decreased clearance, decreased dihydroxyphenyl glycol (DHPG) to NE ratios, and a blunted response to tyramine [11]. The proband and family members carry the heterozygous mutation, A457P (see Fig. 75.2) [12]. Although this is a rare variant

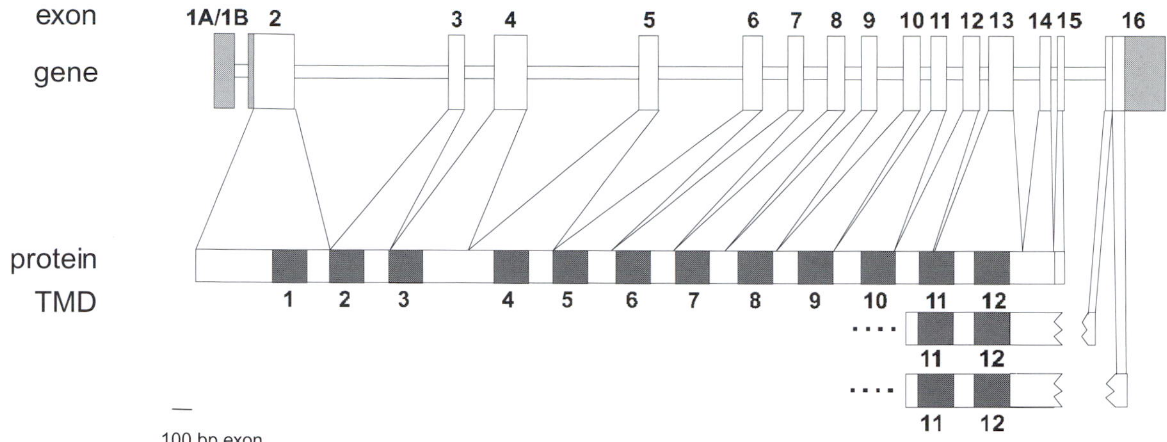

FIGURE 75.1 Exon/intron structure of the human norepinephrine transporter (hNET) gene showing the corresponding regions of the protein encoded by each exon. Untranslated regions of exons are shown in *gray* and protein transmembrane domains (TMD) are shown in *black*. The three protein variants generated by alternative splicing of the hNET gene are depicted. Scale bar = 100 base pair of exon sequence; introns are not drawn to scale.

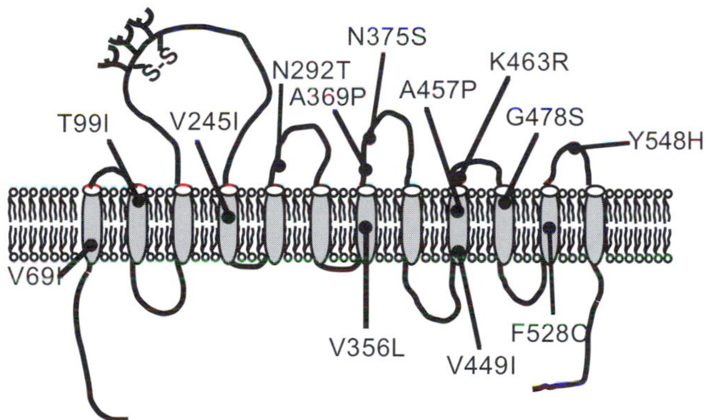

FIGURE 75.2 Human norepinephrine transporter (hNET) amino acid variants generated by nonsynonymous single-nucleotide polymorphisms (SNPs). hNET is depicted as a 12-transmembrane domain-spanning protein with intracellular N- and C-termini. The approximate positions of the variant residues are shown. The number refers to the amino acid position in the protein and is preceded by the single-letter code for the amino acid commonly at that position followed by the single-letter code for the variant. Synonymous SNPs and SNPs in introns and flanking regions are deposited at http://www.ncbi.nlm.nih.gov/SNP.

that has not been found in other kindreds, analysis of the proband's family revealed a significant correlation between A457P and increase in standing-induced heart rate and plasma NE and decreased plasma DHPG-to-NE ratio [12].

Transient transfection of A457P into heterologous expression systems revealed a protein with a near complete loss of transport activity [12] and greatly diminished cell surface expression of the mature, glycosylated form of the transporter (Fig. 75.3) [13]. Furthermore, A457P exerts a dominant negative effect on wild-type hNET uptake activity and suggests that individuals heterozygous for A457P, or other transporter polymorphisms, may be affected to a greater extent than predicted for harboring one mutant allele [13].

CONCLUSIONS

As we found for some patients with OI, other disorders with hyperadrenergic features may be contributed to by hNET polymorphisms. Altered hNET function measured in cardiovascular disease may reflect subsequent damage to the system caused by a distinct insult, but in some cases hNET polymorphisms may be one of the precipitating factors for disease. The presence of hNET regulation at synapses governing cognitive and affective processes provides potential for hNET SNPs to give rise to complex and diverse phenotypes that encompass both autonomic and psychiatric syndromes. hNET SNPs could contribute to a complex interaction between physical illnesses and mental and emotional coping. For example, outcome after heart attack is linked to depression history. Cardiovascular symptoms such as increased heart rate aid in identification of hNET dysfunction in diseases considered primarily psychiatric in nature [14]. For example, the role of NE in cognition and attention through actions in the prefrontal cortex suggests an involvement of this neurotransmitter system in attention-deficit hyperactivity disorder (ADHD). Patients with ADHD with increased standing heart rate might be more likely to harbor hNET SNPs. In this way, hNET dysfunction provides a clue to identifying hNET genetic variation in multiple complex and perhaps disparate disorders.

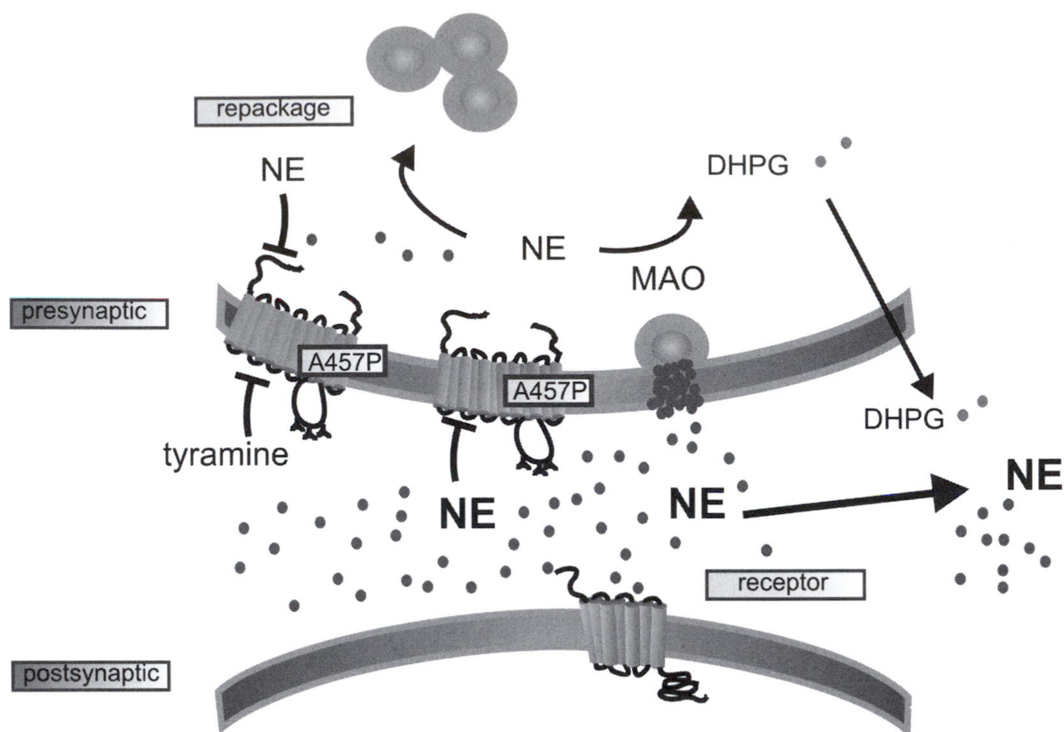

FIGURE 75.3 Schematic representation of A457P function at a noradrenergic synapse. Normally, human norepinephrine transporter (hNET) takes up released norepinephrine (NE) that once in the cytoplasm can be repackaged into exocytotic vesicles or metabolized by monoamine oxidase (MAO) to dihydroxyphenyl glycol (DHPG). Some NE escapes the reuptake process and appears in plasma (when sympathetic nerve terminals are the source of the NE). DHPG can diffuse out of the neuron and also be measured in plasma. The failure of A457P to transport NE generates greater than normal spillover and diminished clearance of NE from the plasma. The lack of uptake diminishes the flux of NE through the MAO degradation pathway and, after release of NE, plasma DHPG levels do not increase as compared with normal. Tyramine is a substrate for hNET and once inside the cell displaces NE from vesicles, thereby increasing cytoplasmic NE level and resulting in the exit of NE from the neuron through a reverse transport mechanism. Tyramine is not able to induce release of NE through reverse transport at A457P.

References

1. Iversen, L. L. 1971. Role of transmitter uptake mechanisms in synaptic neurotransmission. *Br. J. Pharmacol.* 41:571–591.
2. Esler, M. D., G. Wallin, P. K. Dorward, G. Eisenhofer, R. Westerman, I. Meredith, G. Lambert, H. S. Cox, and G. Jennings. 1991. Effects of desipramine on sympathetic nerve firing and norepinephrine spillover to plasma in humans. *Am. J. Physiol.* 260:R817–R823.
3. Bohm, M., K. La Rosee, R. H. Schwinger, and E. Erdmann. 1995. Evidence for reduction of norepinephrine uptake sites in the failing human heart. *J. Am. Coll. Cardiol.* 25:146–153.
4. Hahn, M. K., and R. D. Blakely. 2002. Gene organization and polymorphisms of monoamine transporters: Relationship to psychiatric and other complex diseases. In *Neurotransmitter transporters. Structure, function, and regulation*, ed. M. E. A. Reith, 111–169. Totowa: Humana Press.
5. Xu, F., R. R. Gainetdinov, W. C. Wetsel, S. R. Jones, L. M. Bohn, G. W. Miller, Y. M. Wang, and M. G. Caron. 2000. Mice lacking the norepinephrine transporter are supersensitive to psychostimulants. *Nat. Neurosci.* 3:465–471.
6. Kitayama, S., K. Morita, and T. Dohi. 2001. Functional characterization of the splicing variants of human norepinephrine transporter. *Neurosci. Lett.* 312:108–112.
7. Bauman, P. A., and R. D. Blakely. 2002. Determinants within the C-terminus of the human norepinephrine transporter dictate transporter trafficking, stability, and activity. *Arch. Biochem. Biophys.* 404:80–91.
8. Hahn, M. K., M. S. Mazei, D. Robertson, and R. D. Blakely. 2000. Role of human norepinephrine transporter gene single nucleotide polymorphisms in cardiovascular disease. *Am. J. Med. Genet.* 67: 369.
9. Robertson, D. 1999. The epidemic of orthostatic tachycardia and orthostatic intolerance. *Am. J. Med. Sci.* 317:75–77.
10. Schroeder, C., J. Tank, M. Boschmann, A. Diedrich, A. M. Sharma, I. Biaggioni, F. C. Luft, and J. Jordan. 2002. Selective norepinephrine reuptake inhibition as a human model of orthostatic intolerance. *Circulation* 105:347–353.
11. Jacob, G., J. R. Shannon, F. Costa, R. Furlan, I. Biaggioni, R. Mosqueda-Garcia, R. M. Robertson, and D. Robertson. 1999. Abnormal norepinephrine clearance and adrenergic receptor sensitivity in idiopathic orthostatic intolerance. *Circulation* 99:1706–1712.
12. Shannon, J. R., N. L. Flattem, J. Jordan, G. Jacob, B. K. Black, I. Biaggioni, R. D. Blakely, and D. Robertson. 2000. Clues to the origin of orthostatic intolerance: A genetic defect in the cocaine and antidepressant sensitive norepinephrine transporter. *N. Engl. J. Med.* 342:541–549.
13. Hahn, M. K., D. Robertson, and R. D. Blakely. 2003. A mutation in the human norepinephrine transporter gene (SLC6A2) associated with orthostatic intolerance disrupts surface expression of mutant and wild-type transporters. *J. Neurosci.* 23:4470–4478.
14. Blakely, R. D. 2001. Physiological genomics of antidepressant targets: Keeping the periphery in mind. *J. Neurosci.* 21:8319–8323.

76 Monoamine Oxidase Deficiency

Jacques W. M. Lenders
Department of Internal Medicine
St. Radboud University Medical Center
Nijmegen, The Netherlands

Graeme Eisenhofer
Clinical Neurocardiology Section
National Institutes of Neurological Disorders and Stroke
National Institutes of Health
Bethesda, Maryland

Monoamine oxidase A (MAO-A) and B (MAO-B) catalyze the oxidative deamination of biogenic monoamines. Both mitochondrial isoenzymes are widely expressed among tissues, but some cell types selectively express MAO-B (platelets) and others express MAO-A (skin fibroblasts, catecholaminergic neurons). The two isoenzymes share 70% homology in amino acid sequence and are encoded by two distinct genes with adjacent locations on the human X chromosome (Xp11.23).

The genes encoding MAO-A and MAO-B are located close to the gene for Norrie disease (ND). Exclusive deletion of the ND gene results in X-linked congenital blindness and, in 30 to 50% of patients, progressive hearing loss and mild mental retardation. Several patients have been described with a contiguous chromosomal deletion of MAO-A, MAO-B, and ND genes resulting in a clinical syndrome characterized by severe mental retardation, seizures, hypotonic crises, impaired somatic growth, and altered peripheral autonomic function. Loss of MAO-A and MAO-B activity was reflected neurochemically by severely reduced plasma and urinary concentrations of catecholamine deaminated metabolites, including dihydroxyphenyl glycol (DHPG), the deaminated metabolite of norepinephrine and epinephrine. In contrast, concentrations of the O-methylated metabolites, normetanephrine and metanephrine, were increased. Thus, ratios of plasma normetanephrine to DHPG, which are increased by more than 1000-fold, provide a useful marker for the deficiency (Fig. 76.1). Also increased are platelet contents of 5-hydroxytryptamine and urinary concentrations of phenylethylamine (PE), the respective substrates of MAO-A and MAO-B.

In 1993, a family with X-linked selective and complete MAO-A deficiency was described. The clinical phenotype involved borderline mental retardation and impaired impulse control, including stress-induced aggressive behavior. Carrier female subjects of this syndrome appeared phenotypically normal. The responsible point mutation consisted of a single base pair substitution in the MAO-A gene that introduced a stop codon leading to complete loss of MAO-A activity. The neurochemical phenotype closely resembled that in patients with deletion of both MAO-A and MAO-B genes. In particular, ratios of plasma normetanephrine to DHPG were substantially increased, although less so than in patients with the combined MAO-AB deficiency (see Fig. 76.1). The distinguishing feature in patients with selective MAO-A deficiency was normal urinary PE excretion. The frequency of this mutation must be extremely rare because currently no other patients with selective MAO-A deficiency have been described.

Two patients have been identified with deletions of MAO-B and ND genes, but with the MAO-A gene intact. These subjects showed the usual clinical features of ND and were of normal intelligence and without behavioral abnormalities. The neurochemical phenotype was similarly mild with normal levels of serotonin (5-HT), catecholamines, and catecholamine metabolites, but with increased urinary levels of PE.

The above clinical observations of MAO-A and MAO-B deficiency states closely agree with observations in MAO-A and MAO-B knockout mice. MAO-A knockout mice demonstrated aggressive behavior, probably related to impaired metabolic degradation of 5-HT. These mice showed significantly increased 5-HT levels in several brain areas and architectural alterations in the somatosensory cortex. Both phenomena were reversed by postnatal administration of a 5-HT synthesis inhibitor. As expected from the human findings, MAO-B–deficient mice showed little or only mild phenotypic changes, with the main neurochemical abnormality being increased PE levels.

From the above data, it is clear that MAO-A and MAO-B do not share equal or complementary capacities for the deamination of biogenic monoamines. In particular, catecholamines, including dopamine, are metabolized *in vivo* mainly if not exclusively by MAO-A. Apart from different affinities for monoamine substrate, the importance of MAO-A for catecholamine metabolism likely reflects selective expression of MAO-A in catecholaminergic neurons, the cellular compartment where most catecholamine deamination takes place.

Several polymorphisms of MAO-A or MAO-B genes have been described. Some studies report positive relations between MAO-A polymorphisms and psychiatric or

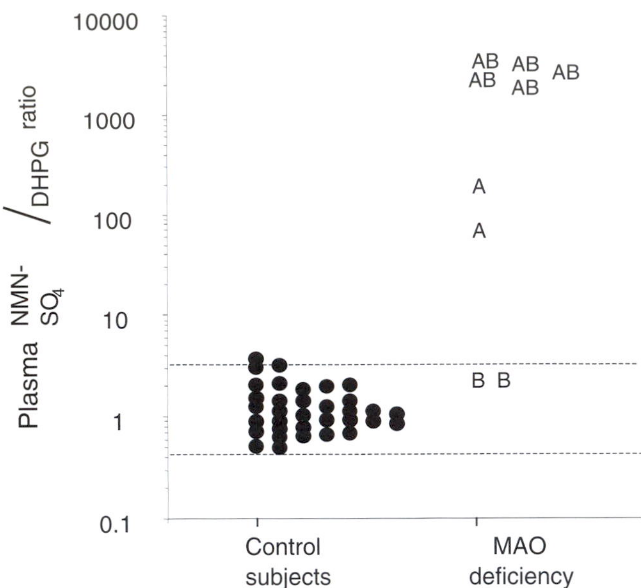

FIGURE 76.1 Plasma normetanephrine to dihydroxyphenyl glycol (DHPG) ratios in control subjects, in two patients with monoamine oxidase A (MAO-A) deficiency (*A*), in two patients with MAO-B deficiency (*B*), and in five patients with MAO-AB deficiency (*AB*). The *dashed lines* represent the 2.5 and 97.5 percentile values of the control subjects. Plasma normetanephrine was measured as the sulfate-conjugated metabolite.

neurologic conditions, including alcoholism, affective disorders, panic disorder, stress-induced aggression, and Parkinson's disease. No study suggests any link of MAO-B polymorphisms to a specific behavioral phenotype. It remains unclear whether any of the reported polymorphisms are of functional significance to monoamine metabolism, as reflected by altered plasma or urinary levels of monoamine metabolites, particularly ratios of plasma normetanephrine to DHPG.

References

1. Kochersperger, L. M., E. L. Parker, M. Siciliano, G. J. Darlington, and R. M. Denney. 1986. Assignment of genes for human monoamine oxidases A and B to the X-chromosome. *J. Neurosci.* 16:601–616.
2. Weyler, W., Y.-P. P. Hsu, and X. O. Breakefield. 1990. Biochemistry and genetics of monoamine-oxidase. *Pharmacol. Ther.* 47:391–417.
3. Murphy, D. L., K. B. Sims, F. Karoum, A. de la Chapelle, R. Norio, E.-M. Sankila, and X. O. Breakefield. 1990. Marked amine and amine metabolite changes in Norrie disease patients with an X-chromosomal deletion affecting monoamine oxidase. *J. Neurochem.* 54:242–247.
4. Brunner, H. G., M. R. Nelen, P. van Zandvoort, N. G. G. M. Abeling, A. H. van Gennip, E. C. Wolters, M. A. Kuiper, H. H. Ropers, and B. A. van Oost. 1993. X-linked borderline mental retardation with prominent behavioral disturbance: Phenotype, genetic localization, and evidence for disturbed monoamine metabolism. *Am. J. Hum. Genet.* 52:1032–1039.
5. Brunner, H. G., M. Nelen, X. O. Breakefield, H. H. Ropers, and B. A. van Oost. 1993. Abnormal behavior associated with a point mutation in the structural gene for monoamine oxidase A. *Science* 262:578–580.
6. Berry, M. D., A. V. Juorio, and I. A. Paterson. 1994. The functional role of monoamine oxidases A and B in the mammalian central nervous system. *Progr. Neurobiol.* 42:375–391.
7. Cases, O., I. Seif, J. Grimsby, P. Gaspar, K. Chen, S. Pournin, U. Müller, M. Aguet, C. Babinet, J. C. Shih, and E. De Maeyer. 1995. Aggressive behavior and altered amounts of brain 5-HT and norepinephrine in mice lacking MAO-A. *Science* 268:1763–1766.
8. Lenders, J. W. M., G. Eisenhofer, N. G. G. M. Abeling, W. Berger, D. L. Murphy, C. H. Konings, L. M. Bleeker Wagemakers, I. J. Kopin, F. Karoum, A. H. van Gennip, and H. G. Brunner. 1996. Specific genetic deficiencies of the A and B isoenzymes of monoamine oxidase are characterized by distinct neurochemical and clinical phenotypes. *J. Clin. Invest.* 97:1–10.
9. Shih, J. C., and M. J. Ridd. 1999. Monoamine oxidase: From genes to behavior. *Ann. Rev. Neurosci.* 22:197–217.
10. Shih, J. C., and R. F. Thompson. 1999. Psychiatric genetics '99. Monoamine oxidase in neuropsychiatry and behavior. *Am. J. Hum. Genet.* 65:593–598.

PART IX

CENTRAL AUTONOMIC DISORDERS

77

Parkinson's Disease

Thomas L. Davis
Department of Neurology
Vanderbilt University
Nashville, Tennessee

Parkinson's disease (PD) is a common idiopathic neurodegenerative disorder that affects an estimated 1% of the population older than 65 years. The cardinal features of PD are resting tremor, bradykinesia, rigidity, and loss of postural reflexes. Signs and symptoms of altered autonomic dysfunction also are frequently present even early in the disease course [1] (Table 77.1).

PD results from a loss of pigmented, dopaminergic nerve cells within the substantia nigra that project to the striatum (putamen and caudate). The diagnosis is made clinically and confirmed only at autopsy when the substantia nigra shows a visible loss of pigment on gross inspection and a markedly reduced population of neurons containing intracytoplasmic inclusions (Lewy bodies) on histologic examination. Lewy bodies, sometimes associated with neuronal loss, may also be found in the preganglionic structures of the sympathetic and parasympathetic nervous system. Shy–Drager syndrome, or multiple system atrophy, characterized by autonomic failure plus parkinsonism or cerebellar ataxia may mimic PD especially early in disease. This difficulty in making a correct early diagnosis complicates any study of the incidence of autonomic failure in PD.

CARDIAC SYMPATHETIC DENERVATION

There is increasing evidence that loss of functional cardiac sympathetic nerve terminals may contribute to the orthostatic hypotension (OH) seen in some patients with PD. To determine the frequency of cardiac sympathetic denervation in PD, Goldstein and colleagues [2] studied 29 patients with PD, 24 patients with multiple system atrophy, 7 patients with pure autonomic failure, 33 control subjects with episodic or persistent orthostatic intolerance without sympathetic neurocirculatory failure, and 19 healthy volunteers [2]. Of the 29 patients with Parkinson disease, 9 with and 11 without sympathetic neurocirculatory failure had low septal 6-[^{18}F]fluorodopamine–derived radioactivity. All six patients with Parkinson disease and decreased 6-[^{18}F]fluorodopamine–derived radioactivity who underwent right heart catheterization had a decreased cardiac extraction fraction of [^{3}H]norepinephrine and virtually no cardiac norepinephrine spillover or venous-arterial increments in plasma levels of dihydroxyphenyl glycol and L-dopa. These findings were unrelated to disease duration, disease severity, or L-dopa treatment and suggest that loss of catecholamine innervation in PD occurs in the sympathetic nervous system in the heart.

TESTS OF SYMPATHETIC FUNCTION

Sympathetic skin responses (SSRs) represent a function of sympathetic sudomotor fibers. Results of studies of SSR in PD have been mixed but suggest that they are abnormal in a minority (0–14%) of patients with PD [3, 4]. Abnormal SSR correlated with duration of disease and with impotence. The abnormality of SSR seen in PD may be caused by intermediolateral column dysfunction. Abnormalities in blood pressure responses to handgrip and standing also have been found in patients with PD as compared with control subjects.

TESTS OF PARASYMPATHETIC FUNCTION

R-R interval variation is primarily indicative of the parasympathetic function of the vagus nerve. Most studies have found mild parasympathetic function in a minority of patients with PD. Spectral analysis of 24-hour ambulatory electrocardiogram have shown that the degree of parasympathetic function correlates with the severity of hypokinesia [5].

ORTHOSTATIC HYPOTENSION

Symptomatic OH may be present as a primary part of PD or as a complication of medications or inactivity [6]. All dopaminergic drugs used to treat PD may exacerbate OH and should be initiated slowly to minimize this effect. Supine hypertension is uncommon in PD and its presence combined with a lack of response to L-dopa suggests the diagnosis of Shy–Drager syndrome. In addition to the general symptomatic measures used to treat OH, the periph-

TABLE 77.1 Autonomic Symptoms in Parkinson's Disease

Bladder dysfunction
Constipation
Dysphagia/drooling
Heat/cold intolerance
Syncope/near syncope
Seborrhea
Sexual dysfunction
Weight loss

eral decarboxylase inhibitor carbidopa (Lodosyn) or the peripheral dopamine antagonist domperidone (Motilium) may be added to a patient's regimen to decrease the peripheral effects of dopamine. Among the available drugs, α_1-adrenergic agonists (mainly midodrine) or plasma volume expanders (mainly fludrocortisone) are the most frequently used [7].

CONSTIPATION

Constipation is eventually seen in almost all patients with PD and is the chief complaint in some cases. The exact mechanism of the constipation remains unknown, but increased transit time probably plays a major role. The antimuscarinic effects of the anticholinergic medications used to treat parkinsonian tremor may also exacerbate constipation. Initially, symptoms may respond to additional dietary fiber and stool softeners, but many patients eventually require a daily bowel regimen that includes an osmotic laxative such as lactulose.

DYSPHAGIA

Dysphagia is seen as a prominent symptom in some patients with PD, usually as part of end-stage disease. It typically occurs earlier in the course of other parkinsonian syndromes such as multiple system atrophy and progressive supranuclear palsy. Although swallowing may improve with dopaminergic therapy, dysphagia is a symptom that is relatively resistant to medication. Anticholinergics lead to drying of the oral mucosa and may make swallowing more difficult. When anticholinergics are necessary for control of parkinsonism, artificial saliva may be used. Some patients may also benefit from a change in diet or speech therapy consultation for swallowing training.

DROOLING

Drooling is a common late manifestation of the disease. Because saliva production is normal, drooling probably arises from the poverty of automatic swallowing. It would therefore be regarded as caused by hypokinesia, a cardinal motor feature, rather than a strictly autonomic manifestation. Use of sugarless gum or hard candy may stimulate swallowing and decrease drooling. It may also respond somewhat to L-dopa. Some investigators have recommend treatment with a peripheral-acting anticholinergic such as propantheline. Direct injection of small amounts of botulinum toxin directly into the salivary glands has been used to treat disabling drooling [8]. Others have suggested that administration of antimuscarinics may further impair swallowing by increasing the viscosity of the saliva.

SEXUAL FUNCTION

Increasing information is becoming available regarding sexual function in PD [9, 10]. A majority of patients report that sexual frequency is less than before they had PD. A decrease in sexual interest was seen in 83% of men and 84% of women. Almost 80% of men were unable to ejaculate, and the majority of women report a decreased frequency of orgasm since the parkinsonism. These changes are not felt to be solely caused by depression. Although dopaminergic medications have been reported to lead to hypersexuality, this is rarely seen. Conversely, these medications are one of the few families of medication not reported to impair sexual function. Erectile dysfunction in men may respond to the use of a vacuum device, papaverine injections, or penile prosthesis. Phosphodiesterase-5 inhibitors may also be effective but should be used with caution in those with OH.

BLADDER DYSFUNCTION

Surveys have suggested that the majority of patients with PD have some degree of bladder dysfunction [9]. This is usually irritative symptomatology caused by involuntary bladder contraction, but obstructive symptoms may also be present. Because the pontine micturition center is spared, these patients have coordinated voiding. Formal urodynamics may be necessary to exclude a coexisting obstructive disorder such as prostatism. Anticholinergics (oxybutynin or tolterodine) may be used to help control symptoms if obstruction is not documented.

References

1. Awerbuch, G. I., and R. Sandyk. 1992. Autonomic functions in the early stages of Parkinson's disease. *Intern. J. Neurosci.* 64:7–14.
2. Goldstein, D. S., C. Holmes, S. T. Li, S. Bruce, L. V. Metman, and R. O. Cannon, III. 2000. Cardiac sympathetic denervation in Parkinson disease. *Ann. Intern. Med.* 133:382–384.
3. De Marinis, M., F. Stocchi, B. Gregori, and N. Accornero. 2000. Sympathetic skin response and cardiovascular autonomic function tests in

Parkinson's disease and multiple system atrophy with autonomic failure. *Mov. Disord.* 15(6):1215–1220.

4. Wang, S. J., J. L. Fuh, D. E. Shan, K. K. Liao, K. P. Lin, C. P. Tsai, and Z. A. Wu. 1993. Sympathetic skin response and R-R interval variation in Parkinson's disease. *Mov. Dis.* 8:151–157.
5. Haapaniemi, T. H., V. Pursiainen, J. T. Korpelainen, H. V. Huikuri, K. A. Sotaniemi, and V. V. Myllyla. 2001. Ambulatory ECG and analysis of heart rate variability in Parkinson's disease. *J. Neurol. Neurosurg. Psychiatry* 70:305–310.
6. Senard, J. M., C. Brefel-Courbon, O. Rascol, and J. L. Montastruc. 2001. Orthostatic hypotension in patients with Parkinson's disease: Pathophysiology and management. *Drugs Aging* 18:495–505.
7. Robertson, D., and T. L. Davis. 1995. Recent advances in the treatment of orthostatic hypotension. *Neurology* 45(Suppl 4):S26–S32.
8. Fang, J., and T. L. Davis. 2002. Botulinum toxin type B for drooling. *Mov. Disord.* 17:S192.
9. Sakakibara, R., H. Shinotoh, T. Uchiyama, M. Sakuma, M. Kashiwado, M. Yoshiyama, and T. Hattori. 2001. Questionnaire-based assessment of pelvic organ dysfunction in Parkinson's disease. *Auton. Neurosci.* 92:76–85.
10. Koller, W. C., B. Vetere-Overfield, A. Williamson, K. Busenbark, J. Nash, and D. Parrish. 1990. Sexual dysfunction in Parkinson's disease. *Clin. Neuropharm.* 13:461–463.
11. Goldstein, D. S. 2003. Dysautonomia in Parkinson's disease: Neurological abnormalities. *Lancet Neurol* 2:669–676.

78

Multiple System Atrophy

Niall Quinn
Sobell Department of Motor Neuroscience and Movement Disorders
Institute of Neurology
London, United Kingdom

Multiple system atrophy (MSA) is a progressive sporadic degenerative disease of the central and autonomic nervous system of unknown cause. Clinically, it manifests as a motor disorder, incorporating parkinsonism or (less frequently) cerebellar or pyramidal features, together with urogenital or cardiovascular autonomic involvement. Pathologically, it involves cell loss and gliosis, in varying combinations, principally in the striatum (mainly putamen), substantia nigra, locus ceruleus, inferior olives, pontine nuclei, cerebellum, and the intermediolateral columns and Onuf's nucleus in the spinal cord. In most of these areas, characteristic oligodendroglial cytoplasmic inclusions (GCIs) are seen, which stain for α-synuclein.

HISTORY, NOSOLOGY, EPIDEMIOLOGY, DEMOGRAPHICS, AND PROGNOSIS

History and Nosology

Cases of MSA have been reported variously as "*olivopontocerebellar degeneration*" or atrophy (OPCA), as Shy–Drager syndrome (SDS) [1], and as "*striatonigral degeneration*" (SND). In 1969, Graham and Oppenheimer [2] first introduced the umbrella term *multiple system atrophy*. It was later emphasized that the combination of parkinsonism and autonomic failure could be caused either by MSA or by Lewy body pathology. The term progressive autonomic failure became frequently attached to descriptions of MSA, but almost imperceptibly the abbreviation PAF then came to be used to signify pure autonomic failure, an even rarer disorder usually associated with Lewy body pathology. Many authors also lumped together genetic with sporadic forms of OPCA or spinocerebellar ataxia (SCA); consequently, chaos reigned. It gradually became apparent that sporadic OPCA (sOPCA) should be considered separately—patients had later onset than hereditary OPCA/SCA cases, their course was more aggressive, and autonomic failure was virtually universal. Later, the term idiopathic late-onset cerebellar ataxia (ILOCA) was introduced for patients with sporadic adult-onset cerebellar ataxia in whom other known causes had been excluded. Currently, genetic testing for various SCAs has reduced this pool, and the most recent estimates are that about 30% of idiopathic late-onset cerebellar ataxia cases will turn out to have MSA.

In 1989, Papp and colleagues [3] described the presence of abundant argyrophilic GCIs in a series of cases clinically labeled as sOPCA, SDS, or SND, which provided a pathologic rationale for "lumping" such cases under the term MSA. In 1998, these inclusions, which are not present in hereditary OPCA/SCA cases, were shown to contain α-synuclein.

Recently, the terms sOPCA, SDS, and SND have largely been jettisoned in favor of describing cases of MSA according to their predominant motor disorder—cerebellar (MSA-C) or parkinsonian (MSA-P).

Epidemiology

The population prevalence of MSA has been estimated at 4/100,000, although with wide confidence intervals. In most reported series, MSA-P cases predominate compared with MSA-C in a ratio of about 4 : 1; however, a few series from "cerebellar" units, and also a large series from Japan, have reported the converse.

Demographics and Prognosis

The incidence regarding sex is approximately equal. No proven case has had onset earlier than age 30 years, the mean age at onset is about 53 years, and onset after age 70 years is uncommon.

The disease is relentlessly progressive and significantly shortens life expectancy. Survival from first symptom (autonomic or motor) averaged 9 to 10 years in one large clinical series [4], but is shorter in pathologic series.

CLINICAL FEATURES

Core clinical features used in published diagnostic criteria include parkinsonism (usually poorly levodopa-responsive), cerebellar features, pyramidal signs, and urogenital (male erectile dysfunction, incontinence, incomplete bladder emptying and retention) and cardiovascular autonomic (particularly orthostatic hypotension) dysfunction.

The parkinsonism is just as often asymmetric as in Parkinson's disease (PD), and although accompanied by a tremor in two thirds of cases (usually irregular and postural/action), less than 10% of cases display a classical pill-rolling tremor of the hands. Frank pyramidal weakness, or a scissors gait, is not seen.

Other clinical features ("red flags") commonly occur and may help to point toward a clinical diagnosis of MSA. These include the frequent, and early, occurrence of rapid eye movement–associated behavior disorder (RBD), the presence of sleep apnea, increased snoring, nocturnal or daytime stridor, inspiratory sighs, contractures, disproportionate antecollis or truncal deviation (Pisa syndrome), myoclonic jerks of the fingers, cold violaceous extremities, sweating disturbances, and emotional incontinence.

CLINICAL DIAGNOSTIC CRITERIA

Quinn [5, 6] introduced the first clinical diagnostic criteria for MSA. These were later operationalized in the (more complex) Consensus Criteria formulated by Gilman and colleagues [7]. A clinicopathologic study in the Queen Square Brain Bank for Neurological Disorders showed a low (13%) rate of false-positive, but an earlier study showed a considerably greater (up to 55%) rate of false-negative, diagnosis in life.

DIFFERENTIAL DIAGNOSIS

The commonest cause for misdiagnoses of MSA in life is PD. Cases of progressive supranuclear palsy (PSP), corticobasal degeneration, and cerebrovascular disease, particularly when it coexists with PD, can sometimes be difficult to differentiate. When the presentation is mainly cerebellar, other conditions entering into the differential diagnosis are SCAs 1, 2, 3, and 6 with an apparently negative family history, late-onset Friedreich's ataxia, and demyelinating disease, especially primary progressive multiple sclerosis.

PARACLINICAL INVESTIGATIONS

MRI may reveal supratentorially putaminal atrophy, posterior putaminal hypointensity or a hyperintense rim at the lateral putaminal border, and infratentorially cerebellar and pontine atrophy, a hyperintense "hot-cross bun" appearance in the pons, and hyperintensity of the middle cerebellar peduncles [8]. However, a normal scan, especially early in the disease course, does not rule out the diagnosis, a "hot-cross bun" may also be seen in SCAs 1 and 3, and pontine atrophy in SCA2. MR spectroscopy tends to show reduced *N*-acetyl aspartate signal in the lentiform nucleus, but this is not specific in individual patients. ^{18}F-fluorodopa positron emission tomography (PET), or dopamine transporter single photon emission computed tomography (SPECT), scans can not reliably distinguish among PD, MSA, and PSP [8]. Reduced D2 receptor binding in striatum on ^{11}C-raclopride PET or IBZM-SPECT may suggest postsynaptic parkinsonism in L-dopa naive patients, but it is much less helpful in treated cases because of down-regulation of postsynaptic D2 receptors by levodopa treatment. Clearcut striatal hypometabolism on ^{18}F-FDG PET scanning argues against PD. The cardiac sympathetic defect in the Lewy body diseases PD and PAF is classically preganglionic, whereas that in MSA is postganglionic. Thus, if cardiac scintigraphy with 123-I-metaiodobenzylguanidine, a precursor of noradrenaline, reveals a clear deficit, Lewy body pathology is much more likely. Conventional cardiovascular autonomic function tests can demonstrate autonomic failure, but not whether it is caused by Lewy body pathology or by MSA [9]. Recordings of urethral and anal sphincter electromyogram may be more helpful. Thus, loss of specialized anterior horn cell neurons in MSA (and also PSP) leads to denervation and reinnervation of the striatal external sphincter muscles, manifesting as increased amplitude, polyphasia, and duration of sphincter muscle potentials. This can be diagnostically helpful provided a number of potential pitfalls are avoided [10]. The growth hormone response to a brief intravenous clonidine infusion is impaired in MSA, but also in some cases with PD. Currently, it appears that a normal response argues against MSA, but that a defective response cannot distinguish between MSA and PD.

MANAGEMENT

It is important to make a definitive diagnosis. Unfortunately, especially early in the disease course, this may not yet be possible, and the diagnosis may need to be reviewed at intervals.

If parkinsonism is prominent, a trial of a levodopa preparation is required. If this causes unacceptable side effects, for example, dystonias/dyskinesias, a trial of a dopamine agonist may be warranted. About 20% of patients benefit from amantadine. There is no effective medical treatment for the cerebellar symptoms. Spasticity and myoclonus rarely need treatment with baclofen, or clonazepam or valproate, respectively. RBD may be helped by clonazepam. Breathing disorders may require continuous positive airway pressure, vocal cord lateralization, or tracheostomy. Emotional incontinence can be helped by selective serotonin reuptake inhibitors or tricyclics. Male erectile dysfunction may be helped by sildenafil, but this can aggravate postural hypotension. Detrusor hyperexcitability can be helped by a peripherally acting anticholinergic such as oxybutynin; but if the residual volume is more than 100 ml, intermittent self-catheterization may also be needed.

For many patients, paramedical intervention—physiotherapy, occupational therapy (including a home visit), speech therapy (including attention to swallowing difficulty) social work, and an expert wheelchair clinic assessment—may give most benefit. Patient organizations such as the Shy–Drager Syndrome/Multiple System Atrophy Support Group (www.shy-drager.com) and the Sarah Matheson Trust for MSA (www.msaweb.co.uk) can provide information and support. In the later stages of the disease, outreach and inpatient care from hospice/palliative care facilities can be invaluable.

References

1. Shy, G. M., and G. A. Drager. 1960. A neurological syndrome associated with orthostatic hypotension. *Arch. Neurol.* 2:511–527.
2. Graham, J. G., and D. R. Oppenheimer. 1969. Orthostatic hypotension and nicotine sensitivity in a case of multiple system atrophy. *J. Neurol. Neurosurg. Psychiatry* 32:28–34.
3. Papp, M. I., J. E. Kahn, and P. L. Lantos. 1989. Glial cytoplasmic inclusions in the CNS of patients with multiple system atrophy (striatonigral degeneration, olivopontocerebellar atrophy and Shy Drager syndrome). *J. Neurol. Sci.* 94:79–100.
4. Wenning, G. K., Y. Ben-Shlomo, M. Magalhaes, S. E. Daniel, and N. P. Quinn. 1994. Clinical features and natural history of multiple system atrophy: An analysis of 100 cases. *Brain* 117:835–845.
5. Quinn, N. 1989. Multiple system atrophy: The nature of the beast. *J. Neurol. Neurosurg. Psychiatry* Jun(Suppl):78–89.
6. Quinn, N. 1994. Multiple system atrophy. In *BIMR Neurology, Vol. 12, Movement Disorders 3*, ed. C. D. Marsden and S. Fahn, 256–275. London: Butterworth-Heinemann.
7. Gilman, S., P. A. Low, N. Quinn, A. Albanese, Y. Ben-Shlomo, C. J. Fowler, H. Kaufmann, T. Klockgether, A. E. Lang, P. L. Lantos, I. Litvan, C. J. Mathias, E. Oliver, D. Robertson, I. Schatz, and G. K. Wenning. 1999. Consensus statement on the diagnosis of multiple system atrophy. *J. Neurol. Sci.* 163:94–98.
8. Wenning, G. K., and N. P. Quinn, eds. 1997. Multiple system atrophy. In *Baillière's clinical neurology, Vol. 6*, 187–200. London: Bailliere Tindall.
9. Riley, D. E., and T. C. Chelimsky. 2003. Autonomic nervous system testing may not distinguish multiple system atrophy from Parkinson's disease. *J. Neurol. Neurosurg. Psychiatry* 74:56–60.
10. Vodusek, D. B. 2001. Sphincter EMG and differential diagnosis of multiple system atrophy. *Mov. Disord.* 16:600–607.

79

Dementia with Lewy Bodies

Gregor K. Wenning
Movement Disorders Section
Department of Neurology
University Hospital
Innsbruck, Austria

Michaela Stampfer
Movement Disorders Section
Department of Neurology
University Hospital
Innsbruck, Austria

CLINICAL ASPECTS AND DIFFERENTIAL DIAGNOSIS

Dementia with Lewy bodies (DLB) represents a still somewhat controversial entity defined by coexistent parkinsonism and progressive cognitive decline accompanied by spontaneous recurrent visual hallucinations and conspicuous fluctuations in alertness and cognitive performance [1]. Affected patients at postmortem examination show numerous Lewy bodies in many parts of the cerebral cortex, particularly neocortical and limbic areas, in addition to the nigral Lewy body degeneration characteristic for Parkinson's disease (PD). Progressive cognitive decline with particular deficits of visuospatial ability and frontal executive function is accompanied by usually only mildly to moderately severe parkinsonism, which is often akinetic–rigid without the classical parkinsonian rest tremor. Recurrent visual hallucinations may occur without exposure to dopaminergic antiparkinsonian agents. Marked diurnal fluctuations in cognitive performance have been the most difficult to define feature of the disease but are often conspicuous to the environment. Current consensus restricts a diagnosis of DLB only to patients with parkinsonism who experience development of dementia within 12 months of the onset of motor symptoms. Patients with PD who experience development of dementia after 12 months of motor onset should be labeled PD dementia (PDD). Whether DLB and PDD are distinct neuropathologically remains a matter of controversy. To improve the differential diagnosis of DLB, consensus criteria have been developed that establish possible and probable levels of diagnostic accuracy [2, 3]. In a prospective validation study these criteria have shown good sensitivity and specificity [2]. Supportive features of DLB according to the criteria developed by McKeith include syncope. Symptomatic orthostatic hypotension (OH) (including syncope) occurs in up to 30% of patients with DLB [1, 4], sometimes as the presenting feature [5]. Syncope may also result from carotid sinus hypersensitivity, which appears to be more common in DLB than Alzheimer disease [6]. Dysautonomic features in DLB may also include urogenital disturbance [4].

PRACTICAL MANAGEMENT

Management of patients with DLB has to be based on a multidimensional approach taking into account the cognitive decline and dementia that form the core clinical syndrome, the characteristic hallucinations and visual delusions present in a majority of cases, as well as in dementia-associated behavioral symptoms and depression. Furthermore, parkinsonism is a therapeutic issue in these patients as are symptoms and signs of autonomic dysfunction and, not infrequently, sleep disorders like rapid eye movement (REM)–associated behavior disorder (RBD).

DEMENTIA

On the basis of one randomized placebo-controlled trial, rivastigmine can be considered efficacious in improving cognitive function and psychotic behavior in DLB [7]. Dosages range between 3 and 12 mg/day with a usual mean target dose close to 10 mg. Main side effects are gastrointestinal with nausea and vomiting, and there is generally no negative impact on motor symptoms. Donepezil, although not tested in randomized controlled fashion, is also likely efficacious in a similar way as rivastigmine. Donepezil is started as a dosage of 5 mg/day and can be increased to 10 mg/day. Side effects are similar to rivastigmine. Tacrine has been poorly studied in DLB and, because of its worse safety profile compared with rivastigmine and donepezil, is not generally recommended.

HALLUCINATIONS AND PSYCHOSIS

Visual hallucinations, delusions, and psychotic behavior may improve when patients with DLB are put on cholinesterase inhibitors like rivastigmine or donepezil. However, add-on treatment with antipsychotics is still frequently needed. As in patients with PD, classic neuroleptics should be avoided because of their potential to significantly worsen motor symptoms. Unfortunately, this is also true for the atypical neuroleptics risperidone and olanzapine. Clozapine with starting bedtime doses of 6.25 mg/day (maintenance dose range between 6.25 and 50 mg/day; rarely 75–150 mg/day) is probably the best current option, although it may be less well tolerated in patients with DLB compared with psychotic patients with PD. Weekly blood count monitoring is cumbersome but inevitable for the first 6 months of the drug regimen (to be followed by biweekly blood count controls). Quetiapine may therefore prove to be an easier to use option with a starting dose of 25 mg, which generally has to be increased in a range between 50 and 150 mg/day. Currently, however, the clinical study data on the use of quetiapine in DLB are limited.

PARKINSONISM

L-Dopa is the gold standard of symptomatic efficacy in PD and also is the drug of choice to treat parkinsonism in DLB. Doses are usually in the low middle range between 300 and 500 mg L-dopa plus decarboxylase inhibitor per day, but may be increased if clinically required. Visual hallucinations and psychotic behavior can be dose limiting. The best compromise between need for improvement of akinesia and rigidity and the risk for increasing psychotic behaviour has to be sought. Dopamine agonists do not offer significant advantages over L-dopa in DLB, but they have a greater risk to induce psychotic side effects.

DYSAUTONOMIA

OH may be a disabling feature of DLB that, if present, frequently exacerbates the disability arising from progressive motor disturbance. A number of simple nonpharmacologic strategies such as elastic support stockings or tights, a high-salt diet, frequent small meals, head-up tilt of the bed at night, and rising slowly from a sitting to a standing position, may all improve orthostatic symptoms and should be tried before resorting to drug therapy. If these measures fail, the mineralocorticoid fludrocortisone may be given at night (0.1–0.3 mg). If orthostatic blood pressure decrease persists, sympathomimetics such as ephedrine (15–45 mg three times daily) or midodrine (2.5–10 mg three times daily) should be added to fludrocortisone. Frequency and urge incontinence often are helped by oxybutynin (2.5–5 mg two to three times daily), but this peripherally acting anticholinergic may precipitate urinary retention. A substantial postmicturition residue of greater than 100 ml is an indication for intermittent self-catheterization (or catheterization by the spouse). In the advanced stages of DLB, a urethral or suprapubic catheter may become necessary. Erectile failure can be improved by oral yohimbine (2.5–5 mg three times daily) or sildenafil (50–100 mg) or by intracavernosal injection of papaverine or a penis implant. RBD is a common cause for disturbed night sleep in patients with DLB. When reasonable suspicion for the presence of RBD emerges from interview with spouses or sleep laboratory studies, a trial of clonazepam starting with 0.5 mg/day may be tried. As with other benzodiazepines, patients should be closely monitored for possible paradoxic reactions and increased anxiety, agitation, or confusion.

References

1. Kuzuhara, S., M. Yoshimura, T. Mizutani, H. Yamanouchi, and Y. Ihara. 1996. Clinical features of diffuse Lewy body disease in the elderly: Analysis of 12 cases. In *Dementia with Lewy bodies: Clinical, pathalogical, and treatment issues*, ed. R. H. Perry, I. G. McKeith, and E. K. Perry, 153–160. Cambridge: Cambridge University Press.
2. McKeith, I. G., C. G. Ballard, R. H. Perry, P. G. Ince, J. T. O'Brien, D. Neill, K. Lowery, E. Jaros, R. Barber, P. Thompson, A. Swann, A. F. Fairbairn, and E. K. Perry. 2000. Prospective validation of consensus criteria for the diagnosis of dementia with Lewy bodies. *Neurology* 54:1050–1058.
3. McKeith, I. G., D. Galasko, K. Kosaka, E. K. Perry, D. W. Dickson, L. A. Hansen, D. P. Salmon, J. Lowe, S. S. Mirra, E. J. Byrne, G. Lennox, N. P. Quinn, J. A. Edwardson, P. G. Ince, C. Bergeron, A. Burns, B. L. Miller, S. Lovestone, D. Collerton, E. N. Jansen, C. Ballard, R. A. de Vos, G. K. Wilcock, K. A. Jellinger, and R. H. Perry. 1996. Consensus guidelines for the clinical and pathologic diagnosis of dementia with Lewy bodies (DLB): Report of the consortium on DLB international workshop. *Neurology* 47:1113–1124.
4. Wenning, G. K., C. Scherfler, R. Granata, S. Bosch, M. Verny, K. R. Chaudhuri, K. Jellinger, W. Poewe, and I. Litvan. 1999. Time course of symptomatic orthostatic hypotension and urinary incontinence in patients with postmortem confirmed parkinsonian syndromes: A clinicopathological study. *J. Neurol. Neurosurg. Psychiatry* 67:620–623.
5. Larner, A. J., C. J. Mathias, and M. N. Rossor. 2000. Autonomic failure preceding dementia with Lewy bodies. *J. Neurol*. 247:229–231.
6. Ballard, C., F. Shaw, I. McKeith, and R. Kenny. 1998. High prevalence of neurovascular instability in neurodegenerative dementias. *Neurology* 51:1760–1762.
7. McKeith, I., T. Del Ser, P. Spano, M. Emre, K. Wesnes, R. Anand, A. Cicin-Sain, R. Ferrara, and R. Spiegel. 2000. Efficacy of rivastigmine in dementia with Lewy bodies: A randomised, double-blind, placebo-controlled international study. *Lancet* 356:2031–2036.

80 Central Disorders of Autonomic Function

Eduardo E. Benarroch
Department of Neurology
Mayo Clinic
Rochester, Minnesota

The central autonomic network includes the insular, anterior cingulate, and orbitofrontal cortex, amygdala, hypothalamus, periaqueductal gray matter, parabrachial nucleus of the pons, nucleus tractus solitarii (NTS), intermediate reticular zone of the medulla including the ventrolateral medulla, and the raphe nuclei and adjacent ventromedial medulla. Disorders involving any of these regions or their connections to the preganglionic sympathetic or parasympathetic nuclei may result in the following: (1) syndromes of autonomic failure, characterized by orthostatic hypotension, anhidrosis, gastrointestinal dysmotility, neurogenic bladder, impotence, and Horner syndrome; or (2) syndromes of autonomic hyperactivity, resulting in cardiac arrhythmias, hypertension, hyperthermia or hypothermia, hyperhidrosis, myocardial damage, or neurogenic pulmonary edema. These manifestations may occur in isolation or in various combinations [1].

DISORDERS OF TELENCEPHALIC AUTTONOMIC REGIONS

Stroke

Hemispheric stroke involving the insular or anterior cingulate cortex can produce cardiac arrhythmias, which are a potential cause of sudden death. Right hemispheric strokes are more frequently associated with supraventricular tachycardia and left hemispheric strokes with ventricular tachyarrhythmias. Infarctions involving the insula may produce hyperhidrosis in the contralateral face and arm. Unilateral or bilateral infarction of the cingulate gyrus can produce urinary and fecal incontinence, tachycardia, and even sudden death [2, 3].

Hydrocephalus and meningioma compressing the medial surface of the frontal lobes commonly produce neurogenic uninhibited bladder.

Seizures

Seizures arising from the amygdala, anterior cingulate cortex, or other limbic–paralimbic areas can produce several autonomic manifestations, frequently misdiagnosed as a primary disorder of the target organ. They may occur during clinical auras, before any recognizable epileptiform discharges in the surface electroencephalogram (EEG) [4]. The most common manifestations are cardiac arrhythmias, particularly ictal sinus tachycardia [5], but atrial fibrillation, premature atrial or ventricular contractions, supraventricular or ventricular tachycardia, and ventricular fibrillation may also occur. Ictal bradycardia is a rare manifestation of temporal or frontotemporal lobe seizures, predominantly from left hemisphere, and may lead to sinus arrest or sinoatrial block [6]. Syncope may be the first manifestation of seizures, and their differentiation may require simultaneous electrocardiogram (ECG)/EEG recordings. Autonomic dysregulation and cardiac arrhythmias may underlie sudden unexpected death in epilepsy. Temporolimbic seizures may also produce mydriasis, flushing, pallor, shivering, sweating, and piloerection, which may be unilateral. Unilateral pilomotor seizures may be a manifestation of ipsilateral temporal lobe lesions. Ictal abdominal pain or vomiting is more common in children than in adults [4].

DISORDERS OF THE DIENCEPHALON

Hypothalamic Disorders

Disorders of the hypothalamus or its connections produce complex autonomic manifestations, commonly associated with disturbances in endocrine, thirst, caloric balance, or sexual functions. Disorders of thermoregulation are an important manifestation of hypothalamic disease. Hypothermia occurs in Wernicke's encephalopathy and may also be a consequence of head injury, mesodiencephalic hematoma, multiple sclerosis, or toluene toxicity. Wernicke's encephalopathy should be suspected in alcoholic or malnourished patients presenting with unexplained hypothermia, and it requires immediate treatment with thiamine. Episodic hyperhidrosis with hypothermia may be the primary manifestation of agenesis of the corpus callosum (Shapiro syndrome) or structural lesions affecting the third ventricle and has been attributed to involvement of the thermoregulatory preoptic anterior hypothalamic region. The episodes may be associated with other manifestations of autonomic hyperactivity and alterations of the level of consciousness; they may vary in duration and may be associated with long-lasting remissions. Anticonvulsants, cyproheptadine, clonidine, or muscarinic antagonists (oxybutynin or glycopyrrolate) may control both hyperhidrosis and hypothermia. Posterior cerebral artery territory infarction involving the hypothalamus and upper brainstem may produce the combination of ipsilateral Horner syndrome and contralateral hyperhidrosis, referred to as hemiplegia vegetativa alterna.

Paroxysmal Sympathetic Storms ("Diencephalic Seizures")

Acute brain lesions may disrupt hypothalamic control of sympathetic function and produce hypertension, tachycardia, hyperthermia or hypothermia, diaphoresis, skin vasodilation, pupil dilation, hyperventilation, shivering, and increased muscle tone [7]. This syndrome of diencephalic autonomic hyperactivity was first described by Penfield in 1929 [8]. It commonly occurs as a complication of closed head injury producing widespread axonal injury and decortication. These patients may respond to opioids and bromocriptine. The other common cause is acute hydrocephalus, which most frequently occurs in the setting of subarachnoid hemorrhage or with mass lesions near the third ventricle [7]. Shunt treatment may completely reverse the episodes.

In intracranial catastrophes, acute sympathoadrenal excitation may produce ECG changes of cardiac ischemia, serious cardiac arrhythmias, and neurogenic pulmonary edema [9].

Fatal Familial Insomnia

Fatal familial insomnia is an autosomal dominant prion disease linked to a point mutation of the prion protein gene. The main manifestations are progressive intractable insomnia, sympathetic hyperactivity (manifested by fever, hyperhidrosis, tachycardia, and hypertension), and abnormal circadian endocrine function. The characteristic pathologic findings are atrophy of the anteroventral and dorsomedial thalamic nuclei, both involved in circuits controlling autonomic function.

DISORDERS OF THE BRAINSTEM

Several neuronal groups of the lower pons and medulla, including the NTS, dorsal vagal, and ambigual nuclei, and intermediate reticular formation and ventrolateral medulla interactively control tonic and reflex vasomotor, cardiovagal, and respiratory functions. Involvement of these nuclei by ischemic, inflammatory, neoplastic, or degenerative disease may produce severe cardiovascular and respiratory disturbances, including excessive sympathoexcitation, baroreflex failure, orthostatic hypotension, syncope, and sleep apnea [1]. Sympathoexcitation reflects stimulation of hypoxia-sensitive neurons of the rostral ventrolateral medulla that excite the preganglionic sympathetic neurons. Baroreflex failure reflects bilateral damage of the NTS, the first relay station of baroreceptor afferents. It resembles clinically a pheochromocytoma with episodes of acute hypertension or excessive lability of blood pressure. Orthostatic hypotension or syncope may occur with tumors or vascular lesions involving the descending sympathoexcitatory projections of the rostral ventrolateral medulla. Central hypoventilation and sleep apnea may reflect involvement of the ventral and dorsal respiratory groups of the medulla or their descending projections to the upper cervical cord.

Vertebrobasilar Disease

Transient ischemic attacks may present with paroxysmal hypertension that precedes any focal neurologic deficit. Bilateral pontomedullary strokes may produce persistent tachycardia, episodic bradycardia, orthostatic hypotension, cardiorespiratory arrest, Ondine's curse, unexplained fever, generalized hyperhidrosis, vomiting, hiccups, dysphagia, aperistaltic esophagus, gastric retention, and urinary retention. Lateral medullary infarction (Wallenberg syndrome) produces Horner syndrome and occasionally profound bradycardia, supine hypotension, acute hypertension, or central hypoventilation. Pulsatile compression of the left ventrolateral medulla by a basilar artery aneurysm or vascular loops has been implicated in neurogenic hypertension. The presence of an arterial loop pressing or distorting the medulla is not a reliable predictor of beneficial response to microvascular decompression in patients with essential hypertension refractory to treatment.

Posterior Fossa Tumors

Posterior fossa tumors, such as cerebellar astrocytoma, hemangioblastoma, medulloblastoma, cerebellopontine angle tumors, and brainstem glioma may initially manifest with orthostatic hypotension, paroxysmal hypertension, or intractable vomiting. Orthostatic hypotension may be the presenting manifestation or may develop after surgical treatment.

Degenerative and Developmental Disorders

Syringobulbia may affect the NTS or its connections with cardiovagal and vasomotor neurons of the ventrolateral medulla [10]. This may produce orthostatic hypotension, impaired cardiovagal function, exaggerated fluctuations of blood pressure and central hypoventilation, contributing to the risk for sudden death. Chiari type I malformation is a common incidental finding with no clinical consequence, but in rare cases it may produce compressive or vascular involvement of the lower medulla, resulting in sleep apnea, cardiorespiratory arrest, or syncope triggered by Valsalva-type maneuvers.

Inflammatory, Toxic, and Metabolic Disorders

Poliomyelitis, brainstem encephalitis, or multiple sclerosis affecting the ventrolateral medulla or NTS may produce hypertension, respiratory arrest, or neurogenic pulmonary edema. Leigh syndrome may produce severe hypertension caused by bilateral involvement of the NTS.

DISORDERS OF THE SPINAL CORD

Traumatic spinal cord lesions above T5 level produce profound abnormalities in control of cardiovascular, thermoregulatory, bladder, bowel, and sexual functions, including the syndrome of autonomic dysreflexia. The autonomic manifestations of spinal cord injury are described in Chapter 81.

Multiple sclerosis can lead to neurogenic bladder with detrusor-sphincter dyssynergia and neurogenic bowel and sexual dysfunction. Abnormal thermoregulatory sweating and subclinical abnormalities in cardiovascular tests, including reduced heart rate response to deep breathing variability and sympathetic vasoconstrictor failure, are frequently found in patients with multiple sclerosis. Devic's neuromyelitis optica produces extensive demyelination and necrosis of the spinal cord, particularly in the thoracic segments, which may result in severe dysautonomia.

Syringomyelia produces interruption of descending autonomic pathways to the intermediolateral cell columns of the spinal cord, either directly by a cervical syrinx or by an associated Chiari malformation [10]. The manifestations include Horner syndrome, sweating abnormalities, and trophic changes in the limbs, especially the hands. Micturition and defecation may be affected at an advanced stage.

Amyotrophic lateral sclerosis may produce subclinical impairment in sudomotor axon reflex in the foot and impaired heart rate response to deep breathing.

Tetanus may produce severe sympathetic and parasympathetic hyperactivity because of both disinhibition of preganglionic neurons and direct damage of brainstem autonomic nuclei. Parasympathetic hyperactivity produces sinus arrest, salivation, and increased bronchial secretions; sympathetic hyperactivity produces tachycardia and other arrhythmias, labile hypertension, fever, and profuse sweating. The stiff-man syndrome, caused by autoantibodies against glutamic acid decarboxylase, may also manifest with paroxysmal sympathetic hyperactivity. This occurs in association with the severe muscle spasms typical of the disease, and both reflect lack of GABAergic inhibition of spinal cord circuits.

References

1. Benarroch, E. E., and F. L. Chang. 1993. Central autonomic disorders. *J. Clin. Neurophysiol.* 10:39–50.
2. Korpelainen, J. T., K. A. Sotaniemi, and V. V. Myllyla. 1999. Autonomic nervous system disorders in stroke. *Clin. Auton. Res.* 9(6):325–333.
3. Oppenheimer, S. M., and V. C. Hachinski. 1992. The cardiac consequences of stroke [Review]. *Neurol. Clin.* 10:167–176.
4. Freeman, R., and S. C. Schachter. 1995. Autonomic epilepsy. *Semin. Neurol.* 15(2):158–166.
5. Blumhardt, L. D., P. E. Smith, and L. Owen. 1986. Electrocardiographic accompaniments of temporal lobe epileptic seizures. *Lancet* 1:1051–1056.
6. Tinuper, P., F. Bisulli, A. Cerullo, R. Carcangiu, C. Marini, G. Pierangeli, and P. Cortelli. 2001. Ictal bradycardia in partial epileptic seizures: Autonomic investigation in three cases and literature review. *Brain* 124:2361–2371.
7. Ropper, A. H. 1997. Management of the autonomic storm. In *Clinical autonomic disorders: Evaluation and management*, 2nd ed., ed. P. A. Low, 791–801. Philadelphia: Lippincott-Raven.
8. Penfield, W. 1929. Diencephalic autonomic epilepsy. *Arch. Neurol.* 22:358–374.
9. Talman, W. T. 1985. Cardiovascular regulation and lesions of the central nervous system. *Ann. Neurol.* 18:1–13.
10. Nogues, M. A., P. K. Newman, V. J. Male, and J. B. Foster. 1982. Cardiovascular reflexes in syringomyelia. *Brain* 105:835–849.

81 Autonomic Disturbances in Spinal Cord Injuries

Christopher J. Mathias
Neurovascular Medicine Unit
Imperial College London at St. Mary's Hospital
& Autonomic Unit
National Hospital for Neurology & Neurosurgery
& Institute of Neurology, University College London
United Kingdom

Normal functioning of the autonomic nervous system is critically dependent on integrity of the spinal cord, because the entire sympathetic outflow (T1–L2/3) and the sacral parasympathetic outflow travel and synapse within the spinal cord, before supplying various target organs (Fig. 81.1). In spinal cord injuries, therefore, autonomic impairment usually occurs, and this depends on the site and the extent of the lesion. In cervical and high thoracic transection, the entire or a large part of the sympathetic outflow, together with the sacral parasympathetic outflow, is separated from cerebral control. Autonomic malfunction may affect the cardiovascular, thermoregulatory, sudomotor, gastrointestinal, urinary, and reproductive systems [1]. The problems are usually worse in those with higher lesions.

Soon after cord injury, there is a transient state of hypoexcitability, described as "spinal shock." There is flaccid paralysis of muscles, lack of tendon reflexes, impairment of spinal autonomic function with atony of the urinary bladder and large bowel, dilation of blood vessels, and lack of spinal autonomic reflexes. This may last from a few days to a few weeks, after which activity in the isolated cord returns. In the chronic phase, with return of isolated spinal function, a different set of autonomic abnormalities occurs.

CARDIOVASCULAR SYSTEM

In recent high injuries, basal blood pressure, especially diastolic, is usually lower than normal. Plasma norepinephrine and epinephrine levels are low, as in the chronic phase. Basal heart rate is usually below normal. In patients with high cervical lesions, who need artificial ventilation because of diaphragmatic paralysis, severe bradycardia and cardiac arrest may occur during tracheal stimulation (Fig. 81.2). This results from increased vagal activity, because efferent muscarinic blockade with atropine prevents bradycardia. Vagal activity is increased by hypoxia and by the absence of sympathetic reflexes; furthermore, there is an inability to reduce vagal activity through the pulmonary inflation reflex because of the inability to breathe. It is necessary to prevent such episodes by adequate oxygenation, treatment of respiratory infection and pulmonary emboli (which contribute to hypoxia), avoidance of cholinomimetic agents such as neostigmine and carbachol, and, if necessary, the use of parenteral atropine or a demand cardiac pacemaker.

In the chronic stage, the levels of basal systolic and diastolic blood pressure are related closely to the level of the spinal lesion—that is, pressure is lower in the high lesions, and increases toward normal as the lesion descends. In tetraplegic patients, plasma norepinephrine levels are about 25% of the levels observed in healthy subjects, and they have reduced basal muscle sympathetic nerve activity, as measured by microneurography. Complicating factors, such as renal damage and failure, can increase blood pressure, regardless of the lesion.

In high lesions, the blood pressure is sensitive to a number of physiologic stimuli. Postural (orthostatic) hypotension is a particular problem in the early stages (Fig. 81.3). It may cause a variety of symptoms, including neck ("coathanger") pain [2] similar to symptoms noted in other forms of chronic autonomic failure. Plasma norepinephrine levels are low and do not increase with head-up postural change, unlike in healthy subjects. There is a marked increase in levels of plasma renin, aldosterone, and vasopressin, which may contribute to the recovery of blood pressure and account for other symptoms, such as reduced urine output. Improvement in symptoms and in postural blood pressure follows repeated head-up tilt, which presumably improves cerebral autoregulation and releases the various hormones that constrict blood vessels, increase intravascular volume, and thus reduce the postural blood pressure decrease. Drugs such as the sympathomimetics ephedrine or midodrine may need to be used.

The reverse, severe hypertension, may occur during autonomic dysreflexia after stimulation below the level of the lesion. This may occur through the skin (such as from complicating pressure sores), from abdominal and pelvic viscera (by contraction of the urinary bladder or irritation from a

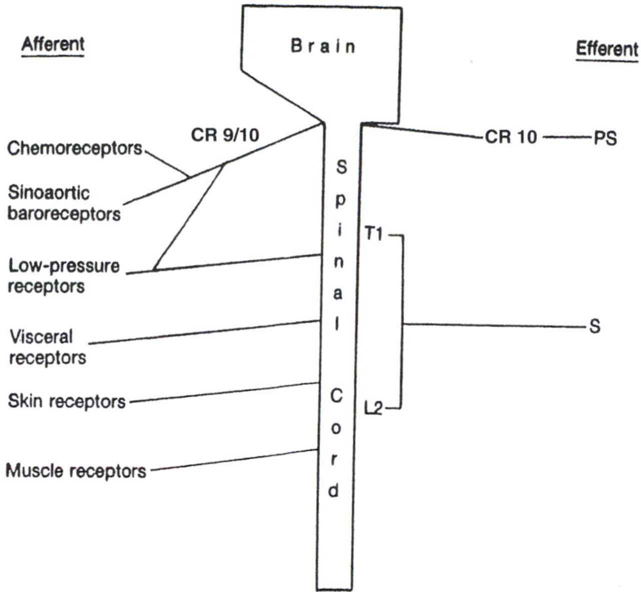

FIGURE 81.1 Schematic outline of the major autonomic pathways controlling circulation. The major afferent input into the central nervous system is through the glossopharyngeal (*CR 9*) and vagus (*CR 10*) nerves by activation of baroreceptors in the carotid sinus and aortic arch. Chemoreceptors and low-pressure receptors also influence the efferent outflow. The latter consists of the cranial parasympathetic (*PS*) outflow to the heart through the vagus nerves, and the sympathetic outflow from the thoracic and upper lumbar segments of the spinal cord. Activation of visceral, skin, and muscle receptors, in addition to cerebral stimulation, influences the efferent outflow. In high spinal cord lesions, therefore, the input from chemoreceptors and baroreceptors is preserved together with the vagal efferent outflow, but there is no connection between the brain and the rest of the sympathetic outflow. The spinal sympathetic outflow may be activated through a range of afferents (visual, skin, and muscle). This occurs through isolated spinal cord reflexes, not controlled by cerebral pathways, as seen normally.

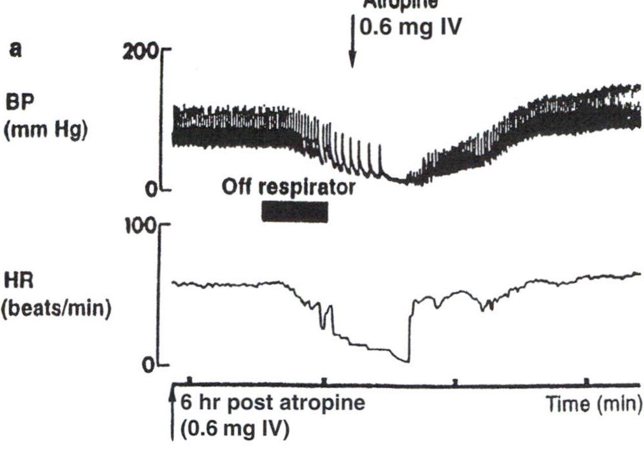

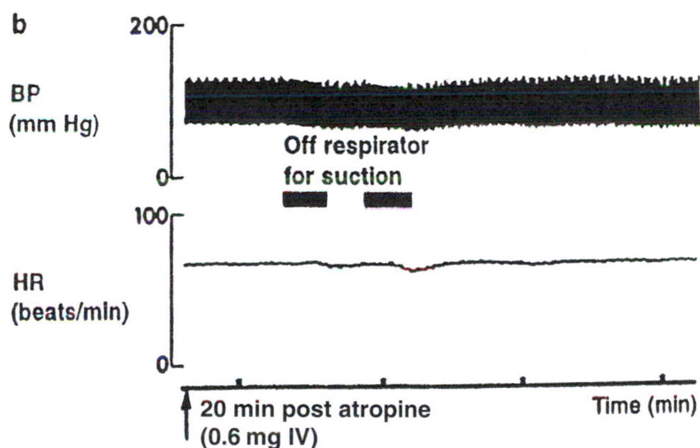

FIGURE 81.2 A, The effect of disconnecting the respirator (as required for aspirating the airways) on the blood pressure (BP) and heart rate (HR) of a recently injured tetraplegic patient (C4/5 lesion) in spinal shock, 6 hours after the last dose of intravenous atropine. Sinus bradycardia and cardiac arrest, also observed in the electrocardiograph, were reversed by reconnection, intravenous atropine, and external cardiac massage. (From Frankel, H. L., C. J. Mathias, and J. M. K. Spalding. 1975. Mechanisms of reflex cardiac arrest in tetraplegic patients. *Lancet* 2:1183–1185.) **B**, The effect of tracheal suction 20 minutes after atropine in the same patient. Disconnection from the respirator and tracheal suction did not decrease either heart rate or blood pressure. (From Mathias, C. J. 1972. Bradycardia and cardiac arrest during tracheal suction—mechanisms in tetraplegic patients. *Eur. J. Inten. Care Med.* 2:147–156.)

urethral catheter) (Fig. 81.4), or through skeletal muscles (during muscle spasms). The paroxysmal increase in blood pressure is the result of increased spinal sympathetic neural activity causing constriction of both resistance and capacitance vessels. These changes occur below the level of the lesion, whereas above the lesion there may be sweating and dilation of cutaneous vessels over the face and neck. Autonomic dysreflexia is accompanied by increased levels of plasma norepinephrine. Plasma norepinephrine levels, even at the height of hypertension, however, are increased only twofold or threefold above the low basal levels and are still within the range of basal levels in healthy subjects; this differs markedly from the levels seen in hypertensive crises caused by a pheochromocytoma.

During autonomic dysreflexia muscle sympathetic nerve activity measured by microneurography shows only a modest increase, suggesting that the pressor response may be caused by increased α-adrenergic receptor sensitivity. This also may explain the increased pressor response to intravenously infused norepinephrine. Other factors, such as impaired baroreflex activity, may be of importance because there is pressor hypersensitivity to a wide range of vasoactive agents of different chemical structures that act on a variety of receptors. Tetraplegic patients also have an enhanced depressor response to vasodilator agents, which further favors baroreflex impairment. Experimental studies indicate the importance of certain neuronal cells with activated nerve growth factors (NGF); furthermore, neutralizing intraspinal NGF prevents the development of autonomic dysreflexia [3].

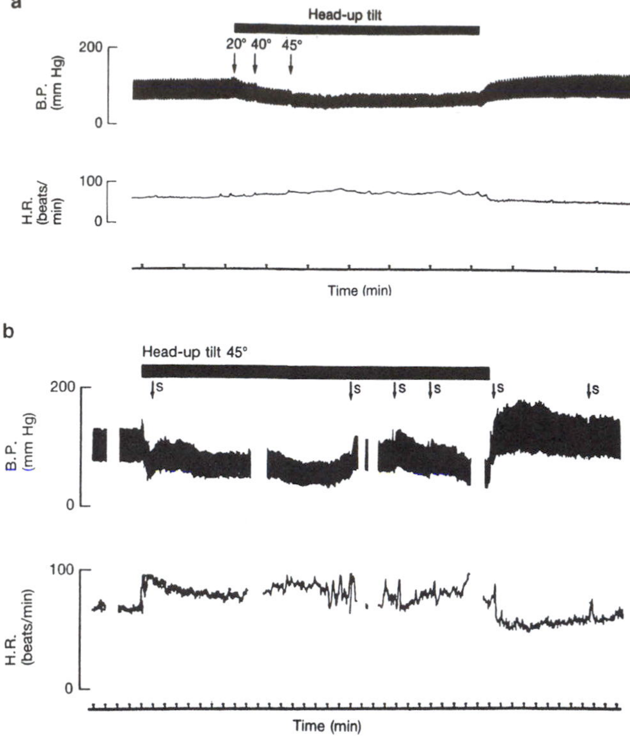

FIGURE 81.3 **A**, Blood pressure (BP) and heart rate (HR) in a tetraplegic patient before and after head-up tilt, in the early stages of rehabilitation, where there were few muscle spasms and minimal autonomic dysreflexia. (From Mathias, C. J., and H. L. Frankel. 1992. The cardiovascular system in tetraplegia and paraplegia. In *Spinal Cord Trauma*, ed. P. J. Vinken, G. W. Bruyn, H. L. Klawans. Vol. 61 of *Handbook of Clinical Neurology*, ed. H. L. Frankel. Elsevier, Science Publishers, Netherlands, 435–456.) **B**, BP and HR in a chronic tetraplegic patient before, during, and after head-up tilt to 45 degrees. BP promptly decreases, but with partial recovery, which in this case is linked to skeletal muscle spasms (*S*) inducing spinal sympathetic activity. Some of the later oscillations may be caused by the increase in plasma renin, which was measured where there were interruptions in the intraarterial record. In the later phases of head-up tilt, skeletal muscle spasms occur more frequently and further increase the BP. On return to the horizontal, BP increases rapidly above the previous level and then returns slowly to horizontal levels. HR usually moves in the opposite direction, except during muscle spasms when there is an initial increase. (From Mathias, C. J., and H. L. Frankel. 1988. Cardiovascular control in spinal man. *Ann. Rev. Physiol.* 50:577–592.)

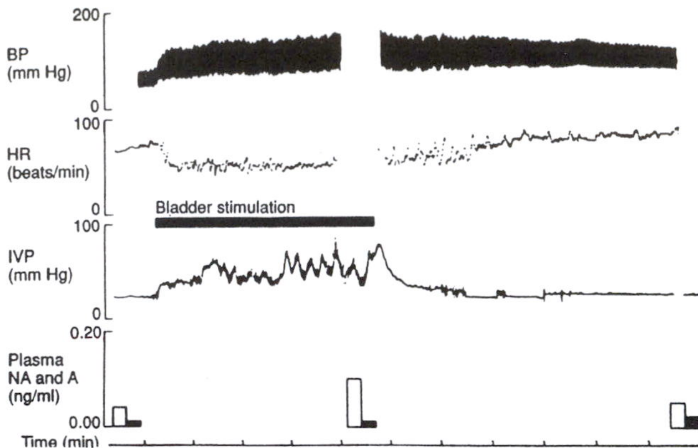

FIGURE 81.4 Blood pressure (BP), heart rate (HR < intravesical pressure [IVP]), plasma norepinephrine (NE) (*open histograms*) and plasma epinephrine (E) (*filled histograms*) in a tetraplegic patient before, during, and after urinary bladder stimulation induced by suprapubic percussion of the anterior abdominal wall. The increase in BP is accompanied by a decrease in HR as a result of increased vagal activity in response to the increased blood pressure. Plasma NE but not E levels increase, suggesting an increase in sympathetic neural activity, independently of adrenomedullary activation. (From Mathias, C. J., and H. L. Frankel. 1986. The neurological and hormonal control of blood vessels and heart in spinal man. *J. Auto. Nerv. Sys.* (suppl):457–464.)

Autonomic dysreflexia is a serious problem. It may result in considerable morbidity, with severe sweating and a throbbing headache, and even mortality as a result of intracranial hemorrhage. The management consists of preventing the initiating factors that increase sympathoneuronal activity. If necessary, a variety of drugs to reduce sympathetic efferent activity can be used.

CUTANEOUS CIRCULATION

In higher lesions, the skin below the lesion is usually warmer and veins appear dilated. There may be extravasation of fluid into subcutaneous tissue that could contribute to skin breakdown and pressure sores. Vasodilation often occurs in the nose (Guttmann's sign); similar changes occur after α-antagonists, reserpine and guanethidine in patients with hypertension.

In spinal shock, the cutaneous responses to the triple or Lewis response are exaggerated, hence, the term *dermatographia rubra*. With the return of spinal cord reflex activity in the chronic phase, there is sympathetic vasoconstriction and skin pallor, hence the term *dermatographia alba*.

THERMOREGULATION AND SUDOMOTOR FUNCTION

Hypothermia may readily occur in high lesions because shivering is diminished and they may be unable to vasoconstrict the cutaneous circulation. The reverse may occur causing hyperthermia because of the inability to sweat and to reflexly vasodilate in the periphery, when heat is lost.

Therefore, maintenance of environmental temperature is of critical importance. With hyperthermia, tepid sponging, increasing airflow with a fan to accelerate heat loss, and, in severe cases, ice-cooled saline by intravenous infusion or urinary bladder irrigation may be needed.

The sympathetic skin response (SSR), a technique that records neurogenic activation of sweat glands, is abnormal in spinal injuries, depending on the level of lesion [4]. Activation of supraspinal centers and descending sudomotor

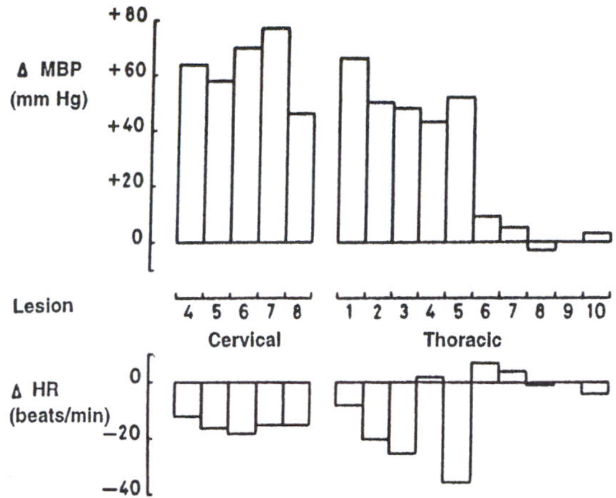

FIGURE 81.5 Changes in mean blood pressure (MBP) and heart rate (HR) in patients with spinal cord lesions at different levels (cervical and thoracic) after urinary bladder stimulation induced by suprapubic percussion of the anterior abdominal wall. In the cervical and high thoracic lesions, there is a marked increase in blood pressure and a decrease in heart rate. In patients with lesions below T5 there are minimal cardiovascular changes. (From Mathias, C. J., and H. L. Frankel. 1986. The neurological and hormonal control of blood vessels and heart in spinal man. *J. Auto. Nerv. Sys.* (suppl):457–464.)

neural pathways in the spinal cord are necessary for the SSR, which is absent in the plantar region in low injuries, and absent in the palmar region in high spinal injuries. Importantly, the presence or absence of the SSR can be a useful marker of spinal cord autonomic involvement, in addition to motor and sensory evaluation, and may improve classification of the extent of spinal functional deficits.

GASTROINTESTINAL SYSTEM

In the early stages of spinal cord injury, there is vagal hyperactivity that may contribute to acid hypersecretion, with gastric ulceration and hemorrhage. H2 receptor antagonists, or allied agents, need to be used prophylactically. In high lesions, paralytic ileus may occur; the mechanisms are unclear and often follow ingestion of solid food, which should be avoided. Large bowel dysfunction is common, and adequate training, together with the use of an appropriate diet, mild laxatives, and stool softeners, may be needed.

URINARY SYSTEM

In the early stages, bladder atony occurs, with urinary retention, bladder distention, and urinary overflow. With recovery of isolated cord function, the bladder can be trained to be an automated reflex or neurogenic bladder. Catheters should ideally be used intermittently in the early stages. Urinary infection in skin, bone, and other tissues may cause secondary amyloidosis, with renal infiltration and serious sequelae.

REPRODUCTIVE SYSTEM

In male patients, sexual function is affected, especially in the early stages, with both erectile and ejaculatory failure. In the chronic phase, priapism may occur during autonomic dysreflexia. Ejaculation, if it occurs, is often retrograde. Various approaches, including electrical stimulation and collection of seminal fluid, have been used for artificial insemination. The phosphodiesterase inhibitor sildenafil (Viagra) is an effectively used drug in spinal injuries; whether it also decreases blood pressure excessively, as it does in other groups with autonomic failure such as multiple system atrophy, is not known [5].

In female patients, menstrual cycle disruption often occurs in the early stages. There is usually recovery within a year, and successful pregnancy has occurred in both tetraplegics and paraplegics. In high lesions, severe autonomic dysreflexia may accompany uterine contractions. Such patients are particularly prone, with the increase of blood pressure, to epileptic seizures and cerebral hemorrhage. It is essential to decrease their blood pressure. A combination of anticonvulsants (such as phenytoin) and agents to reduce spinal cord activity (such as spinal anesthetics) may be needed, together with other agents, to control blood pressure.

References

1. Mathias, C., and H. L. Frankel. 2002. Autonomic disturbances in spinal cord lesions. In *Autonomic failure: A textbook of clinical disorders of the autonomic nervous system,* 4th ed., ed. C. J. Mathias and R. Bannister, 494–513. Oxford: Oxford University Press.
2. Cariga, P., S. Ahmed, C. J. Mathias, and B. P. Gardner. 2002. The prevalence and association of neck (coathanger) pain and orthostatic (postural) hypotension in human spinal cord injury. *Spinal Cord* 40:77–82.
3. Krenz, N. R., S. O. Meaking, A. V. Krassioukov, and L. C. Weaver. 1999. Neutralizing intraspinal nerve growth factor blocks autonomic dysreflexia caused by spinal cord injury. *J. Neurosci.* 19:7405–7414.
4. Cariga, P., M. Catley, G. Savic, H. L. Frankel, C. J. Mathias, P. H. Ellaway. 2002. Organisation of the sympathetic skin response in spinal cord injury. *J. Neurol. Neurosurg. Psychiatry* 72:356–360.
5. Hussain, I. F., C. Brady, M. J. Swinn, C. J. Mathias, and C. Fowler. 2001. Treatment of erectile dysfunction with sildenafil citrate (Viagra) in parkinsonism due to Parkinson's disease or multiple system atrophy with observations on orthostatic hypotension. *J. Neurol. Neurosurg. Psychiatry* 71:371–374.

82 Neuroleptic Malignant Syndrome

P. David Charles
Movement Disorders Clinic
Vanderbilt University
Nashville, Tennessee

Thomas L. Davis
Department of Neurology
Vanderbilt University
Nashville, Tennessee

The neuroleptic malignant syndrome is a rare and potentially fatal syndrome of hyperthermia, rigidity, autonomic instability, and mental status derangement [1]. It is an idiosyncratic reaction to drugs that alter the dopaminergic pathways of the central nervous system. Neuroleptics are the usual inciting agents. These are dopamine antagonists commonly prescribed for the treatment of psychiatric disorders. The incidence of neuroleptic malignant syndrome is estimated to be 0.1 to 2.2% of patients treated with neuroleptics. A similar syndrome can be caused by the sudden withdrawal of dopamine agonists used in the treatment of Parkinson's disease.

CLINICAL FEATURES

The clinical features of neuroleptic malignant syndrome are distinctive, but the four cardinal findings need not occur in every patient. The considerable list of potential symptoms (Table 82.1) can be grouped into the four general areas of hyperthermia, muscular rigidity, mental status changes, and autonomic dysfunction.

Hyperthermia is present in all cases of neuroleptic malignant syndrome and often exceeds 103.0°F. Muscular rigidity is severe and can be associated with tremor and bradykinesia; all three features are caused by extrapyramidal dysfunction. Passive movement of the limbs in all directions (lead pipe rigidity) is resisted. Mental status changes include confusion, delirium, speech disorders, and decreased states of consciousness. Autonomic dysfunction is usually characterized by rapid fluctuations in blood pressure and heart rate. Other autonomic features include sialorrhea, incontinence, and dysphagia. Tachypnea is probably caused by a combination of autonomic instability, muscular rigidity of the chest wall, and aspiration.

The laboratory findings of neuroleptic malignant syndrome are useful in establishing the diagnosis. The sustained muscular contraction causes muscle fiber necrosis and the blood concentration of creatine kinase may exceed 10,000 IU. Other less specific features are a leukocytosis, myoglobinuria, and increased serum concentrations of transaminases, lactic acid dehydrogenase, aldolase, and peripheral catecholamines.

The main morbidity and mortality in patients with neuroleptic malignant syndrome are irreversible brain injury from hyperthermia and renal failure from myoglobinuria secondary to rigidity-induced skeletal muscle necrosis. Other conditions contributing to morbidity and mortality are aspiration pneumonia, myocardial infarction, disseminated intravascular coagulation, and metabolic and electrolyte derangements.

In 1994, the *Diagnostic and Statistical Manual of Mental Disorders-IV (DSM-IV)* [2] recommended diagnostic criteria for neuroleptic malignant syndrome (Table 82.2) with the intention of creating more consistency in diagnosis and facilitating early recognition and intervention, thus reducing morbidity and mortality.

MEDICATIONS AND RISK FACTORS

Neuroleptics are among the most commonly prescribed drugs in the United States. Phenothiazine, thiothixene, and butyrophenones are the agents most commonly implicated in causing neuroleptic malignant syndrome. Haloperidol is the single most common drug associated with the neuroleptic malignant syndrome, most likely because it is one of the most commonly prescribed neuroleptics [3]. The expanding list of implicated drugs now includes amoxapine, tetrabenazine, reserpine, metoclopramide, clozapine, risperidone, olanzapine, monoamine oxidase inhibitors, and tricyclic antidepressants (Table 82.3) [4]. Dopamine antagonism in the central nervous system is the common factor shared by all of these agents; some are more potent dopamine antagonists than others. Intramuscular injection of depot preparations of neuroleptics may increase the risk for neuroleptic malignant syndrome and definitely prolong recovery because prompt drug withdrawal is not possible.

Individuals at increased risk for neuroleptic malignant syndrome cannot be identified before initiating therapy. The onset of symptoms is most often within the first 30 days of starting treatment. Rapid neuroleptic dose escalation,

TABLE 82.1 Clinical Findings in Neuroleptic Malignant Syndrome

Hyperthermia
Often >103°F
Rigidity
Lead pipe in nature
Other extrapyramidal findings
Tremor
Bradykinesia
Dystonic posturing
Mental status changes
Confusion
Obtundation
Mutism
Autonomic instability
Blood pressure lability
Tachycardia
Tachypnea
Sialorrhea
Incontinence
Diaphoresis
Laboratory results
Creatine phosphokinase often >10,000 IU
Leukocytosis
Lactic acid dehydrogenase elevation
Aldolase increase
Transaminase increase

TABLE 82.2 Research Criteria for Neuroleptic Malignant Syndrome

A. The development of severe muscle rigidity and increased temperature associated with the use of neuroleptic medication

B. Presence of two (or more) of the following:
   1. diaphoresis
   2. dysphagia
   3. tremor
   4. incontinence
   5. changes in level of consciousness ranging from confusion to coma
   6. mutism
   7. tachycardia
   8. increased or labile blood pressure
   9. leukocytosis
   10. laboratory evidence of muscle injury (e.g., increased creatine phosphokinase)

C. The symptoms in Criteria A and B are not caused by another substance (e.g., phencyclidine) or a neurologic or other general medical condition (e.g., viral encephalitis)

D. The symptoms in Criteria A and B are not better accounted for by a mental disorder (e.g., mood disorder with catatonic features)

From American Psychiatric Association. 1994. *Diagnostic and statistical manual for mental disorders*, 4th ed., 798. Washington, D.C.

TABLE 82.3 Potential Precipitants: Neuroleptic Malignant Syndrome

Precipitants	Examples
Typical neuroleptics	
Phenothiazine	Fluphenazine, chlorpromazine, thioridazine, promethazine, prochlorperazine, trifluoperazine
Dibenzoxazepines	Pimozide
Butyrophenones	Haloperidol
Dihydroindolones	Molindone
Thioxanthenes	Thiothixene
Dibenzoapines	Loxapine
Atypical neuroleptics	Clozapine, risperidone, olanzapine
Antiemetics	Metoclopramide
Tricyclic antidepressants	Amitriptyline, imipramine, etc.
Benzodiazepines (in overdose and in pharmacy)	Diazepam, lorazepam, etc.
Withdrawal of dopamine agonist	L-Dopa, pergolide, bromocriptine, etc.
Polypharmacy (in combination with neuroleptics)	Alcohol, lithium, cimetidine

dehydration, psychomotor agitation, catatonia, and underlying organic brain disease probably increase the incidence of neuroleptic malignant syndrome in at-risk individuals. A high serum creatinine kinase level during non-neuroleptic malignant syndrome psychotic episodes may also be a risk factor for future neuroleptic malignant syndrome [5]. There is evidence of a genetic predisposition to neuroleptic malignant syndrome in individuals carrying the *Taq*I A polymorphism of the dopamine D2 receptor gene [6]. Other gene polymorphisms have yet to be implicated in the pathogenesis of the syndrome. Neuroleptic malignant syndrome recurs in one third of patients when neuroleptics are reintroduced after recovery from the initial episode. In situations in which the need for neuroleptic therapy outweighs the risk, the chance of a second neuroleptic malignant syndrome episode can be reduced by waiting at least 2 weeks after resolution of symptoms and then using the lowest possible dose of a low-potency agent [4].

DIFFERENTIAL DIAGNOSIS

The differential diagnosis of neuroleptic malignant syndrome includes other syndromes with hyperthermia as a prominent feature, fever complicating Parkinson's disease or other extrapyramidal syndromes, and lethal catatonia. Malignant hyperthermia and neuroleptic malignant syndrome have similar clinical features, but they are distinguishable because malignant hyperthermia is inherited as an autosomal dominant condition and is only triggered by the administration of anesthetic agents [4]. Heat stroke shares some features with neuroleptic malignant syndrome but lacks rigidity and sweating and is characterized by an abrupt onset after physical exercise or exposure to a high ambient temperature. Neuroleptics increase the risk for heat stroke; this may confuse diagnosis in individuals whose history is compatible with both disorders [3]. The clinical features of neuroleptic malignant syndrome can be mimicked in patients with Parkinson's disease whose rigidity worsens at the time of concurrent fever or infection. The same is true for other neurodegenerative disorders of the extrapyramidal system. Common infectious and metabolic disorders must be ruled out before making the diagnosis of neuroleptic malignant syndrome. Lethal catatonia is a rare disorder of psychotic patients known years before the development of neuroleptics. Its clinical features are identical to those of neuroleptic malignant syndrome and the two conditions are only distinguished by the prior use of neuroleptics [7].

PATHOGENESIS

The precise pathogenesis of neuroleptic malignant syndrome is not fully understood. Central dopaminergic hypoactivity has been identified in patients susceptible to neuroleptic malignant syndrome [6]. This supports a hypothesis that dopamine receptor blockade in the basal ganglia and hypothalamus results from treatment with neuroleptics [3]. Disruption of the dopaminergic pathways of the hypothalamus and basal ganglia leads to hyperthermia and rigidity. The experimental infusion of a dopamine agonist on the thermoregulatory center of the hypothalamus causes a dose-dependent decrease in body temperature. Basal ganglia dysfunction commonly produces tremor and other extrapyramidal symptoms in addition to rigidity. The autonomic instability combined with sustained muscle contraction and impaired heat dissipation exacerbates hyperthermia. The cerebrospinal fluid of patients with neuroleptic malignant syndrome shows a persistent reduction of homovanillic acid, the major metabolite of dopamine, supporting the dopamine-blocking hypothesis. Sympathetic nervous system hyperactivity has been recorded in the neuroleptic malignant syndrome active phase, implicating central noradrenergic activity dysregulation in the pathogenesis of neuroleptic malignant syndrome [8]. Other factors must be involved in the pathogenesis of neuroleptic malignant syndrome because its occurrence is rare, whereas the drugs known to induce the syndrome are prescribed to millions of patients each year. Furthermore, the reintroduction of neuroleptic agents in patients with a history of neuroleptic malignant syndrome does not always cause a recurrence.

TREATMENT

Patients with neuroleptic malignant syndrome should be treated in an intensive care unit. Treatment begins with the immediate withdrawal of the offending agent or the reintroduction of the antiparkinson agent that was discontinued. The average time for recovery from neuroleptic malignant syndrome is 10 days, and this is prolonged when depot preparations of neuroleptics were used. Therapy with dopamine agonists, such as bromocriptine, reduces the recovery time of neuroleptic malignant syndrome [7]. They act primarily by restoring the dopaminergic balance in the preoptic area of the hypothalamus and basal ganglia. Levodopa/carbidopa also has been used successfully to reverse the hypodopaminergic state and to reverse hyperthermia [4]. Dantrolene, a skeletal muscle relaxant, reduces the muscle rigidity of malignant hyperthermia and also is useful in neuroleptic malignant syndrome. It is widely accepted that early therapy with bromocriptine/dantrolene can reduce the occurrence of aspiration pneumonia, one of the leading causes of death in neuroleptic malignant syndrome. Benzodiazepines also are useful to treat the agitated mental confusion and the rigidity [4].

Early diagnoses resulting in prompt supportive measures in combination with drug therapy have significantly reduced the mortality from neuroleptic malignant syndrome. Cooling blankets are effective in combating hyperthermia, and vigorous fluid replacement is essential to prevent dehydration. Aspiration is a common complication of neuroleptic malignant syndrome because of decreased chest wall compliance and depressed level of consciousness. Therefore, mechanical ventilation, when indicated, combined with aggressive pulmonary toilet and appropriate antibiotic therapy in the event of pneumonia, is helpful. Renal failure, resulting from muscle breakdown, is the most common and severe complication of neuroleptic malignant syndrome. Fluid replacement and hemodialysis are the primary treatment modalities. The mortality from neuroleptic malignant syndrome increases to 50% if renal failure develops [3].

Electroconvulsive therapy is a last resort when lethal catatonia enters the differential diagnosis [9]. The two syndromes are clinically indistinguishable and lethal catatonia would not respond to the recommended treatment of neuroleptic malignant syndrome.

References

1. Delay, J., and P. Deniker. 1968. Drug-induced extrapyramidal syndromes. In *Handbook of clinical neurology: Disease of the basal ganglia*, ed. P. J. Vinken, and G. W. Bruyn, 248–266. Amsterdam: North-Holland.
2. American Psychiatric Association. 1994. *Diagnostic and statistical manual for mental disorders,* 4th ed., 795–798. Washington, D.C.
3. Adnet, P., P. Lestavel, and R. Krivosic-Horber. 2000. Neuroleptic malignant syndrome. *Br. J. Anaesth.* 85:129–135.
4. Ty, E. B., and A. D. Rothner. 2001. Neuroleptic malignant syndrome in children and adolescents. *J. Child Neurol.* 16:157–163.
5. Hermesh, H., I. Manor, R. Shiloh, D. Aizenberg, Y. Benjamini, H. Munitz, and A. Weizman. 2002. High serum creatinine kinase level:

Possible risk factor for neuroleptic malignant syndrome. *J. Clin. Psychopharmacol.* 22:252–256.

6. Suzuki, A., T. Kondo, K. Otani, K. Mihara, N. Yasui-Furukori, A. Sano, K. Koshiro, and S. Kaneko. 2001. Association of the *Taq*I A polymorphism of the dopamine D_2 receptor gene with predisposition to neuroleptic malignant syndrome. *Am. J. Psychiatry* 158:1714–1716.
7. Guze, B. H., and L. R. Baxter. 1985. Neuroleptic malignant syndrome. *N. Engl. J. Med.* 313:163–166.
8. Gurrera, R. J. 1999. Sympathoadrenal hyperactivity and the etiology of neuroleptic malignant syndrome. *Am. J. Psychiatry* 156:169–180.
9. Caroff, S. N., S. C. Mann, and P. E. Keck, Jr. 1998. Specific treatment of the neuroleptic malignant syndrome. *Biol. Psychiatry* 44:378–381.

PART X

PERIPHERAL AUTONOMIC FAILURE

83

Pure Autonomic Failure

Horacio Kaufmann
Autonomic Nervous System Laboratory
Department of Neurology
Mount Sinai School of Medicine
New York, New York

Irwin J. Schatz
John A. Burns School of Medicine
University of Hawaii at Manoa
Department of Medicine
Honolulu, Hawaii

Pure autonomic failure was first described by Bradbury and Eggleston in 1925 [1]. The disorder has been most frequently referred to as idiopathic orthostatic hypotension (OH). The name pure autonomic failure was introduced by Oppenheimer as one of the primary autonomic failure syndromes. It is a sporadic, adult-onset, slowly progressive, neurodegenerative disorder of the autonomic nervous system characterized by symptomatic OH, bladder and sexual dysfunction, and no somatic neurologic deficits.

Pure autonomic failure affects men slightly more often than women, usually during middle age. Its onset is slow and insidious; the patient may recall that symptoms first presented several years before seeking medical treatment. Unsteadiness, lightheadedness, or faintness on standing, worse in the morning, after meals, during exercise, or in hot weather, usually causes the patient to seek medical advice.

Questioning often reveals aching in the neck or occiput only when standing. Lying down relieves all symptoms. A decreased ability to sweat may be apparent, particularly in hot climates. Men found to have pure autonomic failure may have sought advice about urinary tract symptoms, including hesitancy, urgency, dribbling, and occasional incontinence. Other signs of autonomic disturbance including impotence, erectile and ejaculatory dysfunction, an inability to appreciate orgasm, and retrograde ejaculation may also be apparent. Women may experience urinary retention or incontinence as early symptoms [2, 3]. In contrast to the nausea and pallor that occurs before losing consciousness in patients with neurally mediated syncope, which are prominent signs of autonomic activation, in patients with pure autonomic failure, these signs are noticeably absent and consciousness is lost with little or no warning [2, 3].

Definitive diagnosis of OH as the cause of symptoms is made when symptoms are reproduced while documenting a decline in systolic blood pressure of at least 20 mmHg and diastolic pressure of at least 10 mmHg, within 3 minutes of standing. The diagnosis cannot be excluded with a single measurement of upright blood pressure, which does not fulfill these criteria. Several measurements of orthostatic blood pressure, preferably early in the morning or after a meal, may be necessary. Patients with pure autonomic failure also have decreased sinus arrhythmia and absent blood pressure overshoot during phase IV of Valsalva maneuver, indicating parasympathetic and sympathetic efferent dysfunction. Pure autonomic failure mainly affects efferent postganglionic neurons. Afferent pathways and somatic neurons are not affected.

DIFFERENTIAL DIAGNOSIS

Pure autonomic failure should be distinguished from other forms of neurogenic OH, such as peripheral somatic neuropathies with autonomic involvement (e.g., diabetes and amyloid), multiple system atrophy (MSA), and Parkinson's disease (PD). Patients with pure autonomic failure have no sensory, cerebellar, pyramidal, or extrapyramidal dysfunction. In general, this allows clinical distinction with other forms of neurogenic OH. Early in the course of the disease, the diagnosis of pure autonomic failure is always tentative. After a few years, it is not uncommon that extrapyramidal or cerebellar deficits (frequently both) develop in a patient who appeared to have pure autonomic failure and it turns out that the patient did not have pure autonomic failure but rather MSA. Therefore, a diagnosis of pure autonomic failure may require a five-year history of autonomic dysfunction because other neurologic deficits may develop, thus causing reclassification of the subject's disorder. It is incumbent on physicians to make a meticulous search for central nervous system disorders before diagnosing pure autonomic failure. In PD, clinical evidence of parkinsonism usually precedes the symptoms of autonomic failure by several years but this is not always the case in MSA. Hoarseness (caused by dystonia of the vocal cord abductor) and sleep apnea are highly suggestive of MSA. Pure autonomic failure is less progressive and generally induces less disabling symptoms than do these other syndromes. Patients with pure autonomic failure most often will have a prolonged and sometimes stable course.

CATECHOLAMINE STUDIES

Patients with pure autonomic failure have very low plasma norepinephrine levels when recumbent, whereas plasma norepinephrine levels when recumbent are normal in MSA and variable in patients with PD [4]. On standing, patients with pure autonomic failure, MSA, and some with PD with autonomic failure do not have the expected increase in plasma norepinephrine levels, indicating an inability to normally stimulate the release of catecholamines by baroreflex activation in all these disorders. When norepinephrine is infused into patients with pure autonomic failure, there is an exaggerated increase in blood pressure, reflecting an excessive sensitivity of postsynaptic α-adrenergic receptors to exogenous catecholamines. Patients with MSA and PD have only a mildly increased blood pressure response to infused norepinephrine (Table 83.1), without leftward shift in the dose-response curve. Similarly, β-adrenergic receptor supersensitivity is present to a greater degree in patients with pure autonomic failure than in those with MSA, as shown in a study using intravenous isoproterenol [5].

NEUROENDOCRINE STUDIES

Pure autonomic failure selectively involves efferent autonomic neurons with the postganglionic neurons mainly affected. Afferent pathways are not affected. Baroreceptor-mediated vasopressin release—a measurement of afferent baroreceptor function—is normal in pure autonomic failure, and presumably in PD, but is blunted in MSA [6]. Intravenous clonidine, a centrally active α_2-adrenoceptor agonist that stimulates growth hormone secretion, also tests the function of hypothalamic–pituitary pathways. Clonidine increased serum growth hormone in patients with PD and patients with pure autonomic failure, but not in those with MSA [7]. In summary, neuroendocrine responses to hypotension or centrally acting adrenergic agonists are blunted in patients with MSA, but are preserved in patients with PD and pure autonomic failure because brainstem–hypothalamic–pituitary pathways are only affected in MSA.

TABLE 83.1 Measurement of Plasma Norepinephrine and Response to Exogenous Catecholamines in Pure Autonomic Failure and Multiple System Atrophy

	PAF	MSA
Plasma NE with patient recumbent	Very low	Normal
Plasma NE when patient stands	Minimal or no increase	Subnormal increase
NE infusion	Very marked increase in blood pressure	Modest increase in blood pressure

Adapted from Schatz, I. J. 1986. *Orthostatic hypotension*, 60, Philadelphia: FA Davis, with permission.

MSA, multiple system atrophy; NE, norepinephrine; PAF, pure autonomic failure.

DIAGNOSTIC IMAGING TECHNIQUES

Magnetic resonance imaging (MRI) of the brain and positron emission tomography (PET) of the brain and heart may help in distinguishing among patients with pure autonomic failure, MSA, and PD. In patients with MSA, MRI of the brain frequently shows signal hypointensity in the putamen (relative to pallidum) on T_2-weighted images and atrophy of the brainstem and cerebellum. MRI results of the brain in pure autonomic failure are normal. PET in patients with MSA shows a generalized reduction in glucose utilization rate, indicating hypometabolism, most prominently in the cerebellum, brainstem, striatum, and frontal and motor cortices. None of these findings was present in patients with pure autonomic failure. Sympathetic cardiac innervation, visualized with PET after intravenous infusion of 6-[^{18}F] fluorodopamine, a catecholamine taken up by sympathetic postganglionic neurons and handled similarly to norepinephrine, is selectively affected in PD and pure autonomic failure, but it is intact in MSA. This may turn out to be a useful diagnostic test to distinguish between PD and MSA. Moreover, in a patient with apparent pure autonomic failure, finding normal sympathetic cardiac innervation should indicate a likely development of MSA [10].

NEUROPATHOLOGY

In patients with pure autonomic failure, intracytoplasmic eosinophilic inclusion bodies with the histologic appearance of Lewy bodies, similar to those found in PD, are identified in neurons of the substantia nigra, locus ceruleus, thoracolumbar and sacral spinal cord, and sympathetic ganglia and postganglionic nerves [8].

α-Synuclein, a neuronal protein of unknown function, is a major component of the Lewy body in PD, dementia with Lewy body, and the glial and neuronal cytoplasmic inclusions of MSA. α-Synuclein also is a major component of Lewy bodies in the brain and peripheral autonomic ganglia in patients with pure autonomic failure [9]. Thus, abnormalities in the expression or structure of α-synuclein or associated proteins may cause degeneration of catecholamine-containing neurons [10].

MANAGEMENT

Patient education is an important aspect of treatment. Patients should be encouraged by the relatively benign nature of pure autonomic failure. Treatment of OH with volume expansion and α-adrenergic agonist agents allows for increased standing time and improved quality of life. Bladder management may require intermittent catheterization. See Chapter 109 for a discussion of nonpharmacologic and pharmacologic approaches to therapy.

References

1. Bradbury, S., and C. Eggleston. 1925. Postural hypotension: A report of three cases. *Am. Heart J.* I:75–86.
2. Schatz, I. J. 1984. Orthostatic hypotension. I. Functional and neurogenic causes. *Arch. Intern. Med.* 144:773–777.
3. Bannister, R. 1988. *Autonomic failure: Clinical features of autonomic failure*, 2nd ed. London: Oxford University Press.
4. Polinsky, R. J., I. J. Kopin, M. H. Ebert, and V. Weise. 1981. Pharmacologic distinction of different orthostatic hypotension syndromes. *Neurology* 31:1–7.
5. Baser, S. M., R. T. Brown, M. T. Curras, C. E. Baucom, D. R. Hooper, and R. J. Polinsky. 1991. Beta receptor sensitivity in autonomic failure. *Neurology* 41:1107–1112.
6. Kaufmann, H., E. Oribe, M. Miller, P. Knott, M. Wiltshire-Clement, and M. D. Yahr. 1992. Hypotension-induced vasopressin release distinguishes between pure autonomic failure and multiple system atrophy with autonomic failure. *Neurology* 42:590–593.
7. Kimber, J. R., L. Watson, and C. J. Mathias. 1997. Distinction of idiopathic Parkinson's disease from multiple-system atrophy by stimulation of growth-hormone release with clonidine. *Lancet* 349:1877–1881.
8. Hague, K., S. Lento, S. Morgello, S. Caro, and H. Kaufmann. 1997. The distribution of Lewy bodies in pure autonomic failure: Autopsy findings and review of the literature. *Acta. Neuropathologica* 94: 192–196.
9. Kaufmann, H., K. Hague, and D. Perl. 2001. Accumulation of alpha synuclein in autonomic nerves in pure autonomic failure. *Neurology* 56:980–981.
10. Kaufmann, H. 2000. Primary autonomic failure: Three clinical presentations of one disease. *Ann. Intern. Med.* 133:382–384.

84 Familial Dysautonomia

Felicia B. Axelrod
Dysautonomia Treatment and Evaluation Center
New York University School of Medicine
New York, New York

Max J. Hilz
Department of Clinical Neurophysiology
University of Erlangen-Nuremberg
Nuremberg, Germany
New York University School of Medicine
New York, New York

Familial dysautonomia (FD) is one of the hereditary sensory and autonomic neuropathies that are generally characterized by widespread sensory dysfunction and variable autonomic dysfunction [1]. Sensory abnormalities primarily affect pain and temperature perception. Abnormalities of the autonomic nervous system affect central and peripheral functions. The disorder manifests at birth, slowly progresses with age [2], and cannot be arrested. Symptoms and problems vary with time and there is only preventative, symptomatic, and supportive treatment [3].

GENETICS AND DIAGNOSIS

FD is an autosomal recessive disorder that appears confined to individuals of Ashkenazi Jewish extraction. In this population, the estimated carrier rate is 1 in 30, with a disease frequency of 1 in 3700 live births. Two mutations in the *IKAP* gene, located on chromosome 9 (9q31), were shown to cause FD [4]. The most common mutation is a single-base substitution in intron 20. More than 99% of patients with FD are homozygous for this mutation that affects the splicing of the IKAP transcript. This splicing alteration may be tissue (i.e., neuron) specific [4].

Although penetrance is complete, there is marked variability in expression of the disease. A *de novo* diagnosis is based on clinical recognition and documentation of both sensory and autonomic dysfunction. In addition to lack of emotion overflow tears, there should be four other "cardinal" criteria—absent fungiform papillae (Fig. 84.1), depressed deep tendon reflexes, abnormal histamine test, and pupillary hypersensitivity to parasympathomimetic agents (pilocarpine 0.0625%)—in an individual of Ashkenazi Jewish extraction [1]. Further supportive evidence is provided by findings of decreased response to pain and temperature, orthostatic hypotension, periodic erythematous blotching of the skin, and increased sweating. In addition, there is prominent oromotor incoordination and gastrointestinal dysmotility. Sural nerve biopsy rarely is required because molecular DNA diagnosis is now the definitive confirmatory test.

PATHOLOGY

Sural Nerve

The sural nerve fascicular area is reduced and contains markedly diminished numbers of nonmyelinated and small-diameter myelinated axons [1, 5]. Catecholamine-containing fibers are missing. Even in the youngest subject extensive pathology is evident.

Spinal Cord

The dorsal root ganglia are grossly reduced in size because of decreased neuronal population. Within the spinal cord, lateral root entry zones and Lissauer's tracts are severely depleted of axons. With increasing age, there is further depletion of neurons in dorsal root ganglia and an increase in residual nodules of Nageotte [5]. In addition, loss of dorsal column myelinated axons becomes evident in older patients. Diminution of primary substance P axons in the substantia gelatinosa of spinal cord and medulla has been demonstrated using immunohistochemistry [1, 5].

Sympathetic Nervous System

In adult patients with FD, the mean volume of superior cervical sympathetic ganglia is 34% of the normal size, reflecting a severe decrease in number of neurons [5]. The anatomic defect in the ganglion cells extends to preganglionic neurons as the intermediolateral gray columns of the spinal cord also contain low numbers of neurons. Although clinical, anatomic, biochemical, and pharmacologic data suggest diminution in the numbers of sympathetic neurons in FD, sympathetic ganglia show enhanced staining of cells containing tyrosine hydroxylase, the rate-limiting enzyme in

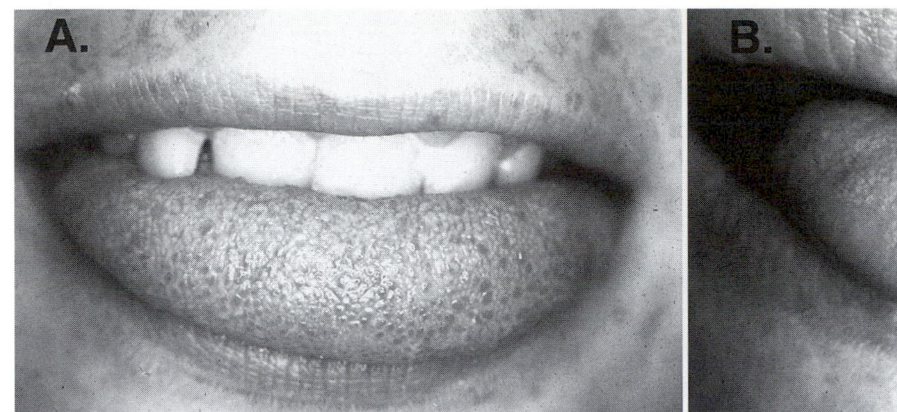

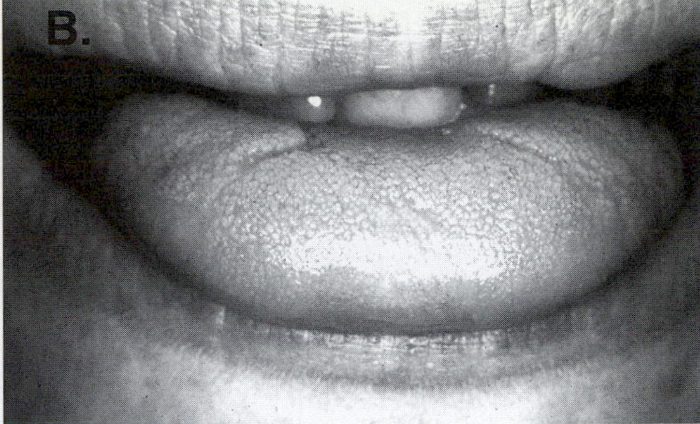

FIGURE 84.1 **A**, Normal tongue with fungiform papillae present on the tip. **B**, Dysautonomic tongue.

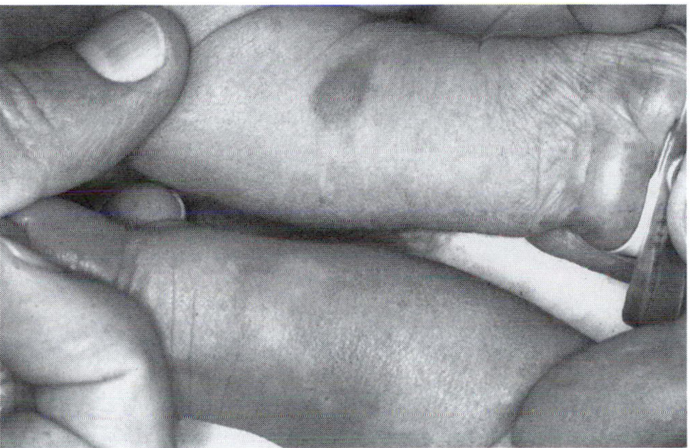

FIGURE 84.2 **A**, Normal histamine test. Reaction displays diffuse axon flare around a central wheal. **B**, Dysautonomic histamine test. Only a narrow areola surrounds the wheal.

catecholamine synthesis [6]. Ultrastructural study of peripheral blood vessels demonstrates the absence of autonomic nerve terminals [1, 7].

Parasympathetic Nervous System

The sphenopalatine ganglia are consistently reduced in size with low total neuronal counts, but the neuronal population is only questionably reduced in other parasympathetic ganglia, such as the ciliary ganglia.

BIOCHEMICAL DATA

Consistent with the decrease in the sympathetic neuronal population, there is a 60% diminution in norepinephrine (NE) synthesis and reduced catabolite excretion. However, dopamine products continue to be excreted in normal amounts resulting in a reduced 3-methoxy-4-hydroxymandelic acid to 3-methoxy-4-hydroxyphenylacetic acid ratios [7]. In addition, plasma levels of NE and dopamine β-hydroxylase (DBH) do not increase when the patient with FD goes from supine to standing position; but during emotional crises, plasma NE and dopamine are markedly increased [8, 9]. During such crises, vomiting usually coincides with high dopamine levels. Increased NE may appear through peripheral conversion of dopamine by DBH. Supine early morning plasma renin activity is increased in patients with FD and the release of renin and aldosterone is not coordinated. In patients with FD with supine hypertension, an increase in plasma atrial natriuretic peptide occurs [8]. The combination of these factors may explain the exaggerated nocturnal urine volume and increased excretion of salt in some patients with FD.

CLINICAL SYMPTOMS AND TREATMENTS

There is a baseline neurologic dysfunction and slow degeneration with age in FD (Table 84.1). In addition, the pervasive nature of the autonomic nervous system results in protean functional abnormalities involving other systems. Frequent manifestations include hypotonia, delayed developmental milestones, oromotor incoordination and gastrointestinal dysmotility, labile body temperature and blood pressure, absence of overflow tears and corneal anesthesia, marked diaphoresis with excitement, breath-holding episodes, and spinal curvature. Patients with FD also are susceptible to periodic autonomic storms, termed *dysautonomic crises* (Table 84.2). The crises are a systemic reaction to stress, either physical or emotional. Currently, the disease process cannot be arrested. Treatment must be directed toward specific problems within each system, which vary considerably among patients, as well as with age.

Signs of the disorder are present from birth. Poor sucking or uncoordinated swallowing is observed in 60% of infants

TABLE 84.1 Neurologic Abnormalities

Sensory system
*Pain loss sparing hands, soles of feet, neck, genital areas, and viscera
*Temperature appreciation abnormal
Deep tendon reflexes depressed
Insensitivity to fractures/Charcot joints
Autonomic system
Oropharyngeal incoordination (feeding problems, especially liquids)
*Esophageal dysmotility, gastroesophageal reflux
Insensitivity to hypoxia and relative insensitivity to hypercapnia
Breath-holding
*Postural hypotension without compensatory tachycardia
*Supine hypertension
Motor system
Hypotonia
Mild/moderate development delay
*Gait often broad-based and progressive ataxia
*Spinal curvature (95%, especially kyphosis)
Cranial nerves
No overflow tears
Taste deficient, especially sweet
Corneal reflexes depressed/corneal ulcerations
*Optic nerve atrophy
Exotropia, myopia
Speech frequently dysarthric and nasal
Intelligence/personality
Usually normal intelligence (verbal skills better than motor)
Tend to be concrete or literal
Skin picking (especially fingers and nose)
*Resistant to change (some patients are phobic)

*Progressive neurologic features.

TABLE 84.2 Autonomic Crisis Features

Excessive sweating of head and trunk
Erythematous blotching of face and trunk
Mottling of peripheral extremities (cutis marmorata)
Hypertension and tachycardia
Nausea/Vomiting
Severe dysphagia/drooling
Irritability
Insomnia
Worsening of tone

in the neonatal period. Oropharyngeal incoordination often persists and puts the patient at risk for aspiration pneumonia, the major cause of lung infections. Gastrostomy often is necessary [3]. If gastroesophageal reflex is present, the risk for aspiration increases. If medical management with prokinetic agents, H2 antagonists, thickening of feeds, and positioning is not successful, then surgical intervention (fundoplication) is performed [3]. Failure of medical management would result in persistence of pneumonia, hematemesis, or apnea.

Crises occur in approximately 40% of patients with FD. Diazepam is the most effective antiemetic for the dysautonomic crisis and can be administered orally, intravenously, or rectally at 0.1 to 0.2 mg/kg per dose. Subsequent doses of diazepam are repeated at 3-hour intervals until the crisis resolves. If diastolic hypotension persists (>90 mmHg) after administering diazepam, then chloral hydrate or clonidine (0.004 mg/kg per dose) is suggested. Clonidine can be repeated at 8-hour intervals [1, 3, 7].

Patients with FD have decreased sensitivity to hypoxia and increased baseline CO_2 levels with rather normal CO_2 sensitivity. Hyperventilation induces prolonged apnea and severe oxygen desaturation. Thus, tachypnea rarely is seen with respiratory infections, and high altitudes and airplane travel can result in syncope and even asystole.

Clinical manifestations of orthostatic hypotension worsen with age and include episodes of lightheadedness, dizzy spells, and leg weakness. Frequently, hypotension is not perceived, although postural changes occur such as a forward list. Unless there is associated hypoxia, hypotension rarely results in syncope. There seems to be an adaptation of cerebrovascular autoregulation to both orthostatic hypotension and chronic supine [10]. Orthostatic hypotension is treated by maintaining adequate hydration, encouraging lower extremity exercise to increase muscle tone and promote venous return, and elastic stockings. Fludrocortisone and midodrine also have been of some benefit [11].

Renal function also appears to deteriorate with advancing age. Pathologic studies reveal excess glomerulosclerosis. Although the cause of the progressive renal disease is not certain, hypoperfusion of the kidney seems a likely explanation. Hypoperfusion could occur because of dehydration, postural hypotension, or vasoconstriction of renal vessels as a result of sympathetic supersensitivity during vomiting crisis.

Sexual maturation is frequently delayed, but primary and secondary sex characteristics eventually develop in both sexes. Women with dysautonomia have conceived and delivered healthy infants. Pregnancies were tolerated well. At time of delivery, blood pressures were labile. One male patient has fathered seven children. All offspring have been phenotypically normal despite their obligatory heterozygote state.

PROGNOSIS

With greater understanding of the disorder and development of treatment programs, survival statistics have markedly improved so that increasing numbers of patients are reaching adulthood. Survival statistics before 1960 reported that 50% of patients died before 5 years of age. Current survival statistics indicate that a newborn with FD has a greater than 50% probability of reaching 30 years of age. Many of the adults have been able to achieve independent function. Causes of death are less often related to pulmonary complications, indicating that more aggressive treatment of aspirations has been beneficial. Still of concern are the patients who succumb to unexplained deaths that may have been the result of unopposed vagal stimulation or a sleep abnormality. A few adult patients have died of renal failure.

References

1. Axelrod, F. B. 1996. Autonomic and sensory disorders. In *Principles and practice of medical genetics*, 3rd ed., ed. A. E. H. Emory, and D. L. Rimoin, 397–411. Edinburgh: Churchill Livingstone.
2. Axelrod, F. B., and C. H. Maayan. 1999. Familial dysautonomia. In *Gellis and Kagen's current pediatric therapy*, 16th ed., ed. F. D. Burg, J. R. Ingelfinger, E. R. Wald, and R. A. Polin, 466–469. Philadelphia: WB Saunders.
3. Slaugenhaupt, S. A., A. Blumenfeld, S. P. Gill, M. Leyne, J. Mull, M. P. Cuajungco, C. E. Liebert, B. Chadwick, M. Idelson, L. Reznik, C. M. Robbins, I. Makalowskia, M. J. Brownsein, D. Krappman, C. Scheidereit, C. H. Maayan, F. B. Axelrod, and J. Gusella. 2001. Tissue-specific expression of a splicing mutation in the IKBKAP gene causes familial dysautonomia. *Am. J. Hum. Genet.* 68:598–604.
4. Axelrod, F. B., K. Iyer, I. Fish, J. Pearson, M. E. Stein, and N. Spielholz. 1981. Progressive sensory loss in familial dysautonomia. *Pediatrics* 65:517–522.
5. Pearson, J., F. B. Axelrod, and J. Dancis. 1974. Current concepts of dysautonomia neurological defects. *Ann. NY Acad. Sci.* 228:288–300.
6. Pearson, J., L. Brandeis, and M. Goldstein. 1979. Tyrosine hydroxylase immunohistoreactivity in familial dysautonomia. *Science* 206: 71–72.
7. Axelrod, F. B. 1999. Familial dysautonomia. In *Autonomic failure*, 4th ed., ed. C. J. Mathias, and R. Bannister, 402–418. New York: Oxford University Press.
8. Axelrod, F. B., L. Krey, J. S. Glickstein, D. Friedman, J. Weider, L. Metakis, V. M. Porges, M. Mineo, and D. Notterman. 1994. Atrial natriuretic peptide and catecholamine response to orthostatic hypotension and treatments in familial dysautonomia. *Clin. Auton. Res.* 4:311–318.
9. Ziegler, M. G., R. C. Lake, and I. J. Kopin. 1976. Deficient sympathetic nervous system response in familial dysautonomia. *N. Engl. J. Med.* 294:630–633.
10. Hilz, M. J., F. B. Axelrod, U. Haertl, C. M. Brown, and B. Stemper. 2002. Transcranial Doppler sonography during head up tilt suggests preserved central sympathetic activation in familial dysautonomia. *J. Neurol. Neurosurg. Psychiatry* 72:657–660.
11. Axelrod, F. B., L. Krey, J. S. Glickstein, J. Weider-Allison, and D. Friedman. 1995. Preliminary observations on the use of midodrine in treating orthostatic hypotension in familial dysautonomia. *J. Auton. Nerv. System* 55:29–35.

85 Hereditary Autonomic Neuropathies

Yadollah Harati
Department of Neurology
Baylor College of Medicine
Houston, Texas

Opas Nawasiripong
Department of Neurology
Baylor College of Medicine
Houston, Texas

There are few inherited peripheral neuropathies in which autonomic dysfunction, whether clinical or subclinical, is detected (Table 85.1).

Autonomic abnormalities are frequent and prominent in familial dysautonomia and amyloidosis (see separate reviews in Chapters 84 and 86). This chapter discusses the remaining inherited neuropathies with autonomic involvement.

FABRY'S DISEASE

Fabry's disease or Anderson–Fabry's disease (angiokeratoma corporis diffusum) is an X-linked recessive, slowly progressive metabolic disorder with protean and nonspecific clinical manifestations. Although the skin, kidney, heart, and peripheral and central nervous system are the most frequently involved organs, autonomic dysfunction also may be present. The clinical manifestations of the disease in the affected hemizygous male individuals result from progressive and widespread accumulation of neutral glycosphingolipids, caused by α-galactosidase A deficiency, in the lysosomes of vascular endothelial, smooth muscle, skin, cornea, neural cells, perineural cells of the autonomic nervous system, ganglia, and body fluids. Heterozygous female carriers are usually asymptomatic; 15%, however, have severe involvement of one or more organs. The classically affected male individuals have no detectable α-galactosidase A activity with the onset of disease manifestation in childhood or adolescence. Variants and milder forms of the disease in which residual enzyme activity may be detected have been reported. The gene for the enzyme has been mapped to the region between Xq21.33 and Xq22 of the long arm of the X chromosome. Currently, more than 30 different small mutations in this gene have been reported.

Clinical Manifestations of Fabry's Disease

The most prominent and frequent clinical presentation of Fabry's disease includes bouts of severe painful burning sensation in the hands and feet; a reddish purple maculopapular rash (angiokeratoma) of lower abdomen, pelvic, genital, upper thigh regions and, at times, in oral mucosa and conjunctive; hypohidrosis; heat intolerance; and lenticular and corneal opacities. Any boy or young man with severe painful sensory neuropathy should be suspected as having Fabry's disease, and careful scrutiny for the skin lesions should be conducted because typical skin lesions are usually sparse and may be easily overlooked.

Triggering factors for the episodic pain include fatigue, exercise, emotional stress, and rapid changes in temperature and humidity. The pathophysiologic events leading to the incapacitating episodes of pain or acroparesthesias have not been clarified.

Early albuminuria, uremia, renal failure, cardiomyopathy, cardiac hypertrophy, conduction abnormalities, aortic degeneration, hypertension, mitral valve thickening, atrioventricular block, and supraventricular arrhythmias may occur. Short P-R interval, ST-T changes, and left ventricular hypertrophy are common electrocardiogram abnormalities of Fabry's disease.

Although cardiac involvement is a constant feature of Fabry's disease, most patients do not experience cardiac symptoms until late in the disease course. Cerebrovascular disease secondary to multifocal abnormalities of large and small vessels may also occur. In young male patients with unexplained cardiovascular abnormalities and a history of acroparesthesia, angiokeratoma, and ophthalmologic findings, the diagnosis of Fabry's disease should always be considered. Ocular manifestations involving the cornea, lens, conjunctiva, and retina are early and prominent, but require slit lamp microscopic evaluation.

Involvement of many other tissues and organs results in a variety of symptoms and signs including gastrointestinal (episodic diarrhea, abdominal cramps, and achalasia), musculoskeletal (bony deformities), hematopoietic (anemia, foamy macrophages, and iron deficiency), pulmonary, vestibular, and auditory symptoms and signs.

Autonomic Involvement

Although there are many reports of structural abnormalities of the autonomic nervous system in Fabry's disease, overt clinical autonomic dysfunction is not commonly

TABLE 85.1 Inherited Peripheral Neuropathies with Dysautonomia

1. Hereditary sensory and autonomic neuropathies types I, II, III* (see Chapter 84), IV, and V
2. Hereditary motor and sensory neuropathy types I and II (Charcot-Marie Tooth disease 1,2)
3. Fabry's disease*
4. Multiple endocrine neoplasia type 2B
5. Amyloidosis* (see Chapter 86)
6. Porphyrias*

*Dysautonomia is prominent and clinically significant.

observed. The contribution of autonomic dysfunction to the overall morbidity of Fabry's disease is unknown.

Anhidrosis or hypohidrosis and possibly the episodic pain are probably caused by the involvement of sympathetic ganglion cells and degeneration of unmyelinated nerve fibers. Both glycosphingolipid accumulation and vascular ischemia appear to play a role in the abnormalities of autonomic ganglia. There is a preferential loss of small myelinated and unmyelinated fibers in the sural nerve biopsies. Detailed clinical autonomic testing has shown involvement of both sympathetic and parasympathetic systems, the latter being more readily demonstrate. Diminished pupillary responses to pilocarpine, impaired gastrointestinal motility, and reduced tear and saliva formation may be observed early in the disease course. Sympathetic dysfunction is evident by the loss of the cutaneous flare response to scratch and histamine and the absence of thermal fingertip wrinkling. Blood pressure, heart rate, and plasma norepinephrine responses to tilt are usually intact. Accumulation of ceramide trihexoside in the myenteric nerve plexuses throughout the gut results in disturbances in peristalsis and gastrocolic reflexes in more than 60% of hemizygous patients. Intestinal dysmotility may produce areas of high intraluminal pressure, allowing the formation of diverticula. Intestinal stasis and bacterial overgrowth will result in diarrhea.

Diagnosis in male patients can be established by measuring α-galactosidase A activity in plasma, leukocytes, or fibroblasts. Laboratory, histologic, and molecular diagnoses identify 100% of hemizygotes and more than 80% of heterozygotes.

Until recently, there was no effective treatment for the autonomic dysfunction observed in Fabry's disease. A recent study has revealed that recombinant α-galactosidase A replacement therapy cleared microvascular endothelial deposits of glycosphingolipid from the kidneys, heart, and skin in patients with Fabry's disease, reversing the pathogenesis of the chief clinical manifestations of this disease. Intravenous Agalsidase β (Fabrazyme) is now approved by the FDA and should be initiated soon after diagnosis. It has been suggested that carbamazepine used in the treatment of episodic pain may result in a dose-dependent aggravation of autonomic dysfunction including urinary retention, nausea, vomiting, and ileus. Fludrocortisone acetate therapy results in a reduction in the frequency of patients' syncopal events.

A successful renal transplantation not only corrects the renal function but may also result in relief from acroparesthesia and pain and a partial restoration of sweating. Enzyme replacement, especially when obtained from human placenta, has been feasibly used in an experimental trial in the treatment of a few patients with Fabry's disease.

PORPHYRIA

Acute hepatic porphyrias (acute intermittent porphyria, variegate porphyria, and hereditary coproporphyria) are a group of autosomal dominant inherited metabolic disorders that manifest as acute or subacute, severe, life-threatening motor neuropathy, abdominal pain, autonomic dysfunction, and neuropsychiatric manifestations. Its gene is thought to be present in 1/80,000 people, although only one-third affected persons ever manifest symptoms of the disease. The basic defect is a 50% reduction in hydroxymethylbilane synthase, previously known as porphobilinogen deaminase activity (acute intermittent porphyria), protoporphyrinogen-IX oxidase (variegate porphyria), and coproporphyrinogen oxidase (coproporphyria), resulting in abnormalities of heme synthesis. In the presence of sufficient endogenous or exogenous stimuli (e.g., drugs, hormones, menstruation, and starvation), this partial deficiency may lead to clinical manifestations.

Clinical Manifestation of Porphyria

The neurologic manifestations of all forms of the acute porphyrias are identical. Symptoms of the acute attack include severe abdominal pain, nausea, vomiting, constipation, diarrhea, urinary frequency and hesitancy, urine discoloration, labile hypertension, tachycardia, pain in limbs and back, and convulsions. Abdominal pain and ileus may occur several days before neurologic manifestations. Porphyria affects predominantly motor nerves, often leading to proximal, facial, and bulbar weakness. It usually develops within 2 to 3 days of the onset of abdominal pain and psychiatric symptoms and may begin in the upper limbs with wrist and finger extensor weakness or with cranial nerve dysfunction. The progression of weakness to trunk and respiratory muscles may resemble Guillain–Barré syndrome, but the ascending pattern of weakness is rare, cerebrospinal fluid is usually normal, and, in some patients, the reflexes remain intact.

The nerve conduction velocities in porphyria are not slowed to the levels observed in demyelinating lesions. The mechanism of the neuropathic changes is poorly understood.

Two hypotheses—the possible neurotoxicity of heme pathway intermediates such as delta-aminolevulinic and porphyrins, and heme deficiency in nervous tissue—have been suggested.

Autonomic Involvement in Porphyria

Autonomic disturbances in sympathetic and parasympathetic systems are prevalent immediately before and during the attacks of porphyrias, suggesting a greater and earlier susceptibility of the autonomic nerves. Persistent sinus tachycardia invariably precedes the development of peripheral neuropathy and respiratory paralysis and, together with labile hypertension, may be explained by damage to vagus or glossopharyngeal nerves, their nuclei, or central connections. Tachycardia and hypertension may be associated with increased catecholamine release and urinary excretion, suggesting increased peripheral sympathetic activity. Patients may have chronic hypertension between the attacks leading to renal function impairment. Orthostatic hypotension may occur in acute attacks of variegate porphyria. Use of a battery of baroreflex tests during the acute attack reveals mostly reversible parasympathetic or sympathetic dysfunction. The parasympathetic tests, however, become abnormal earlier and more frequently than sympathetic tests. Early parasympathetic dysfunction is detected during remission and in late asymptomatic patients. The immediate response of heart rate to standing (30 : 15 ratio) or the Valsalva maneuver may be mildly abnormal in asymptomatic subjects with acute intermittent porphyria, suggesting the occurrence of a subclinical autonomic neuropathy in latent porphyrias.

Gastrointestinal disturbances including abdominal pain, severe vomiting, obstinate constipation, intestinal dilation, and stasis may be explained by the impaired gut motor activity caused by autonomic or enteric nerve damage, or both. Studies on impaired proximal gastrointestinal tract motility and reduced circulating gut peptides in a few patients with acute intermittent porphyria tend to support this hypothesis. Other autonomic dysfunctions observed in acute intermittent porphyrias include sweating disturbances, pupillary dilation, and hesitancy in micturition and bladder distension.

Limited pathologic studies of the autonomic nervous system in acute intermittent porphyrias have revealed lesions of vagus nerve including axonal degeneration and demyelination, and chromatolysis of dorsal nuclei and sympathetic chain, as well as the splanchnic motor cells of the lateral horns and cells of the celiac ganglion. The sympathetic chain ganglia shows a decrease of 50% in the density of ganglion cells and myelinated axons compared with control subjects.

The Watson–Schwartz test is used as a screening test for the detection of porphobilinogen (PBG) in urine during the attack. The laboratory diagnosis of porphyria depends on the measurement of porphyrin precursors in urine. To evaluate the porphyria type, measurement of porphyrins in both urine and feces is required. Enzyme measurements are used to identify asymptomatic family members whose quantitative excretions of porphyrins are normal.

Treatment of Porphyria

The most effective treatment of porphyria attacks is the administration of hematin intravenously. With modern intensive care techniques and the advent of hematin therapy, the mortality rate for acute intermittent porphyrias is less than 10%. Porphyrinogenic drugs avoidance, high glucose intake, vitamin B_6, β-blockers, analgesics, selective anticonvulsants, and hematin therapy (2–5 mg/kg per day intravenously for 3–14 days) are the mainstays of therapy. Phenylephrine and phentolamine are reported to restore normal blood pressure. Recovery from psychiatric and autonomic dysfunction is usually rapid. All at-risk relatives should be screened for the latent disease.

MULTIPLE ENDOCRINE NEOPLASIA TYPE 2B

Multiple endocrine neoplasia type 2 (MEN 2) syndromes are neural crest disorders. The MEN 2 syndromes comprise clinically related autosomal dominant cancer syndromes. MEN 2A (Sipple syndrome) is characterized by medullary thyroid carcinoma, pheochromocytoma in about 50% of cases, and parathyroid hyperplasia or adenoma in about 25% of cases. MEN 2B is similar to MEN 2A but is characterized by earlier age of tumor onset and the developmental abnormalities, which include intestinal ganglioneuromatosis, atypical facies with mucosal neuromas of distal tongue and subconjunctiva, marfanoid habitus, muscle underdevelopment, and bony deformities.

Autonomic manifestations of MEN 2B are not prominent and are generally overshadowed by its other symptoms and signs. They include impaired lacrimation, orthostatic hypotension, impaired reflex vasodilatation of skin and parasympathetic denervation supersensitivity of pupils, with intact sweating and salivary gland function. There are gross and microscopic abnormalities of the peripheral autonomic nervous system with both sympathetic and parasympathetic systems affected. There is disorganized hypertrophy and proliferation of autonomic nerves and ganglia (ganglioneuromatosis). Neural proliferation of the alimentary tract (Auerbach and Meissner's plexus), upper respiratory tract, bladder, prostate, and skin may also be seen. Nerve biopsy shows degeneration and regeneration of unmyelinated fibers.

Genetic linkage studies of MEN have mapped the gene responsible for this syndrome to the pericentromeric region of chromosome 10. This region also contains the RET protooncogene, which codes for a receptor tyrosine kinase.

Different missense mutation within RET protooncogene is thought to be responsible for MEN 2A and 2B.

Diagnosis of and screening for MEN 2A and 2B have been done using pentagastrin stimulation test and plasma calcitonin determinations. Pheochromocytoma is diagnosed by assessing a 24-hour urine collection for metanephrine, vanillylmandelic acid, and fractionated catecholamine levels.

The prognosis in the MEN 2B syndrome is generally poor as a result of an aggressive medullary thyroid carcinoma that develops earlier in life for patients with MEN 2B than those with MEN 2A (5-year survival rate of 78% for MEN 2B and 86% for MEN 2A). This can be improved by regular screening of patients at risk; early diagnosis allows thyroidectomy, adrenalectomy, or both, which are likely to be curative.

HEREDITARY MOTOR AND SENSORY NEUROPATHIES TYPE I AND II (CHARCOT-MARIE TOOTH 1 AND 2)

Clinically significant autonomic dysfunction is not a common feature of Charcot-Marie Tooth disease types 1 and 2 (CMT 1 and 2). When a battery of autonomic function tests are systematically given to patients with well-established CMT abnormalities of sudomotor and local vasomotor responses, heart rate and blood pressure changes, pupillary abnormalities, impairment of sweating, and impaired tear production may be observed, suggesting involvement of postganglionic sympathetic and parasympathetic nerve fibers. Sural nerve biopsies may show abnormalities of unmyelinated nerve fibers, which explains the frequently observed abnormalities of sweat function tests. Pupillary abnormalities are secondary to a parasympathetic denervation of the iris sphincter and ciliary muscle, as shown by a positive methacholic test. Several patients with myotonic pupils received symptomatic relief from 0.025% pilocarpine.

TYPES I, II, IV, AND V HEREDITARY SENSORY AND AUTONOMIC NEUROPATHY

Type I hereditary sensory and autonomic neuropathy (HSAN) with an autosomal dominant gene on chromosome 9q22 and type II with a probable autosomal recessive inheritance pattern exhibit no significant autonomic dysfunction except for hypohidrosis. Types III and IV are autosomal recessive. Type III has preserved and, at times, excessive sweating. Type IV shares some of the features of type II and III, but the patients may have episodes of fever, low IQ, severe hypohidrosis with abnormal or absent sympathetic skin response test, and markedly reduced pain perception. There is a marked loss of small myelinated and unmyelinated nerve fibers. Type V presents with selective loss of extremity pain perception and thermal discrimination and impaired sudomotor function. Sural nerve biopsy reveals selective loss of small myelinated fibers with only a slightly decreased number of larger myelinated fibers.

References

1. Blom, H., C. Andersson, B. O. Olofsson, P. Bjerle, U. Wiklund, and F. Lithner. 1996. Assessment of autonomic nerve function in acute intermittent porphyria: A study based on spectral analysis of heart rate variability. *J. Intern. Med.* 240(2):73–79.
2. Desnick, R. J., and K. Anderson. 1991. Heme biosynthesis and its disorders: The porphyrias and sideroblastic anemias. In *Hematology, basic principles and practice,* ed. R. Hoffman, E. J. Benz, S. J. Shattil, B. Furie, and H. Cohen, 350–367. New York: Churchill Livingstone.
3. Desnick, R. J., R. Brady, J. Barranger, A. J. Collins, D. P. Germain, M. Goldman, G. Grabowski, S. Packman, and W. R. Wilcox. 2003. Fabry disease, an under-recognized multisystemic disorder: Expert recommendations for diagnosis, management, and enzyme replacement therapy. *Ann. Intern. Med.* 138(4):338–346.
4. Dyck, P. J., J. A. Carney, G. W. Sizemore, H. Okazaki, W. S. Brimijoin, and E. H. Lambert. 1979. Multiple endocrine neoplasia, type 2b: Phenotype recognition, neurologic features, and their pathologic basis. *Ann. Neurol.* 6:302–314.
5. Gardner, D. G. 1997. Recent advances in multiple endocrine neoplasia syndromes. *Adv. Intern. Med.* 42:597–627.
6. Harati, Y., and P. A. Low. 1990. Autonomic peripheral neuropathies: Diagnosis and clinical presentation. In *Current neurology,* ed. S. H. Appel, 105–176. St. Louis: Mosby.
7. Ingall, T. J., and J. G. McLeod. 1991. Autonomic function in hereditary motor and sensory neuropathy (Charcot-Marie-Tooth disease). In *Muscle Nerve* 16(1):114–115.
8. Menkes, D. L., T. J. O'Neil, and K. K. Saenz. 1997. Fabry's disease presenting as syncope, angiokeratomas and spoke-like cataracts in young man: Discussion of the differential diagnosis. *Mil. Med.* 162(11):773–776.
9. Thomas, P. K. 1992. Autonomic involvement inherited neuropathies. *Clin. Auton. Res.* 2(1):51–56.
10. Yamamoto, K., N. Suzuki, N. Takahashi, Y. Sasayama, and S. Kikuyama. 1996. Possible mechanism of anhidrosis in a symptomatic female carrier of Fabry's disease: An assessment by skin sympathetic nerve activity and sympathetic skin response. *Clin. Auton. Res.* 6(2):107–110.
11. Eng, C. M., N. Guffon, W. R. Wilcox, D. P. Germain, P. Lee, S. Waldek, L. Caplan, G. E. Linthorst, and R. J. Desnick. 2001. Safety and efficacy of recombinant human α-Galactosidase A replacement therapy in Fabry's disease. *N. Engl. J. Med.* 345(1):9–16.

86 Amyloidotic Autonomic Failure

Hazem Machkhas
Department of Neurology
Baylor College of Medicine
Houston, Texas

Opas Nawasiripong
Department of Neurology
Baylor College of Medicine
Houston, Texas

Yadollah Harati
Department of Neurology
Baylor College of Medicine
Houston, Texas

The term *amyloid* was coined by Rudolph Virchow in 1854 to describe a macroscopic tissue deposit that displayed a positive reaction on staining with iodine. Since then, our knowledge about amyloid and amyloidosis has dramatically expanded. There are now more than 20 different protein molecules that are known to undergo conformational changes leading to the generation of amyloid deposits. These are homogeneous insoluble protein deposits, consisting of polypeptide fibrils, 7.5 to 10 nm in width, arranged in highly ordered aggregates of β-pleated sheets, conferring to them a high degree of stability. Amyloid deposits display a characteristic apple green birefringence when examined under polarized light after staining with Congo red (Fig. 86.1). Amyloidosis refers to a wide spectrum of disorders that result from abnormal extracellular deposits of amyloid. These deposits may be widespread (systemic amyloidosis) or restricted to certain organs (localized amyloidosis). Previous classification of amyloidosis was confusing and ever changing. Refined knowledge about the chemical composition of the amyloid deposits, as well as the recognition of hereditary amyloidosis, has resulted in a much more rational classification (Table 86.1).

The clinical presentation of amyloid deposits depends on the organs involved and the size of the amyloid fibrils. Involvement of the peripheral nervous system is an important feature of the systemic amyloidoses and typically presents with the classical clinical triad of small fiber neuropathy, autonomic neuropathy (AN), and carpal tunnel syndrome (CTS). Autonomic failure is an important feature of immunoglobulin amyloidosis and hereditary systemic amyloidosis and must be considered in all patients with familial or paraproteinemic neuropathies having autonomic dysfunction (especially when CTS coexists). The mechanism of nerve injury is probably the same in all amyloidoses, and it involves physical pressure exerted by amyloid deposits on dorsal root ganglia or autonomic ganglia, or directly on nerve fibers, leading to loss of normal tissue elements and disorientation of tissue architecture. Toxic, ischemic, and immunologic mechanisms have been suggested as alternatives.

The following sections discuss amyloidoses that may demonstrate autonomic involvement.

IMMUNOGLOBULIN AMYLOIDOSIS

The amyloid fibrils in immunoglobulin amyloidosis (AL) amyloidopathy are composed of immunoglobulin light chain proteins or their degradation products. AL is the most common form of systemic amyloidosis. The monoclonal immunoglobulin light chains are produced by monoclonal plasma cells, which may be derived from nonproliferative populations or from a malignant clone, such as in multiple myeloma (MM), Waldenström's macroglobulinemia, non-Hodgkin's lymphoma, and solid tumors like hypernephroma. In nonmalignant AL, the peripheral nervous system is involved in more than 50% of patients and is the presenting symptom in 40% of those cases. In amyloidosis associated with MM, clinical and electrophysiologic evidence of polyneuropathy develops in 13% and 40% of patients, respectively.

The peripheral neuropathy in AL is axonal, distal, symmetric, and sensory with impaired pinprick and temperature more than vibratory and proprioceptive sensations, which is consistent with a small fiber neuropathy. As the disease progresses, large fiber involvement appears. Subtle autonomic abnormalities, as detected by autonomic function tests, seem to be prevalent even in asymptomatic patients. Both sympathetic and parasympathetic systems are affected to different extents. Signs of AN include orthostatic hypotension (OH) with inappropriate heart rate response, impotence, dry mouth, gastrointestinal (GI) autonomic disturbances (dysphagia, early satiety, diarrhea, and constipation), sluggish papillary reaction, impairment of sweating, and bladder dysfunction. Autonomic dysfunction, rather than deposition of amyloid in the mucosa, seems to be a more frequent cause of GI symptoms in these patients. Target organs other than in the peripheral nervous system include the heart, skeletal muscles, liver, intestine, spleen, kidney, tongue, and skin.

Pathogenesis

Pathologic investigations have shown infiltration of dorsal root and sympathetic ganglia in patients with amyloidotic neuropathy early in the course of the disease.

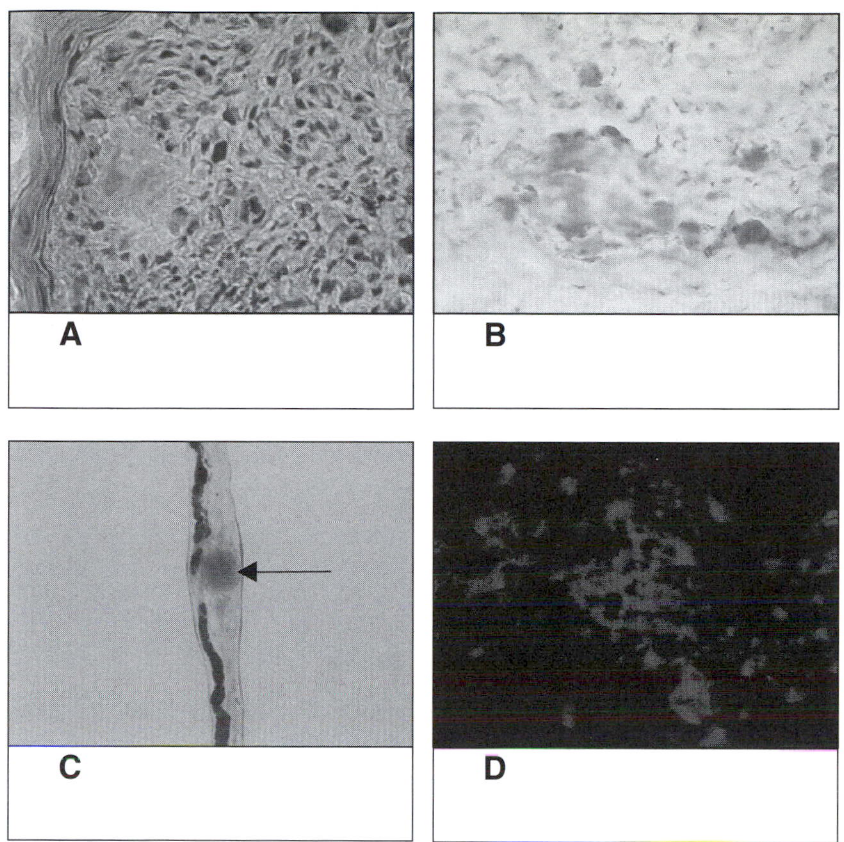

FIGURE 86.1 Amyloid deposits. **A**, Hematoxylin and eosin staining. **B**, Crystal violet. **C**, Teased nerve preparation. **D**, Congo red under fluorescence. (See Color Insert)

Intermediolateral cell column neurons at the T7 level of the spinal cord, which contains the cell bodies of preganglionic sympathetic neurons, may also be reduced.

Diagnosis

Tests of autonomic function are often abnormal. Serum and urine protein electrophoresis detect a monoclonal gammopathy (M protein) in 80% of cases. Lambda light chains are three times as frequent as Kappa. Erythrocyte sedimentation rate is commonly increased. Anemia and proteinuria are common. Congo red is the most specific stain, whereas electron microscopic examination of the amyloid-laden tissues is the most sensitive method of recognizing this disorder. The recently developed iodine-123 serum amyloid P component (^{123}I-SAP) scintigraphy allows for safe and reliable diagnosis and monitoring of progression of disease and response to treatment. Abdominal fat aspiration and rectal biopsy show amyloid in 80% of cases, and bone marrow stains positive for amyloid in 50% of cases. The bone marrow also provides an estimate of the number of plasma cells. In AL without MM, 3 to 5% of the bone marrow cells typically are plasma cells with no malignant features. This is increased in AL with MM to more than 50%, and many plasma cells display malignant features. Sural nerve biopsy provides another tissue source for diagnosis. In patients suspected of having amyloidosis, any tissue obtained during any surgery (e.g., flexor retinaculum during carpal tunnel surgery) may contain amyloid and should be specifically examined for amyloid deposit. Specific antisera currently have been developed that allow the identification of the type of amyloid deposit.

Treatment

Treatment approaches to AL amyloidosis are either specific, geared to suppress or reverse the disease process, or symptomatic. Specific treatments include immunosuppressive or cytotoxic agents. High dose intravenous melphalan with autologous blood stem cell transplantation results in hematologic remission, improved five-year survival, and reversal of amyloid-related disease in a significant number of patients when compared to no treatment. In patients unable to tolerate autologous stem cell transplantation, the combination of high dose dexamethasone and melphalan is an effective therapeutic option. Etanercept may also be used in patients refractory or ineligible to other modalities. In some select cases with specific organ involvement (heart or liver), organ transplantation

TABLE 86.1 Classification of Amyloidosis

	Type	Previous name	Subunit protein	PNS involvement
Systemic amyloidosis	Ig derived (AL)	Primary/myeloma associated	Ig light chain	PN, AN, CTS
	Reactive (AA)	Secondary (acquired)	A protein	PN, AN
	Dialysis associated		B_2-microglobulin	CTS
	Hereditary	Heredofamilial		
		FAP I, II	TTR	PN, AN, CTS
		FAP III	Apolipoprotein	PN
		FAP IV	Gelsolin	PN, CN
		—	Fibrinogen	None
		—	Lysosome	None
Localized amyloidosis	Alzheimer's disease (H,A), HCHA(H), CAA(A), Genitourinary (A), Lichen (A), Cutaneous (H,A), IBM(H,A), Medullary thyroid cancer (H), Bronchopulmonary (A)			

A, acquired; AN, autonomic neuropathy; CAA, cerebral amyloid angiopathy; CN, cranial neuropathy; CTS, carpal tunnel syndrome; FAP, familial amyloid neuropathy; H, hereditary; HCHA, hereditary cerebral hemorrhage with amyloidosis; IBM, inclusion body myopathy; Ig, immunoglobulin; PNS, peripheral nervous system; PN, peripheral neuropathy.

may be successfully attempted, with recovery of organ function. Symptomatic approaches to treatment target various complaints, mostly those associated with autonomic dysfunction. Metoclopramide has been used to treat early satiety, whereas octreotide, a somatostatin analog, has been successfully used to treat amyloidosis-associated diarrhea. Cisapride was reported to be useful in intestinal pseudoobstruction in AL associated with MM. Although fludrocortisone is the mainstay of treatment of OH, midodrine, erythropoietin, and l-threo-3,4-dihydroxyphenylserine (DOPS) are also reported to be helpful. Other therapies for OH include elastic support extending to the waist and instructions to the patients to rise slowly from the lying position and to sit on the edge of the bed for a few minutes before walking. In patients with syncope, investigation of cardiac arrhythmias or heart block can be life-saving. Treatment of the nonneurologic manifestations of this condition also is symptomatic (diuretics, antiarrhythmics, etc.).

Prognosis

The prognosis of AL remains poor. The 5-year survival rate is only 20%. Patients with MM have a poor prognosis with a median survival of 24 to 36 months. Death is attributed to cardiac involvement from congestive heart failure or arrhythmias in 50% of patients. The median survival of patients with AL who have congestive heart failure is only 4 months. The impact of more aggressive therapies, such as autologous stem cell transplantation or organ transplantation, on prognosis is still unclear. AL amyloidosis presenting solely as neuropathy has a better prognosis with a median survival of more than 5 years. The influence of the AN on the evolution of the disease has been evaluated. Median survival from the time of diagnosis of patients with AL with AN was 7.3 months versus 14.8 months for those without AN. Patients with prolonged QT interval on electrocardiogram had even shorter survival periods. The prolonged QT is believed to result from autonomic dysfunction rather than a primary cardiac disorder.

REACTIVE AMYLOIDOSIS

Reactive amyloidosis (AA) is associated with several chronic inflammatory diseases like rheumatoid arthritis, systemic lupus erythematosus, chronic inflammatory bowel disease (especially Crohn's disease), tuberculosis, leprosy, osteomyelitis, Castleman's disease, and suppurative infections. The amyloid in these conditions contains a degradation product of an acute phase serum protein (A protein), which is a nonimmunoglobulin. Renal insufficiency and nephrotic syndrome is seen in 90% of patients. AN has been reported only rarely in association with this type of amyloidosis.

HEREDITARY AMYLOIDOSIS

Hereditary amyloidoses have been linked to various proteins, including transthyretin (TTR), gelsolin, apolipoprotein A1, lysozyme, and fibrinogen. The most common hereditary amyloidosis is familial amyloid polyneuropathy (FAP), associated with mutated TTR, apolipoprotein A1, or gelsolin. The latter two subtypes are exceedingly rare, being restricted to two kindreds in the United States (in Iowa) and Italy (both apolipoprotein A1), and a few kindreds in Finland (gelsolin). Significant autonomic dysfunction has only been described in TTR amyloidosis. A few patients with apolipoprotein A1 amyloidosis have mild gastroparesis as their only sign of autonomic involvement.

TTR is a normal plasma protein tetramer. Each TTR monomer is composed of 127 amino acids synthesized in the liver and choroid plexus. TTR is involved in the transport of vitamin A and thyroid hormones. It is coded by a single gene located on chromosome 18. Most patients with TTR amyloidosis are heterozygous for that gene. Currently, more than 80 TTR point mutations have been described, the most common being the one that substitutes methionine to valine at position 30.

Autonomic involvement in TTR A is common and occurs early with both sympathetic and parasympathetic systems being affected. The severity of autonomic involvement generally correlates with the progression of the disease. Autonomic symptoms include alternating diarrhea and constipation, palpitation caused by cardiac dysrhythmias, anorexia, nausea and vomiting, OH, impotence, urinary and fecal incontinence, and hypohidrosis. Delayed gastric emptying may cause organ distension and anorexia with subsequent cachexia, which may be an important factor in mortality. GI dysfunction is caused by autonomic involvement and direct deposition of amyloid in the intestinal wall. The scalloped pupil deformity has been described in Portuguese and Swedish kindreds and is probably caused by involvement of the ciliary nerves. AN may also cause severe urinary retention with secondary renal damage.

Although diagnosis should not be difficult in typical cases, other hereditary neuropathies like hereditary motor and sensory neuropathies and hereditary sensory and autonomic neuropathies should be excluded. The late onset, predominant sensory symptoms, prominent early autonomic involvement, and frequent association with CTS strongly favor the diagnosis of FAP. Nevertheless, nerve biopsy and DNA analysis may be required for confirmation of diagnosis.

Pathogenesis

Normal TTR is not amyloidogenic, although it is arranged in an extensive β-sheet conformation. Most amyloidogenic mutations increase the content of the β-pleated sheets and result in the production of an insoluble amyloidogenic monomer. Met30 TTR, which is the most common mutation, demonstrated amyloidogenicity in transgenic mice. Amyloid deposits were eventually noted in intestine, kidney, and heart, but not in peripheral nerves (the most common site of involvement in humans). Demonstration of amyloid deposits in dorsal root ganglia and sympathetic chains in FAP is, perhaps, because of the absence of blood–nerve barrier in these structures, allowing easy access of amyloidogenic protein. The mechanism of OH in patients with FAP is not fully understood. Low levels of plasma norepinephrine in patients with OH without significant plasma norepinephrine response to postural changes and low serum dopamine β-hydroxylase activity suggest depletion of peripheral norepinephrine secondary to adrenergic denervation.

Laboratory Data and Diagnosis

Autonomic function tests are abnormal frequently and early in the course of the disease. Amyloid tissue diagnosis is not different from AL. DNA analysis allows the detection of specific mutations and provides valuable information for genetic counseling of family members at risk. This test can be applied to chorionic villi samples for prenatal diagnosis.

Treatment and Prognosis

If left untreated, TTR amyloidosis is invariably fatal, with death occurring within 10 to 15 years. The only available therapeutic approach is orthotopic liver transplantation (OLT). Because the liver is the main source of TTR, OLT is supposed to eliminate the bulk of mutated TTR. Worldwide experience with the procedure currently exceeds 500 cases, with a 5-year survival rate of 80%. In a majority of patients, the progression of neurologic deficits stopped. Whether any significant improvement of symptoms occurs is debatable. For unclear reasons, cardiac amyloidosis may continue to progress despite OLT. The growing experience with OLT has rendered all previous treatment approaches, including plasmapheresis, obsolete.

References

1. Adams, D., D. Samuel, C. Goulon-Goeau, M. Nakazato, P. M. Costa, C. Feray, V. Plante, B. Ducot, P. Ichai, C. Lacroix, S. Metral, H. Bismuth, and G. Said. 2000. The course and prognostic factors of familial amyloid polyneuropathy after liver transplantation. *Brain* 123:1495–1504.
2. Hund, E., R. P. Linke, F. Willig, and A. Grau. 2001. Transthyretin-associated neuropathic amyloidosis, pathogenesis and treatment. *Neurology* 56:431–435.
3. Merlini, G., and V. Bellotti. 2003. Molecular mechanisms of amyloidosis. *N. Engl. J. Med.* 349:583–596.
4. Pepys, M. B. 2001. Pathogenesis, diagnosis and treatment of systemic amyloidosis. *Phil. Trans. R. Soc. Lond.* 356:203–211.
5. Planté-Bordeneuve, V., and G. Said. 2000. Transthyretin related familial amyloid polyneuropathy. *Curr. Opin. Neurol.* 13:569–573.
6. Skinner, M., V. Sanchorawala, D. C. Seldin, L. M. Dember, R. H. Falk, J. L. Berk, J. J. Anderson, C. O'Hara, K. T. Finn, C. A. Libbey, J. Wiesman, K. Quillen, N. Swan, and D. G. Wright. 2004. High-dose meLphalan and autologous stem-cell transplantation in patients with AL amyloidosis: An 8-year study. *Ann. Intern. Med.* 140(2):85–93.

87 Autoimmune Autonomic Neuropathy

Steven Vernino
Department of Neurology
Mayo Clinic
Rochester, Minnesota

Phillip A. Low
Department of Neurology
Mayo Clinic
Rochester, Minnesota

Vanda A. Lennon
Departments of Immunology and
Laboratory Medicine and Pathology
Mayo Clinic
Rochester, Minnesota

Peripheral autonomic dysfunction may result from neurologic autoimmunity. Autoimmune autonomic neuropathy (AAN) typically presents as a subacute panautonomic neuropathy with orthostatic hypotension, gastrointestinal dysmotility, sicca complex, and anhidrosis. The usual course is monophasic worsening followed by incomplete recovery. Some patients experience a chronic progressive course or stable dysautonomia without recovery. Ganglionic acetylcholine receptor (AChR) antibodies are frequently found in patients with AAN, and the level of this antibody correlates with the severity of autonomic signs and symptoms. Currently, there is no proven treatment. The use of intravenous immunoglobulin or plasma exchange is anecdotally effective and may be considered for severe cases of recent onset. Because paraneoplastic autonomic neuropathy can present in a similar fashion, tests for paraneoplastic autoantibodies and evaluation for occult malignancy are warranted in these patients.

Acquired autonomic neuropathy can involve dysfunction of peripheral autonomic nerves or ganglia and can take many forms. Chronic progressive autonomic neuropathy may occur in the context of a more diffuse peripheral neuropathy associated with diabetes, amyloidosis, or other definable causes. A chronic idiopathic presentation without sensorimotor neuropathy has customarily been called pure autonomic failure (PAF, first described by Bradbury and Eggleston), but this arbitrary classification probably encompasses disorders with several different pathophysiologies including chronic AAN. Conversely, most cases of subacute autonomic neuropathy (onset to peak deficit within 3 months) are attributable to neurologic autoimmunity. This also is true for acute autonomic neuropathy when toxic and metabolic causes are excluded. Subacute autonomic neuropathies can be further divided into dysautonomia associated with sensory and motor neuropathy (acute inflammatory neuropathies such as Guillain–Barré syndrome), dysautonomia associated with malignancy (paraneoplastic AAN), or idiopathic AAN. The former two disorders are discussed further in Chapters 89 and 105.

AUTOIMMUNE AUTONOMIC NEUROPATHY

Description

The typical presentation of AAN (formerly known as *acute pandysautonomia*, *idiopathic subacute autonomic neuropathy*, or *autonomic variant of Guillain–Barré syndrome*) is highly characteristic [1]. The typical syndrome occurs in a previously healthy individual in whom autonomic failure develops over the course of a few days or weeks. The most common pattern is severe generalized sympathetic and parasympathetic autonomic failure. Sympathetic failure is manifested as severe orthostatic hypotension and anhidrosis, and parasympathetic failure as dry mouth, dry eyes, sexual dysfunction, constipation, impaired pupillary light response, and fixed heart rate. Gastrointestinal dysmotility is common (70% of patients) and presents with symptoms of anorexia, early satiety, postprandial abdominal pain and vomiting, constipation, or diarrhea. Orthostatic hypotension, anhidrosis, and gastrointestinal dysfunction each occur in more than 50% of patients [1]. Objective autonomic abnormalities are usually obvious and include orthostatic hypotension, tonic pupils, and a fixed heart rate.

The spectrum and severity of dysautonomia, however, varies from patient to patient. Less common presentations include selective cholinergic failure, selective adrenergic neuropathy, or isolated gastrointestinal dysmotility. Motor and sensory nerve abnormalities are minimal or absent. Neuropathic symptoms, such as tingling in distal extremities, are reported by some patients, but these symptoms are not accompanied by objective signs or electrophysiologic evidence of sensory neuropathy.

The concept that subacute autonomic neuropathy is an autoimmune disorder is based on the following observations:

- Clinical associations with lung cancer, myasthenia gravis, and/or thymoma [2],
- Similarity to the autonomic disturbances that can accompany Guillain–Barré syndrome,

- High frequency of organ-specific autoantibodies (thyroid, gastric parietal cell, and glutamic acid decarboxylase antibodies) in patients with AAN compared with patients with degenerative autonomic disorders (V.A. Lennon, unpublished observation),
- Frequent antecedent symptoms consistent with a viral illness (in a review of 27 patients, an antecedent viral syndrome occurred in 59% of cases [1]),
- Increased spinal fluid protein, and
- Individual case reports of benefit from intravenous immunoglobulin therapy [3–5].

The most convincing evidence of an autoimmune pathogenesis is the demonstration of ganglionic nicotinic AChR antibodies in high titer in about 50% of patients [6] (Fig. 87.1). The antibody level correlates with severity of dysautonomia (Fig. 87.2). This observation suggests that some cases of AAN result from an antibody-mediated impairment of synaptic transmission in autonomic ganglia.

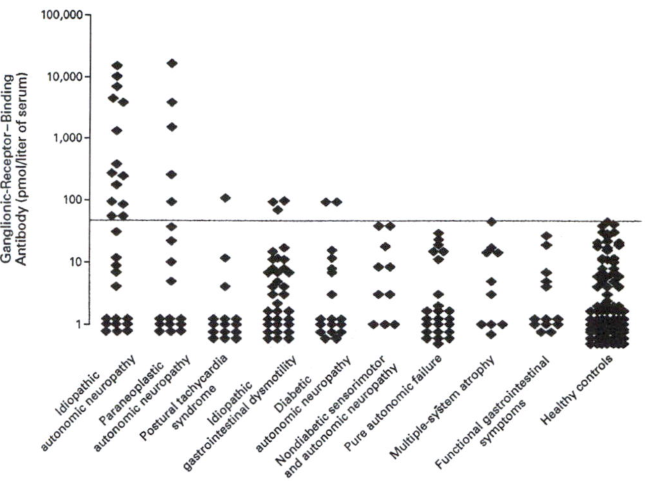

FIGURE 87.1 Serum concentrations of ganglionic–acetylcholine receptor (AChR)–binding antibody in patients with acquired dysautonomia and in control subjects. Values for healthy control subjects and control patients with functional gastrointestinal symptoms were less than 50 pmol/liter. Values for individual patients in each diagnostic group are plotted on a logarithmic scale. Seropositivity was identified in five groups. Ganglionic AChR antibodies were most frequent and of greatest value in patients with idiopathic or paraneoplastic autoimmune autonomic neuropathy (AAN). Antibody values were modestly increased in a minority of patients with postural tachycardia syndrome, idiopathic gastrointestinal dysmotility, or diabetic autonomic neuropathy. In this study, all patients with neurodegenerative autonomic disorders, pure autonomic failure, or multiple-system atrophy (Shy–Drager syndrome) were seronegative. Half the patients with idiopathic AAN were seropositive (i.e., >50 pmol/liter). (Reproduced with permission from Vernino, S., et al. 2000. Autoantibodies to ganglionic acetylcholine receptors in autoimmune neuropathies. *N. Engl. J. Med.* 343:847–855.)

Diagnosis

The diagnosis of idiopathic AAN requires the demonstration of autonomic failure of subacute or acute onset and the exclusion of a toxic or paraneoplastic cause. Patients with paraneoplastic AAN may be clinically indistinguishable from patients with idiopathic AAN until a cancer, usually small cell carcinoma of the lung, is detected (see later). History of an antecedent event (viral syndrome or surgical procedure) or a personal or family history of other autoimmune disorders (such as autoimmune thyroiditis, pernicious anemia, type I diabetes, or myasthenia gravis) supports the diagnosis.

A high serum level of ganglionic AChR antibody is most characteristic of idiopathic AAN. Low values are found in a minority of patients with limited forms of acquired dysautonomia. The serum level of ganglionic AChR antibody cannot distinguish idiopathic from paraneoplastic AAN, and failure to detect this antibody does not rule out the diagnosis of AAN [6].

On the basis of a review of autonomic findings in seropositive patients [7], a particular combination of "cholinergic" autonomic symptoms (neurogenic bladder, impaired pupillary function, gastroparesis, dry eyes, and dry mouth) are most suggestive of AAN.

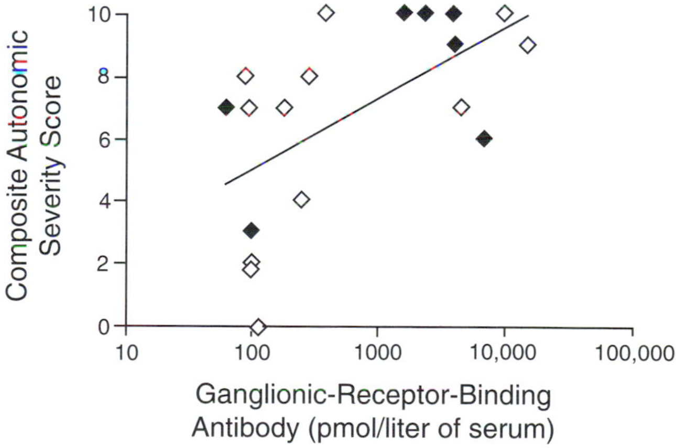

FIGURE 87.2 Correlation of serum levels of ganglionic–acetylcholine receptor (AChR)–binding antibody and severity of autonomic deficits (Composite Autonomic Severity Scale) in 19 seropositive patients with dysautonomia. Antibody values for individual patients are plotted on a logarithmic scale. According to linear regression analysis, higher levels of antibody were significantly associated with greater severity of autonomic dysfunction ($r = 0.59$; $P = 0.007$). Of these 19 patients, 7 also had ganglionic-AChR–blocking antibodies (*solid diamonds*) and 12 did not (*open diamonds*). (Reproduced with permission from Vernino, S., et al. 2000. Autoantibodies to ganglionic acetylcholine receptors in autoimmune neuropathies. *N. Engl. J. Med.* 343:847–855.)

Clinical Course

The original case of acute pandysautonomia reported by Young and colleagues [8] was remarkable for the highly selective autonomic involvement and the patient's complete recovery. Subsequent reports have generally documented only partial improvement. In a clinical series from Mayo Clinic (Rochester, MN) [1], most patients had a distinct

TABLE 87.1 Differentiation of Autoimmune Autonomic Neuropathy, Pure Autonomic Failure, and Multiple System Atrophy

Parameter	AAN	PAF	MSA
Onset	Subacute or insidious	Insidious	Insidious
First symptom	Multiple	Orthostatism	Neurogenic bladder
Gastrointestinal symptom	Common	Absent	Uncommon
Pupillary involvement	Common	Absent	Uncommon
CNS involvement	Absent	Absent	Present
Somatic neuropathy	Mild/minimal*	Absent	Present in 15–20%
Pain	Often present	Absent	Absent
Autonomic findings	Widespread	Limited	Relatively widespread
Progression	Often monophasic	Slow	Inexorably progressive
Prognosis	Relatively good	Relatively good	Poor
Lesion	Postganglionic	Postganglionic	Preganglionic; central
Supine plasma norepinephrine	Reduced	Markedly reduced	Normal
EMG	Usually normal	Normal	Usually normal
Ganglionic AChR antibody	Positive (50%)	Negative†	Negative

*More common in paraneoplastic cases.

†Chronic autoimmune autonomic neuropathy (AAN) may be indistinguishable from pure autonomic failure (PAF) [7].

AChR, acetylcholine receptor; CNS, central nervous system; EMG, electromyogram; MSA, multiple system atrophy.

clinical course with monophasic worsening followed by stabilization or remission without recurrences. Most patients improved spontaneously, but recovery was typically incomplete. Only a third of patients experience major functional improvement of autonomic deficits.

It is now apparent that a subset of patients can present with a more insidious and progressive form of AAN rather than the typical subacute monophasic presentation. Some of these patients are readily identified as having AAN by their pattern of autonomic symptoms or by their serum profile of autoantibodies (ganglionic AChR and other organ-specific antibodies). Some seronegative patients may be difficult to distinguish from degenerative forms of dysautonomia. Features that help to differentiate AAN from PAF and multiple system atrophy are shown in Table 87.1.

Treatment

Treatment for AAN has largely been symptomatic. On the basis of evidence of an autoimmune pathogenesis, it is reasonable to consider plasma exchange or intravenous immunoglobulin. Single case reports of a successful intravenous immunoglobulin therapy [3–5] have all involved early therapeutic intervention. It remains to be determined whether this treatment is effective for patients with a chronic progressive or chronic stable course.

PARANEOPLASTIC AUTOIMMUNE AUTONOMIC NEUROPATHY

Subacute AAN indistinguishable from idiopathic AAN can occur as a remote effect of malignancy (most commonly small cell carcinoma of the lung, less commonly thymoma or other neoplasm). This manifestation of small cell lung carcinoma is less common than sensorimotor neuropathy, polyradiculoneuropathy, or sensory neuronopathy [9]. Paraneoplastic AAN may manifest as pandysautonomia or as severe isolated gastrointestinal dysmotility [10]. More commonly, dysautonomia in these patients is accompanied by symptoms of limbic encephalitis or other elements of a subacute autoimmune neurologic disorder.

Several different autoantibody specificities may be encountered in patients with paraneoplastic autonomic neuropathy. As a group, cation channel autoantibodies are most common (ganglionic or muscle AChR antibodies, voltage-gated N-type or P/Q-type calcium channel antibodies, or neuronal potassium channel antibody). The next most common autoantibody is antineuronal nuclear antibody type 1 (ANNA-1, also known as anti-Hu). A minority of patients will lack any currently recognized autoantibody marker. Small cell lung carcinoma is found in at least 80% of patients who are seropositive for ANNA-1 [9].

References

1. Suarez, G. A., R. D. Fealey, M. Camilleri, and P. A. Low. 1994. Idiopathic autonomic neuropathy: Clinical, neurophysiologic, and follow-up studies on 27 patients. *Neurology* 44:1675–1682.
2. Vernino, S., W. P. Cheshire, and V. A. Lennon. 2001. Myasthenia gravis with autoimmune autonomic neuropathy. *Autonom. Neurosci.* 88:187–192.
3. Heafield, M. T., M. D. Gammage, S. Nightingale, and A. C. Williams. 1996. Idiopathic dysautonomia treated with intravenous gammaglobulin. *Lancet* 347:28–29.
4. Smit, A., M. Vermeulen, J. Koelman, and W. Wieling. 1997. Unusual recovery from acute panautonomic neuropathy after immunoglobulin therapy. *Mayo Clin. Proc.* 72:333–335.

5. Venkataraman, S., M. Alexander, and C. Gnanamuthu. 1998. Postinfectious pandysautonomia with complete recovery after intravenous immunoglobulin therapy. *Neurology* 51:1764–1765.
6. Vernino, S., P. A. Low, R. D. Fealey, J. D. Stewart, G. Farrugia, and V. A. Lennon. 2000. Autoantibodies to ganglionic acetylcholine receptors in autoimmune autonomic neuropathies. *N. Engl. J. Med.* 343: 847–855.
7. Klein, C., S. Vernino, V. A. Lennon, P. Sandroni, R. D. Fealey, L. Benrud-Larson, D. Sletten, and P. A. Low. 2003. The spectrum of autoimmune autonomic neuropathy. *Ann. Neurol.* 53:752–758.
8. Young, R. R., A. K. Asbury, J. L. Corbett, and R. D. Adams. 1975. Pure pan-dysautonomia with recovery. *Brain* 98:613–636.
9. Lucchinetti, C. F., D. W. Kimmel, and V. A. Lennon. 1998. Paraneoplastic and oncologic profiles of patients seropositive for type 1 antineuronal nuclear autoantibodies. *Neurology* 50:652–657.
10. Lennon, V. A., D. F. Sas, M. F. Busk, B. Scheithauer, J. R. Malagelada, M. Camilleri, and L. J. Miller. 1991. Enteric neuronal autoantibodies in pseudoobstruction with small-cell lung carcinoma. *Gastroenterology* 100:137–142.
11. Bradbury, S., and C. Eggleston. 1925. Postural hypotension: A report of three cases. *Ann. Heart J.* 1:73–86.

88 Diabetic Autonomic Dysfunction

Andrew C. Ertl
Division of Diabetes, Metabolism, and Endocrinology
Vanderbilt University
Nashville, Tennessee

Michael Pfeifer
Division of Endocrinology
East Carolina University
Greenville, North Carolina

Stephen N. Davis
Division of Diabetes, Metabolism, and Endocrinology
Vanderbilt University
Nashville, Tennessee

All organ systems innervated by the autonomic nervous system may be impaired in patients with diabetes. The extent of impairment is highly variable from patient to patient, but it is generally related to duration of diabetes as with other complications of diabetes. Nerve impairment can be further complicated by the normal decline in function with age.

Currently, the only preventive treatment for diabetic autonomic dysfunction is maintenance of near-normal blood glucose. Each affected system is reviewed later in this chapter, but, in general, manifestations of autonomic dysfunction are treated symptomatically when appropriate. Often, patient education can avoid many potentially life-threatening problems.

IRIS

Sympathetic nerves, which dilate the iris, show earlier and more extensive impairment than the parasympathetic nerves that constrict the iris. Pupillometry, which is used to measure the ability of pupils to change size, suggests that pilocarpine hypersensitivity demonstrates early parasympathetic autonomic dysfunction in diabetes mellitus before evidence of sympathetic defects. The imbalance between parasympathetic and sympathetic nerves causes an inability to respond quickly to a dark stimulus. Patients will complain of inability to see in dark places such as the movie theater and will have difficulty driving at night. On clinical examination, small, poorly dilated pupils in a dark room combined with the above complaints are indicative. Education about recognition of the problem, reassurance, and proper precautions when in darkness are adequate in most cases. Treatment with sympathetic stimulants or parasympathetic blockers generally is not necessary.

ESOPHAGUS

Dysphagia is the most common presenting symptom of diabetic autonomic dysfunction. This is often confused with cardiac pain, gastric atony, or both. Diagnosis of esophageal and pharyngeal motility dysfunction through barium swallow generally is adequate. Other sources of pain should be ruled out. Currently, an effective drug therapy does not exist.

STOMACH

Signs and symptoms of gastric emptying abnormalities include early satiety, nausea, vomiting, "brittle" diabetes, large fluctuations in blood glucose, and weight loss. Some patients may be asymptomatic. The most effective diagnostic tool for evaluation of gastric emptying abnormality is nuclear medicine solid phase gastric emptying studies. These studies measure both liquid and solid phase emptying, unlike upper gastrointestinal x-ray series, which measure only liquid phase gastric emptying. The use of beef stew or chicken livers is a more adequate test of solid gastric emptying than oatmeal, scrambled eggs, or hard-boiled eggs, which are commonly used. These measure semisolid gastric emptying.

Successful treatment of gastric emptying abnormalities may be complex. Hyperglycemia, *per se*, may result in atonic stomach. Improvement in glucose control has the potential to correct the problem. However, it is difficult, if not impossible, to improve glucose control because of the mismatch between caloric absorption and insulin action onset. Therefore, it may be necessary to initially improve gastric emptying with pharmacologic agents, and then attempt to improve glucose control. Once glucose control is within acceptable limits, it is reasonable to discontinue pharmacologic therapy and evaluate whether glucose control alone is adequate therapy.

Effective pharmacologic therapies with prokinetic action include metoclopramide, bethanechol, cisapride, erythromycin, octreotide, and famotidine. Metoclopramide inhibits the dopaminergic pathway, which inhibits gastric emptying. By inhibiting this pathway, endogenous peristalsis may occur uninhibited. Severe vagal impairment will obviate its efficacy. The usual dose is 10 mg, 30 minutes before meals. Side effects include extrapyramidal symptoms, drooling, and nystagmus.

Bethanechol directly stimulates the stomach through the muscarinic receptors. Thus, it is generally effective in increasing gastric emptying even in cases in which metoclopramide is not effective. To overcome an atonic stomach, bethanechol is given subcutaneously for the first 2 weeks. Beginning dose is 2.5 mg subcutaneously, 30 minutes before each meal, for approximately 3 to 4 days. Subcutaneous bethanechol is increased to 5 mg before each meal and snack for the remainder of the 2 weeks. At the end of this period, patients are switched to 50 mg oral bethanechol, 30 minutes before each meal and snack. Side effects include urinary urgency, sweating, and occasional nausea. If given after or too soon before the meal, it may cause regurgitation.

Cisapride increases smooth muscle activity of the intestines and has some direct ganglionic activity. About 10 to 20 mg is given before meals. Erythromycin works by mimicking motilin. Typically, 250 mg is given every 6 hours. The drawback to this drug is that it often interferes with antibiotic coverage.

Octreotide decreases gut hormone motility inhibitors such as gastric inhibitory polypeptide. As a promotility drug it is not as good as cisapride or bethanechol, but it is not worse than metoclopramide. Typically, 100 µg is given subcutaneously every 6 hours. Famotidine is an unusual H_2 blocker in that it has a neutral effect or some prokinetic effect unlike other H_2 blockers. Doses of 20 to 40 mg are given every 12 to 24 hours. This drug must be adjusted for renal function.

It is recommended that gastric emptying studies be repeated after pharmacologic therapy has begun to verify that emptying has improved. If not, other pharmacologic therapies should be considered. An efficient method to measure efficacy of therapy is to give the drug the gastric emptying study and measure the response. If a patient is unresponsive to any of these therapies, frequent small meals, six times a day, with high-calorie liquid food may be necessary to maintain adequate nutrition.

GALLBLADDER

Diarrhea and the development of gallstones are symptoms of gallbladder atony. Gallstones are much more likely to develop in patients with hypercholesterolemia, as often is seen in patients with diabetes. Gallbladder disease is evaluated by observing the response of the gallbladder to a fatty meal or cholecystokinin. Cholecystectomy may be indicated in some cases.

COLON

The most common gastrointestinal symptom of autonomic neuropathy is constipation. It is evaluated by clinical history. Constipation is treated with a variety of medications including high-fiber products such as psyllium, which is bulk-forming fiber acting to encourage peristaltic activity. Mineral oil and bisacodyl may also be effective. Bisacodyl acts directly on the colonic mucosa to produce normal peristalsis throughout the large intestine.

Diabetic diarrhea is a common result of autonomic dysfunction. However, other causes need to be ruled out. Diabetic diarrhea is characterized by frequent (8–20 bowel movements per day, .300 g of stool per day), watery, persistent bowel movements and is often nocturnal. Mild steatorrhea is common. Treatment is aimed at the cause. Initially a broad-spectrum antibiotic is used to eliminate bacterial overgrowth. Inappropriate spillage of bile salts into the intestines also is a common cause of diarrhea among patients with diabetes. If spillage of bile salts is suspected, bile salt binders should be tried. Pharmacologic therapies include methylcellulose, diphenoxylate hydrochloride with atropine sulphate (10 ml, 6–24 hours), and loperamide hydrochloride (10 ml, 6–24 hours). Octreotide (100 µg subcutaneously every 4–6 hours) has been effective when other treatments have failed.

BLADDER

Both afferent and efferent nerves to the bladder may be affected in patients with diabetes. Afferent neuropathy results in the inability to feel the need to void. Therefore, there is a decrease in frequency of urination, which may be misinterpreted as an improvement in glucose control. The decreased frequency causes bladder stasis and may lead to an increase in the occurrence of urinary tract infections (UTIs). Efferent neuropathy generally occurs later in the course of diabetes causing incomplete voiding, dribbling, and frequent UTIs. Incontinence is a late finding and is rare. Evaluation for bladder dysfunction is considered in male individuals with more than two UTIs per year and in female individuals with more than three UTIs per year. Cystometrogram effectively evaluates both afferent and efferent neuropathy. Having the patient schedule urination every 4 hours generally can treat afferent neuropathy. Efferent neuropathy is treated with bethanechol given orally at a dosage of 30 to 50 mg four times a day. Incontinence may require placement of a suprapubic catheter, permanent catheterization, or both.

PENIS

The incidence of erectile dysfunction (ED), or impotence, which may result from autonomic neuropathy, is nearly three times more common in male patients with diabetes than in age-matched male individuals without diabetes. Signs and symptoms include decreased tumescence and rigidity.

Retrograde ejaculation occurs rarely and may be related to sympathetic dysfunction. The diagnosis of neuropathic ED is one of exclusion (Fig. 88.1).

Treatment is aimed at the cause. Alternative medications for antihypertensive and psychotropic therapy should always be initiated before pharmacologic or mechanical measures are used. Sildenafil has been found to effective in alleviating ED in 50 to 60% of patients with types I or II diabetes mellitus. If the cause is neuropathic, yohimbine occasionally is helpful for patients with early loss of penile rigidity or with pelvic steal syndrome. Suction devices or injections with phentolamine, prostaglandins, or papaverine can be useful. If the above methods fail or are unacceptable, penile prostheses may be useful. Contraindications for use of sildenafil include prior heart attack, atherosclerosis, angina, arrhythmia, chronic low blood pressure problems, and use of organic nitrates. Complications with yohimbine include hypertension. Injections may cause bruising, pain, and priapism. Prostheses often fail to meet the patient's expectations and may be painful.

VAGINA

A dry, thin, atrophic vaginal wall and lack of lubrication characterize vaginal autonomic neuropathy resulting in painful intercourse. Over-the-counter lubricants help to decrease pain during intercourse. However, an estrogen cream not only adds moisture but helps thicken the vaginal wall, thus preventing tearing.

ADRENAL MEDULLA

In patients with severe autonomic neuropathy, there is a loss of the adrenal output of epinephrine and probably of sympathetic tone to the liver resulting in a decreased counter-regulatory response to hypoglycemia. Without the adrenergic signs and symptoms, hypoglycemia may become severe before it is treated. Diagnosis of hypoglycemic unawareness is based on the lack of adrenergic responses such as tachycardia and blood pressure when blood glucose is less than 40 mg/dl. Effective management of this condition requires that the patient, family members, and co-workers be taught to recognize the subtle signs and symptoms of hypoglycemia (mood changes, confusion, slurred speech, fugue-like state, and memory lapses) and how to treat it with glucagon injections and glucose.

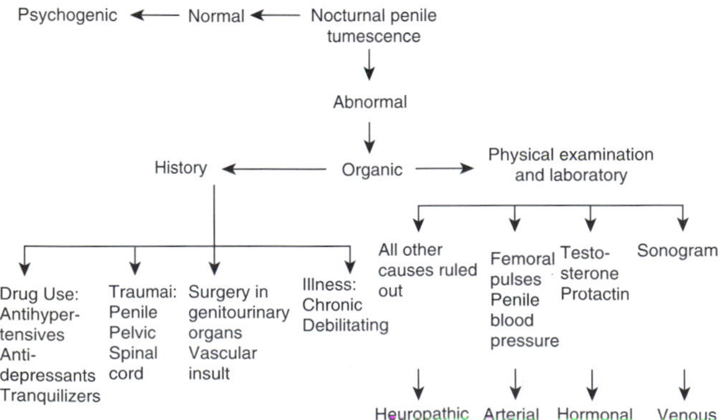

Fig. 88.1 The diagnosis of impotence secondary to diabetic autonomic neuropathy is one of exclusion. The above algorithm is suggested to evaluate the other possible etiologies of impotence.

SUDOMOTOR

Abnormal sweating patterns are commonly found in patients with diabetes. Both upper and lower extremities fail to sweat, whereas the trunk overcompensates. Eventually, complete anhidrosis may occur. The patient generally complains of excessive sweating in the trunk area. Abnormal temperature regulation predisposes to heat stroke and heat exhaustion. Treatment is limited to education. Patients should be warned that they are at increased risk for heat stroke and heat exhaustion and that necessary precautions should be taken.

CARDIOVASCULAR

Clinical manifestations of cardiovascular autonomic neuropathy include exercise intolerance and painless myocardial ischemia. Postural hypotension as a result of vascular autonomic dysfunction is characterized by postural dizziness, nausea, vertigo, weakness, presyncope, or syncope. These signs and symptoms can be misinterpreted as hypoglycemia. Measurement of change in heart rate and blood pressure when moving from sitting or lying to a standing position provide evidence of this condition. This is a diagnosis of exclusion (Fig. 88.2). Treatment of postural hypotension resulting from autonomic neuropathy can be complex because supine hypertension and upright hypotension often occur concurrently. Both the supine hypertension and upright hypotension cannot be treated in the same patient because treatment of one may aggravate the other and vice versa. Keeping the head of the bed in an upright position during sleep often helps the patient adjust to change in position and lessens supine hypertension. The simplest and most efficacious treatment is an atomized spray of 10% phenylephrine hydrochloride (Neo-synephrine). The spray is used approximately every 2 to 4 hours, 3 to 4 sprays per nostril at each dosing. This nearly always results in an improvement in upright hypotension; rare complications include septum perforation and ulceration. Fludrocortisone (0.1–0.5 mg) increases plasma volume and catecholamine

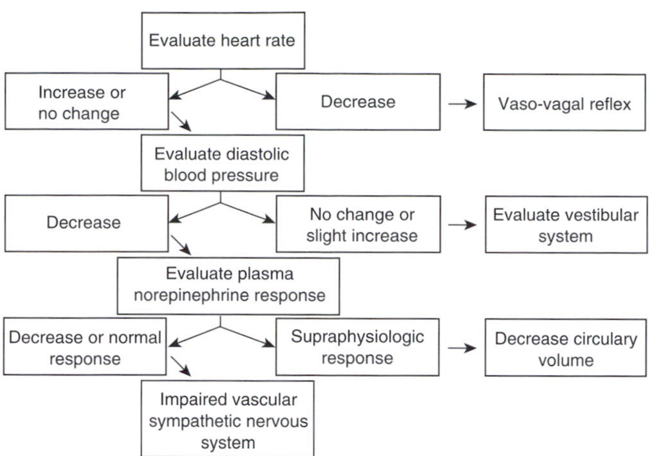

Fig. 88.2 Postural hypotension as a result of vascular autonomic dysfunction is characterized by symptoms that may be misinterpreted as hypoglycemia. The above algorithm may be used to evaluate the etiology of postural hypotension.

sensitivity and often is effective. Sympathetic stimulants (ephedrine and midodrine) also are useful.

Cardiac denervation syndrome, a total loss of innervation to the heart, results in exercise intolerance, poor anesthesia outcome, pregnancy complications, sudden death, and probably cardiomyopathy and painless myocardial ischemia. This syndrome may be evaluated with simple, noninvasive tests such as heart rate variability (R-R variation), heart rate changes during deep breathing at 6 breaths per minute (>15 beat variation is normal for patients younger than 60 years), heart rate ratio during and after a standardized Valsalva maneuver of 40 mmHg for 10 seconds (>1.21 is normal for patients younger than 60 years). Cardiac parasympathetic dysfunction may be evident by decreased heart rate variation to these maneuvers. These heart rate variations decrease with level of dysfunction and age. Awareness of this condition may decrease long-term morbidity and mortality rates. There is no evidence that the occurrence of sudden death and cardiomyopathy can be prevented.

Painless myocardial ischemia, associated with increased morbidity and mortality in patients with diabetes, is more common than in the nondiabetic population. An algorithm to identify those at risk for painless ischemia is provided in Figure 88.3. A study in a small number of patients has shown that approximately 66% of patients screened via this algorithm had ischemia confirmed by stress thallium testing.

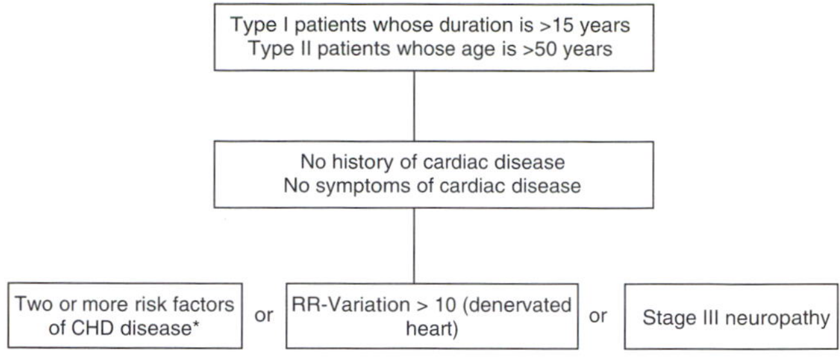

Fig. 88.3 The above criteria are used to identify the patients at risk for painless myocardial ischemia. *, series of risk factors.

Cardiac denervation may also cause exercise intolerance in patients with diabetes. Symptoms may be vague and the patient may present with only fatigue. The American Diabetes Association recommends that all patients with diabetes who are new to an exercise program and are older than 40 years with type II diabetes or have had type I diabetes for more than 15 years should have an exercise tolerance test before initiating an exercise program. There is no known treatment for exercise intolerance, although one study has shown that aldose reductase inhibitors may improve intolerance.

References

1. Ward, J., and Y. Goto, Eds. 1990. *Diabetic neuropathy.* New York: Wiley.
2. Kirby, R. S., C. C. Carson, and G. D. Webster, Eds. 1991. *Impotence: Diagnosis and management of male erectile dysfunction.* Oxford: Butterworth Heinemann.
3. Low, P. A., Ed. 1991. *Clinical autonomic disorders: Evaluation and management.* Boston: Little, Brown.
4. Ewing, D. J., I. W. Campbell, and B. F. Clarke. 1980. The natural history of diabetic autonomic neuropathy. *Q. J. Med.* 193:95–108.

89 Guillain-Barré Syndrome

Phillip A. Low
Department of Neurophysiology
University of South Wales
Liverpool, New South Wales, Australia

James G. McLeod
Department of Neurophysiology
University of South Wales
Liverpool, New South Wales, Australia

Guillain-Barré syndrome (GBS) is a subacute immune-mediated demyelinating neuropathy that may cause profound weakness and respiratory failure. Although the disease affects motor fibers preferentially, paresthesias and pain are common sensory manifestations. Autonomic neuropathy of some degree, particularly involving cardiovascular and gastrointestinal function, is found in two thirds of patients and may be a life-threatening complication of the disease. Autonomic dysfunction in GBS can affect the sympathetic and parasympathetic nervous systems. Autonomic manifestations comprise a combination of autonomic failure and autonomic overreactivity, the latter most commonly being manifested as sinus tachycardia and systemic hypertension. Marked arrhythmias and wide fluctuations in blood pressure may also occur. Gastrointestinal dysmotility is fairly common but rarely progresses to adynamic ileus. Typically, autonomic neuropathy improves in concert with motor and sensory nerve function. Long-term autonomic sequelae are not typical.

CLINICAL FEATURES

The core features of GBS are the acute onset of an ascending, predominantly motor polyradiculoneuropathy associated with areflexia and increased cerebrospinal fluid protein. The disease follows an antecedent bacterial or viral infection in about two thirds of cases. *Campylobacter jejuni* infections are implicated in 17% to 39% of cases in North America and Europe and the frequency is greater in Asian countries [1]. Loss of tendon reflexes is usual. The ascending weakness progresses usually within a couple of weeks. Severe weakness including respiratory paralysis is common.

Although autonomic involvement is not a requirement for diagnosis, autonomic overactivity or underactivity is not uncommon [2–4]. Autonomic dysfunction is relatively common in some series [3]. Patients may have tachycardia, and orthostatic hypotension may alternate with hypertension. Bladder or bowel involvement tends to be mild compared with somatic involvement. Some patients with GBS have life-threatening dysautonomia, which presents most frequently in the acute evolving phase of the disease and tends to correlate with the severity of somatic involvement, being especially common in patients with respiratory failure. In addition to orthostatic hypotension, hypertensive episodes can occur and are usually paroxysmal but occasionally may be sustained [5]. Microneurographic evidence of sympathetic overactivity has been documented, which subsides with recovery from the neuropathy [6]. Sinus tachycardia is present in more than 50% of patients with severe GBS.

Less common autonomic symptoms include constipation, fecal incontinence, gastroparesis, ileus, erectile failure, and pupillary abnormalities. Gastrointestinal dysmotility is fairly common but rarely progresses to severe adynamic ileus. In one study, adynamic ileus occurred in 17 of 114 patients (15%) with severe GBS [7]. Cardiovascular dysautonomia coincided with ileus in only 50 patients. Ileus was thought to be related to mechanical ventilation, immobilization, and preexisting conditions such as prior abdominal surgery or incremental doses of opioids.

Related entities are the autonomic variant, acute motor axonal neuropathy, acute motor and sensory axonal neuropathy, and the Miller–Fisher syndrome (characterized by the triad of ophthalmoplegia, ataxia, and areflexia). These are best considered autoimmune neuropathies with different targets.

INVESTIGATIONS

Tests of autonomic function often are abnormal. Orthostatic hypotension and impaired cardiovagal, sudomotor, and adrenergic vasomotor function have been described. Abnormalities of cardiac rhythm include sinus tachycardia, bradyarrhythmias, heart block, and asystole, and they may necessitate a cardiac pacemaker. Sinus arrest may occur after vigorous vagal stimulation, usually caused by tracheal suction.

ETIOLOGY OR MECHANISMS

The disorder is likely to be immune-mediated, although the antigen is unknown. The evidence is based on the sural nerve biopsy finding of perivascular round cell infiltration, the presence of relevant serum antibodies causing demyelination, frequent antecedent infections, the selectivity of involvement by fiber type, response to immunotherapy, and the overlap with cases of pandysautonomia. The autoimmune basis of GBS and its variants is slowly being unraveled. For example, the Miller–Fisher syndrome is known to have IgG autoantibodies directed at the ganglioside GQ1b in more than 90% of patients [8].

COURSE AND PROGNOSIS

Septic and autonomic complications are the major causes of death in GBS because respiratory failure is usually successfully managed with mechanical ventilation. Typically, autonomic neuropathy in GBS improves in concert with improvement in motor and sensory nerve function. Long-term autonomic sequelae are not typical.

MANAGEMENT

Patients with autonomic instability require close monitoring of heart rate and blood pressure. Paroxysmal hypertension may alternate with hypotension, and patients may be supersensitive to hypotensive and other agents. For these patients, the use of hypotensive drugs is usually best avoided. When sustained hypertension develops, combined α- and β-adrenergic blockade has been suggested, and bradyarrhythmias are probably best treated by the use of a demand pacemaker.

The mainstay of treatment is supportive for the management of orthostatic hypotension and bowel and bladder symptoms. Because there is suggestive evidence of an immune-mediated process, treatment with intravenous immunoglobulin or plasma exchange should be undertaken in patients who have moderate to severe weakness, respiratory compromise, or continue to worsen. Intravenous immunoglobulin is given as 0.4 g/kg (over 4 hours) daily for 5 days, but it has little, if any, effect if administered later than 14 days after onset of the illness [9].

References

1. Koga, M., C. W. Ang, N. Yuki, B. C. Jacobs, P. Herbrink, F. G. van der Meche, K. Hirata, and P. A. van Doorn. 2001. Comparative study of preceding *Campylobacter jejuni* infection in Guillain-Barre syndrome in Japan and The Netherlands. *J. Neurol. Neurosurg. Psychiatry* 70:693–695.
2. Zochodne, D. W. 1994. Autonomic involvement in Guillain-Barre syndrome: A review. *Muscle Nerve* 17:1145–1155.
3. Low, P. A., and J. G. McLeod. 1997. Autonomic neuropathies. In *Clinical autonomic disorders: Evaluation and management*, ed. P. A. Low, 463–486. Philadelphia: Lippincott-Raven.
4. McDougall, A. J., and J. G. McLeod. 1996. Autonomic neuropathy. II: Specific peripheral neuropathies. *J. Neurol. Sci.* 138:1–13.
5. Fagius, J. 1997. Syndromes of autonomic overactivity. In *Clinical autonomic disorders: Evaluation and management*, ed. P. A. Low, 777–789. Philadelphia: Lippincott-Raven.
6. Fagius, J., and B. G. Wallin. 1980. Sympathetic reflex latencies and conduction velocities in patients with polyneuropathy. *J. Neurol. Sci.* 47:449–461.
7. Burns, T. M., N. C. Lawn, P. A. Low, M. Camilleri, and E. F. M. Wijdicks. 2001. Adynamic ileus in severe Guillain-Barre syndrome. *Muscle Nerve* 24:963–965.
8. Yuki, N., S. Sato, S. Tsuji, T. Ohsawa, and T. Miyatake. 1993. Frequent presence of anti-GQ1b antibody in Fisher's syndrome. *Neurology* 43:414–417.
9. Low, P. A., J. C. Stevens, G. A. Suarez, A. J. Windebank, and B. E. Smith. 1995. Diseases of peripheral nerves. In *Clinical neurology, Vol. 4*, ed. R. J. Joynt, 1–193. Philadelphia: Lippincott-Raven.

90

Chagas' Disease

Daniel Bulla
University of Uruguay
Montevideo, Uruguay

Alba Larre Borges
University of Uruguay
Montevideo, Uruguay

Raquel Ponce de Leon
University of Uruguay
Montevideo, Uruguay

Mario Medici
Institute of Neurology
University of Uruguay
Montevideo, Uruguay

Chagas' disease is a trypanosomiasis that is almost entirely limited to the American continents. It has three periods: acute, asymptomatic, and chronic. There is an unusual affinity for involvement of the autonomous nervous system, with pathologic evidence of involvement of virtually all autonomic structures evaluated. The immunopathologic theory is the one most broadly accepted as the cause of those lesions. The heart and gastrointestinal tract (GIT) are the most prominently involved structures, but the disease also involves other organs, such as the urinary tract, eye, and the bronchial tree. Clinical manifestations vary in the different periods, each of which typically lasts many years. Although there is no consensus for specific therapy of the chronic stage, persistence of trypanosoma emphasizes the need to continue treating the parasite once there is clinically significant involvement of these structures. The disease continues to be an experimental model for the study of autoimmune inflammatory autonomic denervation.

Chagas' disease is a trypanosomiasis caused by *Trypanosoma cruzi (T. cruzi)*, occurring almost exclusively in Latin America. The World Health Organization has estimated that 18 million people have been infected by *T. cruzi* and 45,000 of those infected die every year of Chagas' disease. The economic loss because of early mortality and disability exceeds $8 billion per year [1, 2].

There are three relevant routes of transmission: through the vector, through transfusions, and from mother to child. Although vectors are the most important route in Latin America, transfusions are the main source of infection in countries such as the United States and Canada, because of the high immigration rate from endemic regions.

The vector is an insect that belongs to the Hemiptera order, the Reduviidae family, and the Triatominae subfamily. There are 118 classified species, a few of which (those in the domestic habitat) are mainly responsible for transmission to humans [1].

The social and demographic trends observed in recent years, resulting in the movement of persons from rural to urban areas, have resulted in an "urbanization" of the disease. There continue to be sources of these vectors in the poorest areas, and new species of Triatoma tend to occur in areas surrounding these homes.

Blood-borne transmission through transfusions has decreased dramatically thanks to the implementation of mandatory plans for the detection of the disease in blood donors. Countries such as Uruguay and Chile have been declared free from transmission, both by the vector and through transfusions [2].

Almost all autonomic structures may be affected, and there is an acute and a chronic stage. The acute stage is characterized by a high parasitemia with tissue invasion and a distinct neurotropism of *T. cruzi*. There is an inflammatory infiltration of many tissues, especially involving the heart and the autonomic ganglia. Approximately a month after the acute stage, *T. cruzi* practically disappears from blood and tissues and the diagnosis is subsequently serologic. Of the individuals infected, 70% will enter the chronic indeterminate stage, defined as the presence of positive serology in asymptomatic subjects with normal electrocardiogram, chest radiograph, and GIT contrast imaging [3, 4].

A dilated cardiomyopathy develops in approximately 25 to 30% of the infected individuals. It presents as global heart failure, with severe arrhythmias and heart block (right bundle branch block and left anterior hemi-block). There is typically an apical aneurysm. Sudden death is not rare. Autonomic dysregulation may play a significant role in the genesis and maintenance of severe ventricular arrhythmias in this cardiac disease [5, 6].

Koeberle [7] was the first to describe involvement of autonomic structure in Chagas' disease, leading to the neurogenic theory of the cardiomyopathy. Autonomic dysfunction is almost invariable in the chronic stage [8]. Autonomic function tests have shown a predominantly parasympathetic neuropathy. These abnormalities have been demonstrated even in patients in the indeterminate phase. Studies have included heart rate variability, the Valsalva ratio, the blood pressure response to sustained handgrip, and the cardiovascular response to norepinephrine, atropine, and β-blockers [9].

Studies using lower body negative pressure have shown impaired reflexes of the cardiopulmonary receptors in patients with Chagas' disease without cardiac failure. Involvement of the sympathetic cardiac function in the ventricles was shown using meta-iodobenzyl guanidine I_{123} with single photon emission computed tomography [6]. This apparently occurs early in the course of the cardiomyopathy and is related to the regional perfusion of the myocardium [10]. However, orthostatic hypotension is not frequent at any stage of the disease.

The GIT is involved in more than 90% of Chagas' disease cases, but not all patients are symptomatic. Neuron loss leads to the dilation of these structures after several years, resulting in "megaorgans." Megaesophagus and megacolon, the most frequent megaorgans, represent the final stage of autonomic involvement, with more than a 90% loss of Auerbach's and Meissner's parasympathetic plexuses. Motor dysfunction precedes dilation and can be detected through GIT radionuclide studies of motility in a high percentage of patients. The megacolon tests [11] used in experimental models and in patients with Chagas' disease in the chronic, asymptomatic stage show that the esophagus and other segments of the GIT lack any cholinergic innervation, which differs from the idiopathic megacolon seen in Hirschsprung's disease. Functional testing using esophageal manometry and esophageal transit studies with gastric emptying with radiocolloids [12] show early changes in the chronic asymptomatic stage in patients with normal barium studies. There are no follow-up studies of these early changes, considering that the megaformations are less frequent than these, which is evidence of an unequal impairment of the intramural nervous plexuses.

Other portions of the GIT, such as stomach, small bowel, and gall bladder, may also be affected. There are regional differences in the prevalence of these megaformations and myocardial disease. Such organ enlargements are not observed north of the equator, and they are more frequent than myocardial disease in Chile. In Uruguay, the myocardial disease prevails as compared with the enlarged "mega" viscera [5]. Symptoms consist of dysphagia and constipation.

Autonomic changes also have been found in other structures, including the urinary tract, the central nervous system, iris, and bronchia. Scanning with ^{99}m Tc DTPA showed functional disorders in the urinary tract. Abnormal studies were frequently found in patients with chronic undetermined disease [12]: pyelectasia, urethral and pyeloureteral dyskinesias, and unilateral or bilateral flow from bladder to urethra. The same voiding technique showed an increase or reduction of the total residual volume and longer evacuation times.

Therapy includes specific antiparasitic treatment only at the acute stage. The finding of evidence of trypanosomes in tissue has currently posed the need for these drugs at the chronic stage, especially at the first stages when the anatomic changes described earlier are initially seen clinically.

Despite the reduction in the incidence of Chagas' disease as a result of the improved epidemiologic control mentioned earlier, patients infected with *T. cruzi* may proceed with the course of the disease for years after infection, therefore the problem is not solved [6]. The follow-up studies of these changes and the better understanding of their immunopathogenesis have made this an experimental autonomic denervation model; therefore, further research is needed.

References

1. Wendel, S., Z. Brener, M. E. Camargo, and A. Rassi. 1992. Chagas' disease (American trypanosomiasis): Its impact on transfusion and clinical medicine. Sao Paulo, Brazil: ISBT.
2. World Health Organization. Chagas' disease. Annual report 2002: http://www.who.int/ctd/chagas/dates.htm.
3. Bannister, R., and C. Mathias. 1992. *Autonomic Failure*, 3rd ed. Oxford: Oxford University Press.
4. Amorin, D. S. 1984. Cardiopatía chagásica. Modelos experimentales. *Arq. Bras. Cardiología* 42:243–247.
5. Ponce de León, R., D. Bulla, A. Cardozo, A. Pintos, J. Torres, G. Lago, A. Berriolo, C. Heugerot, F. Mut, E. Touya, and M. Franca Rodriguez. 1986. Compromiso del sistema nervioso autónomo en la Enfermedad de Chagas. *Acta. Neurol. Latinoam.* 30:123–131.
6. Marín Neto, J. A., M. Vinicius Simoes, and A. V. Lima Sarabanda. 1999. Chagas' heart disease. *Arq. Bras. Cardiol.* 72(3):264–280.
7. Koberle, F. 1957. Die chronische Chagas Kardiopathie. *Virchows Arch. (Pathol. Anat.)* 330:267–295.
8. Machado, C. R., E. R. Camargos, L. B. Guerra, and M. C. Moreira. 2000. Cardiac autonomic denervation in congestive heart failure, comparison of Chagas' heart disease with other dilated cardiomyopathy. *Hum. Pathol.* 31(1):3–10.
9. Junqueira, L. F., and J. D. Soares. 2002. Impaired autonomic control of heart interval changes to Valsalva manoeuvre in Chagas' disease without other manifestation. *Auton. Neurosci.* 97(1):59–67.
10. Simoes, M. V., A. O. Pintya, G. Bromberg-Marin, A. V. Sarabanda, C. M. Antloga, A. Pazin-Filho, B. C. Maciel, and J. A. Marin-Neto. 2000. Relation of regional sympathetic denervation and myocardial perfusion disturbance to wall motion impairment in Chagas' cardiomyopathy. *Am. J. Cardiol.* 86:975–981.
11. de Rezende, J. M., and U. G. Meneguelli. 2001. A visita ao Brasil de Franz J. Ingelfinger e sua participacao dos conhecimentos sobre o megaesofago chagásico. *Rev. Assoc. Med. Bras.* 47(3):262–268.
12. Ponce de León, R., D. Bulla, and A. Larre Borges. 1996. Estudio del Sistema Nervioso Autónomo cardiovascular en la Enfermedad de Chagas en etapa crónica indeterminada. *Arch. Med. Int.* XVIII(3):103–107.

91 Drug-Induced Autonomic Dysfunction

Neal L. Benowitz
Clinical Pharmacology Unit
University of California, San Francisco
San Francisco, California

Drugs and chemicals induce orthostatic hypotension by interfering with the normal mechanisms of the regulation of blood pressure. Major sites of action include: (1) depletion of blood volume; (2) interference with the function of the sympathetic nervous system at a variety of sites resulting in a failure to maintain vascular resistance, venous tone, or cardiac output with upright posture; (3) direct vasodilation, which decreases vascular resistance, venous tone, or both. Vasodilators may act directly on blood vessels or through interference with the renin-angiotensin system. Table 91.1 describes various drugs and toxins that act on various sites of blood pressure regulation.

In general, when drugs induce orthostatic hypotension by depleting the blood volume or by vasodilation alone, there will be evidence of a compensatory sympathetic neural-reflex response to upright posture—that is, tachycardia, palpations, sweating, increased circulating catecholamines, etc. This presentation may be termed *hyperadrenergic orthostatic hypotension*. When drugs that impair sympathetic function are involved in the pathogenesis of orthostatic hypotension, the expected sympathetic reflex response will be blunted or absent (hypoadrenergic orthostatic hypotension).

Vasovagal syncope may be triggered by drugs, primarily those that produce hyperadrenergic orthostatic hypotension by vasodilation. The typical response in patients with vasovagal syncope is a period of reflex tachycardia after assuming an upright posture, followed after several minutes by sudden bradycardia and hypotension with signs and symptoms of hypoperfusion and increased vagal discharge. The mechanism is believed to be activation of afferent C fibers in ventricular mechanoreceptors, because of the intense myocardial contractile state. Activation of these receptors, similar to the Bezold–Jarisch reflex, produces parasympathetic discharge and inhibits sympathetic responses, resulting in bradycardia and vasodilation with no increase in plasma catecholamines. This type of vagal discharge can be produced in the laboratory by administering isoproterenol to people during upright tilting.

IMPORTANCE OF AGING

The elderly are more susceptible than younger people to drug-induced orthostatic hypotension; and drugs are an important cause of syncope and falls in the elderly. Typically, drug-induced orthostatic hypotension in the elderly results from therapeutic use of drugs such as sedative-hypnotics, diuretics, antihypertensive drugs, cardiac nitrates, and/or antidepressants. The elderly are less able than younger people to compensate for drug-induced disturbances in cardiovascular function. In particular, the elderly may have abnormal baroreceptor function, with less acceleration of the heart rate and cardiac contractility, as well as a diminished ability to conserve sodium and water, compared with younger people. Another contributor to the high incidence of drug-induced orthostatic hypotension is that the elderly often take multiple drugs and therefore are more exposed to adverse drug interactions. Orthostatic hypotension in the elderly may be prevented or minimized by the use of vasoactive drugs in low doses, gradual escalation of doses, and a careful consideration of risk–benefit issues in deciding to use pharmacotherapy with vasoactive drugs in this population.

DRUG INTERACTIONS

Orthostatic hypotension is more likely to occur when the mechanisms of postural blood pressure adjustments are impaired at multiple sites. The most common circumstance predisposing to orthostatic hypotension is probably diuretic-induced hypovolemia. In the presence of hypovolemia, treatment with vasodilators such as angiotensin-converting enzyme inhibitors, α-adrenergic blockers, or cardiac nitrates may induce supine and orthostatic hypotension. Drugs such as β-blockers or postganglionic sympathetic blockers that inhibit sympathetic reflex responses to orthostatic stress may similarly predispose to orthostatic hypotension when vasodilators, including antiarrhymic drugs such as quinidine, antidepressants, or antipsychotic drugs, are administered. These interactions may be minimized by taking

TABLE 91.1 Mechanisms of Chemical-Induced Orthostatic Hypotension

Hypovolaemia
Diuretics
Adrenal insufficiency secondary to discontinuation of chronic glucocorticoid theraphy
Reduced central nervous system sympathetic activity
Barbiturates and other sedative drugs
Methyldopa
L-Dopa
Bromocriptine
Δ^9-THC (marijuana)
Autonomic ganglionic blockade
Trimethaphan
α-Adrenergic blockers
Phentolamine
Phenoxybenzamine
Prazosin
Terazosin
Labetolol
Verapamil
Quinidine
Imipramine and other tricyclic antidepressants
Trazodone
Chlorpromazine
Postganglionic sympathetic blockers
Guanethidine
Debrisoquine
Bretylium
Phenelzine and other MAOIs
Direct vasodilators
Nitrates
Morphine and other opiates
Insulin
Captopril and other ACE inhibitors
Autonomic neuropathy
Alcohol (Wernicke's)
Amiodarone
Vincristine
Cisplatinum
Ciguatera toxin (fish poisoning)
Vacor (rat poisoning)
Release of vasoactivtive substances from microbes
Ivermectine
Diethylcarbamazine
Choroquine and pyrimethamine
Mefloquine and pyrimethamine
Vasovagal
Any hypotension drug reaction with an intact sympathetic response may trigger a vasovagal episode

patients off diuretics for a few days to allow volume repletion before initiation of vasodilator therapy and/or by giving potentially interacting drugs in low doses with a gradual escalation of the dose as tolerated.

AUTONOMIC NEUROPATHY PRODUCED BY SPECIFIC CHEMICALS AND DRUGS

Although most drug-induced orthostatic hypotension occurs when the pharmacology of the drug interferes with vascular homeostasis as described in Table 91.1, several drugs may produce autonomic dysfunction by producing injury to autonomic nerves.

Wernicke's encephalopathy occurs with chronic alcohol abuse and is commonly associated with orthostatic hypotension. Typically, hypotension occurs without an adequate compensatory tachycardia and is associated with an abnormal heart rate response to Valsalva, a subnormal cold pressor response, and hypersensitivity to exogenously infused catecholamines [1]. Hypovolemia often is present, but correction of hypovolemia only transiently improves orthostatic hypotension. On the basis of pathologic findings, the site of the autonomic lesion may be peripheral (peripheral nerves, preganglionic neurons of the intermediolateral cell column of the spinal cord), central (hypothalamus, midbrain tegmentum, fourth ventrical roof nucleus), or both.

Antineoplastic agents including *vincristine* and *cisplatinum* have been associated with autonomic dysfunction. Vincristine is neurotoxic and is known to cause bowel disturbances (severe constipation), bladder dysfunction (urinary retention), and peripheral neuropathy. Vincristine has been associated with orthostatic hypotension caused by autonomic neuropathy, and the affected patients usually have evidence of peripheral neuropathy [2]. Recovery from orthostatic hypotension may occur over several months after vincristine is discontinued. In one patient who was carefully studied, near total loss of urinary norepinephrine excretion with intact afferent and preganglionic responses was found, suggesting the lesion was localized to the postganglionic adrenergic nerves [3]. *Cisplatinum* rarely has been associated with autonomic neuropathy, including severe orthostatic hypotension with a subnormal heart rate response, and in one case gastroparesis with recurrent vomiting. Peripheral neuropathy also is present [4]. Cisplatinum also can cause orthostatic hypotension by inducing the salt-wasting nephropathy and hypovolaemia. In each patient, orthostatic hypotension was aggravated by fluid restrictions and could be ameliorated with fludrocortisone and salt [5].

Ciguatera toxin is produced by dinoflagellates consumed by reef fish. Intoxication—most common after ingestion of barracuda, red snapper, or grouper—typically presents with vomiting, abdominal pain, myalgias, weakness, paresthesias of the mouth, face, and extremities, and pruritus. A peculiar "hot and cold reversal," in which cold objects feel hot and vice versa is reported. Cardiovasular features include bradycardia, hypotension, and in some cases severe orthostatic hypotension [6]. The nature of the autonomic disturbance has been characterized in one patient with severe orthostatic hypotension [7]. This patient had evidence of both increase of vagal tone (the bradycardia and in part orthostatic hypotension was reversed by atropine) and sympathetic insufficiency (low plasma catecholamines and hypersensitivity to the infused noradrenaline). The orthostatic hypotension is reversible in most cases, resolving within 4 to 6 weeks in those cases for which recovery has been documented.

Vacor (N-3-pyridymethyl-N′–p-nitrophenyl urea) is a rodenticide that was sold in packet of cornmeal-like material. Vacor is no longer marketed in the United States, but is still available in some homes and for use by professional exterminators. Vacor ingestion (usually suicidal) produced an unusual syndrome, including irreversible and severe autonomic dysfunction and insulin-dependent diabetes mellitus [8]. Severe orthostatic hypotension developed from 6 hours to 2 days after ingestion of Vacor. The autonomic disturbance in cardiovascular regulation has been characterized as having very low circulating catecholamines at rest without a response to upright posture and hypersensivity to exogenous catecholamines, consistent with destruction of vascular adrenergic neurons. In some patients the response of the heart rate to upright posture is impaired, but in others there is a substantial tachycardia suggesting selective sparing of cardiac autonomic nerves. Other features of intoxication include a peripheral sensory and motor neuropathy and encephalopathy. Other features of the autonomic neuropathy include dysphagia, urinary retention, constipation, lost of sweating, and impotence. These findings suggest generalized peripheral autonomic dysfunction. In many cases the autonomic disturbances and diabetes have been irreversible, but in some cases at least partial recovery occurs, although recovery may take months or years. Treatment of patients with orthostatic hypotension from ingestion of Vacor often has been difficult, but there has been some success with the use of diets high in salt, fludrocortisone, and pressor drugs, including injections of dihydroergotamine.

References

1. Birchfield, R. I. 1964. Postural hypotension in Wernicke's disease: A manifestation of autonomic nervous system involvement. *Am. J. Med.* 36:404–414.
2. Hancock, B. W., and A. Naysmith. 1975. Vincristine-induced autonomic neuropathy. *Br. Med. J.* 3:207.
3. Carmichael, S. M., L. Eagleton, C. R. Ayers, and D. Mohler. 1970. Orthostatic hypotension during vincristine therapy. *Arch. Intern. Med.* 126:290–293.
4. Cohen, S. C., and J. E. Mollam. 1987 . Cisplatin-induced gastric paresis. *J. Neurooncol.* 5:237–240.
5. Hutchinson, F. N., E. A. Perez, L. J. H. Gandara, and G. A. Kaysen. 1988. Renal salt wasting in patients treated with cisplatin. *Ann. Intern. Med.* 108:21–25.
6. Morris, G. J., P. Lewin, N. T. Hargrett, W. C. Smith, P. A. Blake, and R. Schneider. 1982. Clinical feature ciguatera fish poisoning: A study of the disease in the US Virgin Islands. *Arch. Intern. Med.* 142:1090–1092.
7. Geller, R. J., and N. L. Benowitz. 1992. Orthostatic hypotension in ciguatera fish poisoning. *Arch. Intern. Med.* 152:2131–2133.
8. LeWitt, P. A. 1980. The neurotoxicity of the rat poisoning Vacor: A clinical study of 12 cases. *N. Engl. J. Med.* 302:73–77.

PART XI

ORTHOSTATIC INTOLERANCE

92 Neuropathic Postural Tachycardia Syndrome

Phillip A. Low
Department of Neurology
Mayo Clinic
Rochester, Minnesota

Orthostatic hypotension is well recognized but is relatively uncommon. For every patient seen with orthostatic hypotension, there are approximately 5 to 10 patients with orthostatic intolerance, defined as the development on standing of symptoms of cerebral hypoperfusion (e.g., lightheadedness, weakness, and blurred vision) associated with those of sympathetic activation (such as tachycardia, nausea, and tremulousness) and an excessive heart rate increment (≥30 beats/min). The female to male ratio is about 4–5 : 1, and most cases occur between the ages of 15 and 50 years [1].

CLINICAL FEATURES

We prospectively evaluated autonomic symptoms in a large cohort of 108 patients with postural tachycardia syndrome (POTS) using a structured and validated autonomic symptom profile, consisting of 167 questions encompassing 10 autonomic categories of symptoms [2]. About 50% of patients have an antecedent viral illness. Symptoms of dysautonomia were frequent or persistent (64%) and at least moderately severe in the majority and were either unchanged or getting worse in almost all patients (93%) at presentation. Positive family history of similar complaints occurred in 25% of patients. The following orthostatic symptoms occurred in >75% of subjects: lightheadedness/dizziness, lower extremity or diffuse weakness, disequilibrium, tachycardia, and shakiness; hence, the symptoms were caused by a combination of hypoperfusion and autonomic activation. These symptoms were most commonly aggravated by ambient heat, meals, and exertion. Other autonomic symptoms were dry eyes or mouth, gastrointestinal complaints of bloating, early satiety, nausea, pain, and alternating diarrhea and constipation. Fatigue is a significant complaint in about half the patients. Episodic, nonorthostatic symptoms of autonomic surges are common.

QUALITY OF LIFE

In a study of 94 patients (89% female, mean age = 34.2 years), Benrud-Larson evaluated quality of life (36-item Short Form Health Survey [SF-36]) and symptom severity (Autonomic Symptom Profile). Compared with a healthy population, patients with POTS reported impairment in multiple domains of quality of life, including physical, social, and role functioning. Hierarchical regression analyses revealed that symptom severity ($P < 0.001$) and disability status ($P < 0.001$) were independent predictors of the SF-36 physical component score, with all variables accounting for 54% of the variance ($P < 0.0001$).

EVIDENCE OF PERIPHERAL DENERVATION

POTS is heterogeneous; some patients have a limited, presumably autoimmune autonomic neuropathy. Distal anhidrosis affecting the legs is commonly found on the thermoregulatory sweat test and has shown to be postganglionic by the quantitative sudomotor axon reflex test. Peripheral adrenergic denervation is present. There is a loss of baroreflex-mediated reflex vasoconstriction (phase II-L of the Valsalva maneuver) (Fig. 92.1). Leg arteriolar vasoconstriction is impaired [3] because of reduced lower extremity secretion of norepinephrine when compared with the upper extremity [4]. There often is a modest gradual decrease in blood pressure associated with excessive tachycardia (Fig. 92.2). Perivascular round cell infiltration sometimes is seen on nerve biopsy [5], and ganglionic antibody is occasionally positive, especially in the more severely affected patients [6]. Loss of epidermal fibers sometimes is seen on skin biopsy. As a result of peripheral denervation and a reduced edema threshold, venous pooling and leg swelling occurs [3], and hypovolemia develops with continued standing. Pooling may occur in both the abdominal viscera and the legs.

OTHER PATHOPHYSIOLOGIC STUDIES

A mutation in the norepinephrine transporter has been reported [7], but it is rare. There could be an increase in adrenergic tone, evidenced by an increased decline in blood pressure after ganglion blockade [4]. Cerebral hypoperfu-

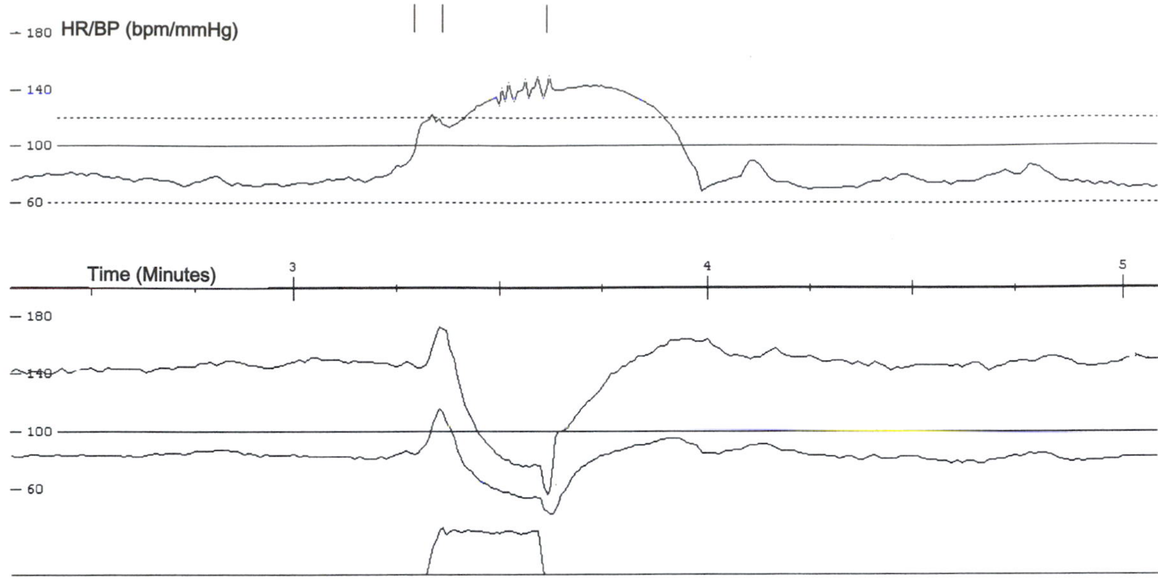

FIGURE 92.1 A 35-year-old woman with neuropathic postural tachycardia syndrome. Heart rate (HR) in beats per minute (bpm) is shown above and blood pressure (BP) in mmHg is shown below. There is a loss of late phase II of the Valsalva maneuver during the Valsalva maneuver.

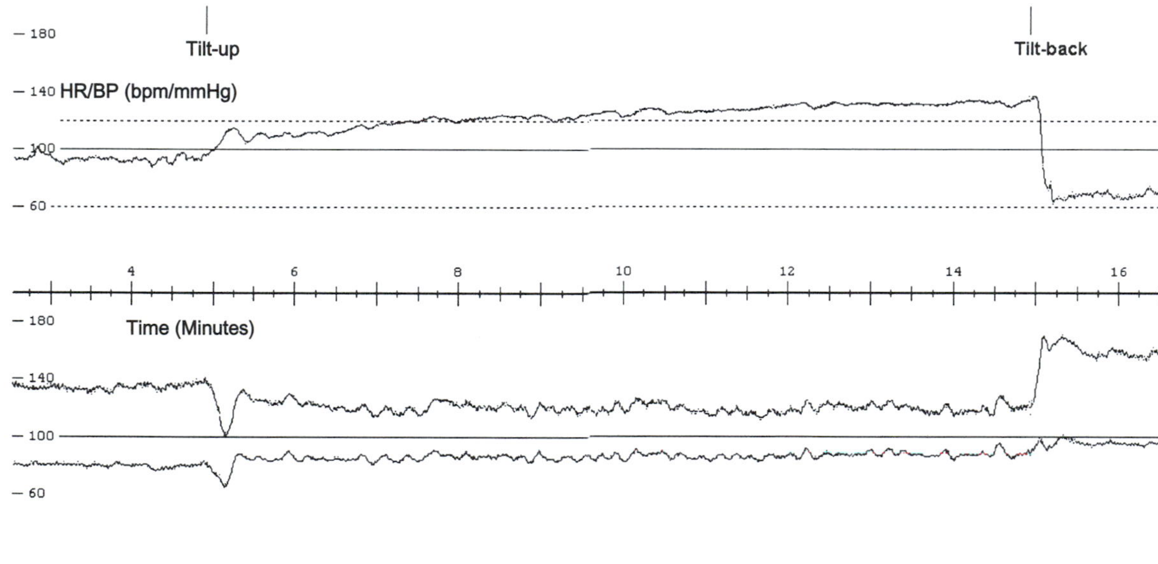

FIGURE 92.2 Same patient as in Figure 92.1. During head-up tilt, there is a progressive and excessive increase in heart rate (HR). Blood pressure (BP) undergoes a transient decrease with recovery in the first half minute followed by a modest gradual decrease in BP.

sion is caused by an increase in cerebral vasoconstrictor tone, partly because of hypocapnia [8].

FOLLOW-UP

On follow-up, 80% of patients showed improvement in their condition and 90% were able to return to work, although only 60% were functionally normal [2]. Some symptoms tend to persist and exercise tolerance is impaired. Patients who had an antecedent event appeared to do better than those with spontaneous POTS. Salt supplementation and β-blockers were the most efficacious therapies.

MANAGEMENT

A variety of approaches have been used to alleviate symptoms in POTS. All patients need volume expansion and a high-salt/high-fluid regimen. Drugs that seem to enjoy the greatest success are midodrine, propranolol, and fludrocortisone. Other measures used include body stockings and physical counter maneuvers. These treatments may influence pathophysiologic mechanisms of POTS such as α-receptor dysfunction, β-receptor supersensitivity, venous pooling, and brainstem center dysfunction. Acutely, we could demonstrate significant improvement after treatment with midodrine and saline [9].

References

1. Low, P. A., T. L. Opfer-Gehrking, S. C. Textor, E. E. Benarroch, W. K. Shen, R. Schondorf, G. A. Suarez, and T. A. Rummans. 1995. Postural tachycardia syndrome (POTS). *Neurology* 45:S19–S25.
2. Sandroni, P., T. L. Opfer-Gehrking, B. R. McPhee, and P. A. Low. 1999. Postural tachycardia syndrome: Clinical features and follow-up study. *Mayo Clin. Proc.* 74:1106–1110.
3. Stewart, J. M. 2002. Pooling in chronic orthostatic intolerance: Arterial vasoconstrictive but not venous compliance defects. *Circulation* 105:2274–2281.
4. Jacob, G., F. Costa, J. R. Shannon, R. M. Robertson, M. Wathen, M. Stein, I. Biaggioni, A. Ertl, B. Black, and D. Robertson. 2000. The neuropathic postural tachycardia syndrome. *N. Engl. J. Med.* 343: 1008–1014.
5. Schondorf, R., and P. A. Low. 1993. Idiopathic postural orthostatic tachycardia syndrome: An attenuated form of acute pandysautonomia? *Neurology* 43:132–137.
6. Vernino, S., P. A. Low, R. D. Fealey, J. D. Stewart, G. Farrugia, and V. A. Lennon. 2000. Autoantibodies to ganglionic acetylcholine receptors in autoimmune autonomic neuropathies. *N. Engl. J. Med.* 343:847–855.
7. Shannon, J. R., N. L. Flattem, J. Jordan, G. Jacob, B. K. Black, I. Biaggioni, R. D. Blakely, and D. Robertson. 2000. Orthostatic intolerance and tachycardia associated with norepinephrine-transporter deficiency. *N. Engl. J. Med.* 342:541–549.
8. Novak, V., J. M. Spies, P. Novak, B. R. McPhee, T. A. Rummans, and P. A. Low. 1998. Hypocapnia and cerebral hypoperfusion in orthostatic intolerance. *Stroke* 29:1876–1881.
9. Gordon, V. M., T. L. Opfer-Gehrking, V. Novak, and P. A. Low. 2000. Hemodynamic and symptomatic effects of acute interventions on tilt in patients with postural tachycardia syndrome. *Clin. Auton. Res.* 10:29–33.
10. Benrud-Larson, L. M., M. S. Dewar, P. Sandroni, T. A. Rummans, J. A. Haythornthwaite, and P. A. Low. 2002. Quality of life in patients with postural tachycardia syndrome. *Mayo Clin. Proc.* 77:531–537.

93 Hyperadrenergic Postural Tachycardia Syndrome

Simi Vincent
Division of Clinical Pharmacology
Vanderbilt University
Nashville, Tennessee

David Robertson
Clinical Research Center
Vanderbilt University
Nashville, Tennessee

Patients with orthostatic intolerance have symptoms on standing that resemble those elicited by inadequate cerebral blood flow. They have heart rate increases on standing of at least 30 beats/min with dizziness, palpitations, poor exercise tolerance, and presyncopal symptoms, although syncope itself is infrequent. There is a 5:1 increased prevalence in women, usually in the 15 to 45 year-old age group. They are usually the most common patient category referred to autonomic clinics. There appear to be dozens, perhaps hundreds, of underlying pathophysiologies, because orthostatic intolerance (postural tachycardia syndrome [POTS]) is a symptom complex rather than a disease entity itself (Table 93.1). There are two major problems in evaluating such patients. First, physical deconditioning (e.g., because of bedrest) can be difficult to distinguish from true pathology; most commonly patients encountered have both an altered pathophysiology plus an overlay of deconditioning. This is one reason elucidation of pathophysiology has moved so slowly. Second, many relatively common diseases have orthostatic intolerance as a rare presentation, and the clinician must exercise special caution that in "diagnosing" POTS the continued importance of ongoing evaluation for the true cause of the illness is not neglected, because there may be important therapeutic implications.

Many of these patients have orthostatic intolerance because of a peripheral cause (see Chapter 92). However, others have a pathophysiology that likely originates in the brain. In this chapter, the term *hyperadrenergic postural tachycardia syndrome*, or *hyperadrenergic orthostatic intolerance*, is used to designate such patients. Unfortunately, it has been difficult for investigators to clearly distinguish between these two pathophysiologies, which are probably themselves heterogeneous. All clinical studies have heretofore included patients with both kinds of orthostatic intolerance mixed together. As our ability to evaluate and define pathophysiology increases, better classification of study subjects should be achieved in future investigations. Perhaps distinguishing clinical signs and symptoms differentiating them will emerge. This chapter considers the evidence for this central form of orthostatic intolerance.

Notably, early investigators observing the tachycardia and "hyperkinetic heart" in these patients generally assumed that enhanced sympathetic activation, or β-adrenoreceptor hypersensitivity, was somehow involved. It was noted early that these patients often had abnormal electrocardiogram tracings, especially ST-T wave changes in the inferior leads (II, III, and AVF) suggestive of ischemia, even though at coronary arteriography no atherosclerosis was noted. It was known that similar hyperadrenergic symptoms were elicited in rare cases of tumors involving the brainstem and in baroreflex failure, and studies in rats showed that destruction of the nuclei of the solitary tracts yielded a profound hyperadrenergic state that culminated in death within hours.

This view was strengthened by the finding that plasma norepinephrine often was increased in POTS and that α_2 agonists, β antagonists, and phenobarbital attenuated the tachycardia or relieved some of the symptoms in patients, or both. Mild baroreflex dysfunction proved to occur commonly. However, it was eventually found that many patients with POTS with mildly increased plasma norepinephrine had neuropathic POTS. Perhaps in such patients there was a combination of compensatory sympathetic activation of still-functioning noradrenergic neurons, especially to the heart, and a slightly reduced clearance of norepinephrine because of a decline in the population of remaining norepinephrine transporters.

One of the most important lines of evidence in support for a central etiology emanates from studies in which both sympathetic and parasympathetic activity have been blocked by the Nn-nicotinic antagonist trimethaphan. With this agent, patients with POTS had greater decreases in sympathetic activity than control subjects; systolic blood pressure decreased by 17 mmHg in patients with POTS but only 4 mmHg in control subjects. Among patients with POTS, the half having the greatest decrease (28 mmHg) after trimethaphan had greater pre-trimethaphan supine systolic blood pressure and greater supine and upright plasma norepinephrine levels. However, supine and upright heart rates were similar in both POTS subgroups.

Analysis of simultaneous peroneal sympathetic nerve traffic (to gauge vascular sympathetic tone) and heart rate (to gauge cardiac sympathetic tone) in patients with POTS showed increased sympathetic tone to the heart but not to the vasculature, a finding confirmed by studies of cardiac norepinephrine spillover, which was increased. This discordance seems robust and may prove to be an important clue to the nature of the central pathophysiology of POTS.

Currently, it is often impossible to identify patients with POTS likely to have enhanced central sympathetic outflow, but some help is afforded by features in Table 93.2 if they are encountered. The use of such tables must be approached cautiously given our limited data and should not be viewed as definitions. In particular, the plasma norepinephrine is limited in that its increase on standing relates in part to the altered blood flow distribution in different postures.

Treatment of hyperadrenergic POTS currently is not very specific (Table 93.3). Physical measures do appear to help. Almost all patients with POTS feel much better for 6 to 48 hours after a saline infusion of 500 to 2000 ml, and even though it is usually impractical to maintain patients on such a regimen, it is sometimes encouraging to a severely affected and frightened patient to see that something can in fact be done to make them feel better.

Low-dose propranolol is the most commonly used agent in our experience, and patients usually describe experiencing fatigue if administered doses greater than 80 mg daily. Yet failures with this agent are common and we often require additional drugs if the simple initial measures fail.

TABLE 93.1 Terms Used for Postural Tachycardia Syndrome

Orthostatic intolerance
Mitral valve prolapse syndrome
Neurocirculatory asthenia
Vasoregulatory asthenia
Hyperkinetic heart syndrome
Postural orthostatic tachycardia syndrome
Orthostatic tachycardia
Effort syndrome
Soldier's heart
Irritable heart

TABLE 93.2 Features of Hyperadrenergic and Neuropathic Postural Tachycardia Syndrome

Features suggestive of hyperadrenergic postural tachycardia syndrome
Plasma norepinephrine levels >1000 pg/ml
Increased muscle sympathetic nerve activity
Increase in low-frequency/high-frequency ratio of heart rate variability
Symptomatic benefit with low-dose clonidine
Features suggestive of neuropathic postural tachycardia syndrome
Plasma norepinephrine levels of high normal to 800 pg/ml
Absent galvanic skin response or abnormal quantitative sudomotor axon reflex test
Other evidence of peripheral neuropathy
Poor response to low-dose clonidine

TABLE 93.3 Treatment of Hyperadrenergic Postural Tachycardia Syndrome

16 oz water 2–3 times daily as needed (acts for ~1 hour only)
10 g sodium diet
Support garment
Propranolol 10–20 mg two to four times daily
Clonidine 0.05–0.10 mg orally twice daily
Methyldopa 125–250 mg half strength or twice daily
Fludrocortisone 0.05–0.30 mg daily
Midodrine 2.5–10 mg three times daily
Phenobarbital 30–100 mg daily

Phenobarbital sometimes helps without worsening fatigue, but many failures occur. Low-dose clonidine or low-dose methyldopa sometimes helps.

References

1. Friesinger, G. C., R. O. Biern, I. Likar, and R. E. Mason. 1972. Exercise electrocardiography and vasoregulatory abnormalities. *Am. J. Cardiol.* 30:733–740.
2. Furlan, R., G. Jacob, M. Snell, D. Robertson, A. Porta, P. Harris, and R. Mosqueda-Garcia. 1998. Chronic orthostatic intolerance: A disorder with discordant cardiac and vascular sympathetic control. *Circulation* 98:2154–2159.
3. Goldstein, D. S., D. Robertson, M. Esler, S. E. Straus, and G. Eisenhofer. 2002. Dysautonomias: Clinical disorders of the autonomic nervous system. *Ann. Intern. Med.* 137:753–763.
4. Hermosillo, A. G., K. Jauregui-Renaud, A. Kostine, M. F. Marquez, J. L. Lara, and M. Cardenas. 2002. Comparative study of cerebral blood flow between postural tachycardia and neurocardiogenic syncope, during head-up tilt test. *Europace* 4:369–374.
5. Hoeldtke, R. D., G. E. Dworkin, S. R. Gaspar, and B. C. Israel. 1989. Sympathotonic orthostatic hypotension: A report of four cases. *Neurology* 39:34–40.
6. Jordan, J., J. R. Shannon, B. K. Black, S. Y. Paranjape, J. Barwise, and D. Robertson. 1998. Raised cerebrovascular resistance in idiopathic orthostatic intolerance: Evidence of sympathetic vasoconstriction. *Hypertension* 32:699–704.
7. Khurana, R. K. 1995. Orthostatic intolerance and orthostatic tachycardia: A heterogeneous disorder. *Clin. Auton. Res.* 5:12–18.
8. Kuchel, O., and J. Leveille. 1998. Idiopathic hypovolemia: A self-perpetuating autonomic dysfunction? *Clin. Auton. Res.* 8:341–346.
9. Low, P. A., V. Novak, J. M. Spies, P. Novak, and G. W. Petty. 1999. Cerebrovascular regulation in the postural orthostatic tachycardia syndrome (POTS). *Am. J. Med. Sci.* 317:124–133.
10. Mano, T., and S. Iwase. 2003. Sympathetic nerve activity in hypotension and orthostatic intolerance. *Acta. Physiol. Scand.* 177:359–365.
11. Miller, J. W., and D. H. Streeten. 1990. Vascular responsiveness to norepinephrine in sympathicotonic orthostatic intolerance. *J. Lab. Clin. Med.* 115:549–558.
12. Novak, V., J. M. Spies, P. Novak, B. R. McPhee, T. A. Rummans, and P. A. Low. 1998. Hypocapnia and cerebral hypoperfusion in orthostatic intolerance. *Stroke* 29:1876–1881.
13. Novak, V., T. L. Opfer-Gehrking, and P. A. Low. 1996. Postural tachycardia syndrome: time frequency mapping. *J. Auton. Nerv. Syst.* 61:628–633.

94

Hypovolemia Syndrome

Fetnat Fouad-Tarazi
Cardiovascular Medicine
Cleveland Clinic Foundation
Cleveland, Ohio

The integrative regulation of the circulation by the autonomic nervous system counterbalances postural stressors. The physiologic response to the redistribution of blood volume is crucial to the maintenance of homeostasis in response to orthostatic stress. In humans, the main effector of this physiologic response is the sympathetic nervous system. During orthostasis, the low-pressure receptors in the cardiopulmonary field and the high-pressure receptors in the large arteries (carotids and aortic arch) sense the initial reduction of cardiac filling and of stroke volume and send impulses to the central autonomic network. The resulting sympathetic vasomotor outflow allows maintenance of mean arterial pressure for a given amount of cardiac filling through an immediate vasoconstriction, venoconstriction, cardiac inotropy, and chronotropy.

Furthermore, there is a regulatory increase of extracellular fluid volume and cardiac filling for a given amount of hydrostatic pooling of blood. Indeed, antinatriuresis and water retention are provoked in the upright posture by the following: (1) decreased renal sodium excretion caused by reflex increase of norepinephrine during orthostasis, which decreases renal blood flow followed by decreased glomerular filtration of sodium, as well as augmentation of reabsorption of the filtered sodium; (2) the increased arginine vasopressin secretion and decreased atrial natriuretic peptide secretion caused by decreased atrial stretch during upright posture; and (3) the stimulation of the renin-angiotensin aldosterone system, which results from decreased renal blood flow and renal perfusion pressure and causes enhancement of sodium/potassium exchange and medication of a delayed vasoconstriction.

In addition, other reflex adjustments take place during orthostatic stress including leg pumping of skeletal muscles, which enhances venous return to the heart, and venoarterial reflex provoked by venous distension, which results in augmentation of arterial vasoconstriction.

Sensors that communicate these perturbations to the central nervous system fall within five categories:

1. Volustat (cardiopulmonary)
2. Arterial barostat
3. Propriostat
4. Vestibular homeostat
5. Engo receptors (change in skeletal muscle tension).

Syncope, presyncope, and orthostatic intolerance represent a disease spectrum and occur as a result of brain hypoxia, which is usually secondary to postural hypotension and reduction of cerebral perfusion pressure beyond the cerebral autoregulation function. Among the causes of syncope, presyncope and orthostatic intolerance are:

1. Cardiovascular causes: cardiac (obstructive or electrophysiologic), vascular (large arterial compliance, small arteriolar reactivity, or venous capacitance causes), and severe hypovolemia
2. Autonomic dysfunction:
   - Peripheral primary autonomic disorders (pure autonomic failure, familial dysautonomia), peripheral secondary autonomic disorders (amyloid autonomic failure, diabetic autonomic failure, paraneoplastic autonomic dysfunction, Guillain–Barré syndrome, Chagas disease, and others)
   - Central autonomic disorders (multiple system atrophy)
   - Neurocardiogenic reflex-mediated postural intolerance
   - Postural tachycardia syndrome (progressive orthostatic tachycardia syndrome [POTS], primary autonomic or secondary to a circulatory provocative mechanism)
   - Specific reflex syncope (e.g., cough and micturition)
   - Others: baroreflex failure, carotid sinus hypersensitivity, drug-related autonomic dysfunction.

It has become more widely recognized that patients with migraine, vertigo, sympathetic dystrophy syndrome, and chronic fatigue syndrome present clinically with homeostatic derangement that operates in parallel to convey new messages to the autonomic nervous system and subsequently present clinically with cardiovascular manifestations of orthostatism.

BLOOD VOLUME AND SYNCOPE

Circulatory volume depletion is usually considered a secondary phenomenon that occurs as a result of fluid loss through the kidney, the gastrointestinal tract, or the skin. Acute circulatory volume depletion also may be caused by hemorrhagic blood loss. Contrary to acute volume depletion, which is characterized by hypotension and compensatory tachycardia, chronic volume depletion presents with clinical features related to the associated hemodynamic and compensatory neurohormonal mechanisms.

Chronic intravascular volume depletion is usually thought to be "secondary" to an underlying event. Patients are interrogated about their dietary habits, salt intake, diuretic use, gastrointestinal losses, excessive diuresis, and nocturia, as well as paroxysmal tachycardia. Search is usually pursued for surreptitious intake of medications, and urine toxicity screening tests are often performed. When no cause can be found, the hypovolemia is labeled idiopathic.

RELATION BETWEEN CHRONIC GLOBAL BLOOD VOLUME DEPLETION AND NEUROCARDIOGENIC RESPONSE TO UPRIGHT POSTURE

The relation between chronic global blood volume depletion (either idiopathic or secondary) and neurocardiogenic response to upright posture is still unclear, probably because of the nonhomogeneous tilt protocols and the differences in the definition of hypovolemia. Indeed, further evaluation of this question is needed to determine if a threshold blood volume is a prerequisite for an abnormal response to orthostatic stress.

Cody and colleagues [1] report orthostatic hypotension after overtreatment with diuretic and converting enzyme inhibition [1]. In 1993, we compared the response to head-up tilt (HUT) among 30 patients with hypovolemia (defined as ≤90% of normal for corresponding sex) and 15 patients with normovolemia; both groups had a similar history of dizziness, syncope, or both [2]. Results showed that variations in blood volume (within the range defined in the study) did not correlate with the occurrence of tilt-induced vasovagal response; however, accentuated orthostatic tachycardia was more prevalent in patients with hypovolemia compared with patients with normovolemia with nonvasovagal response to tilt. In a more recent study [3], we tested the hypothesis that hypovolemia predicts the extent of POTS, as well as the occurrence of secondary neurocardiogenic response (vasovagal reaction/vasodepressor reaction). We evaluated HUT data from 22 patients with a POTS response to HUT who also all had blood volume examination using the ^{125}I-albumin technique [4]. The POTS/VVR group had a more pronounced decrease of systolic blood pressure and a greater increase in heart rate at a shorter duration of the same level of HUT than the POTS/non-VVR group. The plasma volume level and the presence of hypovolemia did not seem to determine the extent of POTS or the occurrence of VVR/VVS in these patients.

Conversely, Jacob and colleagues [5] report that hypovolemia occurred commonly in patients with orthostatic intolerance and is associated with an inappropriately low plasma renin activity. Furthermore, Jacob and colleagues [6] report that idiopathic orthostatic tachycardia (a condition presenting clinically with symptoms of orthostatic intolerance and occasionally with frank syncope) responded acute to saline infusion and to the α_1-adrenoreceptor agonist midodrine; the authors conclude that these findings are consistent with the hypothesis that idiopathic orthostatic tachycardia is principally caused by hypovolemia and loss of adequate lower extremity vascular tone.

DYNAMICS OF POSTURAL BLOOD VOLUME SHIFTS

Less frequently discussed is the distribution of blood volume and the role of the extent of venous pooling on homeostasis. Cardiopulmonary volume influences both cardiac output and low-pressure mechanoreceptors in the cardiopulmonary region. Inadequate cardiac filling is an important cause of postural intolerance and postural tachycardia, and it has been part of the Bezold–Jarisch reflex hypothesis of neurocardiogenic syncope. Increased venous capacitance of various etiologies is an important determinant of cardiac filling [7]. Also, regional autonomic neuropathy [8] was reported as a contributor to the increase of postural heart rate in sympathotonic orthostatic hypotension.

The syndrome of idiopathic hypovolemia is important to recognize because its normal clinical picture may lead to delays in diagnosis and use of appropriate therapy.

CLINICAL FEATURES OF CHRONIC IDIOPATHIC HYPOVOLEMIA

Orthostatic intolerance is a common symptom in patients with chronic idiopathic hypovolemia. However, in contrast with other types of orthostatic intolerance, these patients frequently have episodic clinical manifestations suggestive of adrenergic hyperactivity even in the supine resting posture [9]. Extreme increases in blood pressure have been reported to be associated with symptoms of apprehension and perspiration, simulating pheochromocytoma [9]. The plasma and urinary catecholamines are typically not increased.

Our initial clinical impression was that of an increased prevalence of vasovagal syncope in patients with severe idiopathic hypovolemia. However, this impression was not substantiated by data analysis in 11 such patients [9]; only 1 of the 11 patients experienced development of vasovagal syncope during the HUT, whereas another had vasodepressor syncope without slowing of heart rate.

Marked reduction of pulse pressure may occur in patients with hypovolemia because of the increase of diastolic blood pressure and the accompanying reduction of systolic blood pressure secondary to the reduction of cardiac output. The peripheral radial pulse may be difficult to palpate in such patients. The clinical importance of this phenomenon is to be stressed because it can be misleading clinically and give a false impression of hypotension unless the femoral arterial pulse is palpated or an intraarterial blood pressure recording is obtained [9].

HEMODYNAMIC PROFILE OF CHRONIC IDIOPATHIC HYPOVOLEMIA

Intense vasoconstriction is the most important systemic hemodynamic finding even when blood pressure is normal at rest (Tables 94.1 and 94.2). In our experience, cardiac index was in the low range of normal, whereas left ventricular ejection fraction was normal. The intravascular blood volume was normally distributed between the cardiopulmonary and peripheral segments of the circulation, but the absolute value of the cardiopulmonary volume was reduced compared with that of normal.

NEUROHUMORAL INDEXES OF CHRONIC IDIOPATHIC HYPOVOLEMIA

Patients with severe idiopathic hypovolemia typically have normal baroreceptor reflexes and normal response of the autonomic nervous system to the Valsalva maneuver, cold pressor test, and hyperventilation [9]. Furthermore, supine plasma catecholamines were normal at rest and stimulated adequately during HUT. The heart rate response to graded isoproterenol infusion was increased; however, contrary to patients with hyper-β-adrenergic state [10], there was no excessive anxiety reaction and the only symptomatology was mild palpitation without chest discomfort. Serum electrolytes are normal in patients with idiopathic hypovolemia and unrestricted sodium intake. Supine plasma aldosterone was at the upper limit of normal and normal plasma cortisol was normal. Twenty-four hour urinary sodium excretion ranged from 22 to 236 mEq without correlation to the aldosterone excretion rate.

POSSIBLE MECHANISMS OF CHRONIC IDIOPATHIC HYPOVOLEMIA

The mechanism of volume depletion in patients with idiopathic hypovolemia is difficult to explain. It remains unclear whether the intravascular blood volume contraction induces a reflex hyperadrenergic response or if it is secondary to increased vasoconstriction induced by a primary accentuation of sympathetic activity. Sympathetic overactivity accentuates hypovolemia because of the effects of catecholamine on the venous circulation. The venoconstrictive effect of catecholamines increases capillary hydrostatic pressure and results in transudation of fluid out of the vascular space [11]. Conversely, hypovolemia induced reflex sympathoadrenergic vasoconstriction so that a vicious circle is created. It also has been postulated that the intense vasoconstriction observed in patients with idiopathic hypovolemia could be caused by vascular hyperreaction to a normal adrenergic stimulus affecting both arterial and venous circulation. In our experience, there was no evidence of adrenocortical hypofunction. Although no strict metabolic studies were done, there was no clinical or laboratory evidence of sodium wasting in these patients.

TABLE 94.1 Blood Volume in Patients with Idiopathic Hypovolemia

	Patients with idiopathic hypovolemia (n = 11)	**Healthy subjects* (n = 24)**
TBV (ml/cm)	73 ± 2.3% of normal	29.4 ± 0.81 (male) 23.7 ± 0.54 (female)
CPV (ml/m^2)	277 ± 14†	413 ± 13
CPV/TBV (%)	14.5 ± 0.14†	16.5 ± 0.5
Hematocrit	42 ± 1.0	41 ± 0.6

Data from Fouad, F. M., L. Tadena-Thome, E. L. Bravo, and R. C. Tarazi. 1986. Idiopathic hypovolemia. *Ann. Intern. Med.* 104:298–303.

All values were obtained during normal salt intake and are given as mean ± SE.

*Normal values taken from 12 men and 12 women.

$^\dagger P < 0.05$.

CPV, cardiopulmonary volume; TBV, total blood volume.

TABLE 94.2 Systemic Hemodynamics in Patients with Idiopathic Hypovolemia and Normal Subjects

	Patients (n = 11)	**Healthy subjects (n = 45)**
Age (yr)	23–50	18–66
Systolic blood pressure (mmHg)	129 ± 7.0	117 ± 1.6
Diastolic blood pressure (mmHg)	85 ± 3.0*	78 ± 1.2
Heart rate (beats/min)	76 ± 3.3*	65 ± 1.3
Cardiac index (liters/min/m^2)	2.7 ± 0.1†	2.9 ± 0.07
Total peripheral resistance (U/m^2)	38 ± 1.3‡	32 ± 0.8
Mean transit time (sec)	6.4 ± 0.4‡	8.2 ± 0.3
Ejection fraction (%)	55 ± 1.5	55 ± 1.0

Data from Fouad, F. M., L. Tadena-Thome, E. L. Bravo, and R. C. Tarazi. 1986. Idiopathic hypovolemia. *Ann. Intern. Med.* 104:298–303.

All values are given as mean ± SE.

$^* P < 0.02$, $^\dagger P < 0.05$, and $^\ddagger P < 0.01$ from healthy subjects.

RESPONSE TO THERAPY

The syndrome of idiopathic hypovolemia is important to recognize because of its important therapeutic implications. Unlike patients with hyper-β-adrenergic state, patients with idiopathic hypovolemia did not manifest improvement of symptoms when treated with β-blockers. Conversely, acute expansion of blood volume using human serum albumin led to obvious improvement of symptoms; the increase in blood volume was associated with an increase in cardiac output, a reduction of systemic vascular resistance, and an attenuation of the tilt-induced accentuated tachycardic response.

Chronic blood volume expansion was difficult to maintain in our patients. Treatment with fludrocortisone and a high-sodium diet led to some relief of symptoms in four of six patients who received this treatment [9]. Addition of clonidine proved helpful in three of four patients, probably by toning down the sympathetic nervous system and buffering heart rate response to upright posture. Another mechanism of action of clonidine could be an increase of transcapillary transfer of fluid into the venous system [12].

Contrary to what would be generally conceived, the episodic hypertension in patients with idiopathic hypovolemia has been primarily treated with volume expansion, which shuts off the excessive hyperreactive sympathoadrenal and/or vascular mechanisms induced by the hypovolemic state. Indeed, it was previously reported that blood pressure response to treatment with ganglion blockers is inversely related to the extent of intravascular blood volume, which was thought to explain the increased sensitivity of patients with hypovolemia to neural blocking drugs [13]; accentuation of the hypotensive reaction in these patients may be attributed to sudden inhibition by the neural blocking agent of the venoconstriction that would have been induced by secondary adrenergic activation during uncorrected hypovolemia. Consequently, a marked decrease of venous return would be associated with an accentuated hypotensive response.

Thus, idiopathic hypovolemia is a definite syndrome characterized by orthostatic intolerance, disabling orthostatic tachycardia, and episodes of paroxysmal supine hypertension. The pathophysiologic mechanism of the syndrome is still unclear. Favorable clinical response has been observed when patients are treated with blood volume expansion, either alone or in combination with clonidine therapy.

FUTURE CONSIDERATIONS

Standardization of the definition of hypovolemia is necessary. Normal blood volume in humans has been shown to vary with the degree of leanness or obesity of an individual rather than linearly with body mass [14, 15]. It also has been shown to be related primarily to the tissue mass of individuals rather than surface area.

Feldschuh and Enson [16] demonstrated that blood volume can be most precisely predicted in relation to degree of deviation from ideal weight. Normal blood volume varies from 105 to 41 ml/kg in extremely obese individuals. Feldschuh and Enson's published algorithms using height and weight, although significantly more precise, were difficult to calculate and were not widely used.

Blood volume measurements also have been hampered by the technical requirements in preparing precisely matched injectants and standards for tracers. Chromated red cells (for red cell measurements) are a particularly complex procedure that involves multiple steps and requires retransfusion of the patient's autologous blood sample.

Radiolabeled iodine has been commonly used as a plasma tracer. In 1999, the U.S. Food and Drug Administration approved a new semiautomated system, the Daxor BVA-100, that included the use of a prepackaged injectate, matching standards, and collection kit. The kit uses an albumin I-131 tracer and enables a 4- to 5-point postinjection sampling to be collected from a single venipuncture site. The system has an accuracy of ±2.5% for the blood volume measurement. It was shown that the system also can be used to measure red cell volume precisely [17, 18]. The system also incorporated the published algorithms for using degree of deviation from ideal weight for predicting individual normal blood volumes. More precise individual predicted normal values permit a sharper differentiation between individual normal and abnormal blood volume measurements.

Preliminary data from our laboratory (unpublished) using this technique of blood volume determination in 611 patients with a history of orthostatic intolerance confirmed that hypovolemia is present in a large number of patients. Normal blood volume was considered to be ±8% of ideal (for sex, height, and body weight). As a group, hypovolemia was more common than hypervolemia; 15.7% of the group was more than 16% hypovolemic; only 7.1% were 16% or more hypervolemic. Furthermore, for the 611 patients as a group, there was a finding of overall incomplete plasma compensation in response to decreased red cell volume. In our previously reported study, we focused on plasma volume diminution in regard to hypovolemia. In our much larger series, it is apparent that plasma volume abnormalities must be considered in the context of their relation to red cell volume. A patient, for example, who has a significant anemia, may have a normal or an expanded plasma volume, yet may be significantly hypovolemic. In contrast, a patient with syncope with an identical degree of plasma volume expansion and a normal red cell volume is not hypovolemic and has primarily a disturbance of the autonomic nervous system.

Use of blood volume measurement in conjunction with tilt-table testing provides for the first time a clearer understanding of patients with identical symptoms whose underlying pathology may be very different and who require different treatments.

Further evaluation is needed to determine if a critical threshold blood volume is a prerequisite for an abnormal response to orthostatic stress. Also, it is essential to include the dynamics of blood volume shifts when addressing postural changes, exercise, postprandial conditions, and other situational issues. Furthermore, the interaction between volume factors, autonomic reflexes, and the renin-angiotensin aldosterone system needs more in-depth evaluation.

References

1. Cody, R. J., E. L. Bravo, F. M. Fouad, and R. C. Tarazi. 1981. Cardiovascular reflexes during long-term converting enzyme inhibition and sodium depletion. The response to tilt in hypertensive patients. *Am. J. Med.* 71:422–426.
2. Jaeger, F. J., J. D. Malone, L. W. Castle, and F. M. Fouad-Tarazi. 1993. Is absolute hypovolemia a risk factor for vasovagal syncope. *Pacing Clin. Electrophysiol.* 16:743–750.
3. Ali-Hasan, S., J. Hammel, and F. Fouad-Tarazi. 2001. Is hypovolemia a determinant of postural tachycardia syndrome and its sequelae? *Pacing Clin. Electrophysiol.* 24:574.
4. Tarazi, R. C., M. M. Ibrahim, H. P. Dustan, and C. M. Ferrario. 1974. Cardiac factors in hypertension. *Circ. Res.* 34,35(Suppl 1):I213–I221.
5. Jacob, G., D. Robertson, R. Mosqueda-Garcia, A. Ertl, R. M. Robertson, and I. Biaggioni. 1997. Hypovolemia in syncope and orthostatic intolerance. Role of the renin-angiotensin system. *Am. J. Med.* 103:128–133.
6. Jacob, G., J. R. Shannon, B. Black, I. Biaggioni, R. Mosqueda-Garcia, R. M. Robertson, and D. Robertson. 2000. Neuropathic postural tachycardia syndrome. *N. Engl. J. Med.* 343:1008–1014.
7. Abi-Samra, F., J. D. Maloney, F. M. Fouad-Tarazi, and L. W. Castle. 1988. The usefulness of head-up tilt testing and hemodynamic investigations in the workup of syncope of unknown origin. *Pacing Clin. Electrophysiol.* 11:1202–1214.
8. Hoeldtke, R. D., S. R. Dworkin, and B. C. Israel. 1989. Sympathotonic orthostatic hypotension: A report of four cases. *Neurology* 39:34–40.
9. Fouad, F. M., L. Tadena-Thome, E. L. Bravo, and R. C. Tarazi. 1986. Idiopathic hypovolemia. *Ann. Intern. Med.* 104:298–303.
10. Frohlich, E. D., R. C. Tarazi, and P. Dustan. 1969. Hyperdynamic beta-adrenergic circulatory state. *Arch. Intern. Med.* 117:614–619.
11. Cohn, J. N. 1966. Relationship of plasma volume changes to resistance and capacitance vessel effects of sympathomimetic amines and angiotensin in man. *Clin. Sci.* 30:267–278.
12. Onesti, G., A. B. Schwartz, K. E. Kim, V. Paz-Martinez, and D. Swartz. 1971. Antihypertensive effect of clonidine. *Circ. Res.* 28:53–69.
13. Tarazi, R. C., and R. W. Gifford, Jr. 1974. Systemic arterial pressure. In *Pathologic physiology: Mechanisms of diseases*, ed 5, ed. W. A. Sodeman, Jr., and W. A. Sodeman, 177–205. Philadelphia: WB Saunders.
14. Gregersen, M. I., and J. L. Nickerson. 1950. Relation of blood volume and cardiac output to body type. *J. Appl. Physiol.* 3:329.
15. Moore, F. D. 1960. *Metabolic care of surgical patients.* 139–161. Philadelphia: WB Saunders.
16. Feldschuh, J., and Y. Enson. 1977. Prediction of the normal blood volume? Blood volume and body habitus. *Circulation* 56:605–612.
17. Fairbanks, V. F., G. G. Klee, G. A. Wiseman, J. D. Hoyer, A. Tefferi, R. M. Petitt, and M. N. Silverstein. 1996. Measurement of blood volume and red cell mass: Re-examination of Cr-51 and I-125 methods. *Blood Cells Mol. Dis.* 22:169–186.
18. Fairbanks, V. F. 2000. Commentary: Should whole body red cell mass be measured or calculated. *Blood Cells Mol. Dis.* 26:32–36.

P A R T XII

OTHER CLINICAL CONDITIONS

95

Disorders of Sweating

Robert D. Fealey
Department of Neurology
Mayo Clinic
Rochester, Minnesota

Sweating, an important thermoregulatory activity under autonomic control, can be disturbed by disorders resulting in excessive (hyperhidrosis) or deficient (hypohidrosis and anhidrosis) sweating. The distribution of abnormal sweating can be ascertained through established autonomic tests and inferences regarding the pathophysiology of the disorder made. Sweating excess of the hands (essential hyperhidrosis) and global anhidrosis with heat intolerance and hyperthermia are examples of disorders that are readily recognized and treated.

Hyperhidrosis is defined as sweating that is excessive for a given stimulus. Some of the physiologic factors that increase the sweat response normally are mentioned in Table 95.1. When sweating exceeds these physiologic considerations, pathologic responses or conditions need to be considered.

Hyperhidrosis can be generalized or localized, which presents the physician with a challenging differential diagnosis (Tables 95.2 and 95.3).

Generalized hyperhidrosis can be primary (as in episodic hypothermia with hyperhidrosis or Shapiro syndrome) or secondary and caused by general medical disorders. The hyperhidrosis is usually episodic rather than continuous with most disorders. In pheochromocytoma, high circulating levels of catecholamines may stimulate normal thermoregulatory structures to produce cholinergic sudomotor activity. Tumors may produce cytokines (especially interleukin-6), which are pyrogenic, causing prostaglandin E_2 release, intermittent fever, and eventually sweating. Anticholinergics, H_2 receptor antagonists, plasma exchange, and prostaglandin inhibitor drug therapy can be effective in these disorders. In hyperthyroidism, inappropriate heat production and increased autonomic nerve sensitivity to circulating epinephrine may cause increased body temperature and sweating, and β-adrenergic blockade can be effective treatment.

Localized hyperhidrosis of the hands, soles, and axillae with normal sweating elsewhere is a common disorder known as essential hyperhidrosis, by far the most commonly encountered. Evidence suggests an abnormal, regional increased activity of the adrenergic component of sweat gland innervation, coupled with overactivity of sympathetic fibers passing through the T2–T4 ganglia, may be partially responsible. This is a disorder that occurs in adolescents and young adults. A familial tendency is present 25 to 50% of the time. Axillary hyperhidrosis may present without other areas involved and vice versa. Essential hyperhidrosis is frequently socially and occupationally disabling and requires treatment. Commonly used therapeutic modalities with the details of treatment are given in Table 95.4.

Another fairly common localized hyperhidrosis occurs in postmenopausal women and primarily affects the head and upper trunk. Multiple factors including age and hormonal-hypothalamic set-point alterations are likely involved. A disorder known as idiopathic paroxysmal localized hyperhidrosis, which occurs in men and women, may be related because both conditions are responsive to clonidine, a centrally acting α_2-adrenergic receptor agonist.

Otherwise, localized hyperhidrosis is usually the result of autonomic nervous system lesions, which are associated with compensatory or perilesional hyperhidrosis. Not uncommonly the patient's attention is given to the excessive sweating area when the abnormality is the widespread anhidrosis elsewhere! Diabetic autonomic failure, pure autonomic failure (Bradbury–Eggleston syndrome), Ross syndrome, harlequin syndrome, and chronic idiopathic anhidrosis are examples in which the phenomenon may occur. Both gustatory sweating and the auriculotemporal (Frey's) syndrome represent examples of localized hyperhidrosis caused by aberrant regeneration of autonomic nerves damaged either surgically or by neuropathy.

Rare cases of essential hyperhidrosis occur in which the acral (distal) parts sweat heavily whereas other body parts do not exhibit any thermoregulatory sweating. Contralateral hyperhidrosis after cerebral infarction has been described as an uncommon complication possibly because of interruption of descending inhibitory pathways.

Patients with cervical and upper thoracic complete spinal cord traumatic transections are frequently troubled with localized hyperhidrosis of the head and upper trunk when noxious stimuli below the level of their lesion cause autonomic hyperreflexia. When accompanied by paroxysmal hypertension, this syndrome can be confused with pheochromocytoma. Often, the causative stimulus is a distended bladder or rectum. Increased spinal α-adrenoreceptors and peripheral microvascular adrenoreceptors, accumulation of substance P, and reduction of inhibitory transmitters below the cord lesion may be causative. In syringomyelia, the excessive sweating is segmental and often appears in dermatomes where sensation is later disturbed.

Hyperhidrosis with partial nerve trunk injury occurs as part of a complex regional pain syndrome and may be because of an obvious lesion or an occult problem such as paraspinal metastatic deposits affecting the sympathetic chain or white rami.

TABLE 95.1 Normal (Physiologic) Factors Affecting Sweating

Parameter	Comments
Age and sex effects	Threshold lower and gland output higher in men Higher sweat output per gland in young vs. old individuals
Acclimatization	Increased output with endurance training, chronic heat, or greater humidity exposure
Circadian rhythm	Threshold temperature to sweat varies often lowest from midnight to 4 AM
Posture	Lying on side produces a contralateral hyperhidrosis and ipsilateral hypohidrosis
Stress and eating	Stress can augment sweating in palms, axillae, feet forehead; some healthy subjects have symmetric gustatory sweating with spicy foods

HYPOHIDROSIS AND ANHIDROSIS

Hypohidrosis is reduction in sweating and anhidrosis is the absence of sweating in response to an appropriate thermoregulatory or pharmacologic stimulus. Physiologic hypohidrosis occurs in skin over bony prominences, in proximal extremities in the elderly, and in dehydrated states in which delayed sweat onset and generalized hypohidrosis is observed.

Pathologic hypohidrosis and anhidrosis may produce symptoms of heat intolerance and dry skin; for example, a patient may recognize that exercise in hot weather causes exhaustion but not sweating or that their feet are dry and stockings no longer wet at day's end. More often, patients are unaware of specific symptoms, therefore trophic skin changes or other signs and symptoms of autonomic neuropathy should be sought. Areas of compensatory, excessive sweating may be noted rather than the anhidrotic regions. The distribution and severity of pathologic sweat loss can be characterized by tests of sympathetic sudomotor function (Table 95.5). These tests may provide clues as to the

TABLE 95.2 Pathologic Hyperhidrosis: Differential Diagnosis and Some Causes of Generalized Hyperhidrosis

Condition	Pathophysiologic mechanism
Pheochromocytoma	Physiologic response to inappropriate catecholamine-induced thermogenesis; inhibited by anticholinergics
Thyrotoxicosis	Physiologic response to inappropriate heat production–induced thermogenesis; inhibited by β-blockers
Acromegaly	Growth hormone–induced increase in sweat gland secretion rate; treated with somatostatin analogs, and dopamine agonists especially with prolactin cosecretion
Malignancy and chronic infection	Night sweats; ? related to altered hypothalamic set-point temperature and effects on prostaglandin E_2 or other thermogenic cytokines like interleukin (IL)-1β, tumor necrosis factor, IL-6; probably vagal afferent "pyrogenic" pathways activated by complement factors
Episodic hypothermia and hyperhidrosis: Shapiro syndrome	Developmental abnormalities of central thermoregulatory nuclei/corpus callosum usually present; clonidine, cyproheptadine, anticonvulsants, oxybutynin, glycopyrrolate may be effective prescriptions
Other causes	Severe anxiety, hypoglycemia, hypotension, cholinergic agents, diencephalic epilepsy

TABLE 95.3 Pathologic Hyperhidrosis Differential Diagnosis and Some Causes of Localized Hyperhidrosis

Condition	Pathophysiologic mechanism of sweating
Essential hyperhidrosis	Excessive physiologic and emotional sweating affecting hands, feet, and axillae; type 1: rest of body sweats normally; type 2: coexists with large areas of anhidrosis; probably contribution from adrenergic-mediated sweating as well as cholinergic; symmetric distribution
Perilesional and compensatory hyperhydrosis	Central and/or peripheral denervation of large numbers of sweat glands produces increased sweat secretion in those remaining innervated; often asymmetric distribution
Gustatory sweating	Resprouting of secremotor axons to supply denervated sweat glands
Postcerebral infarct	Loss of contralateral inhibition with cortical and upper brainstem infarction
Autonomic dysreflexia	Uninhibited segmental somatosympathetic reflex; recent drug prescription; includes nifedipine and sublingual captopril
Complex regional pain syndromes	Localized sympathetic sudomotor hyperactivity; probably axon reflex vs. direct irritation/infiltration of sympathetic preganglionic or postganglionic fibers
Paroxysmal localized hyperhidrosis	Idiopathic; ? transiently decreased hypothalamic set-point temperature; responsive to clonidine, a centrally acting, α_2-adrenergic agonist

TABLE 95.4 Treatment Measures for Primary Hyperhidrosis

Treatment	Details of treatment	Side effects/Complications
Topical Rx	20% Aluminum chloride hexahydrate in anhydrous ethyl alcohol (Drysol). Apply to dry skin daily or every other day half-strength wash off, AM.	Irritation of skin; less effect on palms and soles, which may require occlusive (plastic wrap) technique
Tanning Rx.	Glutaraldehyde (2–10%) solution; apply 2–4 times/week as needed	Stains skin brown; for soles of feet only
Iontophoresis	For palms/soles; 15–30 ma. current 20 min. at start. Drionic battery-run unit or galvanic generator needed. 3–6 treatments/week for total of 10–15 treatments initially; 1–2 treatments/week maintenance	Shocks, tingling may occur Difficult to use in axilla Drionic unit not effective when batteries low
Anticholinergic	Glycopyrrolate (Robinul/Robinul Forte) at 1–2 mg orally three times daily as needed; for intermittent/adjunctive treatment	Dry mouth, blurred vision Contraindicated: glaucoma GI or GU tract obstruction
Clonidine	Useful for paroxysmal, localized (e.g., hemibody) hyperhidrosis 0.1–0.3 mg orally three times daily or as TTS patch (0.1–0.3 mg/day) weekly	Somnolence, hypotension, constipation, nausea, rash, impotence, agitation
Excision	2nd and 3rd thoracic ganglionic sympathectomy (palmar hyperhidrosis), sweat glands (axillary liposuction); recent preference is for T2 sympathectomy to limit compensatory hyperhidrosis	Horner syndrome, dry skin, transient dysesthetic pain Postoperative scar or infection Compensatory hyperhidrosis of trunk, pelvis, legs, and feet
BOTOX	50 to 100 mU of botulinum toxin A into each axilla or body area treated; high doses 200 mU prolong effect; can be repeated	Injection discomfort, variable, duration of effect 3–12 months, expensive, mild grip weakness when palm is treated; contraindicated in pregnancy, NMJ disease

GI, gastrointestinal; GU, genitourinary; mU, mouse units; NMJ, neuromuscular junction; Rx, prescription.

TABLE 95.5 Some Tests of Sympathetic Sudomotor Function

Test	Method	Use
TST (thermoregulatory sweat test)	Whole body heating; Alizarin red indicator of sweating and nonsweating skin	Good screen for focal or generalized lesions; determine preganglionic vs. postganglionic when used with a postganglionic test; body surface anhidrosis can be quantitated
QSART (quantitative sudomotor axon reflex test)	Iontophoresis of 1% acetylcholine; record indirect axon reflex response	Quantitative response from one or more sites; determine sweat volume and latency of response; test of postganglionic axons
Pilocarpine sweat test	Iontophoresis of 1% pilocarpine solution; record sweat rate or volume output	Quantitative response from one or more sites; determine sweat output from directly activated glands; test of postganglionic axons and sweat glands
Silastic imprint method	Iontophoresis of pilocarpine; count sweat glands directly activated	Quantitative response from one or more sites; determine sweat drop size, density test of postganglionic axons and sweat glands
Q-TST (quantitative thermoregulatory sweat test)	Analyzes frequency sweat expulsion and local sweat rate	Quantitative response from one or more sites; determine sweat volume and latency of response; test for postganglionic lesions frequency of sweat expulsions with TRH and heating tests central control
PASP (peripheral autonomic skin potential)	Measures change in sweating indirectly by change in skin resistance	Dynamic, semiquantitative; adaptable to EMG equipment; complex, multisynaptic somatosympathetic loop with CNS and PNS components

ACh, acetylcholine; CNS, central nervous system; EMG, electromyography; PNS, peripheral nervous system; TRH, thyrotropin-releasing hormone.

underlying pathophysiology, and the common distributions of anhidrosis are discussed in the following sections.

Distal Anhidrosis

Distal anhidrosis refers to sweat loss affecting the peripheral (acral) portions of the extremities, the lower anterior abdomen, and the central forehead. The feet by far are the most commonly affected and the lesion is usually a postganglionic denervation as occurs in peripheral neuropathy.

Global Anhidrosis

A global anhidrosis pattern denotes near total body (>80%) sweat loss. This can occur in central lesions (i.e., multiple system atrophy [MSA-parkinsonism and MSA-cerebellar], hypothalamic tumor, cervical spinal cord transection); at times, residual acral (distal) sweating will be present in MSA. Large areas of sweat loss that are shown to be preganglionic or central in origin characterize early MSA. Tests such as the thermoregulatory sweat test show global anhidrosis, whereas postganglionic sweat tests such as quantitative sudomotor axon reflex test (QSART) often are normal.

Global anhidrosis combined with minute islands of preserved sweating and absent QSART is most often caused by a widespread postganglionic lesion (i.e., panautonomic neuropathy). Recently, reversible global anhidrosis has been observed in some cases of autoimmune autonomic neuropathy associated with α_3 acetylcholine receptor ganglionic antibodies.

Dermatomal, Focal, or Multifocal Anhidrosis

Dermatomal, focal, or multifocal anhidrosis refers to sweat loss within the distribution of a peripheral nerve(s) or its branches or root(s) of origin (T1 to L2 or L3 ventral roots). Mononeuritis multiplex produces a multifocal pattern. Focal abnormalities also can occur with skin disorders that damage sweat glands or plug their ducts.

Segmental Anhidrosis

This pattern occurs when large, contiguous body areas of sweat loss with sharply demarcated borders conforming to sympathetic dermatomes are present. Sympathectomy produces such a pattern. When borders are not well defined and anhidrosis is not contiguous a regional pattern is said to exist. Both postganglionic and preganglionic lesions may produce these distributions.

Hemianhidrosis

Sweat loss over one half of the body caused by a lesion of the descending sympathetic efferents in the brainstem or upper cervical cord is called hemianhidrosis. Often the pattern is incomplete. Strokes, tumors, demyelinating lesions, and trauma are frequently causative. Mixed patterns of anhidrosis (i.e., distal with focal) often occur (e.g., in diabetic neuropathy).

Examples of most of the distributions described above are shown in Figure 95.1. Many disorders cause disturbances in sweating and characteristic abnormalities of tests of sudomotor function. Primary autonomic disorders, central and peripheral nervous system lesions, iatrogenic causes, and disorders of skin can be implicated. Table 95.6 summarizes some of these disorders.

Hyperthermia, heat intolerance, heat prostration, and heat stroke may occur with widespread failure of thermoregulatory sweating, whereas local skin trophic changes occur with chronic postganglionic sudomotor neuropathy. Observing some preventative guidelines can lessen heat prostration and dangerous hyperthermia with heat stroke can be successfully

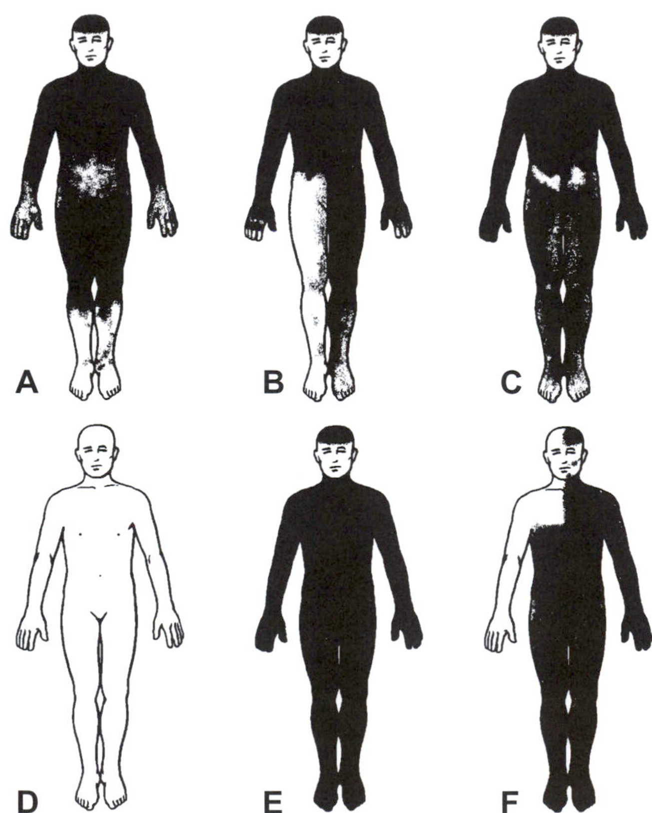

FIGURE 95.1 Examples from patients with diabetes mellitus (**A–E**); patient in **F** had Pancoast's syndrome (apical lung tumor) on the right. Shown are distal (**A**), segmental (**B** and **F**), focal (multifocal, dermatomal) (**C**), global (**D**), normal (**E**), and mixed (**C**; showing multifocal and distal patterns). Sweating in *dark shaded areas*. Note how pattern of anhidrosis can suggest the pathophysiology: the glove and stocking pattern (**A**) in length-dependent neuropathy, the unilateral limb loss (**B** and **F**) with sympathetic chain lesions, and the curvilinear dermatomal anhidrosis in diabetic truncal radiculopathy (**C**).

TABLE 95.6 Sweating Disorders: Typical Findings on Tests of Sudomotor Function

Clinical disorder	Pattern/Site of lesion on the basis of TST/QSART data
Primary autonomic disorders	
PAF; CIA, Ross syndrome	Global or segmental anhidrosis without acral sparing; probably ganglionic neuron or preganglionic synapse or postganglionic axon
Multiple system atrophy (both MSA-P and MSA-C)	Global, segmental, or regional widespread anhidrosis with or without acral sparing; early preganglionic (IML cell column) involvement, both preganglionic and postganglionic later stages
Acute pandysautonomia (panautonomic neuropathy); subacute, paraneoplastic, other autoimmune autonomic neuropathies	Segmental or distal (or both) anhidrosis without acral sparing but with scattered islands of preserved sweating; global at times; ganglionic neuron, axon, or preganglionic synaptic involvement; may show dramatic improvement in months; may show associated α_3-ganglionic AChR antibodies
Neurogenic chronic idiopathic intestinal pseudoobstruction	Often normal studies; occasional distal or more widespread regional postganglionic involvement
Central nervous system lesions	
Tumors: hypothalamic, parasellar, pineal, posterior fossa (brainstem), spinal cord	Global or segmental with or without acral sparing; preganglionic involvement
Cerebral infarction	Contralateral hyperhidrosis occurs (most prominent acutely) with cortical lesions and ipsilateral anhidrosis with brainstem stroke; preganglionic
SCI; syringomyelia; demyelinating myelopathy	Global anhidrosis with cervical cord level; segmental loss below level with thoracic, little, or no anhidrosis with lumbar complete cord lesions; preganglionic
Parkinson's disease, progressive supranuclear palsy	Often sweating is normal; distal loss in feet and regional loss in lower extremities can occur and is usually a postganglionic lesion
Dysautonomia of advanced age	Regional affecting proximal extremities, lower trunk; preganglionic (IML cell loss) and sweat gland (atrophy)
Peripheral nervous disorders	
Diabetic neuropathy Primary systemic and familial amyloidosis Hereditary sensory and autonomic neuropathy	Distal (length-dependent) postganglionic anhidrosis most common; focal (dermatomal), segmental (head and neck), unilateral lower limb occur; global loss at times with profound autonomic involvement; usually postganglionic lesion
Guillain-Barré syndrome; Lambert-Eaton myasthenic syndrome	Can be global without acral sparing; regional, segmental, and distal occur; postganglionic; partial recovery not unusual
Vincristine, propafenone, heavy metal, uremic, nutritional idiopathic small fiber neuropathies	Distal (length-dependent) anhidrosis; postganglionic
Connective tissue diseases	Focal, multifocal, dermatomal anhidrosis (forearm common); postganglionic axonal and skin involvement
Tangier and Fabry's diseases	Distal, focal, multifocal; segmental affecting head and upper extremities; postganglionic except preganglionic in Tangiers's disease and sweat gland in Fabry's disease
Leprosy	Multifocal affecting cooler areas of body; scattered islands of anhidrosis to widespread distal, postganglionic sweat loss depending on type
Iatrogenic causes	
Drug induced: (phenothiazines, butyrophenones, tricyclic antidepressants, anticholinergic/antiparkinson drugs nicotinic and muscarinic anticholinergics	Block central and peripheral autonomic pathway receptors; antimuscarinics can reduce QSART responses for up to 48 hours depending on half-life, dose TST shows mild, generalized, symmetrically reduced sweating
Surgical sympathectomy	Segmental loss preganglionic and postganglionic; compensatory hyperhidrosis elsewhere common but depends on extent of sympathectomy
Cutaneous disorders	
Cholinergic urticaria	Focal loss/postganglionic or sweat gland
Psoriasis and miliaria rubra	Focal loss related to skin-sweat duct inflammation, blockage
Hypohidrotic ectodermal dysplasia	Scattered areas to global anhidrosis; absence of sweat glands
Radiation injury	Sharp bordered (often rectangular), areas of anhidrosis conforming to radiation ports; affects sweat glands

AChR, acetylcholine receptor; CIA, chronic idiopathic anhidrosis; IML, intermediolateral cell column of spinal cord; MSA-C, multiple system atrophy with cerebellar dysfunction presentation; MSA-P, multiple system atrophy with parkinsonian features; PAF, pure autonomic failure; QSART, quantitative sudomotor axon reflex text; SCI, spinal cord injury; TST, thermoregulatory sweat test.

TABLE 95.7 Heat Intolerance and Heat Stroke Management

Management of heat intolerance	Heat stroke management
Avoid exercise in hot/humid conditions Plan outdoor activities for early AM or late PM	Heat stroke is a medical emergency! Diagnosis: CBT > 41°C (105.8°F), central nervous system disturbances (incoordination, confusion, coma), ashen or pink skin
Decrease house thermostat setting Wear head covering and loose, lightweight, breathable clothing outdoors	Immediately remove from hot environment, loosen and remove clothing Circulatory collapse, seizures, hypoxia are common; tracheal intubation, IV isotonic fluids through central line, IV anticonvulsants (diazepam 5- to 10-mg doses) may be necessary
Stay well hydrated (2–2.5 liters of fluid/day), drink water, sports drinks; an aspirin can decrease core "set-point" temperature of sweat onset Avoid alcohol, diuretics, caffeine, benzodiazepines, barbiturates, anticholinergic and neuroleptic drugs	Surface cooling using tepid water sponging and fanning is preferred method; cool to achieve core temperature of 39.0°C; massaging skin with ice bags or ice water immersion are less preferred methods Avoid shivering, use IV diazepam if shivering occurs
Gradually acclimate to a hot environment over weeks before attempting strenuous activity outdoors	Give 5% dextrose in water in IV fluids as hypoglycemia is common; be prepared for evacuation to treat disseminated intravascular coagulation, prolonged shock, renal failure, rhabdomyolysis
Cease any activity and cool down if heat edema, heat syncope, heat cramps, or heat exhaustion occur	Phenothiazines and dantrolene have been advocated to reduce core temperature

CBT, core body temperature; IV, intravenous.

treated. Table 95.7 provides the therapeutic measures for these clinical situations.

References

1. Fealey, R. D. 1997. Thermoregulatory sweat test. In *Clinical autonomic disorders*, 2nd ed., ed. P. A. Low, 245–257. Philadelphia: Lippincott-Raven.
2. Fealey, R. D. 2000. Thermoregulatory failure. In *Handbook of clinical neurology: The autonomic nervous system. Part II, Dysfunctions*, ed. O. Appenzeller, 53–84. Amsterdam: Elsevier Science BV.
3. Fealey, R. D., P. A. Low, and J. E. Thomas. 1989. Thermoregulatory sweating abnormalities in diabetes mellitus. *Mayo Clin. Proc.* 64:617–628.
4. Khurana, R. K. 1993. Acral sympathetic dysfunctions and hyperhidrosis. In *Clinical autonomic disorders (evaluation and management)*, ed. P. A. Low, 767–775. Boston: Little, Brown.
5. Kihara, M., R. D. Fealey, A. Takahashi, and D. James. 1995. Sudomotor dysfunction and its investigation. In *Handbook of autonomic nervous system dysfunction*, ed. A. Korczyn, 523–533. New York: Marcel Dekker.
6. Low, P. A., and R. D. Fealey. 1999. Sudomotor neuropathy. *Diabetic neuropathy,* 2nd ed., ed. P. J. Dyck and P. K. Thomas, 191–199. Philadelphia: WB Saunders.
7. Quinton, P. M. 1983. Sweating and its disorders. *Ann. Rev. Med.* 34:429–452.
8. Togel, B., B. Greve, and C. Raulin. 2002. Current therapeutic strategies for hyperhidrosis: A review. *Eur. J. Dermatol.* 12:219–223.

96

Male Erectile Dysfunction

Douglas F. Milam
Department of Urologic Surgery
Vanderbilt University
Nashville, Tennessee

Impotence is defined by inability to attain penile rigidity sufficient for vaginal penetration or inability to maintain rigidity until ejaculation. Individuals with autonomic dysfunction are markedly more prone to development of impotence than those without autonomic dysfunction. Of men in the population at large, at age 40, approximately 5% never have penile rigidity sufficient for vaginal penetration [1]. By age 70, at least 15% of men experience complete erectile dysfunction (ED), whereas approximately 50% have varying degrees of ED. Age and physical health are the most important predictors of the onset of ED. Smoking was the most important lifestyle variable and ED did not correlate with male hormone levels.

These figures contrast sharply with the prevalence of impotence in the autonomic dysfunction population. Patients with Parkinson's disease and multiple system atrophy (MSA) both have a high rate of impotence. Impotence is a common early finding in MSA, whereas patients with Parkinson's disease usually experience development of impotence later in their disease. Singer and colleagues [2], in a population of older patients with Parkinson's disease, demonstrated that 60% of men were affected compared with 37.5% of age-matched control subjects. Beck and colleagues [3] evaluated 62 patients with MSA for impotence. Their data indicate that 96% of the men were impotent and 37% appeared to have impotence as the initial symptom of autonomic dysfunction. Other studies have demonstrated similar results [4].

MECHANISM OF ERECTION

Psychogenic or tactile sexual stimulation, or both, is the initial point in the pathway leading to penile erection. Nerve signals are carried through the pelvic plexus, a portion of which condenses into the cavernous nerves of the penile corpora cavernosa. The pelvic plexus receives input from both the sympathetic and parasympathetic nervous system. Sympathetic fibers originate in the thoracolumbar spinal cord, condense into the hypogastric plexus located immediately below the aortic bifurcation, and course into the pelvic plexus. Parasympathetic fibers originate in sacral spinal cord segments 2–4 and join the pelvic plexus. Discrete nerves carrying both sympathetic and parasympathetic fibers innervate the organs of the pelvis. In 1982, Walsh and Donker [5] demonstrated that nerves coursing immediately lateral to the urethra continue on to innervate the corpora cavernosa. It is now known that branches of those nerves are the principal innervation of the neuromuscular junction where arterial smooth muscle controls penile blood flow.

Sexual stimulation causes the release of nitric oxide (NO) by the cavernous nerves into the neuromuscular junction (Fig. 96.1). NO activates guanylyl cyclase, which converts guanosine-5′-triphosphate into cyclic guanosine monophosphate (cGMP). Protein kinase G is activated by cGMP and, in turn, activates several proteins that decrease intracellular calcium (Ca^{2+}) concentration. Decreased smooth muscle Ca^{2+} concentration causes muscular relaxation, cavernosal artery dilation, increased blood flow, and subsequent penile erection. The control of blood flow on the venous outflow side is less well understood.

ETIOLOGIC FACTORS OF ERECTILE DYSFUNCTION

The anatomic site currently believed to be the most common cause of ED is the neuromuscular junction where the cavernosal nerves meet the smooth muscle of the deep cavernous penile arteries. This is where NO and cGMP play a critical role in regulating penile blood flow [6]. Neurologic diseases also can produce discrete lesions in central or peripheral nerves that cause ED. In particular, MSA, multiple sclerosis, and other processes affecting the spinal cord can produce decreased erectile rigidity, failure of emission, or retrograde ejaculation. Other causes of impotence include drug-induced ED, endocrine disorders, vascular disease, and venogenic ED.

NEUROMUSCULAR JUNCTION DISORDERS

NO is released from cavernosal nerves causing activation of guanylyl cyclase within the corpus cavernosum. Figure 96.1 illustrates that there are several steps that, if not

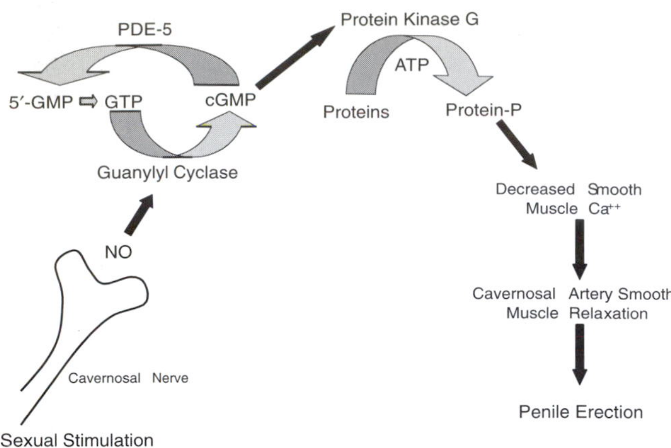

FIGURE 96.1 Erectile pathway.

functioning properly, could impede erectile function. Most work currently is focused on generation of NO by the cavernous nerves. Further understanding of all the steps in the erectile pathway will likely implicate other biochemical reactions as causes of ED. That at least 50% of patients with decreased rigidity from all causes other than trauma or medical treatment respond to phosphodiesterase type-5 (PDE-5) inhibition is strong evidence supporting the inference that biochemical dysfunction at the neuromuscular junction is by far the most common cause of impotence.

NEUROGENIC ERECTILE DYSFUNCTION

Pure neurogenic ED is a frequent cause of erectile failure. Interruption of either somatic or autonomic nerves or their end units may cause ED. These nerves control the flow of blood into and likely out of the corpora cavernosa. Afferent somatic sensory signals are carried from the penis through the pudendal nerve to sacral segments 2–4. This information is routed both to the brain and to spinal cord autonomic centers. Parasympathetic autonomic nerves originate in the intermediolateral gray matter of sacral segments 2–4. These preganglionic fibers exit the anterior nerve roots to join with the sympathetic fibers of the hypogastric nerve to form the pelvic plexus and cavernosal nerves. The paired cavernosal nerves penetrate the corpora cavernosa and innervate the cavernous artery and veins. Parasympathetic ganglia are located distally near the end organ.

Sympathetic innervation also originates in the intermediolateral lateral gray matter but at thoracolumbar levels T10-L2. Sympathetic efferents course through the retroperitoneum and condense into the hypogastric plexus located anterior and slightly caudal to the aortic bifurcation. A concentration of postganglionic sympathetic fibers forms the hypogastric nerve, which is joined by parasympathetic efferents. Adrenergic innervation appears to play a role in the process of detumescence. High concentrations of norepinephrine have been demonstrated in the tissue of the corpora cavernosa and tributary arterioles. In addition, the α-adrenergic antagonist, phentolamine, is routinely used for intracorporal injection therapy to produce erection.

Afferent signals capable of initiating erection can either originate within the brain, as is the case with psychogenic erections, or result from tactile stimulation. Patients with spinal cord injury often respond to tactile sensation, but usually require medical therapy to maintain the erection through intercourse. There is no discrete center for psychogenic erections. The temporal lobe appears to be important, however; other locations such as the gyrus rectus, the cingulate gyrus, the hypothalamus, and the mammillary bodies also appear to be important.

ENDOCRINE DISORDERS

Testosterone plays a permissive role in erectile function. Androgen replacement (testosterone cipionate 200 mg every 2–3 weeks or daily topical testosterone preparations) is expected to induce return of erectile function in patients with very low or undetectable serum testosterone concentrations because of hypogonadism. These patients are relatively uncommon, however. More commonly, the impotent patient will have normal or mildly decreased levels of circulating androgens. Testosterone replacement rarely restores erectile function in those with mildly decreased serum testosterone levels and should not be routinely given for that indication. Testosterone supplementation is never indicated for patients with normal circulating androgen levels.

The most common endocrine disorder affecting erectile ability is diabetes mellitus. The most important effect diabetes has on erectile ability appears to relate to loss of function of long autonomic nerves. Erection is partially mediated by efferent parasympathetic cholinergic neural stimuli. Loss of long cholinergic neurons results in interruption of the efferent side of the erectile reflex arc. Diabetes also appears to produce dysfunction of the neuromuscular junction at the level of arterial smooth muscle in the penile corpora cavernosa. Studies have indicated markedly decreased acetylcholine and NO concentrations in the trabeculae of the corpora cavernosa in patients with diabetes [7]. These findings probably represent a combination of neural loss and neuromuscular junction dysfunction.

MEDICAL AND SURGICAL TREATMENT

Effective oral medical therapy has changed the work-up and treatment of ED. Diagnostic tests such as plasma testosterone often are deferred to medical therapy failures if the patient has normal libido, no gynecomastia, and testes of normal size and consistency.

Current medical therapy is based on inhibition of PDE-5 [8]. Figure 96.1 illustrates that cGMP is broken down to inactive 5′-GMP by PDE-5. Sildenafil, vardenafil, and tadalafil competitively inhibit PDE-5 breakdown of cGMP by binding to the catalytic domain of PDE-5. Use of a PDE-5 inhibitor results in improved erectile rigidity even in patients with decreased NO or cGMP synthesis. Generally, 60% of patients overall and 80% with ED caused by spinal cord injury respond to PDE-5 inhibition.

A study examined the response to sildenafil in patients with Parkinson's disease and MSA [9]. Patients with Parkinson's disease experienced improved erectile rigidity similar to patients with idiopathic ED. They did not experience significant orthostatic hypotension. One hour after medication, the standing mean blood pressure decreased 9 mm Hg, compared with 6 mmHg in healthy volunteers. However, this was not the case for patients with MSA. Six patients had been enrolled before the study was halted because of profound hypotension. Three patients who had stable blood pressures at study entry experienced standing blood pressure decreases of 128/85 to 65/55, 104/60 to 56/32, and 115/70 to 55/39 1 hour after taking medication. PDE-5 inhibitors should be used with caution in patients with MSA.

Other therapeutic interventions including pharmacologic injection of prostaglandin E_1, intraurethral delivery of prostaglandin E_1, vacuum erection devices, and inflatable penile implants produce excellent results in selected patients. Patients who have good performance status should be offered urologic referral if initial medical therapy does not achieve adequate penile rigidity.

References

1. Feldman, H. A., I. Goldstein, D. G. Hatzichristou, R. J. Krane, and J. B. McKinlay. 1994. Impotence and its medical and psychosocial correlates: Results of the Massachusetts Male Aging Study. *J. Urol.* 151:54–61.
2. Singer, C., W. J. Weiner, J. R. Sanchez-Ramos, and M. Ackerman. 1989. Sexual dysfunction in men with Parkinson's disease. *J. Neurol. Rehab.* 3:199–204.
3. Beck, R. O., C. D. Betts, and C. J. Fowler. 1994. Genitourinary dysfunction in multisystem atrophy: Clinical features and treatment in 62 cases. *J. Urol.* 151:1336–1341.
4. Wenning, G., Y. Ben Shlomo, M. Magalhaes, S. E. Daniel, and N. P. Quinn. 1994. Clinical features and natural history of multisystem atrophy. *Brain* 117:835–845.
5. Walsh, P. C., and P. J. Donker. 1982. Impotence following radical prostatectomy: Insight into etiology and prevention. *J. Urol.* 128:492, 1982.
6. Kim, N., K. M. Azadzoi, I. Goldstein, I. Saenz de Tejada. 1991. A nitric oxide-like factor mediates nonadrenergic, noncholinergic neurogenic relaxation of penile corpus cavernosum smooth muscle. *J. Clin. Invest.* 88:112, 1991.
7. Blanco, R., I. Saenz de Tejada, I. Goldstein, R. J. Krave, H. H. Wotiz, and R. H. Cohen. 1990. Dysfunctional penile cholinergic nerves in diabetic impotent men. *J. Urol.* 44:278–280.
8. Turko, I. V., S. A. Ballard, S. H. Francis, and J. D. Corbin. 1999. Inhibition of cyclic GMP-binding cyclic GMP-specific phosphodiesterase (Type 5) by sildenafil and related compounds. *Mol. Pharmacol.* 56:124–130.
9. Hussain, I. F., C. M. Brady, M. J. Swinn, C. J. Mathias, and C. J. Fowler. 2001. Treatment of erectile dysfunction with sildenafil citrate (Viagra) in parkinsonism due to Parkinson's disease or multiple system atrophy with observations on orthostatic hypotension. *J. Neurol. Neurosurg. Psychiatry* 71:371–374.

97 Sleep-Disordered Breathing and Autonomic Failure

Sudhansu Chokroverty
St. Vincent's Catholic Medical Center
New York, New York

Autonomic nervous system (ANS), sleep, and breathing are closely interrelated. Sleep has a profound effect on the functions of the ANS and the control of breathing. The basic ANS changes during sleep include increased parasympathetic tone and decreased sympathetic activity with intermittent increase of sympathetic activity during phasic rapid eye movement (REM) sleep. Respiratory homeostasis becomes unstable during normal sleep, causing a few periods of apneas and hypopneas, particularly at sleep onset and during REM sleep. The nucleus tractus solitarius (NTS), located in the dorsal medulla, can be considered a central station in the central autonomic network with its reciprocally connected ascending projections to the hypothalamus, the limbic system, and other supramedullary regions, as well as the descending projections to the ventral medulla and intermediolateral neurons of the spinal cord. Furthermore, the peripheral respiratory receptors, the central respiratory and the sleep-promoting neurons in the preoptic-anterior hypothalamic region, and the NTS are intimately linked by the ANS. Therefore, it is logical to expect sleep-disordered breathing (SDB) in patients with autonomic failure (AF). This chapter briefly summarizes such respiratory arrhythmias in AF.

Two separate and independent systems control breathing during wakefulness and sleep: the metabolic (the automatic or autonomic) and the voluntary (or behavioral) systems. These two systems behave differently during wakefulness and two states of sleep (e.g., non–rapid eye movement (NREM) and REM sleep determined on the basis of electroencephalogram criteria). During NREM sleep, respiration is controlled entirely by the metabolic controlling system, whereas during wakefulness both the voluntary and the metabolic systems remain active, and during REM sleep, the voluntary system also is partly active. Therefore, a failure of the metabolic controlling system in the medulla as a result of pathology in the ascending, descending, or afferent projections of the central autonomic network or brainstem lesions will cause sleep apnea and other respiratory arrhythmias during sleep (Ondine's curse). During normal sleep, there is mild hypoventilation as a result of decreased number of functioning respiratory units, decreased sensitivity of the medullary chemoreceptors, and increased upper airway resistance. This physiologic sleep-related hypoventilation becomes prolonged during pathologic alteration.

SLEEP-DISORDERED BREATHING IN AUTONOMIC FAILURE

SDB including sleep apnea has been described in many patients with AF. AF can be primary or secondary to a variety of central or peripheral neurologic or other medical disorders and familial dysautonomia. The best known condition with primary AF is multiple system atrophy (MSA) with progressive AF (also known as the Shy-Drager syndrome). MSA is a multisystem neurodegenerative disease characterized initially by dysautonomic manifestations (e.g., the four most important manifestations consist of orthostatic hypotension, urinary sphincter dysfunction, hypohidrosis or anhidrosis, and impotence in men) followed by a parkinsonian–cerebellar syndrome, and upper motor neuron and lower neuron dysfunction. A number of sleep-related respiratory arrhythmias have been noted in most of these patients (Fig. 97.1) in the intermediate stage of the illness, which lasts on an average about 9 years. Polysomnographic (PSG) recordings confirmed the presence of sleep apnea and other respiratory arrhythmias in many reports.

The most common respiratory disturbances in MSA are sleep apnea or hypopnea, dysrhythmic breathing, and nocturnal stridor. Sleep apnea can be three types: central (CA), upper airway obstructive (OA), and mixed type (MA). During CA, there is cessation of both airflow and effort (i.e., no diaphragmatic or intercostal muscle activities), whereas during OA there is no airflow but the effort continues (see Fig. 97.1). MA is characterized by an initial period of CA followed by OA (see Fig. 97.1). Hypopnea has the same significance as apnea and is manifested by a reduction of the tidal volume by one half of the value of the preceding respiratory cycle with or without oxygen desaturation or arousal. To be significant, apnea or hypopnea must last at least 10 seconds, and apnea or hypopnea index (number of episodes per hour of sleep) or respiratory disturbance index (total number of apneas and hypopneas per hour of sleep) should be five or more.

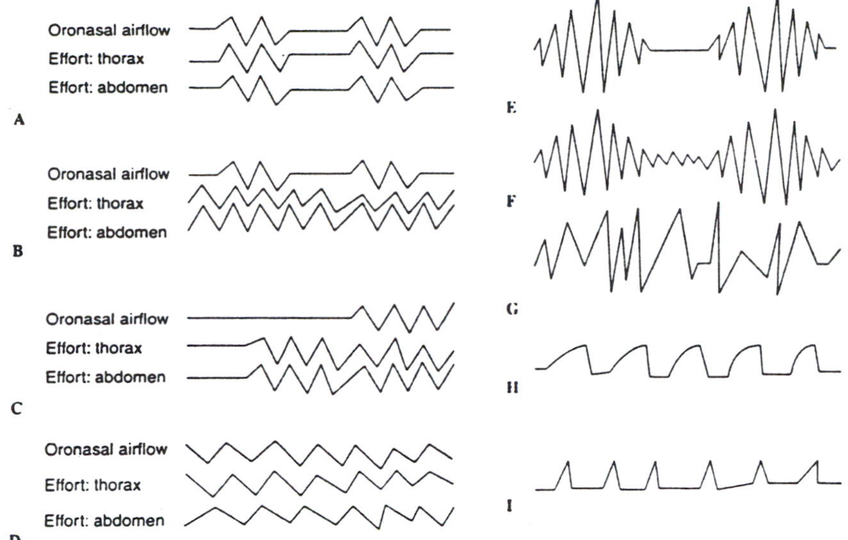

FIGURE 97.1 Schematic diagram showing different respiratory patterns in multiple system atrophy. **A**, Central apnea. **B**, Upper airway obstructive apnea. **C**, Mixed apnea. **D**, Paradoxic breathing. **E**, Cheyne–Stokes breathing. **F**, Cheyne-Stokes variant pattern. **G**, Dysrhythmic breathing. **H**, Apneustic breathing. **I**, Inspiratory gasp. (Reproduced with permission from Chokroverty, S. 1999. Sleep, breathing and neurological disorders. In *Sleep disorders medicine: Basic science, technical consideration and clinical aspects.* S. Chokroverty, Ed, 509–571. Boston: Butterworth-Heinemann.)

Apneic–hypopneic episodes are accompanied by oxygen desaturation, repeated arousals throughout the night causing a reduction of slow wave and REM sleep, and increased wakefulness after sleep onset. These nocturnal episodes of repeated oxygen desaturation and arousals may cause daytime somnolence, daytime fatigue, intellectual deterioration, impotence in men, and occasionally early morning headache, and they also may lead to systemic or pulmonary hypertension, congestive cardiac failure, or cardiac arrhythmias. Hypercapnic ventilatory responses may be impaired in some of these patients, suggesting impairment of central respiratory chemoreceptors in the brainstem. Dysrhythmic breathing, characterized by a pattern of nonrhythmic respiration of irregular rate, rhythm, and amplitude (see Fig. 97.1), more apparent during sleep than during wakefulness and often accompanied by short periods of apneas or hypopneas, is common in MSA. Normal hypercapnic ventilatory responses in some patients and dysrhythmic breathing imply a defect in the respiratory pattern generators in the brainstem. In many patients with MSA, nocturnal stridor is a common feature causing marked inspiratory breathing difficulty and is associated with laryngeal abductor paralysis, severe snoring, and upper airway obstruction. Less commonly, the patients with MSA may have other respiratory disturbances, which may include alveolar hypoventilation, paradoxic breathing (opposing chest wall and abdominal movements denoting upper airway obstruction), apneustic breathing with a prolonged inspiration and an increase in the ratio of inspiratory to expiratory time, inspiratory gasps, Cheyne-Stokes or Cheyne-Stokes variant breathing (see Fig. 97.1), which is a type of CA, and sudden respiratory arrest, often during sleep at night leading to sudden death.

Neuropathologic findings in MSA comprise those noted in striatonigral and olivopontocerebellar degeneration, a distinctive argyrophilic oligodendroglial cytoplasmic inclusion in the cortical motor, premotor and supplementary motor areas, extrapyramidal and corticocerebellar systems, brainstem reticular formation, and supraspinal autonomic systems and their targets. In addition, there is neuronal loss in the same regions and in the intermediolateral column of the spinal cord. Respiratory arrhythmias probably result in part from direct involvement of the brainstem region containing respiratory neurons in addition to other mechanisms.

Sleep apneas accompanied by oxygen desaturation also have been noted in patients with familial dysautonomia (Riley–Day syndrome). Familial dysautonomia is a recessively inherited disorder confined to the Jewish population. In addition to the dysautonomic manifestations of fluctuating postural hypotension and paroxysmal hypertension, defective lacrimation, impaired sweating, and vasomotor instability, the patient presents a variety of cardiovascular, skeletal, renal, neuromuscular, and respiratory abnormalities. PSG recordings in several reports of familial dysautonomia documented central and upper airway obstructive sleep apneas.

Sleep apneas and hypopneas have been described in Parkinson's disease (PD) and chronic renal failure associated with AF and acquired polyneuropathies, particularly diabetic autonomic neuropathies (DANs), and occasionally in amyloidosis and Guillain-Barré syndrome. Patients with PD may have SDB characterized by laryngeal stridor, diaphragmatic dyskinesias, OA, CA, MA, and upper airway dysfunction with tremor-like oscillations. Unlike patients with MSA, those with PD do not have vocal cord abductor paralysis. Autonomic dysfunction in idiopathic PD is less severe than in MSA. A poor response to levodopa and abnormal urethral sphincter electromyography may distinguish MSA from idiopathic PD. Sleep apneas also have been described in many patients with chronic renal failure and autonomic dysfunction. In DAN, PSG recordings have documented a variety of SDB including CA and OA, and respiratory irregularities associated with esophageal reflux during sleep causing frequent awakenings. Sleep apnea in DAN may have an adverse effect on insulin resistance. However, the mechanism of SDB in DAN is poorly understood. Patients with congenital central hypoventilation syndrome and neonatal Hirschsprung disease (intestinal aganglionosis) with dysautonomia may also present with SDB. A few scattered reports of autonomic dysfunction including cardiac arrhythmias have been described in patients with upper airway obstructive sleep apnea syndrome, a common primary sleep disorder.

DIAGNOSIS

First and foremost in the diagnosis of AF is the clinical manifestation of dysautonomia followed by autonomic function tests. For secondary AF, appropriate tests to establish the primary cause should be performed. To document the presence, type, and severity of sleep apnea, it is essential to perform overnight PSG consisting of simultaneous recording of electroencephalogram, electrooculogram, electromyogram, electrocardiogram, recording of respiration by oronasal thermistors and preferably by nasal pressure cannula to record airflow and respiratory effort by piezoelectric or mercury strain gauges or respiratory inductive plethysmography, and oxygen saturation by finger oximetry. All patients with reports of excessive daytime sleepiness should have a PSG preformed. Daytime nap studies are not adequate because REM sleep is usually not recorded and the severity and presence of sleep apnea are difficult to assess.

Multiple sleep latency test during daytime may be obtained to objectively document propensity to sleepiness. A mean sleep latency of less than 5 minutes is consistent with excessive sleepiness. Pulmonary function tests including ventilatory functions, measurement of lung volumes, gas distribution, arterial blood gases, and assessment of chemical control of breathing by determining hypercapnic and hypoxic ventilatory responses and mouth occlusion pressure (P.01) are important to exclude intrinsic pulmonary diseases and to identify impairment of chemical control of breathing. Electromyogram of the laryngeal and urethral sphincter muscles may be indicated in selected patients with MSA. In patients with nocturnal stridor, upper airway endoscopy and laryngoscopy may be needed to detect laryngeal paralysis. Newer techniques of autonomic monitoring such as heart rate variability, spectral frequency of heart rate, and pulse transit time may also be used during PSG recording.

TREATMENT

Only symptomatic measures for sleep apnea or other respiratory arrhythmias and treatment of the primary condition causing secondary AF are available. MSA is an inexorably progressive neurologic disease pursuing a relentless course despite improvement of orthostatic hypotension and other dysautonomic manifestations following symptomatic treatment that may improve the quality of life temporarily.

GENERAL MEASURES AND MEDICAL TREATMENT

General measures include avoidance of alcohol and sedative–hypnotics, which may depress respiration. Medical treatment of sleep apnea is not generally satisfactory, but protriptyline, a nonsedative tricyclic, and selective serotonin reuptake inhibitors in mild cases of CA and OA and acetazolamide in CA may have some limited usefulness.

MECHANICAL TREATMENT

In moderate to severe cases of upper airway obstructive sleep apnea, nasal continuous positive airway pressure (CPAP) by using a nasal mask throughout the night is useful. After such treatment, sleep quality often will improve and daytime somnolence will be eliminated because of reduction or elimination of sleep-related OAs or MAs or oxygen desaturation. However, the natural history of MSA will not be altered by such treatment. The benefit of nasal CPAP in MSA has not been as dramatic as in patients with primary obstructive sleep apnea syndrome because of the natural history of inexorable progression of the illness despite all symptomatic measures. A sufficient number of studies of such disorders using CPAP treatment have not been made. In acquired autonomic neuropathies, CPAP treatment is an excellent therapy for OAs. Several types of home CPAP units are available.

SURGICAL TREATMENT

Tracheostomy remains the only effective emergency treatment for severe respiratory dysfunction in patients with laryngeal stridor caused by laryngeal abductor paralysis and in patients who have been resuscitated from respiratory arrest. However, the decision to perform tracheostomy in a progressive neurodegenerative disease with AF with an overall unfavorable prognosis must be carefully weighed before pursuing this therapy. Palliative measures, however, should be used to improve a patient's quality of life temporarily.

References

1. Chokroverty, S. 1999. Sleep, breathing and neurological disorders. In *Sleep disorders medicine: Basic science, technical consideration and clinical aspects,* ed. S. Chokroverty, 509–571. Boston: Butterworth-Heinemann.
2. Chokroverty, S. 1997. Sleep apnea and autonomic failure. In *Clinical autonomic disorders,* ed. P. A. Low, 633–647. Boston: Little, Brown.
3. Shy, G. M., and G. A. Drager. 1960. A neurological syndrome associated with orthostatic hypotension. *Arch. Neurol.* 2:511–527.
4. Bannister R., and C. J. Mathias. 1999. Clinical features and evaluation of the primary chronic autonomic failure syndromes. In *Autonomic failure: A textbook of clinical disorders of the autonomic nervous system,* 4th ed., ed. C. J. Mathias, and R. Bannister, 307–316. Oxford: Oxford University Press.
5. Low, P. A. 1997. Laboratory evaluation of autonomic failure. In *Clinical autonomic disorders*, ed. P. A. Low, 179–208. Boston: Little, Brown.
6. Gilman, S., R. D. Chervin, R. A. Koeppe, F. B. Consens, R. Little, H. An, L. Junck, and M. Heumann. 2003. Obstructive sleep apnea is related to a thalamic cholinergic deficit in MSA. *Neurology* 61:35–39.

98

Hypoadrenocorticism

David H. P. Streeten[†]

The autonomic nervous system has important relations with the function of the adrenal cortex (1) in the actions of sympathetic nervous function on adrenocortical secretion, and (2) in the profound effects of cortisol and aldosterone deficiency on the efficacy of sympathetic nervous activity in maintaining the blood pressure, especially during stress.

EFFECTS OF AUTONOMIC ACTIVITY ON ADRENOCORTICAL SECRETION

There is convincing evidence from animal studies that the hypothalamic-pituitary-adrenal (HPA) system is stimulated at various central sites, resulting in an increase in corticotropin-releasing hormone (CRH) secretion and the release of adrenocorticotrophic hormone (ACTH) from pituitary corticotropes *in vitro* [1]. Conversely, measurements in the human subject have shown that increasing plasma norepinephrine (NE) levels by NE infusions, into the range seen in moderate stress, had no effect on the ACTH or cortisol response to CRH administration [2]. Although these observations fail to show any direct action of NE on the pituitary response to CRH, they do not rule out the possibility that autonomic neuronal activity within the hypothalamus might increase CRH or vasopressin release and consequently cortisol secretion in human subjects. In patients with multiple system atrophy (MSA) and idiopathic orthostatic hypotension, insulin-induced hypoglycemia, normally a potent stimulus to the sympathetic nervous system, frequently fails to stimulate epinephrine release from the adrenal medullae, but does not fail to increase HPA function, as indicated by a normal increase in cortisol secretion [3]. These important observations strongly suggest that diffuse autonomic insufficiency has little, if any, effect on adrenocortical secretion in response to hypoglycemic stress in humans. In contrast with these findings related to the release of cortisol, there is little doubt that autonomic failure, through the loss of β-adrenergic stimulation of renin release from the juxtaglomerular apparatus, which it induces, profoundly reduces the adrenocortical section of aldosterone. Hyporeninemic hypoaldosteronism may arise either centrally in patients with MSA or peripherally in patients with diabetic or other forms of peripheral neuropathy. It may cause hyperkalemia and hypovolemia, which are reversible with fludrocortisone administration. It also contributes to the severity of the orthostatic hypotension that results predominantly from the direct effect of autonomic failure on vascular contractility, and this is somewhat ameliorated, but not completely corrected, by fludrocortisone in these patients.

[†]Deceased.

EFFECTS OF HYPOADRENOCORTICISM ON AUTONOMIC FAILURE

Cortisol, secreted by the cells of the zona fasciculata, reaches the zona medullaris through the adrenal portal venous circulation to create an usually high concentration of the steroid within the adrenal medulla. This increased cortisol concentration is required for induction of the enzyme phenylethanolamine *N*-methyltransferase, which normally methylates norepinephrine to form epinephrine. The deficiency of epinephrine production that one would, therefore, expect to result from adrenocortical insufficiency may play an important role in the excessive susceptibility of patients with primary or secondary hypocortisolism to fasting or insulin-induced hypoglycemia. There is no clear evidence that adrenocortical deficiency has other direct effects on the function of autonomic neurons.

Cortisol and other glucocorticoids do have essential functions in sensitizing the vasoconstrictive response of the peripheral vasculature to norepinephrine. This phenomenon was first demonstrated in the experiments of Fritz and Levine [4], who found that the sensitivity of the meso-appendicular arterial supply of the rat to locally applied NE was strikingly reduced *in vivo* by previous bilateral adrenalectomy. This requirement of the vasculature for adequate concentrations of glucocorticoid is of great clinical importance. It probably underlies the orthostatic hypotension that is so reliable as an early clinical manifestation of cortisol deficiency, and it causes recumbent hypotension and shock in patients with adrenocortical deficiency during stress. The common stress-induced hypotension that is unresponsive to intravenous infusions of phenylephrine, norepinephrine, epinephrine, and dopamine is certainly caused by hypocortisolism in many patients. In these individuals, glucocorticoid administration rapidly restores normal vascular responsiveness to sympathomimetic drugs and is followed by restoration of normotension.

References

1. Vale, W., J. Vaughan, M. Smith, G. Yamamoto, J. Rivier, and C. Rivier. 1983. Effects of synthetic bovine corticotropin-releasing factor, glucocorticoids, catecholamines, neurohypophyseal peptides, and other substances on cultured corticotropic cells. *Endocrinology* 113:1121–1131.
2. Milson, S. R., R. A. Donald, E. A. Espiner, M. G. Nichols, and J. H. Livesey. 1986. The effect of peripheral catecholamine concentrations on the pituitary-adrenal response to corticotrophin releasing factor in man. *Clin. Endocrinol.* 25:241–246.
3. Polinsky, R. J., I. J. Kopin, M. H. Ebert, V. Weisse, and L. Recant. 1981. Hormonal responses to hypoglycemia in orthostatic hypotension patients with adrenergic insufficiency. *Life Sci.* 29:417–425.
4. Fritz, I., and R. Levine. 1951. Action of adrenal cortical steroids and norepinephrine on vascular responses to stress in adrenalectomized rats. *Am. J. Physiol.* 165:456–465.

99

Mastocytosis

L. Jackson Roberts, II
Division of Clinical Pharmacology
Vanderbilt University
Nashville, Tennessee

Although mastocytosis is not a disorder of the autonomic nervous system, some of the symptoms and signs of the disease may be interpreted as consistent with autonomic dysfunction. Thus, it is important for physicians involved in the evaluation of patients suspected of having disorders of the autonomic nervous system to recognize the hallmarks of mastocytosis.

MASTOCYTOSIS AND ALLIED ACTIVATION DISORDERS OF THE MAST CELL

Mastocytosis is a disease characterized by an abnormal proliferation of tissue mast cells. The cause of the overproliferation of mast cells remains unknown. Although unusual forms of the disease can occur primarily in children (e.g., a localized mastocytoma), the disease in adults exists primarily in two forms: the abnormal proliferation of mast cells appears to be either limited to the skin (cutaneous mastocytosis) or involves multiple tissues throughout the body (systemic mastocytosis) [1, 2].

In recent years, an allied activation idiopathic disorder(s) of mast cells also has been identified in which patients experience episodes of systemic mast cell activation in the absence of any evidence of abnormal mast cell proliferation [3]. An allergic basis for the activation of mast cells may be suspected in some patients, whereas in others the cause remains unclear. Whereas mastocytosis is an uncommon disease, idiopathic activation disorders of the mast cell are encountered more frequently.

SYMPTOMS AND SIGNS

The symptoms of both mastocytosis and systemic activation disorders of the mast cell are attributed primarily to episodic release of mast cell mediators [3]. The episodes of mastocyte activation can be brief, lasting several minutes, or protracted, lasting a few hours. These episodes frequently occur without any identifiable inciting cause. However, exposure to heat, exertion, and emotional upset are commonly identified as precipitating factors by many patients. The major symptoms experienced by these patients are listed in Table 99.1. Probably the most important clinical clue that should lead to the suspicion of a diagnosis of systemic mast cell disease is flushing. In some patients, cutaneous vasodilation is not appreciated, but patients will usually note that they feel very warm. Unlike allergic anaphylaxis, bronchospasm, angioedema, and urticaria are uncommon manifestations. Characteristically, after an episode of mastocyte activation, patients experience extreme fatigue and lethargy, which can last for hours.

Hemodynamic alterations frequently occur during episodes of systemic mast cell activation [3]. Characteristically, the blood pressure decreases and the heart rate increases. At times the reduction in blood pressure can be profound, resulting in severe lightheadedness or frank syncope. The reduction in blood pressure is accentuated in the upright position, and patients note that lightheadedness is improved on assuming the supine position. However, in some patients, the blood pressure increases, at times dramatically, during episodes of mast cell activation. The increase in blood pressure also is accompanied by an increase in heart rate. The basis for the increase in blood pressure in some patients remains speculative.

MAST CELL MEDIATORS RESPONSIBLE FOR THE SYMPTOMS AND SIGNS

The hemodynamic alterations and symptoms experienced by patients with mastocytosis had previously been attributed to the release of excessive quantities of histamine from mast cells. However, treatment with antagonists of histamine H_1 and H_2 receptors had not been found to prevent episodes of vasodilation in these patients. In 1980, the discovery of marked overproduction of prostaglandin D_2, a potent vasodilator, in patients with mastocytosis was reported. Subsequently, it was found that treatment of patients with mastocytosis with inhibitors of prostaglandin biosynthesis in addition to antihistamines can be effective in ameliorating episodes of vasodilation in these patients [3]. However, a subset of patients with disorders of systemic mast cell activation are "aspirin hypersensitive" and administration of

TABLE 99.1 Symptoms of Systemic Mast Cell Activation

1. Flushing (and/or a feeling of warmth)
2. Palpitations
3. Dyspnea (usually without wheezing)
4. Chest discomfort
5. Headache
6. Lightheadedness and occasionally syncope
7. Gastrointestinal symptoms
   A. Nausea and occasionally vomiting
   B. Abdominal cramps and occasionally diarrhea
8. Profound lethargy after the attack

any prostaglandin inhibitor, even in small doses, can provoke a severe episode of mastocyte activation. Thus, great caution must be exercised in treating patients with disorders of systemic mast cell activation with inhibitors of prostaglandin biosynthesis. The pathogenesis of "aspirin hypersensitivity" remains poorly understood.

DIAGNOSIS

The diagnosis of systemic disorders of the mast cell is not always straightforward [4]. Patients with mastocytosis frequently have small pigmented cutaneous lesions, termed *urticaria pigmentosa*. Urticaria pigmentosa lesions characteristically urticate when stroked (Darier's sign). When visible cutaneous clues to the diagnosis are absent, the diagnosis relies on the recognition of a compatible clinical history. In patients with mastocytosis, a diagnosis may be made histologically by demonstrating abnormal mast cell proliferation in the skin or bone marrow. In patients with activation disorders of the mast cell in the absence of abnormal mast cell proliferation, the diagnosis relies entirely on demonstrating a release of increased quantities of histamine and prostaglandin D_2 during episodes of suspected mastocyte activation. In patients with systemic mastocytosis, increased urinary excretion of metabolites of histamine and prostaglandin D_2 can usually be demonstrated even at quiescent times. Conversely, in patients with idiopathic activation disorders of the mast cell, increased excretion of metabolites of histamine and prostaglandin D_2 can only be demonstrated in fractional urine collected during episodes of mastocyte activation.

SUMMARY

Patients with disorders of systemic mast cell activation may be encountered more frequently than previously thought, and some of the symptoms and signs manifested by these patients (e.g., orthostatic hypotension, during episodes of mastocyte activation) are not unlike some of those experienced by some patients with autonomic dysfunction. Specifically, a patient with "spells" characterized by flushing that may be precipitated by heat, exertion, or emotional upset accompanied by lightheadedness and either a reduction or increase in blood pressure and tachycardia should lead the astute clinician to consider the possibility of a disorder of systemic mast cell activation.

References

1. Metcalfe, D. D. 1991. Classification and diagnosis of mastocytosis: Current status. *J. Invest. Dermatol.* 96:2S–4S.
2. Soter, N. N. 1991. The skin in mastocytosis. *J. Invest. Dermatol.* 96:32S–39S.
3. Roberts II, L. J., and J. A. Oates. 1992. Disorders of vasodilator hormones: The cardioid syndrome and mastocytosis. In *Williams textbook of endocrinology*, 3rd ed., ed. J. D. Wilson, and D. W. Foster, 1619–1633. Philadelphia: WB Saunders.
4. Roberts, L. J., and J. A. Oates. 1991. The biochemical diagnosis of systemic mast cell disorders. *J. Invest. Dermatol.* 96:19S–25S.

100

Cocaine Overdose

Wanpen Vongpatanasin
Division of Hypertension
University of Texas Southwestern Medical Center
Dallas, Texas

Ronald G. Victor
Division of Hypertension
University of Texas Southwestern Medical Center
Dallas, Texas

Cocaine abuse has reached epidemic proportions in the United States and has emerged as a major cause of life-threatening cardiovascular emergencies. The cardiovascular complications induced by cocaine has been attributed to inhibition of norepinephrine (NE) reuptake in peripheral sympathetic nerve terminals, leading to increased NE concentration in the synaptic cleft [1]. However, this hypothesis was based on *ex vivo* rodent experiments with little supporting evidence from studies in intact animals or humans. Our data from series of experiments in humans not only indicated that peripheral NE reuptake inhibition is much less important than previously assumed, but also underscored the role of central sympathoexcitatory effect of cocaine, the neural stimulus for NE release [2].

EFFECTS OF COCAINE ON THE PERIPHERAL CIRCULATION

Until recently, cocaine was thought to increase blood pressure (BP) only by inhibition of peripheral NE reuptake. However, this is unlikely to be the only mechanism, because other drugs such as tricyclic antidepressants, which are more effective than cocaine at blocking the NE transporter, do not increase BP [3]. Furthermore, in healthy humans, intranasal cocaine increases BP and activates baroreceptor reflexes, thereby reflexively decreasing sympathetic nerve activity (SNA), the neural stimulus for NE release [4]. If there is little stimulus for NE release into the synaptic cleft, there should be little NE available for reuptake by the transporter, and thus little transporter activity to be blocked by cocaine. Indeed, administration of small doses of intranasal cocaine used in rhinolaryngologic procedures had no effect on plasma NE levels in cocaine-naïve healthy individuals, whereas the intrabrachial administration of cocaine that matched the same venous concentration caused a substantial increase in venous forearm NE in the same subjects [2]. Failure of intranasal cocaine to increase plasma NE is because of baroreflex-mediated withdrawal of SNA during systemic cocaine counterbalancing the inhibition of peripheral NE reuptake. When SNA was clamped during systemic cocaine administration by the concomitant infusion of intravenous nitroprusside to minimize the increase in BP and baroreflex activation (Fig. 100.1), however, the increase in venous NE concentrations also was restored, matching the increase seen with intrabrachial cocaine.

Therefore, our studies in healthy cocaine-naïve subjects indicated that baroreceptor reflexes play a key role in buffering the sympathomimetic actions of cocaine in the human peripheral circulation. The degree of peripheral vasoconstriction induced by a given dose of cocaine is critically dependent on the ambient level of central sympathetic outflow, which is suppressed in individuals with intact baroreceptor function. In this regard, patients with impaired baroreceptor reflexes such as those with long-standing hypertension or heart failure would experience augmented risk for hypertensive crisis and other catastrophic cardiovascular complications from cocaine because of unrestrained central sympathetic outflow coupled with inhibition of peripheral NE reuptake.

AUTONOMIC EFFECTS OF COCAINE ON THE HEART

Effects of cocaine on the heart rate, myocardial contractility, and coronary tone also are assumed to be related to inhibition of the cardiac NE reuptake [1]. However, studies in humans challenged this hypothesis because these excitatory effects of cocaine were seen only with the systemic route of administration. Intranasal cocaine increased heart rate and caused α-adrenergic–mediated coronary vasoconstriction in humans, whereas infusion of cocaine directly into the coronary circulation, even at the dose that produced very high local concentration, did not produce the same effects [5]. Similarly, intranasal cocaine acutely increased left ventricular contractility [6], whereas intracoronary cocaine did not increase ejection fraction [7]. These data suggest a central rather than peripheral site of action of cocaine to increase sympathetic outflow to the heart. Although direct measurement of SNA to the heart is not feasible in humans, our previous study indicates that intranasal cocaine stimulates

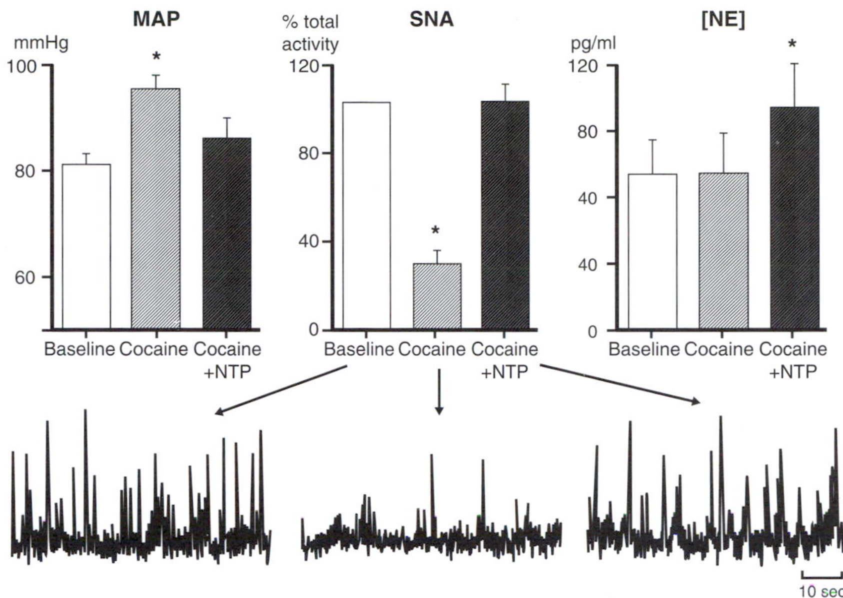

FIGURE 100.1 The role of baroreflexes in buffering sympathomimetic effects of cocaine. Summary data of five healthy subjects showing mean arterial pressure (MAP), sympathetic nerve activity (SNA), and venous NE concentration (*top*) and original recordings of muscle SNA in one subject (*bottom*) at baseline, after intranasal cocaine alone, and after intranasal cocaine plus intravenous nitroprusside. With intranasal cocaine alone, MAP increased and muscle SNA decreased reflexively, whereas forearm venous NE concentration was unchanged. When SNA was carefully returned to the baseline level by attenuating the cocaine-induced increase in MAP with nitroprusside, a significant increase in venous NE concentration was observed. $^{*}P = 0.01$ vs baseline.

central sympathetic outflow, as measured by intraneuronal recordings of SNA to the cutaneous circulation. Furthermore, the increase in SNA is accompanied by a parallel increase in heart rate that is abolished by β-adrenergic receptor blockade but unaffected by muscarinic receptor blockade, indicating sympathetic rather than parasympathetic mediation. This sympathetic-mediated increase in the heart rate is a potent effect of cocaine because it can overcome the opposing influence of baroreceptors to activate parasympathetic outflow to the sinus node. In humans, this central sympathoexcitatory effect of cocaine on the heart rate is the main mechanism by which cocaine increases BP (Fig. 100.2), because other determinants of BP such as systemic vascular resistance and stroke volume remain unchanged after systemic administration of cocaine [6].

EFFECTS OF COCAINE ON THERMOREGULATION

Hyperthermia is a well-known complication of cocaine overdose, which further amplifies its cardiovascular toxicity. Fatal cocaine overdose typically is associated with high blood cocaine levels (3–6 mg/liter), but cocaine-related deaths also can occur at 10 to 20 times lower blood levels when hyperthermia is present [8]. The hyperthermic properties of cocaine have been attributed largely to a hypermetabolic state (agitation with increased locomotor activity) that increases heat production. However, we recently demonstrated that impaired heat dissipation is another major mechanism by which cocaine increases body temperature [8]. When healthy cocaine-naïve individuals were subjected to passive heating, pretreatment with even a small dose of intranasal cocaine impaired both sweating and cutaneous vasodilation, the major autonomic adjustments to thermal stress (Fig. 100.3) [8]. The precise mechanism by which cocaine impairs both cutaneous vasodilation and sweating is still unknown, but it is likely to be a central mechanism of action because heat perception also is impaired. This was a dramatic effect because subjects experienced less thermal discomfort even though core temperature was greater than with placebo (Fig. 100.4). In addition, heat perception is the key trigger for behavioral adjustments such as seeking a cooler environment or adjusting the thermostat on the air conditioner, which, in humans, constitute the most powerful thermoregulatory responses [9].

TREATMENT OF COCAINE OVERDOSE

Treatment of cocaine-induced acute hypertension should be targeted to minimize the increase in cardiac output. Because cocaine causes a sympathetic increase in heart rate, a β-blocker theoretically should be the treatment of choice. However, unopposed β-adrenergic blockade can exacerbate cocaine-induced coronary vasoconstriction, and thus should be avoided. Combined β- and α-adrenergic receptor blockers such as labetalol have the advantage over pure β-blockers in abolishing BP-increasing effects of cocaine, but still do not reverse cocaine-induced coronary vasoconstriction [1]. Whether antihypertensive medications that decrease central sympathetic discharge such as the α_2 agonist clonidine will be effective in antagonizing cocaine-induced acute hypertension and coronary ischemia remains to be seen.

Treatment of cocaine-induced myocardial ischemia should include nitroglycerin, aspirin, oxygen, morphine, and

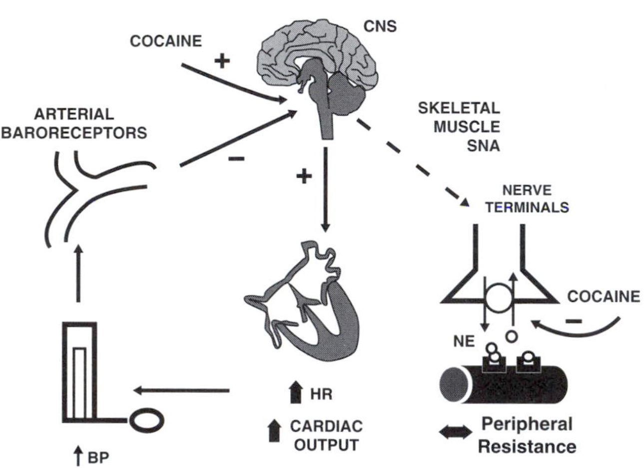

FIGURE 100.2 Diagram showing how cocaine increases blood pressure (BP) in humans. Cocaine increases sympathetic nerve discharge to the heart causing tachycardia and increased BP. The increase in BP activates arterial baroreceptors, which, in turn, trigger sympathetic withdrawal to the skeletal muscle vasculature. Although cocaine can inhibit the peripheral NE transporter, this mechanism is not effective in increasing NE levels at the synaptic cleft because the muscle SNA, the neural stimulus for NE release, is suppressed.

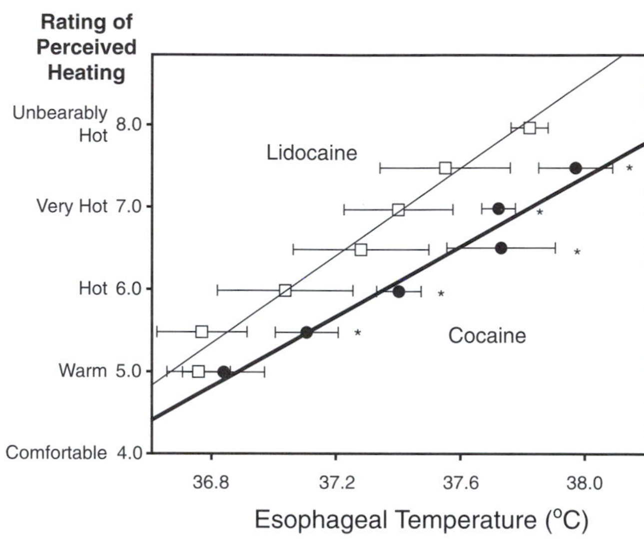

FIGURE 100.4 Effects of cocaine on thermal perception. Esophageal temperature at each rating of thermal sensation for both heat stresses. Values are displayed as mean ± SEM. At any given esophageal temperature greater than 37°C, the rating scores of perceived heating were significantly lower during cocaine trials (*closed circles*) than lidocaine or placebo trials (*open squares*), and these differences became even larger as esophageal temperature increased progressively, suggesting that cocaine impaired thermal perception (*$P < 0.05$ vs. lidocaine).

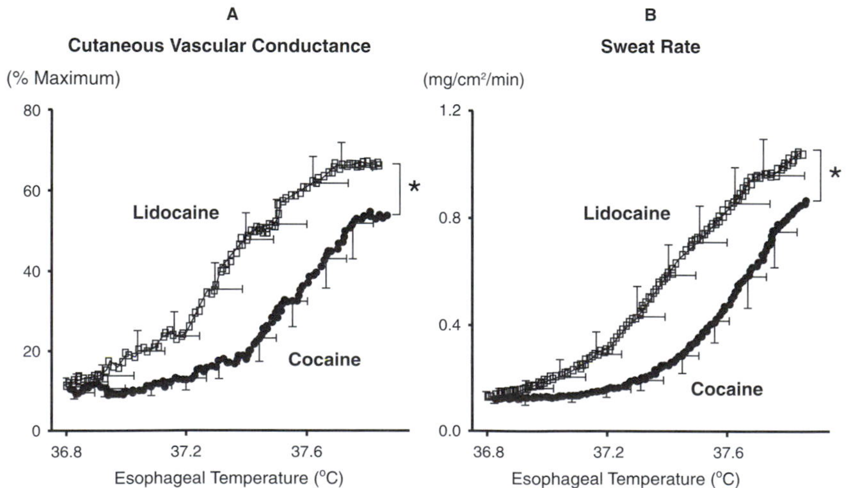

FIGURE 100.3 Effects of cocaine on autonomic adjustments to heat stress. Changes in cutaneous vascular conductance (**A**) and sweat rate (**B**) relative to esophageal temperature during both stresses (cocaine: *closed circles*; lidocaine or placebo: *open squares*). Data are mean ± SEM. Cocaine significantly increased the esophageal temperature threshold for the onset of cutaneous vasodilation ($P = 0.01$) and sweating ($P < 0.001$) without affecting the slope of the elevation in cutaneous vascular conductance or sweat rate relative to the increase in esophageal temperature. At any given esophageal temperature, cutaneous vascular conductance and sweat rate were significantly reduced for the cocaine trial (*$P < 0.01$ cocaine vs lidocaine trials).

benzodiazepine. Phentolamine and verapamil also are effective in reversing cocaine-induced coronary vasoconstriction [1]. Propranolol is contraindicated.

Patients with cocaine-induced hyperthermia should be taken into a cool environment to promote heat dissipation. Patients with agitation and increased motor activity should be treated with sedatives and anxiolytics to minimize heat production. Systemic administration of clonidine has been shown to decrease skin sympathetic vasoconstrictor activity in humans and to prevent postoperative shivering in patients undergoing surgery [10]. Its usefulness in the treatment of cocaine-induced hyperthermia requires further investigation.

References

1. Lange, R. A., and L. D. Hillis. 2001. Cardiovascular complications of cocaine use. *N. Engl. J. Med.* 345:351–358.
2. Tuncel, M., Z. Wang, D. Arbique, P. J. Fadel, R. G. Victor, and W. Vongpatanasin. 2002. Mechanism of the blood pressure-raising effect of cocaine in humans. *Circulation* 105:1054–1059.
3. Schroeder, J. S., A. V. Mullin, G. R. Elliot, H. Steiner, M. Nichols, A. Gordon, and M. Paulos. 1989. Cardiovascular effects of desipramine in children. *J. Am. Acad. Child Adolesc. Psychiatry* 28:376–370.
4. Jacobsen, T. N., P. A. Grayburn, R. W. I. Snyder, J. Hansen, B. Chavoshan, C. Landau, R. A. Lange, L. D. Hillis, and R. G. Victor. 1997. Effects of the intranasal cocaine on sympathetic nerve discharge in humans. *J. Clin. Invest.* 99:628–634.
5. Daniel, W. C., R. A. Lange, C. Landau, J. E. Willard, and L. D. Willis. 1996. Effects of the intracoronary infusion of cocaine on coronary arterial dimensions and blood flow in humans. *Am. J. Cardiol.* 78:288–291.
6. Boehrer, J. D., D. J. Moliterno, J. E. Willard, R. W. Snyder, R. P. Horton, D. B. Glamann, R. A. Lange, and L. D. Hillis. 1992. Hemodynamic effects of intranasal cocaine in humans. *J. Am. Coll. Cardiol.* 20:90–93.
7. Pitts, W. R., R. A. Lange, J. E. Cigarroa, and L. D. Hillis. 1997. Cocaine-induced myocardial ischemia and infarction: Pathophysiology, recognition and management. *Prog. Cardiovasc. Dis.* 40:65–76.
8. Crandall, C. G., W. Vongpatanasin, and R. G. Victor. 2002. Mechanism of cocaine-induced hyperthermia in humans. *Ann. Intern. Med.* 136:785–791.
9. Sessler, D. I. 1997. Mild perioperative hypothermia. *N. Engl. J. Med.* 336:1730–1737.
10. Kirno, K., S. Lundin, and M. Elam. 1993. Epidural clonidine depresses sympathetic nerve activity in humans by a supraspinal mechanism. *Anesthesiology* 78:1021–1027.

101 Sympathetic Nervous System and Pain

Wilfrid Jänig
Physiologisches Institut
Christian-Albrechts-Universität zu Kiel
Kiel, Germany

Normally the sympathetic nervous system is involved in various protective body reactions that are associated with pain or impending pain [1–4], but not in the generation of pain by activation of afferent neurons [5–7]. Under certain biologic and pathophysiologic conditions it may also be involved in the *generation* of pain. These conditions have been defined by quantitative investigations conducted on patients with pain depending on the sympathetic nervous system and on animal behavioral models. On the basis of these quantitative data, hypotheses have been developed to test experimentally the mechanisms underlying the role of the (efferent) sympathetic nervous system in the generation of pain.

SYMPATHETIC–AFFERENT COUPLING DEPENDING ON ACTIVITY IN SYMPATHETIC NEURONS: HYPOTHESES DRIVEN BY CLINICAL OBSERVATIONS

Pain dependent on activity in sympathetic neurons is called *sympathetically maintained pain* (SMP) [8, 9]. SMP is a symptom and includes generically spontaneous pain and pain evoked by mechanical and cold stimuli. It may be present in the complex regional pain syndrome type I and type II and in other neuropathic pain syndromes [8]. The idea about the involvement of the (efferent) sympathetic nervous system in pain is based on various clinical observations, which have been documented in the literature for decades [10–14]. Representative for these multiple observations on patients with SMP are quantitative experimental investigations conducted recently [15–19]. These experiments demonstrate the following: (1) sympathetic postganglionic neurons can be involved in the generation of pain; (2) blockade of the sympathetic activity can relieve the pain; and (3) norepinephrine injected intracutaneously is able to rekindle the pain.

The interpretation of these data is: Nociceptors are excited and possibly sensitized by norepinephrine released by the sympathetic fibers. Either the nociceptors have expressed adrenoceptors and/or the excitatory effect is generated indirectly—for example, through changes in blood flow. Sympathetically maintained activity in nociceptive neurons may generate a state of central sensitization/hyperexcitability leading to spontaneous pain and secondary evoked pain (mechanical and cold allodynia) [20, 22].

The coupling between sympathetic postganglionic neurons and primary afferent neurons that underlies SMP can occur in several ways. First, it may occur after trauma with nerve lesions at the lesion site, along the nerve, and in the dorsal root ganglion. The afferent activation is mediated by norepinephrine released by the postganglionic axons and by α-adrenoceptors expressed by the afferent neurons. It may also occur indirectly by changes in the micromilieu of the lesioned primary afferent neurons (e.g., by changes of blood flow in the dorsal root ganglion). Second, after trauma without nerve lesion the sympathetic activity may be mediated indirectly to the afferent neurons (i.e., through the vascular bed). Experiments supporting both general ideas have been performed on human models, on animal behavioral models, and on reduced animal models *in vivo* and *in vitro* [6, 7, 14, 20–24].

ROLE OF SYMPATHETIC NERVOUS SYSTEM IN GENERATION OF PAIN AND HYPERALGESIA DURING INFLAMMATION: HYPOTHESES DEVELOPED ON THE BASIS OF EXPERIMENTS IN BEHAVIORAL ANIMAL MODELS

Ideas that the sympathetic nervous system also may be involved in the generation of pain during inflammation have been developed from experiments using animal behavioral models. These hypotheses are not yet directly linked to and anchored in clinical observations. The hypothetical mechanisms by which the sympathetic nervous system might be involved in inflammatory pain are different from those underlying pain after trauma with nerve lesion (neuropathic pain). Behavioral signs of hyperalgesia elicited by mechanical or heat stimulation will generically be called (mechanical or heat) hyperalgesia.

Cutaneous Mechanical Hyperalgesia Elicited by the Inflammatory Mediator Bradykinin

In rats, the paw withdrawal threshold to mechanical stimulation is dose-dependently decreased by intracutaneous injection of bradykinin (BK) [25]. BK reacts with BK_2 receptors and leads to release of a prostaglandin, which sensitizes nociceptors for mechanical stimulation; sensitization is blocked by the cyclooxygenase inhibitor indomethacin [26, 27]. After surgical sympathectomy (performed ≥8 days before the behavioral measurements), mechanical hyperalgesia after intracutaneous BK injection disappears. However, it does not change after decentralization of the lumbar sympathetic trunk (leaving the postganglionic neurons in the paravertebral ganglia intact). It is hypothesized that the cutaneous nociceptors are sensitized for mechanical stimulation by a prostaglandin (possibly prostaglandin E_2), which is released either from the sympathetic terminals or from other cells in association with the sympathetic terminals in the skin. This novel function of the sympathetic innervation of skin is independent of its activity and norepinephrine release [24, 27].

Cutaneous Hyperalgesia Generated by Nerve Growth Factor

Systemic injection of nerve growth factor (NGF) is followed by a transient thermal and mechanical hyperalgesia in rats [28, 29] and humans [30]. During experimental inflammation (evoked by Freund's adjuvant in the rat hind paw), NGF increases in the inflamed tissue paralleled by the development of thermal and mechanical hyperalgesia [31, 32]. Both are prevented by anti-NGF antibodies [29, 32]. The mechanisms responsible are sensitization of nociceptors through high-affinity NGF receptors (trkA receptors) and an induction of increased synthesis of calcitonin gene–related peptide and substance P in the afferent cell bodies by NGF taken up by the afferent terminals and transported to the cell bodies. The NGF-induced sensitization of nociceptors also seems to be mediated indirectly by the sympathetic postganglionic terminals. Heat and mechanical hyperalgesia generated by local injection of NGF into the skin is prevented or significantly reduced after chemical or surgical sympathectomy [33, 34]. These experiments suggest that NGF released during inflammation by inflammatory cells acts on the sympathetic terminals through high-affinity trkA receptors, inducing the release of inflammatory mediators, and subsequently sensitization of nociceptors for mechanical and heat stimuli [24, 35, 36].

MECHANICAL HYPERALGESIC BEHAVIOR GENERATED BY ACTIVATION OF THE SYMPATHOADRENAL SYSTEM (ADRENAL MEDULLA)

Activation of the sympathoadrenal system (adrenal medulla; e.g., by release of the central sympathetic circuits from vagal inhibition), but not of the sympathoneural system, generates mechanical hyperalgesia and enhances BK-induced mechanical hyperalgesia (decrease of paw withdrawal threshold to mechanical stimulation of the skin). Both develop over 7 to 14 days after activation of the adrenal medullae and reverse slowly after denervation of the adrenal medullae [27, 37]. Application of epinephrine through a minipump over days simulates the slow development of mechanical hyperalgesia (S. G. Khasar, July 2003, personal communication).

The results of this experiment are interpreted in the following way: Epinephrine released by persistent activation of the adrenal medullae sensitizes cutaneous nociceptors for mechanical stimuli. This sensitization of nociceptors and its reversal are slow and take days to develop. The slow time course implies that the nociceptor sensitization cannot be acutely blocked by an adrenoceptor antagonist given intracutaneously. Epinephrine probably does not act directly on the cutaneous nociceptors, but rather on cells in the microenvironment of the nociceptors inducing slow changes that result in nociceptor sensitization. Candidate cells may be mast cells, macrophages, or keratinocytes [24, 37, 38]. This novel mechanism of pain and hyperalgesia involving the sympathoadrenal system may operate in ill-defined pain syndromes such as irritable bowel syndrome, functional dyspepsia, fibromyalgia, chronic fatigue syndrome, and others [39–41].

References

1. Bandler, R., and M. T. Shipley. 1994. Columnar organization in the midbrain periaqueductal gray: Modules for emotional expression? *Trends Neurosci.* 17:379–389.
2. Jänig, W. 1995. The sympathetic nervous system in pain. *Eur. J. Anaesthesiol.* 12(Suppl 10):53–60.
3. Jänig, W., and H. J. Häbler. 1995. Visceral-autonomic integration. In *Visceral pain. Progress in pain research and management, Vol 5*, ed. G. F. Gebhart, 311–348. Seattle, WA: IASP Press.
4. Jänig, W., and H. J. Häbler. 2000. Specificity in the organization of the autonomic nervous system: A basis for precise neural regulation of homeostatic and protective body functions. *Prog. Brain Res.* 122:351–367.
5. Jänig, W., and M. Koltzenburg. 1991. What is the interaction between the sympathetic terminal and the primary afferent fiber? In *Towards a new pharmacotherapy of pain*, ed. A. I. Basbaum, and J.-M. Besson, 331–352. Chichester, UK: Dahlem Workshop Reports, John Wiley & Sons.
6. Jänig, W., J. D. Levine, and M. Michaelis. 1996. Interactions of sympathetic and primary afferent neurons following nerve injury and tissue trauma. *Prog. Brain Res.* 112:161–184.

7. Jänig, W., and E. M. McLachlan. 1994. The role of modifications in noradrenergic peripheral pathways after nerve lesions in the generation of pain. In *Pharmacological approaches to the treatment of pain: New concepts and critical issues. Progress in pain research and management, Vol 1*, ed. H. L. Fields, and J. C. Liebeskind, 101–128. Seattle, WA: IASP Press.
8. Stanton-Hicks, M., W. Jänig, S. Hassenbusch, J. D. Haddox, R. Boas, and P. Wilson. 1995. Reflex sympathetic dystrophy: Changing concepts and taxonomy. *Pain* 63:127–133.
9. Jänig, W., and M. Stanton-Hicks, Eds. 1996. *Reflex sympathetic dystrophy: A reappraisal.* Seattle, WA: IASP Press.
10. Sweet, W. H., and J. C. White. 1969. *Pain and the neurosurgeon.* Springfield, IL: Charles C. Thomas.
11. Baron, R., H. Blumberg, and W. Jänig. 1996. Clinical characteristics of patients with complex regional pain syndrome in Germany with special emphasis on vasomotor function. In *Progress in pain research and management, Vol 6. Reflex sympathetic dystrophy: A reappraisal,* ed. M. Stanton-Hicks, and W. Jänig, 25–48. Seattle, WA: IASP Press.
12. Blumberg, H., and W. Jänig. 1994. Clinical manifestations of reflex sympathetic dystrophy and sympathetically maintained pain. In *Textbook of pain*, ed. P. D. Wall, and R. Melzack, 685–697. Edinburgh: Churchill Livingstone.
13. Bonica, J. J. 1990. Causalgia and other reflex sympathetic dystrophies. In *The management of pain*, ed. J. J. Bonica, 220–243. Philadelphia: Lea and Febinger.
14. Harden, R. N., R. Baron, and W. Jänig, Eds. 2001. *Complex regional pain syndrome.* Seattle, WA: IASP Press.
15. Ali, Z., S. N. Raja, U. Wesselmann, P. N. Fuchs, R. A. Meyer, and J. N. Campbell. 2000. Intradermal injection of norepinephrine evokes pain in patients with sympathetically maintained pain. *Pain* 88: 161–168.
16. Baron, R., J. Schattschneider, A. Binder, D. Siebrecht, and G. Wasner. 2002. Relation between sympathetic vasoconstrictor activity and pain and hyperalgesia in complex regional pain syndromes: A case-control study. *Lancet* 359:1655–1660.
17. Price, D. D., S. Long, B. Wilsey, and A. Rafii. 1998. Analysis of peak magnitude and duration of analgesia produced by local anesthetics injected into sympathetic ganglia of complex regional pain syndrome patients. *Clin. J. Pain.* 14:216–226.
18. Torebjörk, H. E., L. K. Wahren, B. G. Wallin, R. Hallin, and M. Koltzenburg. 1995. Noradrenaline-evoked pain in neuralgia. *Pain* 63:11–20.
19. Wahren, L. K., T. Gordh, Jr., and H. E. Torebjörk. 1995. Effects of regional intravenous guanethidine in patients with neuralgia in the hand: A follow-up study over a decade. *Pain* 62:379–385.
20. Jänig, W., and R. Baron. 2001. The role of the sympathetic nervous system in neuropathic pain: Clinical observations and animal models. In *Neuropathic pain: Pathophysiology and treatment*, ed. P. T. Hansson, H. L. Fields, R. G. Hill, and P. Marchettini, 125–149. Seattle: IASP Press.
21. Jänig, W., and R. Baron. 2002. Complex regional pain syndrome is a disease of the central nervous system. *Clin. Auton. Res.* 12:150–164.
22. Jänig, W., and R. Baron. 2003. Complex regional pain syndrome: Mystery explained? *Lancet* 2:687–697.
23. Jänig, W. 1999. Pain in the sympathetic nervous system: Pathophysiological mechanisms. In *Autonomic failure*, ed. R. Bannister, and C. J. Mathias, 99–108. New York: Oxford University Press.
24. Jänig, W., and H. J. Häbler. 2000. Sympathetic nervous system: Contribution to chronic pain. *Prog. Brain Res.* 129:451–468.
25. Taiwo, Y. O., and J. D. Levine. 1988. Characterization of the arachidonic acid metabolites mediating bradykinin and noradrenaline hyperalgesia. *Brain. Res.* 458:402–406.
26. Khasar, S. G., F. J. P. Miao, and J. D. Levine. 1995. Inflammation modulates the contribution of receptor-subtypes to bradykinin-induced hyperalgesia in the rat. *Neuroscience* 69:685–690.
27. Khasar, S. G., F. J. P. Miao, W. Jänig, and J. D. Levine. 1998. Modulation of bradykinin-induced mechanical hyperalgesia in the rat by activity in abdominal vagal afferents. *Eur. J. Neurosci.* 10:435–444.
28. Lewin, G. R., A. M. Ritter, and L. M. Mendell. 1993. Nerve growth factor-induced hyperalgesia in the neonatal and adult rat. *J. Neurosci.* 13:2136–2148.
29. Lewin, G. R., A. Rueff, and L. M. Mendell. 1994. Peripheral and central mechanisms of NGF-induced hyperalgesia. *Eur. J. Neurosci.* 6:1903–1912.
30. Petty, B. G., D. R. Cornblath, B. T. Adornato, V. Chaudhry, C. Flexner, M. Wachsman, D. Sinicropi, L. E. Burton, and S. J. Peroutka. 1994. The effect of systemically administered recombinant human nerve growth factor in healthy human subjects. *Ann. Neurol.* 36:244–246.
31. Donnerer, J., R. Schuligoi, and C. Stein. 1992. Increased content and transport of substance P and calcitonin gene-related peptide in sensory nerves innervating inflamed tissue: Evidence for a regulatory function of nerve growth factor in vivo. *Neuroscience* 49:693–698.
32. Woolf, C. J., B. Safieh-Garabedian, Q.-P. Ma, P. Crilly, and J. Winter. 1994. Nerve growth factor contributes to the generation of inflammatory sensory hypersensitivity. *Neuroscience* 62:327–331.
33. Andreev, N. Y., N. Dimitrieva, M. Koltzenburg, and S. B. McMahon. 1995. Peripheral administration of nerve growth factor in the adult rat produces a thermal hyperalgesia that requires the presence of sympathetic post-ganglionic neurones. *Pain* 63:109–115.
34. Woolf, C. J., Q.-P. Ma, A. Allchorne, and S. Poole. 1996. Peripheral cell types contributing to the hyperalgesic action of nerve growth factor in inflammation. *J. Neurosci.* 16:2716–2723.
35. McMahon, S. B. 1996. NGF as a mediator of inflammatory pain. *Philos. Trans. R Soc. Lond. B Biol. Sci.* 351:431–440.
36. Woolf, C. J. 1996. Phenotypic modification of primary sensory neurons: The role of nerve growth factor in the production of persistent pain. *Philos. Trans. R Soc. Lond. B Biol. Sci.* 351:441–448.
37. Khasar, S. G., F. J. P. Miao, W. Jänig, and J. D. Levine. 1998. Vagotomy-induced enhancement of mechanical hyperalgesia in the rat is sympathoadrenal-mediated. *J. Neurosci.* 18:3043–3049.
38. Jänig, W., S. G. Khasar, J. D. Levine, and F. J. P. Miao. 2000. The role of vagal visceral afferents in the control of nociception. *Prog. Brain. Res.* 122:273–287.
39. Goebell, H., and G. Holtmann, Eds. 1998. *Functional dyspepsia and irritable bowel syndrome.* Lancaster: Kluwer Academic Publishers.
40. Mayer, E. A., and H. E. Raybould, Eds. 1993. *Basic and clinical aspects of chronic abdominal pain. Pain research and clinical management, Vol 9.* Amsterdam: Elsevier Science Publishers BV.
41. Wolfe, F., H. A. Smythe, M. B. Yunus, R. M. Bennett, C. Bombardier, D. L. Goldenberg, P. Tugwell, S. M. Campbell, M. Abeles, and P. Clark. 1990. The American College of Rheumatology 1990 Criteria for the classification of fibromyalgia. Report of the Multicenter Criteria Committee. *Arthritis Rheum.* 33:160–172.

102

Baroreflex Functioning in Monogenic Hypertension

Friedrich C. Luft
Franz Volhard Klinik
HELIOS Klinikum
Berlin, Germany

Essential hypertension has a strong genetic component; however, the genes involved are not known. Presumably, many genes are involved. Rare forms of monogenic hypertension exist in which only one gene is responsible for the hypertensive phenotype. Elucidating the function of such genes has given us much insight into hypertensive mechanisms. Examples include glucocorticoid-remediable aldosteronism, apparent mineralocorticoid excess, pseudo-hypoaldosteronism, Liddle syndrome, and pseudohypoaldosteronism type 2. A chimeric, adrenocorticotrophic hormone–regulated gene causing increased aldosterone production, a defective 11 β-hydroxysteroid dehydrogenase gene, a gain-of-function mutation in the mineralocorticoid receptor, a mutated b or g subunit of the epithelial sodium channel, and mutated with no lysine (WNK) kinases are responsible for these syndromes [1]. All of these monogenic forms feature salt-sensitive hypertension. Diuretic therapy and decreased salt in the diet are effective treatments. Because the mechanism of the hypertension in these forms of monogenic hypertension is so well elucidated, baroreflex regulation has drawn relatively little attention. We have been investigating a monogenic form of hypertension that has not yet been elucidated. Perhaps because the molecular genetic approach has not brought us to a solution and our attempts to clone the responsible gene have been unsuccessful, we have concerned ourselves with clinical clues that might help us in terms of candidate genes. Our subjects have undergone extensive clinical testing.

AUTOSOMAL-DOMINANT HYPERTENSION WITH BRACHYDACTYLY

Bilginturan first described autosomal dominant hypertension syndrome in 1973 [2]. He and his associates identified a family residing on the Black Sea coast in eastern Turkey. Affected persons had severe hypertension and died of stroke before age 50 years. Interestingly, all affected persons also had brachydactyly and were about 10 cm shorter than nonaffected family members. No further investigations were possible at that time.

We had the opportunity to revisit this family with Bilginturan more than 20 years later. We confirmed the presence of severe hypertension and brachydactyly. The two phenotypes were associated in every case. No clinical studies in eastern Turkey were possible at that time. To study the hypertension further, we invited affected and nonaffected family members to come to our clinical research center in Berlin [3]. We confirmed that affected adults were 10 to 15 cm shorter than unaffected individuals; however, their body mass index (27 kg/m^2) was not different. Blood pressure increased steeply with age in the affected people so that by age 40 years, they had a mean blood pressure of 140 mm Hg, compared with 92 mmHg in unaffected individuals. Complete clinical, roentgenographic, and laboratory evaluation was performed in six subjects, including 24-hour blood pressure measurements and humoral determinations before and after volume expansion with 2 liters normal saline over 4 hours, followed by volume contraction on the following day with a 20-mmol sodium diet and 40 mg furosemide at 8 AM, 12 PM, and 4 PM. Two affected men aged 46 and 31 years; three affected women aged 40, 31, and 30 years; and one unaffected man aged 29 years were studied.

The systolic pressures ranged from 170 to 250 mmHg, and diastolic pressures ranged from 100 to 150 mm Hg in affected people; the unaffected man had a blood pressure of 120/70 mmHg. Thyroid, adrenal, and renal functions were normal; electrolyte and acid-base status was normal. Calcium and phosphate homeostasis was normal. Day–night circadian blood pressure rhythm was preserved. The subjects were not salt sensitive; renin, aldosterone, and catecholamine values reacted appropriately to volume expansion and contraction. Affected persons had mild cardiac hypertrophy and increased radial artery wall thickness. Fibroblasts from affected people grew more rapidly in culture than from unaffected people. We concluded that this novel form of inherited hypertension resembles essential hypertension. The most remarkable finding in our view was that, in contrast to all the other monogenic hypertension forms described, our syndrome did not cause salt-sensitive hypertension. Genomic DNA from affected and nonaffected individuals enabled us to perform a linkage analysis. We showed that the responsible gene lies on the short arm of chromosome 12 [4]. Our LOD score (logarithm of the odds ratio) was greater than 9, indicating strong evidence for linkage.

At the beginning we were faced with an area of interest spanning 10 cM. We ruled out some promising candidate genes, including the genes for parathyroid hormone–related peptide and the sulfonyl urea receptor type 2. We then returned to the patients for more clues. We reasoned that perhaps clinical pharmacology might help us and that blood pressure might be more responsive to a particular pharmacologic agent [5]. Thus, we performed a randomized double-blind, crossover trial of six regimens, β-blocker, hydrochlorothiazide, angiotensin-converting enzyme inhibitor, calcium channel blocker, a centrally acting imidazole receptor agonist, and placebo. All the drugs decreased blood pressures about 10 mmHg compared with placebo. No single agent was superior. β-Blockade decreased heart rate and hydrochlorothiazide decreased serum potassium levels as expected. Thus, the patients indeed resembled individuals with essential hypertension. However, the pharmacologic phenotype did not help us further in the identification of candidate genes.

NEUROVASCULAR CONTACT

The notion that hypertension might be initiated by neurovascular contact between the posterior inferior cerebellar artery and the ventrolateral medulla (VLM) stems from Jannetta and colleagues [6]. They observed that patients with trigeminal neuralgia who underwent vascular decompression surgery often were relieved of their hypertension and their pain [6]. Jannetta and colleagues [7] subsequently performed animal investigations in baboons, which had a small balloon implanted into the region of the VLM. This balloon was connected by a catheter to a second balloon in the thoracic aorta. The aortic balloon caused the balloon impinging on the VLM to pulsate. The pulsatile impulse was conducted over days in the baboons and was associated with an increase in blood pressure sufficient to induce an increase in heart size. Because Bilginturan had found "tortuous vessels" on cerebral arteriography in one of the patients years earlier, we asked affected and nonaffected family members to undergo magnetic resonance angiography [8]. We studied 15 hypertensive affected and 12 normotensive nonaffected family members. We then tested for linkage between the hypertension–brachydactyly phenotypes and the presence of neurovascular contact. All 15 affected family members had evidence for neurovascular contact. All had left-sided posterior inferior cerebellar artery or vertebral artery loops, whereas six had bilateral neurovascular contact. None of the nonaffected family members had neurovascular contact. The phenotypes were linked with an LOD score of 9.2 given a penetrance of 99%. We next embarked on investigations of baroreflex function in this family.

BAROREFLEX TESTING

We first performed a "field study" using a Portapres device (sample rate 100 Hz) to measure pulse intervals and finger blood pressure [9]. Brachial arterial blood pressure was measured oscillometrically. After a supine baseline period of 15 minutes, the subjects stood up and measurements were continued for another 5 minutes. The Ewing coefficient was calculated as the coefficient of the longest and shortest R-R interval immediately after standing as the RR30/15 ratio. The Valsalva maneuver was performed to permit determination of the Valsalva ratio and blood pressure responses. We studied 17 hypertensive affected and 12 normotensive nonaffected family members. Overall, baroreflex sensitivity (BRS) calculated using the cross-spectral (low-frequency BRS, high-frequency BRS) and sequence techniques (BRS^+, BRS^-) was not different between the groups. However, in younger family members, BRS^+ was 12 and 22 msec/mmHg in affected and in nonaffected family members, respectively. Figure 102.1 shows the BRS calculated using the sequence technique for up slopes (BRS^+). Figure 102.2 shows the up slopes plotted against mean arterial blood pressure. In nonaffected family members, the BRS decreased with increasing mean arterial blood pressure, which was not the case in affected persons. The decline in BRS with age and with increasing blood pressure was absent in affected family members. Thus, noninvasive testing showed impaired baroreflex control of heart rate at a young age. The reduced BRS in young family members with moderate arterial hypertension suggested to us that the impaired baroreflex function is not secondary to the hypertension, but it might be a primary abnormality, which aggravates the progression of hypertension.

INVASIVE BAROREFLEX TESTING

To study the possible autonomic abnormalities in this family further, we studied five patients in Berlin under complete ganglionic blockade with trimethaphan and also performed microneurography [10]. The blood pressure during complete ganglionic blockade was 134/82 and 90/49 mmHg in patients and in control subjects, respectively. During ganglionic blockade, plasma vasopressin concentration increased 24-fold in control subjects and less than 2-fold in the patients. In the patients, cold pressor testing, handgrip testing, and upright posture all increased blood pressure excessively. In contrast, muscle sympathetic nerve activity was not increased at rest or during cold pressor testing. The phenylephrine dose that increased systolic blood pressure

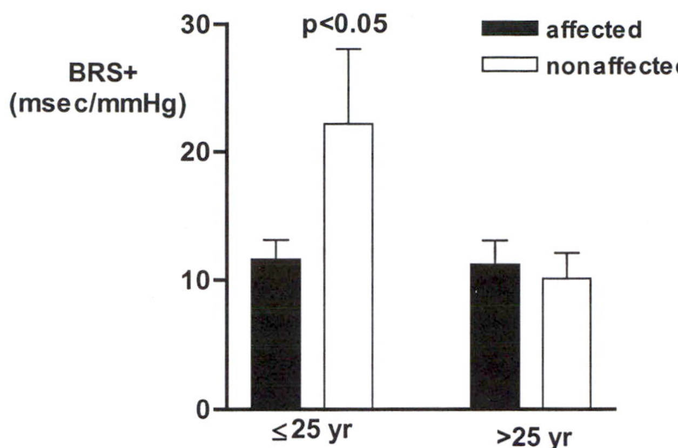

FIGURE 102.1 Baroreflex sensitivity through the sequence technique for up slopes (BRS⁺) presented as mean ± SEM for younger and older affected and nonaffected subjects.

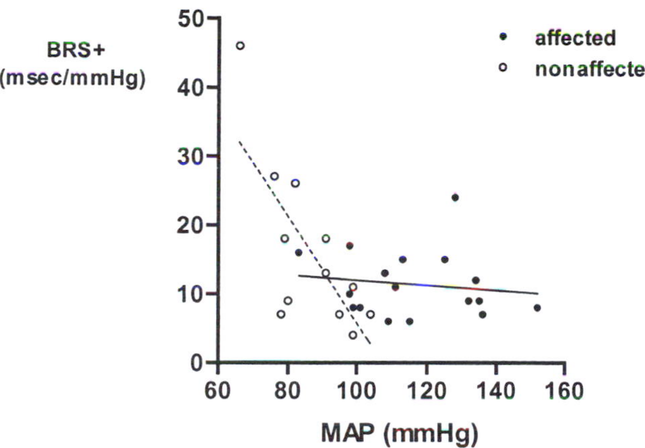

FIGURE 102.2 Baroreflex sensitivity (BRS) calculated using the sequence technique for up slopes (BRS⁺) plotted against mean arterial blood pressure. In nonaffected family members, BRS decreased with increasing blood pressure. In affected members, no relation was observed.

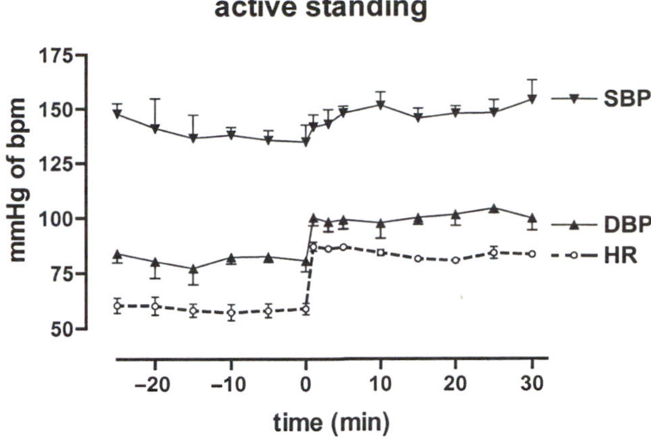

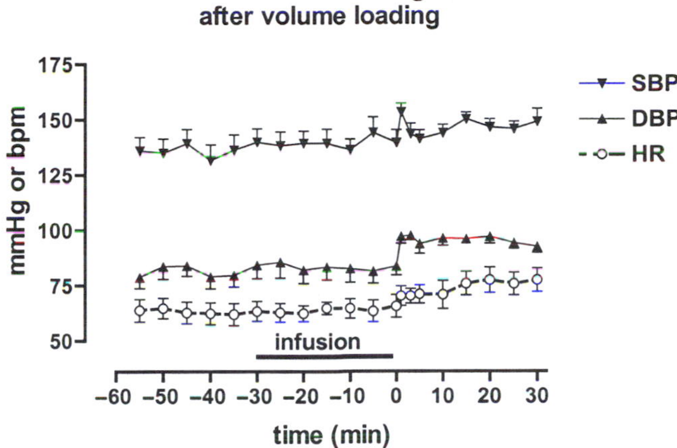

FIGURE 102.3 Affected persons showed orthostatic hypertension that was ameliorated with volume expansion, suggesting a sympathetic mechanism.

12.5 mmHg was 8 µg in patients and 135 µg in control subjects before ganglionic blockade and 5 µg in patients and 13 µg in control subjects during ganglionic blockade.

Figure 102.3 shows the orthostatic hypertension that we observed in the patients. The orthostatic hypertension was ameliorated by volume expansion. Figure 102.4 shows the blood pressure increases with phenylephrine in patients and control subjects with or without ganglionic blockade. When ganglionic blockade was performed, results for patients and control subjects were similar. The patients were also hypersensitive to nitroprusside. Interestingly, their spontaneous muscle sympathetic nerve activity was no different than control subjects. We interpreted these data as indicating that baroreflex blood pressure buffering and baroreflex-mediated vasopressin release are severely impaired in these subjects.

COMPARISONS WITH PATIENTS WHO HAVE ESSENTIAL HYPERTENSION

We, of course, had no evidence that neurovascular contact is responsible for these responses; however, we elected to investigate the issue further. Because neurovascular contact also occurs in patients with essential hypertension, we decided to recruit individuals with hypertension with neurovascular contact who did not have monogenic hypertension [11]. Patients were screened with magnetic resonance angiography, and those with neurovascular contact were invited to participate. Six patients with neurovascular contact and essential hypertension were compared with the five patients with monogenic hypertension and brachydactyly. The responses to incremental phenylephrine doses were assessed before and during ganglionic blockade with trimethaphan. The supine blood pressure was 172/89 mmHg before ganglionic blockade in the patients with essential hypertension. Their blood pressure decreased

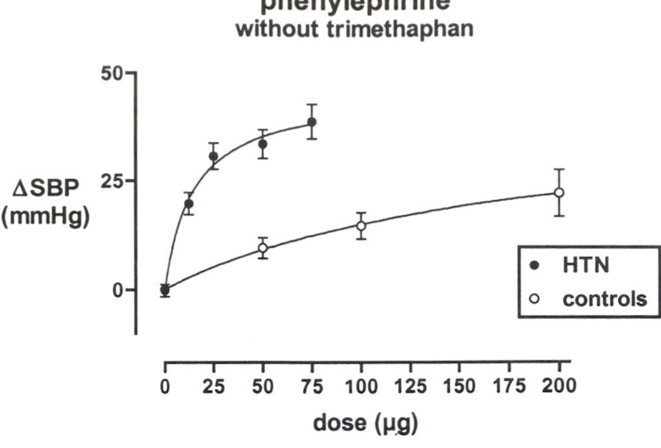

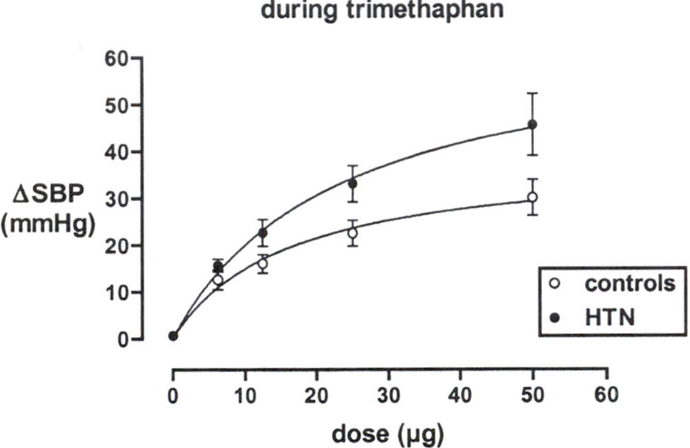

FIGURE 102.4 **Top**, Substantial increase in blood pressure to incremental doses of phenylephrine in patients compared with control subjects. **Bottom**, With ganglionic blockade, this difference was sharply reduced.

by 47/18 mmHg with trimethaphan, which was more than was observed in the patients with monogenic hypertension. Before ganglionic blockade, 25 μg phenylephrine increased systolic blood pressure by 17 mm Hg in patients with essential hypertension, compared with 30 mmHg in patients with autosomal dominant hypertension. Thus, the patients with essential hypertension and neurovascular contact did not resemble the patients with monogenic hypertension and neurovascular contact. We interpreted the findings as suggesting no proof for a causative association between neurovascular contact and absent baroreflex buffering of blood pressure.

Our microneurography data are not in accord with an observation by Schobel and colleagues [12]. Although we found no increase in muscle sympathetic nerve activity in our patients with monogenic hypertension and brachydactyly, Schobel and colleagues [12] report that patients with essential hypertension and neurovascular contact had increased muscle sympathetic nerve activity, compared with patients with essential hypertension who had no signs of neurovascular contact. Schobel and colleagues [12] believe that neurovascular contact may stimulate sympathetic nerve activity and elicit hypertension through stimulation of the VLM. Because we found no evidence for increased sympathetic nerve activity in our subjects with monogenic hypertension, compared with nonhypertensive healthy subjects, we have elected not to perform measurements of muscle sympathetic nerve activity in our patients with essential hypertension and neurovascular contact. We are aware that patients with hypertension with neurovascular contact are being subjected to decompression surgery [13]. However, the results, although intriguing, are uncontrolled. We do not believe it is justified to recommend surgery to our patients with monogenic hypertension until we have a better understanding of their disease on a molecular basis.

LESSONS FROM MONOGENIC HYPERTENSION

We have not yet cloned the gene for monogenic hypertension and brachydactyly. A deletion syndrome on chromosome 12p and three additional (non-Turkish) families have enabled us to sharply reduce our area of interest from 12 cM to about 3 cM. We have experienced frustrations and misadventures in the molecular genetics laboratory, but are convinced that we will achieve our goal. In contrast, we believe that our clinical studies have taught us a great deal about baroreflex buffering of blood pressure. We have compared patients with idiopathic orthostatic intolerance, patients with essential hypertension, patients with monogenic hypertension, patients with multiple system atrophy, and healthy control subjects in terms of sensitivity to phenylephrine and nitroprusside, with and without ganglionic blockade [14]. Figure 102.5 shows systolic blood pressure changes with phenylephrine, potentiation of the phenylephrine pressor effect under ganglion blockade, and baroslopes in the five groups. Blood pressure increased more in patients with monogenic hypertension and multiple systems atrophy. These two groups also exhibited the weakest potentiation of the pressor effect with ganglion blockade and had the smallest baroslope. Furthermore, they showed the greatest decrease in blood pressure in response to nitroprusside. These findings suggest that patients with multiple system atrophy and patients with this form of monogenic hypertension both have severely impaired baroreflex buffering of blood pressure. We also learned that the sensitivity to vasoactive drugs was much more a function of baroreflex buffering and much less a function of vascular sensitivity. Both heart rate and sympathetic vasomotor tone contribute to blood pressure buffering. We suggest that even minor changes in baroreflex function can greatly influence the sensitivity to vasoactive medications.

In conclusion, we are still far removed from understanding monogenic hypertension with brachydactyly

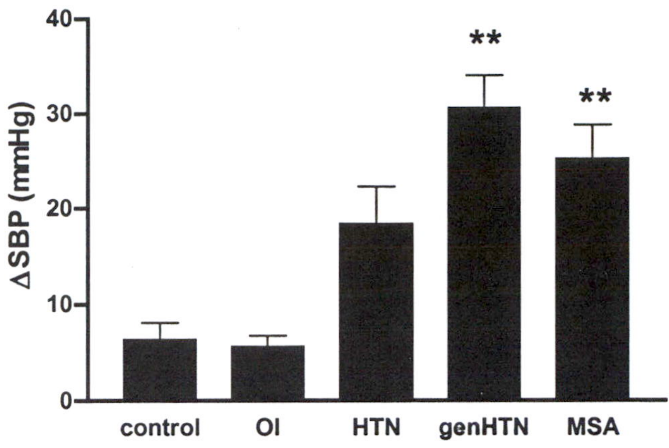

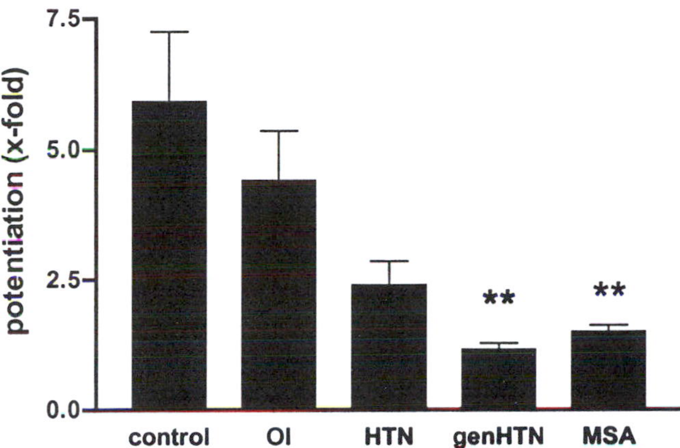

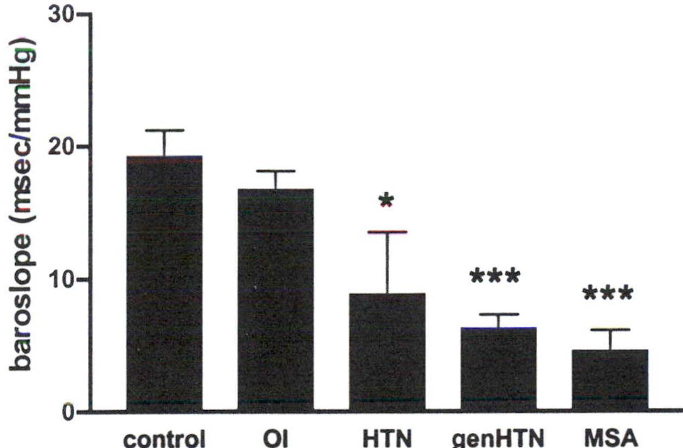

FIGURE 102.5 **Top**, Change in systolic blood pressure with 25 μg phenylephrine in control subjects, subjects with orthostatic intolerance (OI), patients with essential hypertension (HTN), patients with monogenic (genHTN) hypertension, and patients with multiple system atrophy (MSA). The patients with genHTN and the patients with MSA were the most sensitive. **Middle**, Potentiation of the pressor effect after complete ganglionic blockade. Again, the genHTN and MSA subjects showed the least potentiation. **Bottom**, The baroslope was most reduced in these same groups.

mechanistically. Nevertheless, our investigations have contributed much to our understanding of baroreflex buffering in other conditions. Elucidation of hypertension on a molecular level hopefully will clarify the baroreflex defect further.

References

1. Toka, H. R., and F. C. Luft. 2002. Monogenic forms of human hypertension. *Semin. Nephrol.* 22:81–88.
2. Bilginturan, N., S. Zileli, S. Karacadag, and T. Pirnar. 1973. Hereditary brachydactyly associated with hypertension. *J. Med. Genet.* 10:253–259.
3. Schuster, H., T. F. Wienker, H. R. Toka, S. Bahring, E. Jeschke, O. Toka, A. Busjahn, A. Hempel, C. Tahlhammer, W. Oelkers, J. Kunze, N. Bilginturan, H. Haller, and F. C. Luft. 1996. Autosomal dominant hypertension and brachydactyly in a Turkish kindred resembles essential hypertension. *Hypertension* 28:1085–1092.
4. Schuster, H., T. E. Wienker, S. Bahring, N. Bilginturan, H. R. Toka, H. Neitzel, E. Jeschke, O. Toka, D. Gilbert, A. Lowe, J. Ott, H. Haller, and F. C. Luft. 1996. Severe autosomal dominant hypertension and brachydactyly in a unique Turkish kindred maps to human chromosome 12. *Nat Genet.* 13:98–100.
5. Schuster, H., O. Toka, H. R. Toka, A. Busjahn, O. Oztekin, T. F. Wienker, N. Bilginturan, S. Bahring, F. Skrabal, H. Haller, and F. C. Luft. 1998. A cross-over medication trial for patients with autosomal-dominant hypertension with brachydactyly. *Kidney Int.* 53:167–172.
6. Jannetta, P. J., R. Segal, and S. K. Wolfson, Jr. 1985. Neurogenic hypertension: Etiology and surgical treatment. I. Observations in 53 patients. *Ann. Surg.* 201:391–398.
7. Jannetta, P. J., R. Segal, S. K. Wolfson, M. Dujovny, and A. Semba. 1985. Neurogenic hypertension: Etiology and surgical treatment. II. Observations in an experimental nonhuman primate model. *Ann Surg.* 201:254–261.
8. Naraghi, R., H. Schuster, H. R. Toka, S. Bahring, O. Toka, O. Oztekin, N. Bilginturan, H. Knoblauch, T. F. Wienker, A. Busjahn, H. Haller, R. Fahlbusch, and F. C. Luft. 1997. Neurovascular compression at the ventrolateral medulla in autosomal dominant hypertension and brachydactyly. *Stroke* 28:1749–1754.
9. Tank, J., O. Toka, H. R. Toka, J. Jordan, A. Diedrich, A. Busjahn, and F. C. Luft. 2001. Autonomic nervous system function in patients with monogenic hypertension and brachydactyly: A field study in northeastern Turkey. *J. Hum. Hypertens.* 15:787–792.
10. Jordan, J., H. R. Toka, K. Heusser, O. Toka, J. R. Shannon, J. Tank, A. Diedrich, C. Stabroth, M. Stoffels, R. Naraghi, W. Oelkers, H. Schuster, H. P. Schobel, H. Haller, and F. C. Luft. 2000. Severely impaired baroreflex-buffering in patients with monogenic hypertension and neurovascular contact. *Circulation* 102:2611–2618.
11. Jordan, J., J. Tank, H. Hohenbleicher, H. Toka, C. Schroder, A. M. Sharma, and F. C. Luft. 2002. Heterogeneity of autonomic regulation in hypertension and neurovascular contact. *J. Hypertens.* 20:701–706.
12. Schobel, H. P., H. Frank, R. Naraghi, H. Geiger, E. Titz, and K. Heusser. 2002. Hypertension in patients with neurovascular compression is associated with increased central sympathetic outflow. *J. Am. Soc. Nephrol.* 13:35–41.
13. Geiger, H., R. Naraghi, H. P. Schobel, H. Frank, R. B. Sterzel, and R. Fahlbusch. 1998. Decrease of blood pressure by ventrolateral medullary decompression in essential hypertension. *Lancet* 352: 446–449.
14. Jordan, J., J. Tank, J. R. Shannon, A. Diedrich, A. Lipp, C. Schroder, G. Arnold, A. M. Sharma, I. Biaggioni, D. Robertson, and F. C. Luft. 2000. Baroreflex buffering and susceptibility to vasoactive drugs. *Circulation.* 105:1459–1464.

103

Carcinoid Tumors

Kenneth R. Hande
Division of Medical Oncology
Vanderbilt University
Nashville, Tennessee

Carcinoid tumors arise from neuroendocrine cells. They are composed of monotonously similar cells with round nuclei, pink granular cytoplasm, and few mitosis [1]. Electron microscopy shows granules of various size and shape that contain many biologic amines including serotonin, histamine, dopamine, substance P, neurotensin, prostaglandins, gastrin, kallikrein, somatostatin, corticotrophin, and neuron-specific enolase [2]. When released into the systemic circulation, these neuropeptides may cause flushing, diarrhea, wheezing, heart disease, and rarely hypotension (the carcinoid syndrome).

Carcinoid tumor can arise anywhere in the body (Table 103.1). About 70% originate within three organs: the appendix, the small intestine, and the rectum [3]. Most appendiceal carcinoids are small, do not cause symptoms, and are diagnosed incidentally during appendectomy [4]. Larger tumors are found more frequently with small bowel than with appendiceal carcinoids. Most small bowel carcinoids occur in the ileum. Carcinoids may cause mesenteric fibrosis with partial bowel obstruction. Patients may have abdominal symptoms for months before diagnosis [5]. Half of rectal carcinoids are found incidentally at routine sigmoidoscopy. Rectal carcinoids do not secrete serotonin and are not associated with the carcinoid syndrome.

Less commonly, carcinoids may originate in the stomach, colon, or bronchus. Gastric carcinoids can be divided into three types: (1) those associated with chronic atrophic gastritis type A (CAG-A), (2) those associated with multiple endocrine neoplasm-1 or Zollinger–Ellison syndrome, and (3) those of the sporadic type [1, 6]. Gastric atrophy results in hypergastrinemia leading to hyperplasia of multiple benign carcinoids. Sporadic gastric carcinoids are more aggressive than CAG-A tumors and are associated with an atypical carcinoid syndrome mediated by histamine and 5-hydroxytryptophan. The flush of the atypical carcinoid syndrome consists of patchy, serpiginous areas of erythema with defined bonders rather than the common diffuse rash of most carcinoids. Pulmonary carcinoids usually present with symptoms of bronchial obstruction (pneumonia, cough, and hemoptysis). They can secrete adrenocorticotrophic hormone, growth hormone, or serotonin resulting in Cushing' syndrome, acromegaly, or carcinoid syndrome (5% of cases).

"Carcinoid syndrome" describes the humoral manifestations of carcinoid tumors (Table 103.2). Most patients with the carcinoid syndrome have hepatic metastasis [1–3]. The association between hepatic metastases and carcinoid syndrome is caused by efficient inactivation by the liver of amines released into the portal circulation by primary gastrointestinal tumors. In contrast, venous drainage from metastatic hepatic tumors goes directly into the systemic circulation.

The typical paroxysmal flushing of the carcinoid syndrome is manifested by transient episodes of erythema usually limited to the face, neck, and the upper trunk [2]. Patients may experience a sensation of warmth during flushing and sometimes palpitations. Although severe flushing and hypotension can occur, most episodes are brief (1–2 minutes) and do not cause dizziness or palpitations. Rare, severe attacks of flushing may be accompanied by shock and syncope. Flushing over a long period can cause a constant facial erythema and persistent cutaneous telangiectasia. Flushing usually occurs spontaneously in the absence of any evident precipitating cause. Serotonin is not the mediator of the flushing. Bradykinin is released in some patients during flushing, but the absence of detectable bradykinin release in other patients suggests that it is not a universal mediator of the flush. Production of the vasodilator prostaglandin E_2 is not increased in patients with the carcinoid syndrome. With tumors of the midgut, tachykinins are believed to be mediators of the flushing. Tachykinins are a family of structurally related peptides that exert similar biologic effects, such as vasodilation and contraction of various types of smooth muscle. These peptides include substance P, substance K (neurokinin α), and neuropeptide K (an extended form of substance K).

Diarrhea varies from 2 to 30 stools a day. It is usually a discomfort and an annoyance, but is not disabling. Occasionally, voluminous diarrhea may cause malabsorption and fluid and electrolyte imbalance. Diarrhea is frequently accompanied by abdominal cramping. A variety of carcinoid tumor products (serotonin, substance P, histamine, etc.) stimulate peristalsis. Small and large bowel transit times are two and six times faster in patients with carcinoid syndrome than healthy subjects [7]. Bronchospasm may occur with episodes of flushing. Pellagra from excess tryptophan

TABLE 103.1 Characteristics of Carcinoid Tumors

	Foregut*	Midgut†	Hindgut‡
Carcinoids, %	20%	60%	15%
Argentaffin stain	Negative	Positive	+/–
Urine excretion	5-HTP, histamine	5-HIAA	negative
Metastasis frequency	20%	5–35%	3%
Carcinoid syndrome	Atypical type	Typical type	Rare

*Respiratory tract, pancreas, stomach, and proximal duodenum.
†Jejunum, ileum, appendix, cecum, and ovary.
‡Distal colon and rectum.
5-HIAA, 5-hydroxyindole acetic acid; 5-HTP, 5-hydroxytryptophan.

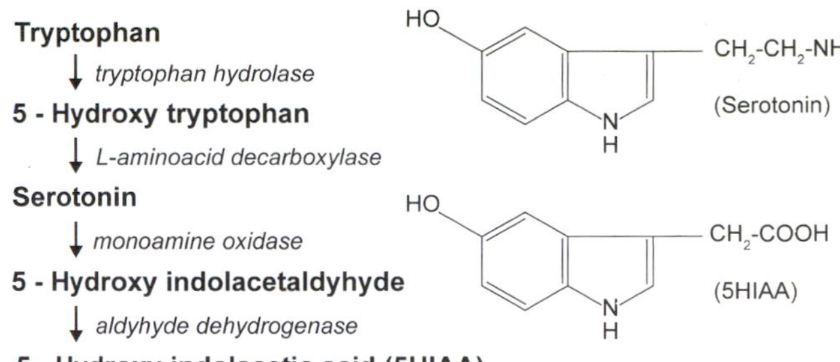

FIGURE 103.1 Metabolism and structure of serotonin and 5-hydroxy indolacetic acid.

TABLE 103.2 Clinical Features of Carcinoid Syndrome

Feature	Frequency
Diarrhea	70–80%
Flushing	60–75%
Heart disease	20–40%
Telangiectasia	20–25%
Wheezing	10–20%
Pellagra	1–2%

catabolism is uncommon. Carcinoid heart disease is manifest pathologically by plaquelike thickening on the endocardium of heart leaflets. Tricuspid regulation and tricuspid stenosis occurs in 92% and 27% of patients with carcinoid heart disease, respectively. Left-sided lesions are rare. Carcinoid heart disease is associated with high plasma serotonin concentrations [8].

The most dramatic manifestation of carcinoid tumors is the carcinoid crisis. This is observed in patients who have the more intense syndromes associated with foregut carcinoids or patients who have greatly increased 5-hydroxyindole acetic acid (5-HIAA) levels (>200 mg/24 hr). Carcinoid crisis is frequently precipitated by physically stressful situations, particularly by induction of anesthesia. Patients will develop an intense generalized flush that persists for hours or days. There may be severe diarrhea. Central nervous system symptoms are common, ranging from mild light-headedness or vertigo through somnolence to deep coma. There are usually associated cardiovascular abnormalities including tachycardiac, rhythm irregularity, hypertension, or severe hypotension.

Urinary excretion of 5-HIAA, the end metabolite of serotonin metabolism (Fig. 103.1), is used to confirm the diagnosis of carcinoid syndrome. Normal excretion is less than 10 mg/24 hr. Values of more than 25 mg/24 hr are essentially diagnostic of carcinoid syndrome. A sensitivity of 73% and a specificity of 100% have been reported for increased urinary 5-HIAA in metastatic carcinoid tumors. Serine chromogranin A is increased in 60 to 80% of carcinoid tumors and appears to correlate with tumor mass. Somatostatin receptor scintography (^{111}In-pentreotide) is useful in tumor localization with 65 to 80% sensitivity in detecting metastatic disease [6].

Treatment of localized carcinoid tumors is surgical resection. Carcinoids smaller than 2 cm are usually cured [5, 9]. Therapy for patients with metastatic disease is usually palliative. It is important to remember that carcinoid tumors have an indolent growth pattern and patients may live many years even with metastatic disease (median survival >5 years). Somatostatin analogues have a central role in the treatment of patients with carcinoid syndrome. Somatostatin is a 14-amino acid peptide that inhibits the secretion of a broad range of hormones. Somatostatin binds to somatostatin receptors expressed on 80% of carcinoid tumors. Somatostatin analogues, such as octreotide, are effective in relieving the symptoms of carcinoid syndrome in 90% of patients and decrease urinary 5-HIAA excretion in 72%. Long-acting preparations of somatostatin analogs (Lanreotide, Octreotide-LAR) can be administered once a month [10]. Chemotherapy has shown only minimal benefit in treatment of carcinoid tumors. Hepatic artery embolization can be used for hepatic metastases. Urinary 5-HIAA excretion and symptoms improve in up to 80% of patients after tumor embolization. Survival benefit from embolization procedures has not been documented.

References

1. Kulke, M. H., and R. J. Mayer. 1999. Carcinoid tumors. *N. Engl. J. Med.* 340:858–868.
2. Caplin, M. E., J. R. Buscombe, A. J. Hilson, A. L. Jones, A. F. Watkinson, and A. K. Burroughs. 1998. Carcinoid tumor. *Lancet* 352:799–805.
3. Modlin, I. M., and A. Sandor. 1997. An analysis of 8305 cases of carcinoid tumors. *Cancer* 79:813–829.
4. Moertel, C. G., L. H. Weiland, D. M. Nagorney, and M. B. Dockerty. 1987. Carcinoid tumor of the appendix: Treatment and prognosis. *N. Engl. J. Med.* 317:1699–1701.
5. Moertel, C. G. 1987. Karnofsky Memorial Lecture: An odyssey in the land of small tumors. *J. Clin. Oncol.* 10:1502–1522.

6. Oberg, K. 2002. Carcinoid tumors: Molecular genetics, tumor biology, and update of diagnosis and treatment. *Curr. Opin. Oncol.* 14:38–45.
7. Von Der Ohe, M. R., M. Camilleri, L. K. Kvols, and G. M. Thomforde. 1993. Motor dysfunction of the small bowel and colon in patients with the carcinoid syndrome and diarrhea. *N. Eng. J. Med.* 329:1073–1078.
8. Robiolio, P. A., V. H. Rigolin, J. S. Wilson, J. K. Harrison, L. L. Sanders, T. M. Bashore, and J. M. Feldman. 1995. Carcinoid heart disease: Correlation of high serotonin levels with valvular abnormalities detected by cardiac catheterization and echocardiography. *Circulation* 92:790–795.
9. Soreide, J. A., J. A. van Heerden, G. B. Thompson, J. K. Harrison, L. L. Sanders, T. M. Bashore, and J. M. Feldman. 2000. Gastrointestinal carcinoid tumors: Long-term prognosis for surgically treated patients. *World J. Surg.* 24:1431–1436.
10. Rubin, J., J. Ajani, W. Schirrmer, A. P. Venook, R. Bukowski, R. Pommier, L. Saltz, P. Dandona, and L. Anthony. 1999. Octreotide acetate long acting formulation verses open-label subcutaneous octreotide acetate in malignant carcinoid syndrome. *J. Clin. Oncol.* 17:600–606.

104 Chronic Fatigue and the Autonomic Nervous System

Roy Freeman
Center for Autonomic and Peripheral Nerve Disorders
Beth Israel Deaconess Medical Center
Boston, Massachusetts

Chronic fatigue syndrome (CFS) is a heterogeneous disorder. Features of autonomic dysfunction manifesting as autonomic symptoms and signs, autonomic test abnormalities, a predisposition to neurally mediated syncope, orthostatic intolerance, and postural tachycardia are present in some patients. The prevalence of autonomic dysfunction in CFS is unknown.

CFS is characterized by disabling fatigue accompanied by multiple systemic symptoms. The cause of the syndrome is unknown and there are no validated diagnostic tests. A case definition for CFS was developed under the leadership of the U.S. Centers for Disease Control and Prevention in 1988 and was revised in 1994 [1]. Autonomic features are not listed in this case definition. Nevertheless, signs and symptoms referable to the autonomic nervous system have appeared repeatedly in case studies of sporadic and epidemic CFS [2, 3]. Features of autonomic dysfunction have included orthostatic hypotension and tachycardia, episodes of sweating, pallor, sluggish pupillary responses, constipation, and frequency of micturition [2, 3].

Streeten and Anderson [4] first drew attention to the possibility that fatigue and exhaustion in some patients with the CFS might be caused by failure to maintain blood pressure in the erect posture. Although numerous studies have confirmed the association between autonomic dysfunction and CFS, the prevalence of autonomic dysfunction is not known, and it is not known in what ways patients with CFS with and without autonomic manifestations differ.

This subgroup of patients with CFS, however, is well recognized and was classified as subtype "orthostatic intolerant predominant" by the Name Change Workgroup of the federal CFS Coordinating Committee of the Department of Health and Human Services.

CHRONIC FATIGUE SYNDROME, ORTHOSTATIC INTOLERANCE, AND NEURALLY MEDIATED SYNCOPE

Rowe and colleagues [5] were first to address systematically the relation between CFS and orthostatic intolerance proposed by Streeten and Anderson [4]. They suggested, based on tilt-table studies of patients with CFS, that neurally mediated hypotension might be an unrecognized cause of chronic fatigue [5]. These investigators documented a positive tilt-table test in 97% of patients with CFS and suggested that a predisposition to neurally mediated syncope (also called neurocardiogenic, vasovagal syncope, and neurally mediated hypotension) may underlie some of the symptoms of CFS [5, 6]. Several follow-up studies [7–10] (with some exceptions [11, 12]) confirmed the presence of tilt-table abnormalities in patients with chronic fatigue and documented other autonomic abnormalities. The incidence of neurally mediated syncope in patients with CFS in these studies, however, was somewhat less than that documented by Rowe and co-workers [5]. Furthermore, the incidence of neurally mediated syncope in control subjects was somewhat greater [7–10] For example, we observed that 25% of patients with CFS and 0% of control subjects had neurally mediated syncope provoked by tilt-table testing [7]. Studies from other centers report similar results. Stewart and colleagues [9] reported 8% of adolescent subjects with CFS exhibited neurally mediated syncope on tilt-table testing in comparison with 31% of control subjects; whereas Schondorf and colleagues [8] reported that 34% of subjects with CFS exhibited neurally mediated syncope in comparison with 17% of control subjects.

Confounding variables that are responsible for the differences among studies include the clinical heterogeneity of patients with CFS and control subjects studied, but more importantly differences in tilt-test protocols. Intravenous cannulation, fasting, and isoproterenol use all increase the likelihood of a positive test result. Our current studies underscore this phenomenon. When patients with CFS were tested after an overnight fast and with intravenous cannulation, the incidence of neurally mediated syncope was not different from that in control subjects.

Despite these exciting initial observations, which raised the possibility of rational pharmacologic treatment for some patients with CFS, well designed therapeutic interventions in patients with chronic fatigue, even those with documented autonomic features, have not met consistent success. Several factors may be responsible. First, the pathophysiology of the autonomic dysfunction in CFS remains incompletely understood. Second, it is probable that there is dysfunction at several sites of the nervous and cardiovascular systems, thus a single intervention may not be sufficient. Third, although it is currently well accepted that there is heterogeneity in patients with chronic fatigue, it is likely that heterogeneity also exists in chronic fatigue patients with autonomic manifestations.

CHRONIC FATIGUE SYNDROME, POSTURAL TACHYCARDIA, AND ORTHOSTATIC INTOLERANCE

A postural tachycardia with associated orthostatic intolerance is the autonomic marker that, in our and other studies, is observed most frequently in individuals with CFS. The pathologic basis of the postural tachycardia and its relation to the features of CFS is unknown, although of all autonomic symptoms and signs associated with CFS it seems most likely to have a primary role in symptoms and to be amenable to therapeutic intervention [13].

The relation between CFS and postural tachycardia was first noted in a study of five subjects with symptoms of orthostatic intolerance and postural tachycardia on tilt-table testing. All subjects fulfilled criteria for CFS [14]. Other studies in the ensuing years documented a strong association between CFS and postural tachycardia. There also is a high prevalence of chronic fatigue in cohorts of patients selected for postural tachycardia. Furthermore, the two conditions have other features in common. Female predominance, light headedness, dizziness, palpitations, exercise intolerance, chest pain, gastrointestinal symptoms, anxiety, antecedent viral infection, and dependent skin changes are characteristic features in patients with postural tachycardia and also frequently occur in patients with CFS [15–17].

PATHOPHYSIOLOGY OF POSTURAL TACHYCARDIA

The physiologic basis of the postural tachycardia syndrome is unresolved. Investigators, studying the disorder from different standpoints, have documented baroreflex dysfunction, α-adrenoreceptor and β-adrenoreceptor supersensitivity, hypovolemia, reduced erythrocyte volume, venous system abnormalities, increased venous plasma norepinephrine levels at rest and on standing, lower norepinephrine spillover in the legs than the arms to the arms, and, presumably a rare association, a deficiency in norepinephrine transport because of a functional mutation in the gene encoding the norepinephrine transporter. These deficits may underlie the symptoms of orthostatic intolerance that occur despite normal blood pressure. It is not known which of these pathophysiologies occurs more frequently or how they contribute to the clinical features of patients with CFS [13].

CONCLUSION

On the basis of our current understanding, it seems likely that CFS is a heterogeneous disorder and that autonomic dysfunction, frequently manifesting as orthostatic intolerance, plays a role in its pathophysiology in some patients. To date, no epidemiologic studies have defined the prevalence of orthostatic intolerance in CFS. Similarly, although it is estimated that 500,000 individuals in the United States have orthostatic intolerance [18], it is not known how many of these individuals have chronic fatigue or satisfy Fukuda criteria for CFS [1]. Future studies are likely to elucidate the relation between autonomic dysfunction and CFS, and thereby contribute to our understanding of CFS in general.

References

1. Fukuda, K., S. E. Straus, I. Hickie, M. C. Sharpe, J. G. Dobbins, and A. Komaroff. 1994. The chronic fatigue syndrome: A comprehensive approach to its definition and study. International Chronic Fatigue Syndrome Study Group. *Ann. Intern. Med.* 121:953–959.
2. Ramsay, A. M. 1978. Epidemic neuromyasthenia. *Postgrad. Med. J.* 54:718–721.
3. Parish, J. G. 1978. Early outbreaks of epidemic neuromyasthenia. *Postgrad. Med. J.* 54:711–717.
4. Streeten, D. H., and G. H. J. Anderson. 1992. Delayed orthostatic intolerance [see comments]. *Arch. Intern. Med.* 152:1066–1072.
5. Rowe, P. C., I. Bou-Holaigah, J. S. Kan, H. Calkins. 1995. Is neurally mediated hypotension an unrecognized cause of chronic fatigue? *Lancet* 345:623–624.
6. Bou-Holaigah, I., P. C. Rowe, J. Kan, and H. Calkins. 1995. The relationship between neurally mediated hypotension and the chronic fatigue syndrome. *JAMA*. 274:961–967.
7. Freeman, R., and A. L. Komaroff. 1997. Does the chronic fatigue syndrome involve the autonomic nervous system? *Am. J. Med.* 102:357–364.
8. Schondorf, R., J. Benoit, T. Wein, and D. Phaneuf. 1999. Orthostatic intolerance in the chronic fatigue syndrome. *J. Auton. Nerv. Syst.* 75:192–201.
9. Stewart, J. M., M. H. Gewitz, A. Weldon, and J. Munoz. 1999. Patterns of orthostatic intolerance: The orthostatic tachycardia syndrome and adolescent chronic fatigue. *J. Pediatr.* 135:218–225.
10. Stewart, J. M. 2000. Autonomic nervous system dysfunction in adolescents with postural orthostatic tachycardia syndrome and chronic fatigue syndrome is characterized by attenuated vagal baroreflex and potentiated sympathetic vasomotion. *Pediatr. Res.* 48:218–226.
11. Soetekouw, P. M., J. W. Lenders, G. Bleijenberg, T. Thien, J. W. van der Meer. 1999. Autonomic function in patients with chronic fatigue syndrome. *Clin. Auton. Res.* 9:334–340.
12. LaManca, J. J., A. Peckerman, J. Walker, W. Kesil, S. Cook, A. Taylor, and B. H. Natelson. 1999. Cardiovascular response during head-up tilt in chronic fatigue syndrome. *Clin. Physiol.* 19:111–120.
13. Freeman, R. 2002. The chronic fatigue syndrome is a disease of the autonomic nervous system. Sometimes. *Clin. Auton. Res.* 12:231–233.

14. De Lorenzo, F., J. Hargreaves, and V. V. Kakkar. 1996. Possible relationship between chronic fatigue and postural tachycardia syndromes. *Clin. Auton. Res.* 6:263–264.
15. Schondorf, R., and P. A. Low. 1993. Idiopathic postural orthostatic tachycardia syndrome: An attenuated form of acute pandysautonomia? *Neurology* 43:132–137.
16. Furlan, R., G. Jacob, M. Snell, D. Robertson, A. Porta, P. Harris, R. Mosqueda-Garcia. 1998. Chronic orthostatic intolerance: A disorder with discordant cardiac and vascular sympathetic control. *Circulation* 98:2154–2159.
17. Jacob, G., F. Costa, J. R. Shannon, R. M. Robertson, M. Wathen, M. Stein, I. Biaggioni, A. Ertl, B. Black, and D. Robertson. 2000. The neuropathic postural tachycardia syndrome. *N. Engl. J. Med.* 343:1008–1014.
18. Robertson, D. 1999. The epidemic of orthostatic tachycardia and orthostatic intolerance. *Am. J. Med. Sci.* 317:75–77.

105 Paraneoplastic Autonomic Dysfunction

Ramesh K. Khurana
Division of Neurology
Union Memorial Hospital
Baltimore, Maryland

Paraneoplastic autonomic dysfunction (PAD), as a result of the tumor's remote effect on the autonomic nervous system, is rare, but it is extremely important to recognize for the following reasons: (1) it may be the initial manifestation of an underlying malignancy; (2) it may be more devastating than the tumor itself; (3) it may simulate metastatic disease or other conditions such as B_{12} deficiency and multiple system atrophy (MSA); (4) it may be confirmed with serologic tests; and (5) early treatment of the tumor may arrest the progression or improve the autonomic dysfunction. PAD may be immune-mediated or nonimmune-mediated. The latter (inappropriate diuresis, Cushing syndrome, neoplastic fever, etc.), attributed to the ectopic production of hormones and cytokines, is not included in this review. Immune-mediated PAD is discussed later and in Table 105.1; see Table 105.2 for supplemental details.

BRAINSTEM DYSFUNCTION SYNDROME

Brainstem dysfunction syndrome is a rare syndrome characterized by dilated and nonreactive pupils, which are supersensitive to dilute epinephrine and methacholine, hypoalacrima, sudomotor abnormality, daytime somnolence, labile pressure, and fatal sleep apnea. Autopsy of one case showed neuronal loss in the regions of Edinger–Westphal nucleus, the locus ceruleus, the dorsal motor nucleus, and the brainstem reticular formation.

MORVAN SYNDROME

Clinical features of Morvan syndrome include muscle stiffness, cramps, myokymia, weakness, pseudomyotonia, hallucinations, complex nocturnal behavior, insomnia, hyperhidrosis, increased salivation and lacrimation, tachycardia, abnormal hormonal circadian rhythm, severe constipation, and urinary incontinence. Electromyography shows spontaneous firing of motor units as doublet, triplet, or multiple discharges occurring at irregular intervals with a high intraburst frequency. The passive transfer of neuromyotonia IgG (voltage-gated potassium channel [VGKC] antibody) increases neuronal excitability in mice. Antibodies against VGCKs have been demonstrated in the serum and on neuronal dendrites in the hippocampus, thalamic neurons, and peripheral nerves. Patients show improvement after plasma exchange and immunosuppression with prednisone and azathioprine.

SUBACUTE SENSORY NEURONOPATHY

First described by Denny Brown in 1948, subacute sensory neuronopathy is characterized by subacute onset and asymmetric distribution of dysesthesia, lancinating pains, and numbness affecting the limbs, face, and tongue. Loss of proprioception, sensory ataxia, pseudo-athetosis, and areflexia are common, whereas motor strength is spared. This syndrome may mimic subacute combined degeneration or tabes dorsalis. Autonomic dysfunction is present in more than one third of cases. Tests show local or widespread sympathetic and parasympathetic insufficiency. Hu antigens are expressed throughout the central nervous system, sensory and sympathetic ganglia, and cancer cells. Anti-Hu/type 1 anti-neuronal nuclear autoantibodies (ANNA-1) is the serologic marker.

ENTERIC NEURONOPATHY

Pseudoobstruction of bowels, a distinguishing feature of enteric neuronopathy, may precede or follow the diagnosis of tumor. Postural dizziness, syncope, and other symptoms may follow. Somatic neurologic findings are of variable severity and affect the peripheral or central nervous system. The syndrome may mimic MSA, but pseudoobstruction of bowels in MSA is rare. Myenteric plexus neurons display lymphocytic infiltration and progressive loss.

AUTONOMIC NEUROPATHY

Autonomic dysfunction may occur with minimal or no somatic involvement. There is subacute onset of orthostatic, gastrointestinal, genitourinary, and papillary symptoms. Autonomic tests show widespread parasympathetic and sympathetic dysfunctions. The patients may be seropositive for ganglionic acetylcholine receptor autoantibodies, and ANNA-1.

LAMBERT–EATON MYASTHENIC SYNDROME

Patients with Lambert–Eaton myasthenic syndrome (LEMS) present with symmetric proximal weakness, reduced or absent reflexes, and ptosis. Autonomic symptoms (subclinical, except dry mouth) occur in about three fourths of patients. Autonomic tests show widespread cholinergic and adrenergic abnormalities. The electrophysiologic hallmarks LEMS are low amplitude of the compound muscle action potentials, decremental responses on 2- to 5-Hz nerve stimulation, and augmentation greater than 100% on 20- to 50-Hz stimulation. Almost all patients show autoantibody against PQ-type voltage-gated calcium channels (VGCC). The following evidence proves the pathogenicity of the VGCC antibodies: expression of VGCC antigen cancer cells, passive transfer of the human disorder to mice with the injection of LEMs IgG, antibody binding to the active zone particles (AZPs) of the presynaptic calcium channels, reduced number and disorganization of AZPs demonstrated by freeze-fracture studies of the patient's neuromuscular junction, reduced presynaptic quantal release of acetylcholine, and relatively rapid improvement after removal of antibodies with plasma exchange. Immunoglobulin G in LEMS, found to impair transmitter release from parasympathetic (bladder) and sympathetic (vas deferens) neurons, is probably responsible for autonomic dysfunction. However, contribution of other factors such as antibodies against neuronal ganglionic acetylcholine receptor cannot be excluded.

TABLE 105.1 Classification of Immune-Mediated Paraneoplastic Autonomic Dysfunction

I. Involving the central nervous system
   A. Brainstem dysfunction syndrome
II. Involving both the central nervous system and peripheral nervous system
   A. Morvan syndrome
   B. Sensory neuronopathy
   C. Enteric neuronopathy
III. Involving the peripheral nervous system
   A. Autonomic neuropathy
IV. Involving the neuromuscular junction
   A. Lambert–Eaton myasthenic syndrome

DIAGNOSIS

Paraneoplastic disorder should be suspected in patients with progressive autonomic symptoms such as orthostatic

TABLE 105.2 Paraneoplastic Neurologic Syndromes: Clinical and Immunologic Features and Associated Tumors

PNS	Distinguishing clinical feature	Antibodies	Common tumor type	Other tumors
Brainstem dysfunction	Sleep apnea and hypoventilation	Cytotoxic antineuroblastoma Immunoglobulins	Ganglioneuroma	—
Morvan syndrome	Pseudomyotonia, myokymia, abnormal EKG	Anti-VGKC	Thymoma	SCLS, Hodgkin's disease
Sensory neuronopathy	Progressive and severe proprioceptive deficit	Anti-Hu/ANNA-1 Antiamphiphysin	SCLC	GIT, breast, adrenal glands, uterus, prostate, lymphoma, neuroblastoma, testicular seminoma, embryonal carcinoma
Enteric neuronopathy	Intestinal pseudoobstruction	Anti-Hu/ANNA-1, enteric neuronal, ganglionic acetylcholine receptor, N-type calcium channel	SCLC	Pulmonary carcinoid, undifferentiated epithelioma
Autonomic neuropathy	Widespread autonomic failure with little somatic involvement	Anti-Hu/ANNA-1	SCLC	Pancreas, bladder, rectum, prostate, thymus, Hodgkin's disease
Lambert–Eaton myasthenic syndrome	Proximal weakness improves with exercise, abnormal repetitive nerve stimulation test	Anti-VGCC, ganglionic acetylcholine receptor	SCLS	Breast, GIT, GU tract, prostate, gallbladder, lymphosarcoma

ANNA-1, antineuronal nuclear antibody; EKG, electrocardiogram; GIT, gastrointestinal tract; GU, genitourinary; PNS, paraneoplastic neurologic syndrome; SCLC, small cell lung cancer; VGCC, voltage-gated calcium channel; VGKC, voltage-gated potassium channel.

TABLE 105.3 Algorithm

Autonomic symptoms with or without
Somatic neurologic symptoms
↓
Neurological examination
Brain MRI with contrast
CSF examination, nerve conduction studies
Autonomic evaluation
↓
Autonomic dysfunction with a distinguishing feature (i.e., intestinal pseudoobstruction in patients with enteric neuropathy)
↓
Exclude other causes with similar presentation
Using appropriate laboratory tests
Obtain antibody/antibodies titers against the most frequent tumor/tumors
↓
If serology positive, work-up for commonly
Suspected tumor. If serology negative,
↓
Screen for others tumors
↓
If work-up negative, longitudinal follow-up and repeat studies

hypotension, dry mouth, urinary retention, and constipation (Table 105.3). Occurrence of sleep apnea, pseudomyotonia, myokymia, pseudoobstruction of bowels, or progressive proprioceptive deficit should strengthen this suspicion. The diagnosis is made by exclusion of other causes of autonomic dysfunction, by electrophysiologic studies in patients with neuromyotonia or suspected LEMS, and by serologic studies indicating the presence of Anti-Hu/ANNA-1, enteric neuronal antibodies, and/or ganglionic acetylcholine receptor autoantibodies. These antibodies constitute a diagnostic tool and may suggest the likely location of the neoplasm, but their pathogenetic role (except in LEMS and Morvan syndrome) remains unclear. These antibodies may also serve as markers of antigen expression in tumors. Because tumors producing paraneoplastic manifestations are usually small, a diligent search with appropriate tests is mandatory. Close longitudinal follow-up and repeat studies may be necessary to diagnose the tumor.

TREATMENT

A proper diagnosis can spare the patients unnecessary surgery in cases of pseudoobstruction of the bowels. Treatment may be directed at the tumor, the antibodies, and the symptoms. An early surgical and cytotoxic reduction of the tumor may diminish autonomic dysfunction in some patients. Use of steroids, plasmapheresis, intravenous immunoglobulin, or immunosuppression with cyclophosphamide to reduce the antibody may provide benefit. For example, plasma exchange results in clinical and electrophysiologic improvements in patients with LEMS or Morvan syndrome. The patients with LEMS show symptomatic benefit from drugs such as guanidine and 3,4-diaminopyridine, which enhance cholinergic function. Symptomatic improvement of orthostatic hypotension with fludrocortisone, dry mouth with artificial saliva, neoplastic fever with naproxen, etc., can symptomatically improve the quality of life.

References

1. Khurana, R. K. 2000. Neoplasia and the autonomic nervous system. In *Handbook of clinical neurology: The autonomic nervous system. Part II. Vol 75,* ed. O. Appenzeller, 527–549. Amsterdam: Elsevier Science BV.
2. Khurana, R. K. 1994. Cholinergic dysfunction in Shy-Drager syndrome: Effect of the parasympathetomimetic agent, bethanechol. *Clin. Auton. Res.* 4:5–13.
3. Liguori, R., A. Vincent, L. Clover, P. Avoni, G. Plazzi, P. Cortelli, A. Baruzzi, T. Carey, P. Gambetti, E. Lugaresi, and P. Montagna. 2001. Morvan's syndrome: Peripheral and central nervous system and cardiac involvement with antibodies to voltage-gated potassium channels. *Brain* 124:2417–2426.
4. Hart, I. K. 2000. Acquired neuromyotonia: A new antibody-mediated neuronal potassium channelopathy. *Am. J. Med. Sci.* 319(4):209–216.
5. Dalmau, J., F. Graus, M. K. Rosenblum, and J. B. Posner. 1992. Anti-Hu associated paraneoplastic encephalomyelitis/sensory neuronopathy. A clinical study of 71 patients. *Medicine (Baltimore)* 71:59–72.
6. Lennon, V. A., D. F. Sas, M. F. Busk, B. Scheithauer, J.-R. Malagelada, M. Camilleri, and L. J. Miller. 1991. Enteric neuronal antibodies in pseudoobstruction with small-cell lung carcinoma. *Gastroenterology* 100:137–142.
7. Vernino, S., P. A. Low, F. D. Fealey, J. D. Steward, G. Farrugia, and V. A. Lennon. 2000. Autoantibodies to ganglionic acetylcholine receptors in autoimmune autonomic neuropathies. *N. Engl. J. Med.* 343: 847–855.

106

Panic Disorder

Murray Esler
Baker Medical Research Institute
Melbourne, Australia

Marlies Alvarenga
Department of General Practice
Monash University
Melbourne, Australia

David Kaye
Baker Medical Research Institute
Melbourne, Australia

Gavin Lambert
Baker Medical Research Institute
Melbourne, Australia

Jane Thompson
Baker Medical Research Institute
Melbourne, Australia

Jacqui Hastings
Baker Medical Research Institute
Melbourne, Australia

Rosemary Schwarz
Royal Women's Hospital
Melbourne, Australia

Margaret Morris
Department of Pharmacology
Melbourne University
Melbourne, Australia

Jeff Richards
Department of General Practice
Monash University
Melbourne, Australia

Some people are subject to episodes of recurring, often inexplicable anxiety. These attacks typically are unpleasant and are accompanied by physical symptoms such as sweating, palpitations, tremor, and a sensation of suffocation. There may be a precipitating cause, such as being in a confining space (as in claustrophobia) or in public places (as in agoraphobia), but in many cases the occurrence of the panic attacks is unexpected. Recurring attacks over a period of months, or in many cases years, forms the basis for the diagnosis of panic disorder [1]. This is a distressing and often very restricting condition, and it can lead to social avoidance behavior in some cases so extreme that the affected individuals never leave their home.

Until recently, it has been thought that although panic disorder was distressing and disabling, it did not constitute a risk to life. Affected individuals often fear that they have heart disease, because of the nature of their symptoms, but have been reassured that this is not the case. Understanding autonomic nervous system responses during a panic attack has been seen as relevant clinically, because this might provide a rational basis for understanding the symptoms, and through this, for facilitating treatment, which can be based in part on patient self-knowledge, as with cognitive behavior therapy [2].

Epidemiologic studies, however, indicate that there is an increased risk for myocardial infarction and sudden death in patients with panic disorder [3, 4]. Although this is a significantly increased risk, it is, of course, still small in individual sufferers, and applies not only in men who may be of such an age that unrecognized underlying coronary artery disease may be present, but also in premenopausal women with low coronary risk. The cause is not known, but possibly involves activation of the sympathetic nerves of the heart, predisposing to disturbances of cardiac rhythm and possibly coronary artery spasm. Accordingly, studying the mediating autonomic mechanisms of cardiac risk in patients with panic disorder is pertinent, both in terms of devising strategies for primary heart attack prevention in them [5, 6] and, in a broader context, for exploring the larger issue of the ways by which mental stress might contribute to cardiac risk [7].

RESTING SYMPATHETIC NERVOUS SYSTEM FUNCTION IN PANIC DISORDER

Sympathetic Nervous Activity and Epinephrine Secretion Rates

Sympathetic nerve firing rates measured directly by microneurography, in the sympathetic outflow to the skeletal muscle vasculature, and rates of norepinephrine spillover from the sympathetic nerves of the whole body are normal in untreated, resting patients with panic disorder, as is the spillover of norepinephrine measured selectively for the sympathetic nerves of the heart [5]. Similarly, adrenal medullary secretion of epinephrine, measured by isotope dilution, typically is normal [5].

Epinephrine Cotransmission in Sympathetic Nerves

Release of epinephrine from the sympathetic nerves of the heart, as an accessory neurotransmitter, has been demonstrated in patients with panic disorder (Fig. 106.1). Sympathetic nerves have the capacity to extract circulating

Panic Disorder: Epinephrine release from the sympathetic nerves of the heart

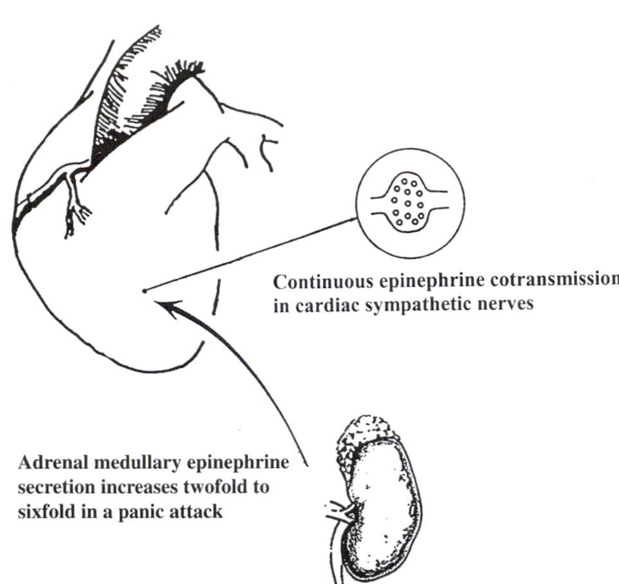

FIGURE 106.1 Adrenal medullary secretion of epinephrine increased twofold to sixfold during a panic attack. Uptake of epinephrine from plasma into the sympathetic nerves of the heart during epinephrine surges increases the neuronal epinephrine stores, leading to continuous release of epinephrine, as a sympathetic cotransmitter.

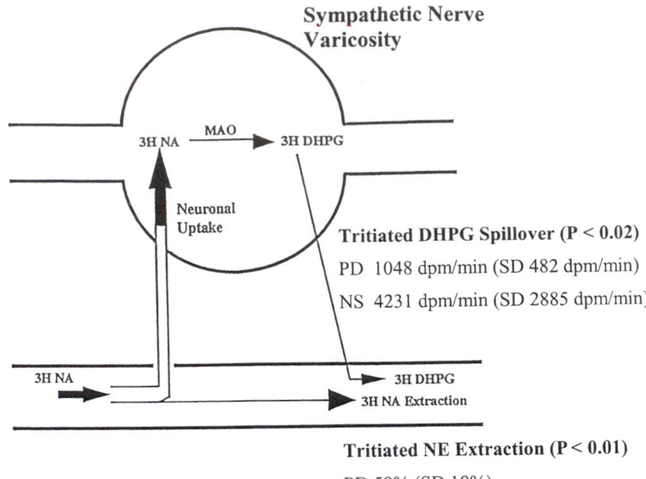

FIGURE 106.2 Representation of transcardiac processing of tritiated norepinephrine (3H NE). The majority of titrated norepinephrine is removed from plasma through a clearance mechanism involving neuronal uptake by sympathetic nerves. Within sympathetic nerves, 3H NE is metabolized to tritiated 3,4-dihydroxyphenylglycol (3H DHPG) by monoamine oxidase (MAO), with some subsequent release into the venous circulation. Tritiated norepinephrine uptake by the heart was reduced in 10 patients with panic disorder (PD), 59% (SD 19%) compared with 82% (SD 5%) in healthy subjects (NS) ($P < 0.01$). In parallel, release of tritiated DHPG into the coronary sinus venous drainage of the heart was lower, 1048 dpm/min (SD 482 dpm/min), than in healthy subjects, 4231 dpm/min (SD 2885 dpm/min) ($P < 0.02$). This provides strong phenotypic evidence of impaired neuronal norepinephrine reuptake in panic disorder.

epinephrine from plasma [8]. During the surges of epinephrine secretion accompanying panic attacks, this process loads the sympathetic neuronal vesicles with epinephrine, which is continuously coreleased with norepinephrine in the interim periods between attacks (see Fig. 106.1) [5].

Reduction in Neuronal Norepinephrine Reuptake by Sympathetic Nerves

Each pulse of the sympathetic neural signal is terminated in tissues primarily by reuptake of the released norepinephrine into the sympathetic varicosity through the norepinephrine transporter [8]. The processes of neuronal reuptake of norepinephrine can be quantified in humans during the course of an infusion of tritiated norepinephrine by analysis of the disposition and intraneuronal processing of the tracer [8] (Fig. 106.2). In untreated patients with panic disorder, there is evidence that the process of neuronal reuptake of norepinephrine is impaired (see Fig. 106.2). Such an abnormality, possibly genetic in nature [9], would be expected to magnify sympathetically mediated responses, particularly in the heart, where norepinephrine inactivation is so dependent on neuronal reuptake [8], causing sensitization to symptom development and predisposition to the development of panic disorder.

AUTONOMIC NERVOUS CHANGES DURING A PANIC ATTACK

Heart rate and blood pressure increase during a panic attack, primarily because of sympathetic nervous system activation and adrenal medullary secretion of epinephrine [5] (Figs. 106.1 and 106.3).

Sympathetic Nerve Firing and Secretion of Epinephrine

When recorded directly by microneurography, the size of sympathetic bursts increases remarkably during a panic attack, without any increase in firing rate [5] (see Fig. 106.3), presumably by recruitment of additional firing fibers. This response is qualitatively different from that seen during laboratory mental stress with stimuli such as difficult mental arithmetic, where muscle sympathetic nerve activity increases little, if at all [8]. During a panic attack, the secretion of epinephrine increases twofold to sixfold [5].

PANIC ATTACKS

Sympathetic Nervous Activation

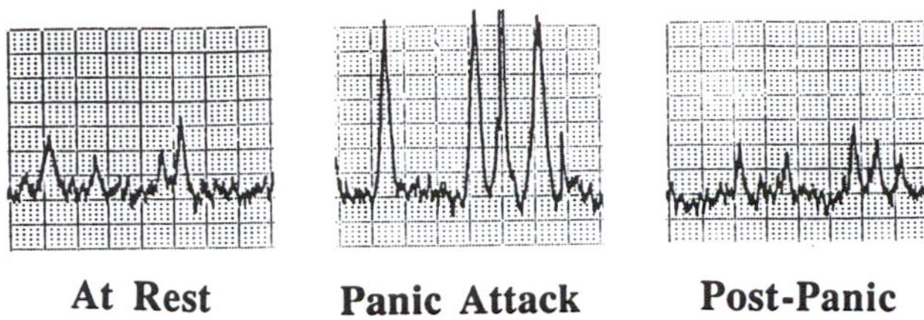

Cardiac Release of NPY

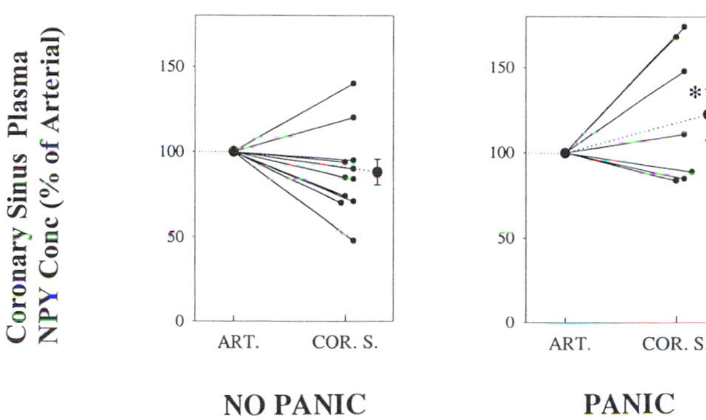

FIGURE 106.3 **Top**, Multifiber sympathetic nerve firing in the sympathetic outflow to the skeletal muscle vasculature in a patient with panic disorder, measured by clinical microneurography. During a panic attack, there was a large increase in the amplitude of sympathetic "bursts," without any increase in burst frequency. **Bottom**, The arterial and coronary sinus concentration of the sympathetic cotransmitter, neuropeptide Y (NPY), is shown in patients with panic disorder at rest and during a panic attack. There was no net release of NPY from the sympathetic nerves of the heart into the coronary sinus at baseline, but a panic attack evoked measurable release of the sympathetic cotransmitter. $*P < 0.05$.

Release of Neuropeptide Y

With the pronounced activation of the cardiac sympathetic outflow occurring during a panic attack, neuropeptide Y (NPY) is coreleased from the cardiac sympathetic nerves and appears in measurable quantities in coronary sinus venous blood (see Fig. 106.3).

MEDIATING AUTONOMIC MECHANISMS OF CARDIAC RISK DURING A PANIC ATTACK

Epidemiologic studies indicate that there is an increased risk for sudden death and myocardial infarction in patients with panic disorder (a threefold to sixfold increase) [3, 4]. Our own extensive clinical experience with the cardiologic management of patients with panic disorder has provided case material encompassing the range of cardiac complications that occur. Those patients with typical, severe anginal chest pain during panic attacks, who are in the minority, appear to be at cardiac risk. During panic attacks in such patients, we have documented various triggered cardiac arrhythmias (Fig. 106.4), recurrent emergency room attendances with angina and electrocardiogram changes of ischemia [6], coronary artery spasm during panic attacks occurring at the time of coronary angiography (see Fig. 106.4), and myocardial infarction associated with coronary spasm and thrombosis [6]. Our research findings suggest that release of epinephrine as a cotransmitter from cardiac sympathetic nerves and activation of the sympathetic nervous system during panic attacks may be mediating mechanisms.

Panic Disorder: Coronary Spasm

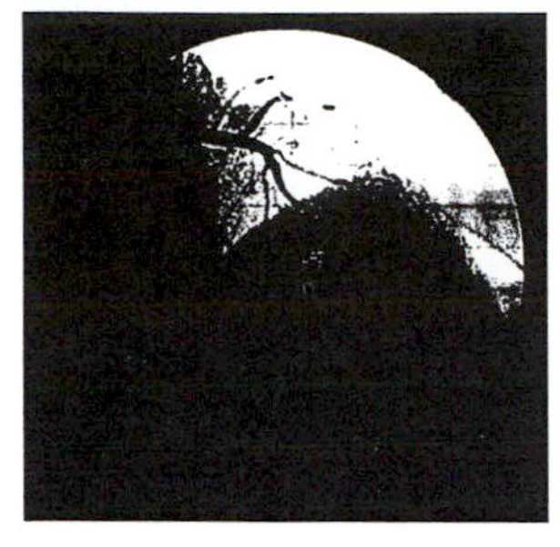

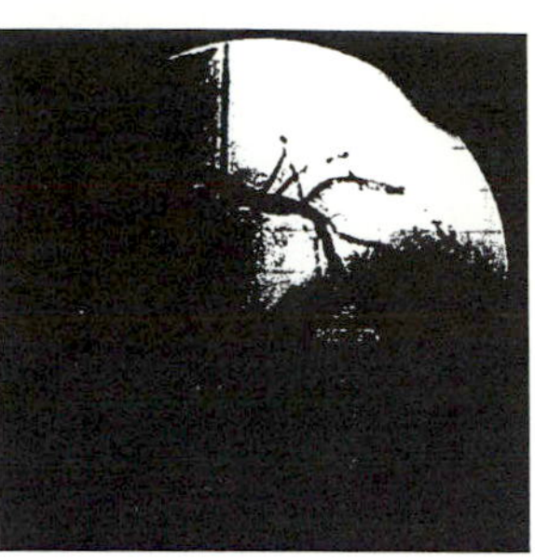

LAD Coronary Spasm   Post GTN

Panic Disorder: Atrial Fibrillation

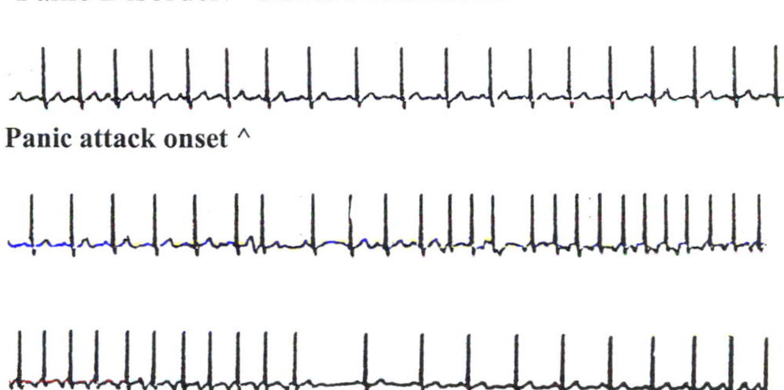

FIGURE 106.4 **Top**, Coronary angiograms in a patient with panic disorder, performed because of recurrent angina. During a panic attack occurring during angiography, spasm occurred in the left anterior descending coronary artery (LAD). The arterial spasm was reversed by administration of glyceryl trinitrate (GTN). **Bottom**, Atrial fibrillation precipitated by a panic attack.

In this context, release of NPY from the sympathetic nerves of the heart into the coronary sinus during the sympathetic activation accompanying panic attacks is an intriguing finding, given the capacity of NPY to cause coronary artery spasm [10]. A better understanding of the mechanism of coronary artery spasm in panic disorder would facilitate therapeutic intervention. Currently, we treat patients with panic disorder and clinical evidence of coronary spasm with drugs and other measures aimed at preventing or minimizing their panic attacks, a dihydropyridine calcium channel blocker as a nonspecific antispasm measure and low-dose aspirin as prophylaxis against coronary thrombosis during spasm [6]. NPY antagonists are not yet available for clinical testing.

References

1. American Psychiatric Association. 1994. *Diagnostic and Statistical Manual of Mental Disorders, IV,* 4th ed. Washington, DC: American Psychiatric Association.
2. Richards, J. C., N. Bickley, C. S. Rees, and P. Beros. 1997. An investigation of the mechanisms of change in the cognitive behavioural treatment of panic disorder. *Health Perspect.* 1:35–44.
3. Kawachi, I., D. Sparrow, P. S. Vokanas, and S. T. Weiss. 1994. Symptoms of anxiety and coronary heart disease: The normative aging study. *Circulation* 90:2225–2229.
4. Kawachi, I., G. A. Colditz, A. Ascherio, E. B. Rimm, E. Giovannucci, M. J. Stampfer, and W. C. Willett. 1994. Prospective study of phobic anxiety and risk of coronary heart disease in men. *Circulation* 89:1992–1997.
5. Wilkinson, D. J. C., J. M. Thompson, G. W. Lambert, G. L. Jennings, R. G. Schwarz, D. Jefferys, A. G. Turner, and M. D. Esler. 1998. Sympathetic activity in patients with panic disorder at rest, under laboratory mental stress and during panic attacks. *Arch. Gen. Psychiatry* 55:511–520.
6. Mansour, V. M., D. J. C. Wilkinson, G. L. Jennings, R. G. Schwarz, J. M. Thompson, and M. D. Esler. 1998. Panic disorder: Coronary spasm as a basis for coronary risk? *Med. J. Aust.* 168:390–392.
7. Esler, M. D. 1998. Mental stress, panic disorder and the heart. *Stress Med.* 14:237–243.
8. Esler, M., G. Jennings, G. Lambert, I. Meredith, M. Horne, and G. Eisenhofer. 1990. Overflow of catecholamine neurotransmitters to the circulation: Source, fate and functions. *Physiol. Rev.* 70:963–985.
9. Shannon, J. R., N. L. Flattem, J. Jordan, G. Jacob, B. K. Black, I. Biaggioni, R. D. Blakely, and D. Robertson. 2000. Orthostatic intolerance and tachycardia associated with norepinephrine-transporter deficiency. *N. Engl. J. Med.* 342:541–549.
10. Hass, M. 1998. Neuropeptide Y: A cardiac sympathetic cotransmitter? In *Catecholamines—bridging basic science with clinical medicine*, ed. D. S. Goldstein and R. McCarthy, 129–132. San Diego: Academic Press.

P A R T XIII

MANAGEMENT OF AUTONOMIC DISORDERS

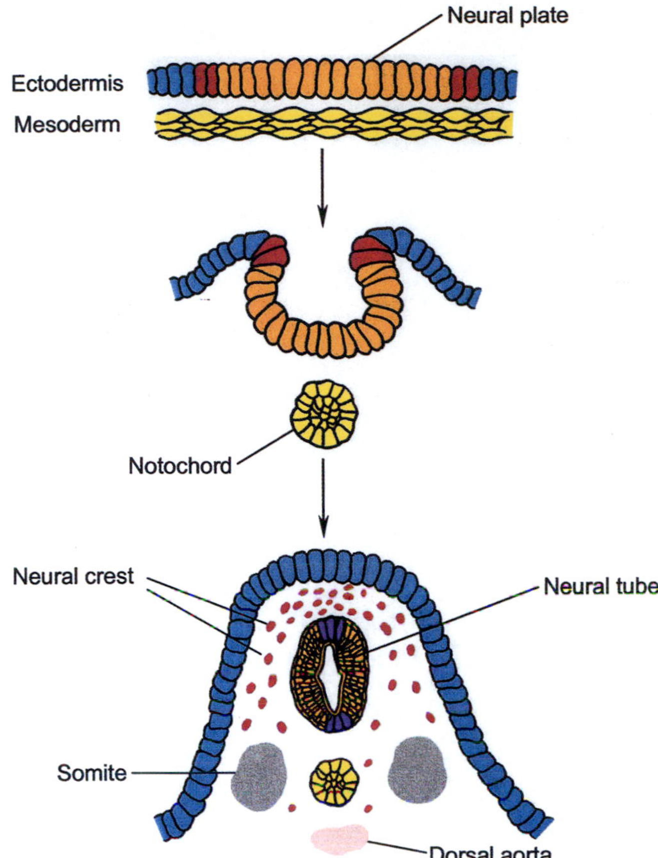

FIGURE 2.1 All cell types of the autonomic nervous system (ANS) are derived from neural crest cells. Neural crest cells are formed at the dorsal neural tube and migrate along diverse routes. Depending on their specific routes and interactions with the target tissues, they differentiate into a variety of cell types including pigment cells, different types of neurons and glia of the ANS, and parts of the adrenal gland.

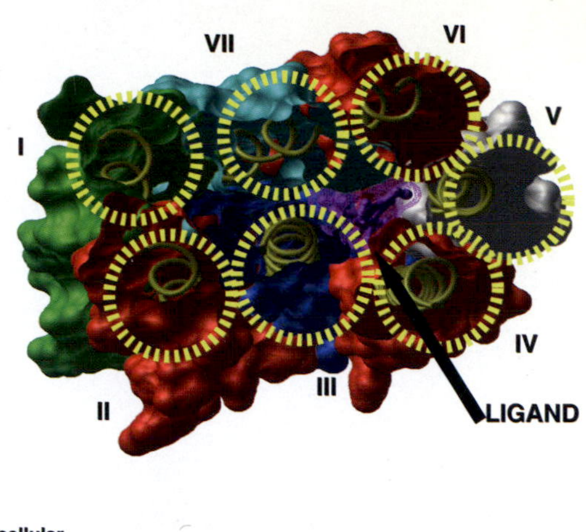

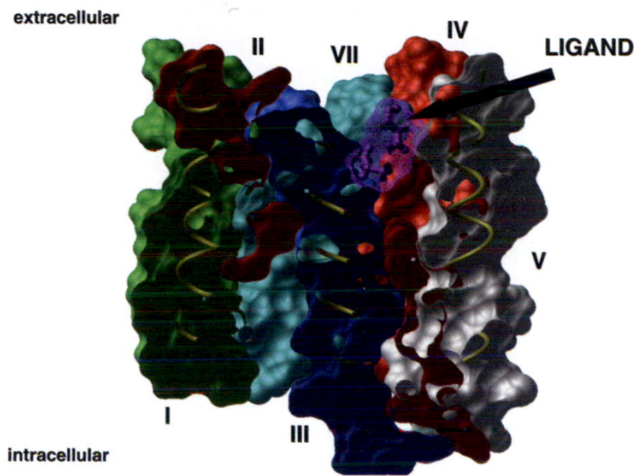

FIGURE 11.2 Cutaway three-dimensional model of the hamster α_{1B}-AR, showing the seven α-helical transmembrane domains indicated by *Roman numerals* and by *dashed circles* and backbone ribbons (*yellow corkscrews*), with the catecholamine agonist, epinephrine (*magenta ball and stick model with surrounding dot surface*), modeled in its binding pocket. **Top**, Top view (looking down onto the plane of the membrane). **Bottom**, Side view. This model was kindly provided by Dr. J. Novotny.

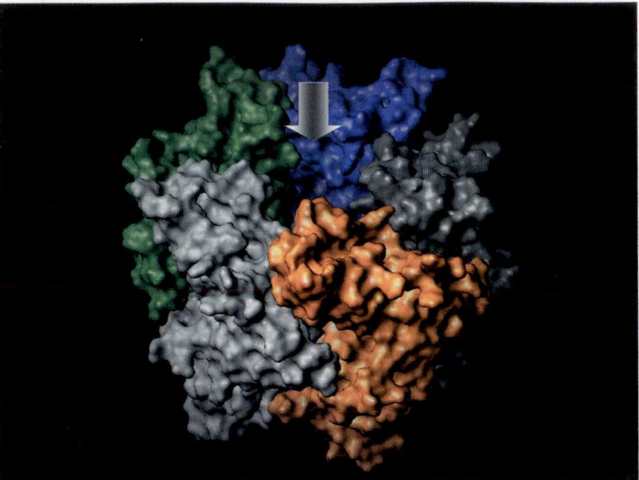

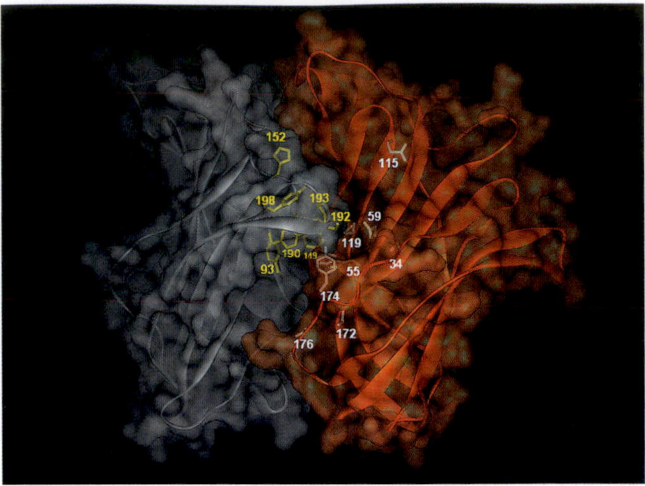

FIGURE 17.3 X-ray crystallographic structure of the acetylcholine binding protein. The structure was produced from crystallographic coordinates of Sixma and colleagues [4, 5]. Surfaces are represented as Connolly surfaces. **Left**, Colors are used to delineate the subunit interfaces in the homomeric pentamer. The vestibule on the extracellular surface that represents the entry to the internal channel in the receptor is shown by the *arrow*. **Right**, A single subunit interface. Note the residues that have been found to be determinants in the binding of agonists and alkaloid and peptidic antagonists to the receptor. Hence, the numbers (yellow, α subunit; white, γ subunit) delineate the probable binding surface(s) for large and small antagonists. These residues come from seven distinct segments of amino acid sequence in the subunit, as determined from extensive mutagenesis and labeling studies [6].

FIGURE 18.1 Mechanism of acetylcholine (ACh) hydrolysis by acetylcholinesterase (AChE). AChE contains a "catalyptic triad" in the active site formed by a serine (Ser$_{200}$), a histidine (His$_{440}$), and a glutamic acid (Glu$_{327}$). Ser$_{200}$ activated by His$_{440}$ and Glu$_{327}$ forms a nucleophilic attack on the carbonyl group of ACh (step 1) and the quaternary transition state (step 2) decomposes, resulting in the intermediate acetyl enzyme (step 3). Hydrolysis of the acetyl enzyme reactivates the enzyme.

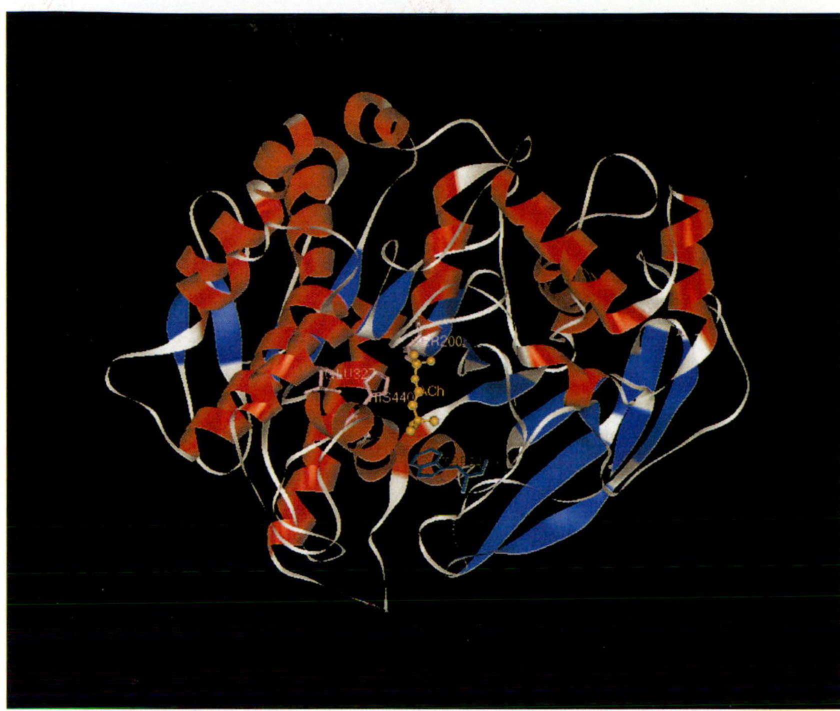

FIGURE 18.2 Ribbon scheme of the three-dimensional structure of acetylcholinesterase (AChE) from *Torpedo californica. Light blue arrows* represent β-strands, and *red coils* represent α-helices. The side chains of the catalytic triad (Ser_{200}, His_{440}, and Glu $_{327}$) and the peripheral site (Trp_{84}) in the active site gorge are indicated as stick figures. Acetylcholine (ACh) docked manually is represented in *yellow* as ball stick figure. Source: PDB ID: 2ACE (Sussman et al. 1991).

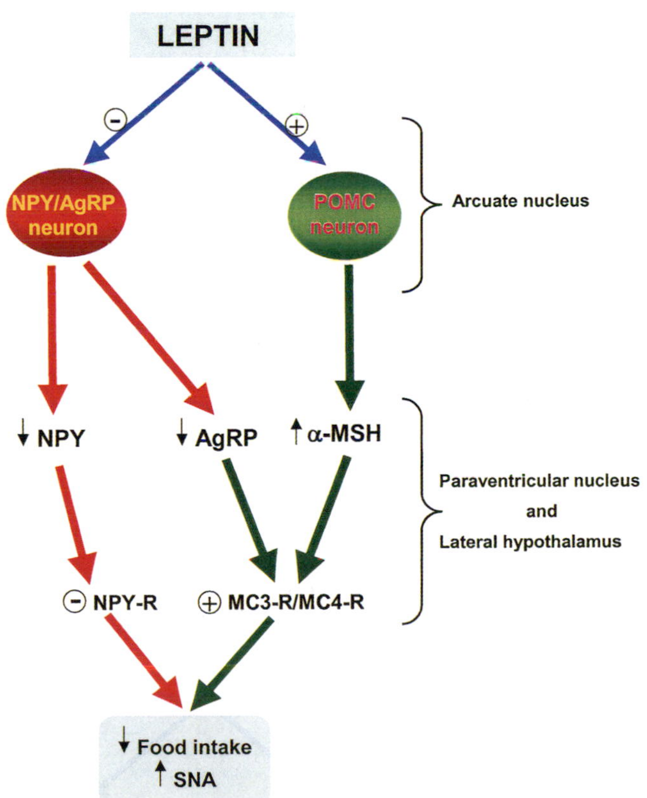

FIGURE 21.3 Interaction of leptin with neuropeptide Y (NPY)/agouti-related protein (AgRP)- and proopiomelanocortin (POMC)-containing neurons in the hypothalamic arcuate nucleus. Increased action of leptin inhibits the NPY/AgRP anabolic pathway and stimulates the POMC catabolic pathway, leading to decrease in food intake and increase in sympathetic nerve activity (SNA). MC3-R, melanocortin-3 receptor; MC4-R, melanocortin-4 receptor; α-MSH, α-melanocyte–stimulating hormone.

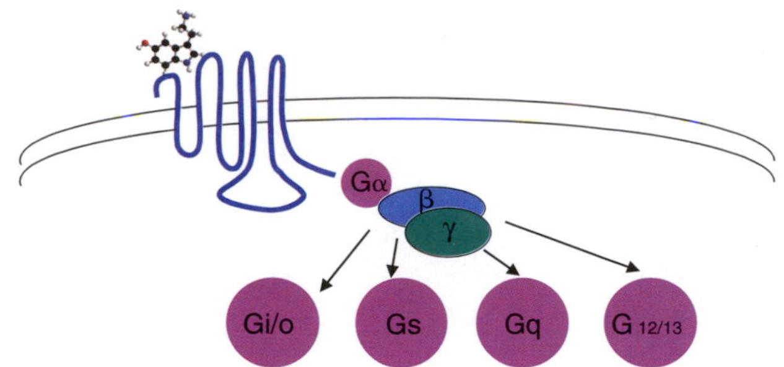

FIGURE 23.3 Serotonin (5-hydroxytryptamine [5-HT]) receptors couple to multiple G proteins. G proteins are classified on the basis of their α subunits. 5-HT receptors have been definitively shown to couple to four different families of G proteins.

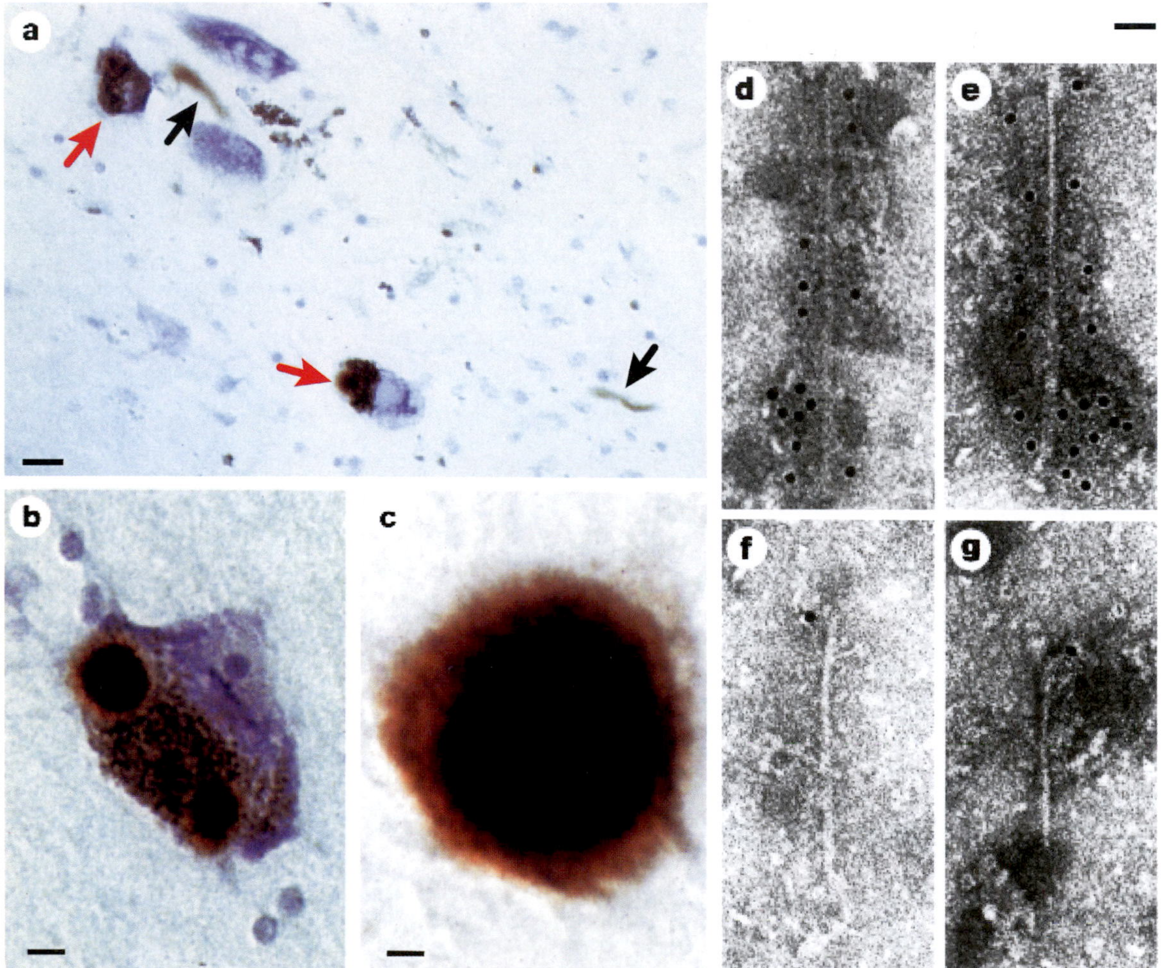

FIGURE 54.1 The α-synuclein pathology of Parkinson's disease. Lewy bodies and Lewy neurites in the substantia nigra and several other brain regions define Parkinson's disease at a neuropathologic level. These entities are shown here at the light (**A–C**) and electron microscopic (**D–G**) levels, labeled by α-synuclein antibodies. **A**, Two pigmented nerve cells, each containing an α-synuclein–positive Lewy body (*red arrows*). Lewy neurites (*black arrows*) also are immunopositive. Scale bar = 20 µm. **B**, Pigmented nerve cell with two α-synuclein–positive Lewy bodies. Scale bar = 8 µm. **C**, α-Synuclein–positive extracellular Lewy body. Scale bar = 4 µm. **D–G**, Isolated filaments from the substantia nigra of patients with Parkinson's disease are decorated with an antibody directed against the carboxyl-terminal (**D** and **E**) or the amino-terminal (**F** and **G**) region of α-synuclein. The gold particles conjugated to the second antibody appear as *black dots*. Note the uniform decoration in **D** and **E**, and the labeling of only one filament end in **F** and **G**. Scale bar (For D–G) = 100 nm.

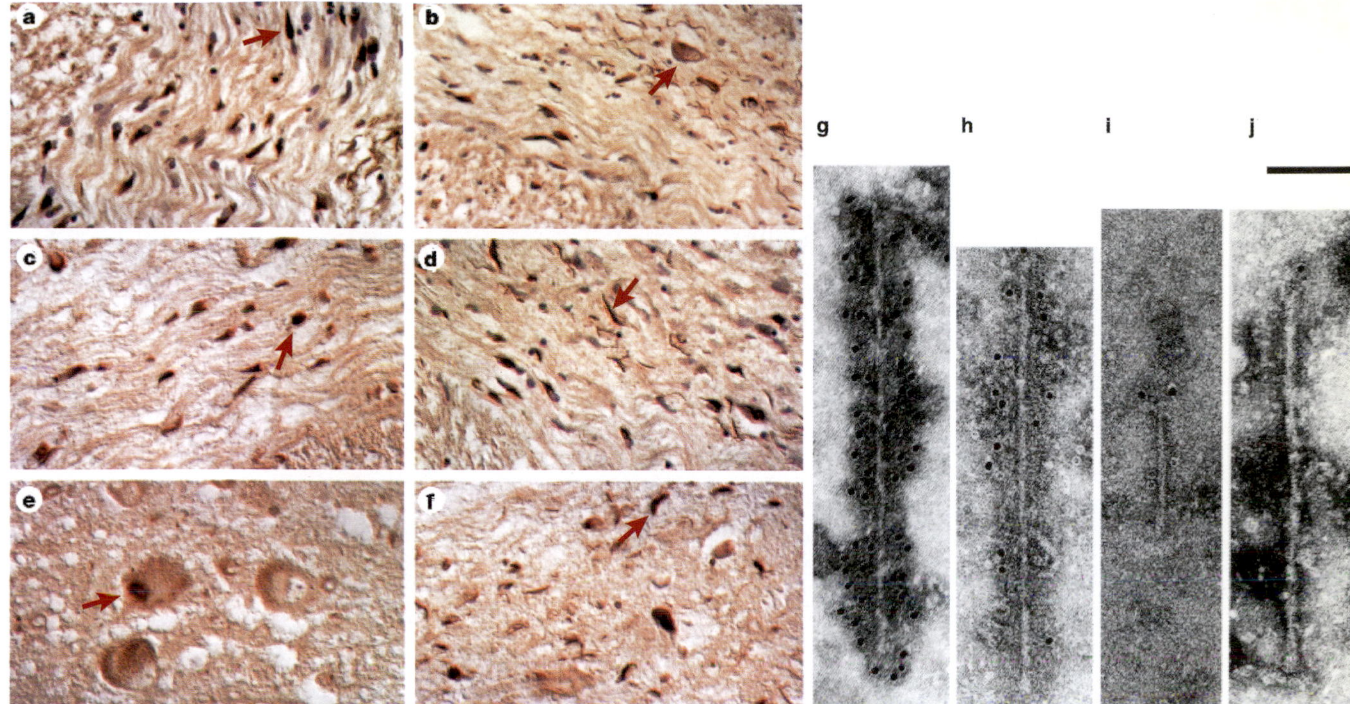

FIGURE 54.2 The α-synuclein pathology of multiple system atrophy. Glial cytoplasmic inclusions in several brain regions define multiple system atrophy at a neuropathologic level. Similar inclusions also are present in the nucleus of some glial cells, the cytoplasm and nucleus of some nerve cells, and in nerve cell processes. Here, these entities are shown at the light (**A–F**) and electron microscopic (**G–J**) levels, labeled by α-synuclein antibodies. **A–D**, α-Synuclein–immunoreactive oligodendrocytes and nerve cells in white matter of pons (**A**, **B**, and **D**) and cerebellum (**C**). **E** and **F**, α-Synuclein–immunoreactive oligodendrocytes and nerve cells in gray matter of pons (**E**) and frontal cortex (**F**). *Arrows* identify examples of each of the characteristic lesions stained for α-synuclein: cytoplasmic oligodendroglial inclusions (**A** and **F**), cytoplasmic nerve cell inclusions (**B**), nuclear oligodendroglial inclusion (**C**), neuropil threads (**D**), and nuclear nerve cell inclusion (**E**). Scale bars = 33 μm (**E**); 50 μm (**A–D**, **F**). **G–J**, Isolated filaments from the frontal cortex and cerebellum of patients with multiple system atrophy are decorated with an antibody directed against the carboxyl-terminal (**G** and **H**) or the amino-terminal (**I** and **J**) region of α-synuclein. The gold particles conjugated to the second antibody appear as *black dots*. Note the uniform decoration in **G** and **H**, and the labeling of only one filament end in **I** and **J**. A "twisted" filament is shown in **G**, whereas **H** shows a "straight" filament. Scale bar = 100 nm.

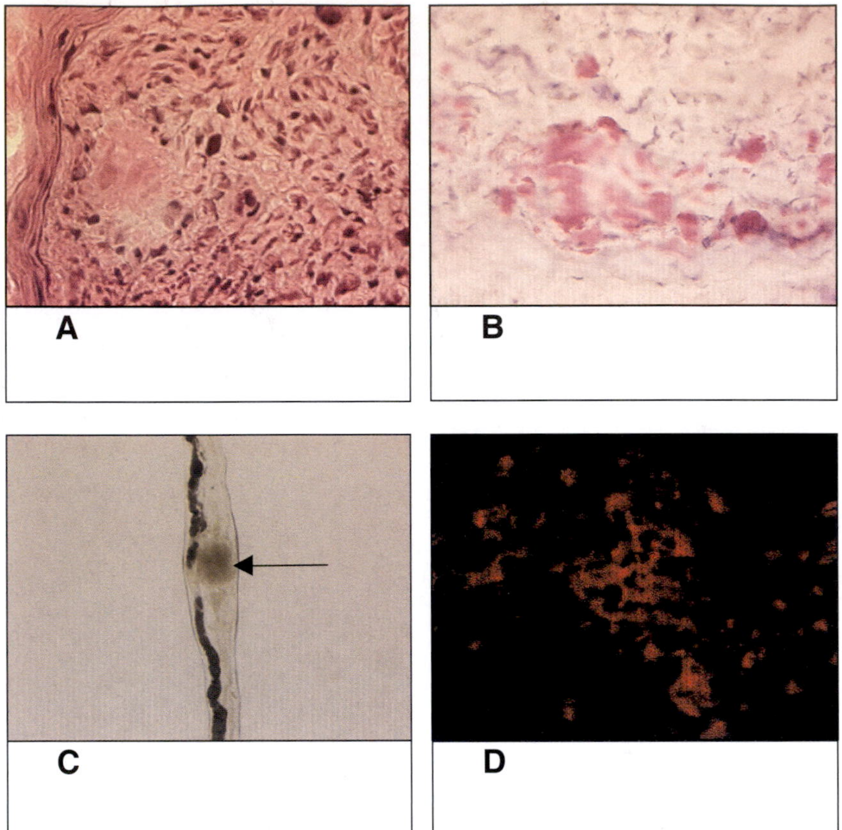

FIGURE 86.1 Amyloid deposits. **A**, Hematoxylin and eosin staining. **B**, Crystal violet. **C**, Teased nerve preparation. **D**, Congo red under fluorescence.

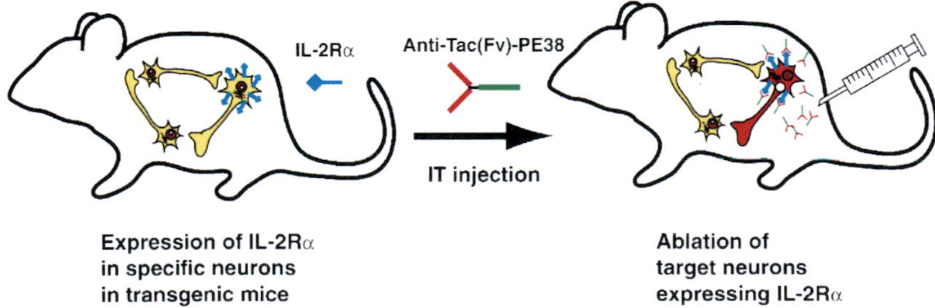

FIGURE 119.1 Strategy for immunotoxin-mediated cell targeting. Human interleukin-2 receptor α-subunit (IL-2Rα) is expressed in specific cell types in transgenic mice under the control of an appropriate tissue-specific gene promoter. Adult transgenic mice are treated with anti-Tac-based immunotoxin (IT), and the cells bearing the receptor are disrupted by the cytotoxic activity of the IT.

107 Hypoglycemic Associated Autonomic Dysfunction

Darleen A. Sandoval
Division of Diabetes, Endocrinology, and Metabolism
Vanderbilt University
Nashville, Tennessee

Stephen N. Davis
Division of Diabetes, Endocrinology, and Metabolism
Department of Medicine
Vanderbilt University School of Medicine and
Nashville Veterans Affairs Medical Center
Nashville, Tennessee

INTRODUCTION

The hallmark study, the Diabetes Control and Complications Trial, found that type 1 diabetes mellitus (DM) patients who maintained glucose levels close to the normal range slowed the progression or prevented microvascular diabetes complications (e.g. nephropathy, retinopathy and neuropathy [1]. Unfortunately, along with these important benefits came a threefold greater incidence of severe hypoglycemia (blood sugar < 2.9 mM; 50 mg/dl) [2]. Hypoglycemia impairs cognitive function, which may contribute to an increase in life threatening accidents, and if untreated can lead to seizures, coma and even death. Under normal circumstances, autonomic and neuroendocrine systems (termed counterregulatory mechanisms) are able to prevent hypoglycemia and maintain glucose homeostasis. Dysfunction in either of these counterregulatory systems would lead to serious inabilities in maintaining glucose levels. This chapter discusses how dysfunction of the autonomic nervous system (ANS) contributes to an increase in the incidence of hypoglycemia in type 1 DM.

Maintenance of Glucose Homeostasis

The autonomic nervous system (ANS) plays an integral role in defending the body against hypoglycemia. Both sympathetic and parasympathetic branches of the ANS are activated during hypoglycemia. Sympathetic nervous system (SNS) activation leads to increased circulating levels of norepinephrine and epinephrine. This increase in SNS drive leads to increases in heart rate, blood pressure, fat metabolism and glucose output by the liver and kidney. Importantly, glucose utilization by peripheral tissues (e.g. muscle) is significantly reduced by SNS activation. Increased SNS drive and/or increased plasma epinephrine levels can increase glucagon secretion from the pancreas. Glucagon is an important fast acting mediator of glucose output by the liver and is thus an important defender of glucose homeostasis. Together epinephrine (via the ANS) and glucagon are the primary factors that defend against hypoglycemia during physical stress.

However, after approximately five years disease duration, type 1 DM patients, lose the ability to release glucagon in response to hypoglycemia. Therefore, type 1 DM patients become dependent on autonomic counterregulatory responses to prevent hypoglycemia.

Hypoglycemic Associated Autonomic Dysfunction

Unfortunately, repeated hypoglycemia, similar to that occurring with intensive glucose control, compromises ANS function during subsequent physiological stress. Heller and Cryer [3] provided the first comprehensive study illustrating this dysfunction. They showed that norepinephrine, epinephrine, pancreatic polypeptide (a plasma marker for the parasympathetic nervous system) and hypoglycemic symptoms initiated by the ANS were all substantially reduced one day after two episodes of antecedent hypoglycemia. Several other studies [4, 5, 6] including our own [7, 8, 9] have shown similar results in type 1 DM and non-diabetic subjects. In fact, type 2 DM patients have also been discovered to have reduced ANS responses during hypoglycemia [10]. Cryer described the acute reduction of the ANS responses in defending against recurrent hypoglycemia as hypoglycemia-associated autonomic failure [11]. We have coined the term hypoglycemic associated autonomic dysfunction (HAAD) both because it is acute (within hours, [8] and because it is reversible with strict avoidance of hypoglycemia [12, 13]. Importantly, these factors also distinguish HAAD from classical diabetic autonomic neuropathy, which occurs due to the effect of chronic hyperglycemia on autonomic neurons.

Frequency, Intensity and Duration of Antecedent Hypoglycemia

Understanding the frequency, intensity and duration of antecedent hypoglycemia necessary to induce HAAD is of considerable clinical importance. Two 90 minute antecedent bouts of hyperinsulinemic hypoglycemia (~2.9 mM; 50 mg/dl) causes an approximate 50% blunting of plasma catecholamine, pancreatic polypeptide and muscle sympathetic nerve activity during next day hypoglycemia [7, 9]. Interestingly, we have seen a similar effect within hours after the first exposure to hypoglycemia. Plasma epinephrine (~50%), norepinephrine (~33%), and pancreatic polypeptide (~50%) responses to afternoon hypoglycemia were blunted two hours after a single episode of morning hypoglycemia [8]. Thus, one episode of hypoglycemia of 2.9 mM (50 mg/dl) may be enough to induce HAAD and therefore increase the cycle of hypoglycemia in type 1 DM.

We have also investigated the depth and duration of antecedent hypoglycemia needed to induced HAAD [7, 9]. Two-90 min episodes of mild day 1 antecedent hypoglycemia (3.9 mM; 70 mg/dl) was enough to significantly blunt epinephrine and muscle sympathetic nerve activity while deeper levels of antecedent hypoglycemic (3.3 and 2.9 mM; 60 and 50 mg/dl) further and significantly blunted epinephrine, norepinephrine, and pancreatic polypeptide responses to next day hypoglycemia (~2.9 mM; 50 mg/dl) [9]. In addition, a minimal duration of antecedent hypoglycemia may induce HAAD. Two five-minute episodes of antecedent hypoglycemia at 2.9 mM (50 mg/dl) significantly blunted epinephrine and muscle sympathetic nerve activity by a similar extent as compared to two 90-minute episodes of equivalent hypoglycemia. Thus, it seems that minimal duration (~5 min) and frequency (one previous episode on the same day) are necessary for development of HAAD.

Exercise May Also Induce HAAD

Until recently it was thought that autonomic dysfunction could only be induced by hypoglycemia and was not general to other types of stress such as exercise [14]. However, data from our laboratory has demonstrated that two 90 minute antecedent bouts of hypoglycemia (2.9 mM; 50 mg/dl) significantly blunt plasma catecholamine and pancreatic polypeptide responses to subsequent moderate intensity exercise (~50% VO_{2max}) in healthy non-diabetic [15] and type 1 DM [16] subjects. Furthermore, we have found a reciprocal effect in that two 90-minute bouts of exercise blunt plasma catecholamine, pancreatic polypeptide, and muscle sympathetic nerve activity (Figure 1) responses to next day hypoglycemia in non-diabetics [17]. McGregor et al. [18] showed qualitatively similar results using a shorter duration (60 vs. 90 min) and higher intensity of exercise (70 vs. 50% VO_{2max}). Interestingly, we have also found that morning exercise (90 minutes at ~50% VO_{2max}) will not only increase insulin sensitivity but will also blunt plasma catecholamine and pancreatic polypeptide responses to subsequent afternoon exercise (90 minutes at ~50% VO_{2max}) occurring three hours later [16]. Thus, although exercise has many potential therapeutic benefits to type 1 DM patients (i.e. reductions in cardiovascular risk factors, weight maintenance, and stress relief), the combination of increased insulin sensitivity and blunted autonomic function may increase the incidence of hypoglycemia up to one day after a prolonged exercise bout. A summary graph of the effects of antecedent hypoglycemia on epinephrine and muscle sympathetic nerve activity on day 2 exercise, or antecedent exercise on responses to day 2 hypoglycemia are summarized in Figure 2. It remains unknown how duration and intensity of prior exercise impact these responses.

Mechanisms for HAAD

The cause for HAAD remains unknown at this time. Several mechanisms including antecedent elevations in lactate and ketone bodies [19] or cortisol [20, 21] have been implicated in causing HAAD. Infusion of lactate, reaching levels equivalent to that of intense exercise, and millimolar levels of betahydroxybutyrate, both reduced the catecholamine response to hyperinsulinemic induced hypoglycemia [19]. These substrates have been postulated to provide an alternative fuel to the brain leading to reduced sympathetic drive and thus may explain the incidence of HAAD. However, it should be noted that the levels achieved with these infusions are greater than levels typically seen during a hypoglycemic episode (~5 vs. 1.4 mM for lactate and ~1600 vs. 14 µM for betahydroxybutyrate). Thus, it remains unclear whether elevations of these substrates during antecedent hypoglycemia would be high enough to elicit HAAD.

Elevations in cortisol during antecedent hypoglycemia may be another mechanism by which HAAD occurs. Infusions of cortisol blunted norepinephrine synthesis and release to a similar extent as repeated immobilization stress in rats [22]. In humans, we have also found that antecedent infusion of cortisol during a hyperinsulinemic euglycemic clamp reduces plasma catecholamine, pancreatic polypep-

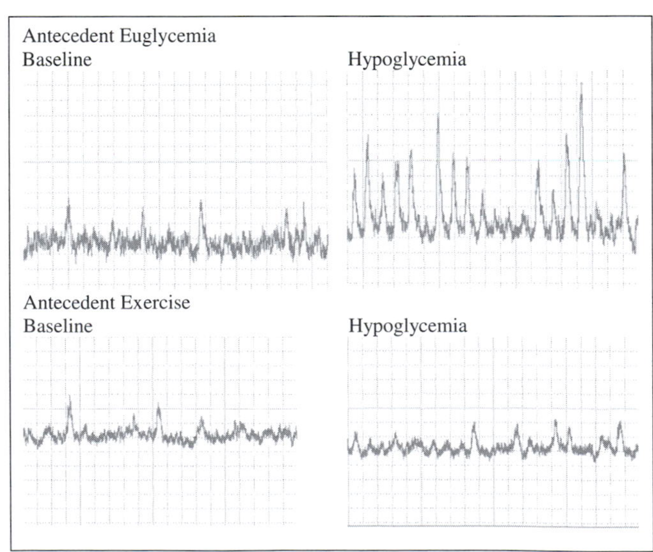

FIGURE 107.1 Changes in muscle sympathetic nerve activity from a representative type 1 DM patient during day 2 responses to hypoglycemia after prior euglycemia or 90 minutes of exercise at 50% VO_{2max}.

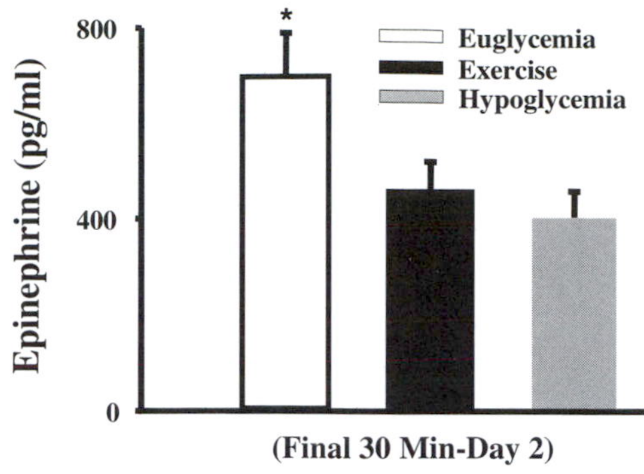

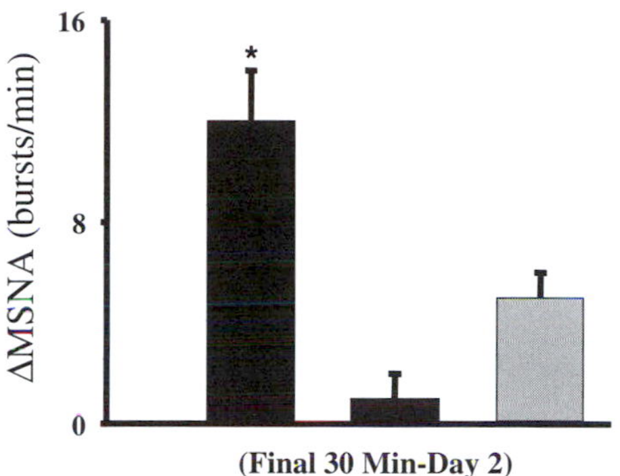

FIGURE 107.2 Day 2 responses of epinephrine and muscle sympathetic nerve activity to 2 hours of clamped hypoglycemia (50 mg/dl) or exercise (90 minutes at 50% VO_{2max}) after day 1 euglycemia, exercise or hypoglycemia, respectively. Reprinted with permission from the American Physiological Society (Galassetti, et al. 2001. Effect of antecedent prolonged exercise on subsequent counterregulatory responses to hypoglycemia. *Am. J. Physiol.* 280:E908–E917).

tide, and muscle sympathetic nerve responses to subsequent hypoglycemia [21]. In addition, Addison's patients, who are unable to release cortisol, have been found to have similar responses of plasma catecholamine, pancreatic polypeptide and muscle sympathetic nerve activity during repeated episodes of hypoglycemia [20]. More recently, McGregor et al. [23] infused ACTH to increase endogenous cortisol levels on day 1 and also saw blunted epinephrine, norepinephrine, and pancreatic polypeptide responses to day 2 hypoglycemia. These data strongly support a role for antecedent elevations of cortisol in causing HAAD during subsequent episodes of hypoglycemia.

Conclusions

Type 1 DM patients who tightly regulate their blood glucose levels can suffer from repeated episodes of hypoglycemia. Fear of hypoglycemia limits widespread implementation of this intensive glucose treatment. This fear may prevent patients from realizing the benefits of intensive glycemic control in reducing diabetes related complications such as retinopathy, nephropathy, and neuropathy. Although hyperinsulinemia clearly plays a role in the incidence of hypoglycemia, HAAD magnifies the incidence. In addition, despite the beneficial therapeutic effects of exercise, exercise may independently increase incidence of hypoglycemia through similarly blunted autonomic function. The cause of HAAD may be due to antecedent elevations of cortisol. Further research examining how cortisol may blunt the ANS responses to stress may aid in the development of interventions to reduce HAAD and thus remove a major obstacle to intensive glucose treatment in patients with DM.

References

1. The Diabetes Control and Complications Trial Research Group. 1993. The effect of intensive treatment of diabetes on the development and progression of long-term complications in insulin-dependent diabetes mellitus. *N. Engl. J. Med.* 329:977–986.
2. The Diabetes Control and Complications Trial Research Group. 1997. Hypoglycaemia in the diabetes control and complication trial. *Diabetes* 46:271–286.
3. Heller, S. R., and P. E. Cryer. 1991. Reduced neuroendocrine and symptomatic responses to subsequent hypoglycemia after one episode of hypoglycemia in nondiabetic humans. *Diabetes* 40:223–226.
4. Davis, M. R., and H. Shamoon. 1991. Counterregulatory adaptation to recurrent hypoglycemia in normal humans. *J. Clin. Endocrinol. Metab.* 73:995–1001.
5. Davis, M. R., and H. Shamoon. 1992. Impaired glucose disposal following mild hypoglycemia in nondiabetic and type 1 diabetic humans. *Metabolism* 41:216–223.
6. Widom, B., and D. Simonson. 1992. Intermittent hypoglycemia impairs glucose counterregulation. *Diabetes* 41:1597–1602.
7. Davis, S. N., S. Mann, P. Galassetti, R. A. Neill, D. Tate, A. C. Ertl, and F. Costa. 2000. Effects of differing durations of antecedent hypoglycemia on counterregulatory responses to subsequent hypoglycemia in normal humans. *Diabetes* 49:1897–1903.
8. Davis, S. N., and D. Tate. 2001. Effects of morning hypoglycemia on neuroendocrine and metabolic responses to subsequent afternoon hypoglycemia in normal man. *J. Clin. Endocrinol. Metab.* 86: 2043–2050.
9. Davis, S. N., C. Shavers, R. Mosqueda-Garcia, and F. Costa. 1997. Effects of differing antecedent hypoglycemia on subsequent counterregulation in normal humans. *Diabetes* 46:1328–1335.
10. Segel, S. A., D. S. Paramore, and P. E. Cryer. 2002. Hypoglycemia-associated autonomic failure in advanced type 2 diabetes. *Diabetes* 51:724–733.
11. Cryer, P. E. 1992. Iatrogenic hypoglycemia as a cause of hypoglycemia-associated autonomic failure in IDDM. *Diabetes* 41: 255–260.
12. Fanelli, C., L. Epifano, A. M. Rambotti, S. Pampanelli, A. Di Vincenzo, F. Modarelli, M. Lepore, B. Annibale, M. Ciofetta, and P. Bottini. 1993. Meticulous prevention of hypoglycemia normalizes the glycemic thresholds and magnitude of most of neuroendocrine responses to, symptoms of, and cognitive function during hypoglycemia in intensively treated patients with short-term IDDM. *Diabetes* 42:1683–1689.
13. Fanelli, C., S. Pampanelli, L. Epifano, A. M. Rambotti, A. Di Vincenzo, F. Modarelli, M. Ciofetta, M. Lepore, B. Annibale, and E. Torlone. 1994. Long-term recovery from unawareness, deficient counterregulation and lack of cognitive dysfunction during hypoglycaemia, following institution of rational, intensive insulin therapy in IDDM. *Diabetologia* 37:1265–1276.
14. Rattarasarn, C., S. Dagogo-Jack, J. Zachwieja, and P. E. Cryer. 1994. Hypoglycemia-induced autonomic failure in IDDM is specific for stim-

ulus of hypoglycemia and is not attributable to prior autonomic activation. *Diabetes* 43:809–818.

15. Davis, S. N., P. Galassetti, D. H. Wasserman, and D. Tate. 2000. Effects of antecedent hypoglycemia on subsequent counterregulatory responses to exercise. *Diabetes* 49:73–81.
16. Galassetti, P., D. Tate, R. A. Neill, P. G. Morris, and S. N. Davis. 2001. Effect of antecedent hypoglycemia on neuroendocrine responses to subsequent exercise in Type 1 Diabetes. *Diabetes* 50:A54.
17. Galassetti, P., S. Mann, D. Tate, R. A. Neill, F. Costa, D. H. Wasserman, and S. N. Davis. 2001. Effect of antecedent prolonged exercise on subsequent counterregulatory responses to hypoglycemia. *Am. J. Physiol.* 280:E908–E917.
18. McGregor, V. P., J. S. Greiwe, S. Banarer, and P. Cryer. 2001. Limited impact of vigorous exercise on defenses against hypoglycemia: relevance to hypoglycemia-associated autonomic failure. *Diabetes* 40:A138.
19. Veneman, T., A. Mitrakou, M. Mokan, P. E. Cryer, and J. E. Gerich. 1994. Effects of hyperketonemia or hyperlacticacidemia on symptoms, cognitive dysfunction, and counterregulatory hormone responses during hypoglycemia in normal humans. *Diabetes* 43:1311–1317.
20. Davis, S. N., C. Shavers, and F. Costa. 1997. Prevention of an increase in plasma cortisol during hypoglycemia preserves subsequent counterregulatory responses. *J. Clin. Invest.* 100:429–438.
21. Davis, S. N., C. Shavers, F. Costa, and R. Mosqueda-Garcia. 1996. Role of cortisol in the pathogenesis of deficient counterregulation after antecedent hypoglycemia in normal man. *J. Clin. Invest.* 98: 680–691.
22. Kventansky, R., K. Fukuhara, K. Pacak, D. Goldstein, and I. J. Kopin. 1993. Endogenous glucocorticoids restrain catecholamine synthesis and release at rest and during immobilization stress in rats. *Endocrinology* 133:1411–1419.
23. McGregor, V. P., S. Banarer, and P. E. Cryer. 2002. Elevated endogenous cortisol reduces autonomic neuroendocrine and symptom responses to subsequent hypoglycemia. *Am. J. Physiol. Endocrinol. Metab.* 282:E770–E777.

108 Surgical Sympathectomy

Emily M. Garland
Division of Clinical Pharmacology
Vanderbilt University
Nashville, Tennessee

The history of surgical sympathectomy as a treatment strategy originated in 1889, the same year that Gaskell and Langley described the anatomy of the sympathetic ganglia. The sympathetic ganglia are located in two chains that run along both sides of the vertebral column. Each chain consists of 3 cervical, 12 thoracic, 3 to 5 lumbar, and 3 to 4 sacral ganglia. Destruction of parts of the sympathetic chain (sympathectomy) has been used to treat a variety of disorders, initially because no other effective treatment could be found. The first cervical sympathectomy was performed in 1889 for epilepsy. During the next 20 years, this operation was performed without success to treat exophthalmos, glaucoma, trigeminal neuralgia, optic nerve atrophy, and angioma of the external carotid artery. Finally, in the early 1920s, sympathectomy that included excision of the upper thoracic ganglia was found to be of benefit for hyperhidrosis, vasospastic conditions, and angina pectoris.

In the 1930s and 1940s, open thoracolumbar sympathectomy was used in the treatment of hypertension and angina. Unfortunately, the benefits were outweighed by an operative mortality rate of 5 to 10%. The extent of the surgery was variable; the procedure, introduced by Smithwick, which included a splanchnicectomy and removal of the sympathetic ganglia from T6–9 to L1–2, was found to optimize efficacy whereas minimizing morbidity and mortality. Although largely replaced by medical therapy or cardiovascular surgery, sympathectomy was still recognized as an effective treatment for essential hypertension into the 1950s. A 10-year follow-up study published in 1960 reported a long-term decrease in blood pressure in about one third of the 100 patients. Improvement was presumably related to vasodilation of the arteries and veins in the denervated area. Other investigators reported a return toward preoperative blood pressure levels after 2 years and a less favorable long-term outcome. In addition to reduction in blood pressure, other benefits included increased longevity, relief of congestive failure, angina pectoris and headache, improvement in electrocardiogram, and disappearance of papilledema and retinopathy. Renal insufficiency was a contraindication to surgery. Many complications were related to fluid or air accumulation in the chest cavity. Pain and impotence also were common. Orthostatic hypotension occurred in essentially everyone immediately after surgery, but it was reported to disappear over time. Some investigators recommended a total or subtotal adrenalectomy in combination with a less extensive sympathectomy (T12 to L2) to be as effective as Smithwick's procedure, but with less postoperative morbidity and disability.

Endoscopic sympathectomy procedures were introduced in the 1940s. Thoracoscopic sympathectomies have been performed since then to treat several neurologic and vascular conditions, including palmar hyperhidrosis, Raynaud's syndrome, Buerger's disease, reflex sympathetic dystrophy, refractory cardiac arrhythmia, and intractable visceral pain.

Surgical sympathectomy (T1–T3) has sometimes been found to be helpful in the treatment of pain syndromes, including reflex sympathetic dystrophy (no significant nerve injury) and causalgia (nerve involvement). Both types of pain are likely to be related to increased sensitivity of primary afferent sensory fibers to catecholamines and have been reported to improve after sympathectomy in patients who experienced good, although temporary, pain relief from sympathetic block. However, these studies have not included a placebo control and the recurrence of pain may necessitate additional surgery. Furthermore, postsympathectomy pain, unrelated to the pain for which surgery was performed, occurs in 30 to 50% of patients undergoing sympathectomy for chronic pain. Because pathways for upper abdominal visceral pain involve the splanchnic nerves, a thoracoscopic sympathetic–splanchnicectomy has been performed, with at least short-term benefit, in patients with upper abdominal pain related to cancer.

Peripheral vascular disease has been prominent in the history of surgical sympathectomy. Interruption of sympathetic pathways reduces peripheral resistance and increases blood flow. In the mid-twentieth century, it was commonly agreed that lumbar sympathectomy reduced the need for amputation because of ischemic rest pain and ulceration in the lower extremities. Even after it had largely been replaced by direct arterial surgery (bypass), sympathectomy was still recommended for the subgroup of patients with a relatively high ankle: brachial systolic pressure ratio, and less advanced skin changes. Sympathectomy also has been recommended for treatment of severe or refractory Raynaud syndrome. Despite the recurrence of symptoms, their frequency and severity are reduced. Intermittent claudication is not benefited by surgical sympathectomy, and this procedure has been replaced by medical treatment and smoking cessation in the treatment of Buerger's disease.

A major indication for endoscopic thoracic (T2 and T3) sympathectomy, for the past three decades, is essential hyperhidrosis and facial blushing. Hyperhidrosis is caused by localized overactivity of sympathetic fibers, leading to excessive sweating in specific parts of the body. Long-term improvement has been reported in more than 90% of patients with palmar hyperhidrosis treated by thoracoscopic sympathectomy. This procedure is not recommended for hyperhidrosis of the feet because destruction of that part of the sympathetic chain can result in impotence.

Over the years, the procedures for sympathectomy have been varied to maximize the chances of success and to minimize the number of postoperative complications. The extent of the sympathectomy used to treat hypertension resulted in failure of ejaculation, increased colonic motility, impaired perception of pain, pain, and postural hypotension. By limiting surgery to T2–T3 for palmar hyperhidrosis and adding only T4 for axillary hyperhidrosis, many side effects can be avoided. Mild short-term postoperative complications are more common than severe complications and include atelectasis, pneumonia, pneumothorax, and hemothorax. Neuralgia, Horner syndrome, and compensatory sweating are possible long-term complications. The risk for Horner syndrome can be minimized by leaving the lower part of the stellate ganglion untouched. The most common side effect of thoracodorsal sympathectomy is compensatory sweating, the occurrence of which can be reduced to 20 to 25% by limiting the surgery to T2 and the portions of the chain between T2 and adjoining ganglia. Other side effects might prove to be beneficial in some patients. The sympathetic fibers passing through the T2 and T3 ganglia also affect cardiac autonomic activity. Endoscopic thoracic sympathectomy has been found to reduce resting heart rate and to moderate the stimulus of heart rate elicited by exercise testing. Accordingly, endoscopic transthoracic sympathicotomy has been applied with improvement to patients with severe angina pectoris, who are not suitable for coronary artery bypass grafting or angioplasty.

References

1. Drott, C. 1994. The history of cervicothoracic sympathectomy. *Eur. J. Surg. Suppl.* 572:5–7.
2. Ahn, S. S., C. K. Wieslander, and K. M. Ro. 2000. Current developments in thoracoscopic sympathectomy. *Ann. Vasc. Surg.* 14(4): 415–420.
3. Evelyn, K. A., M. M. Singh, W. P. Chapman, G. A. Perera, and H. Thaler. 1960. Effect of thoracolumbar sympathectomy on clinical course of primary (essential) hypertension: A ten-year study of 100 sympathectomized patients compared with individually matched, symptomatically treated control subjects. *Am. J. Med.* 28:188–221.
4. Zintel, H. A., A. M. Sellers, W. A. Jeffers, J. A. Mackie, J. H. Hafkenschiel, and M. A. Lindauer. 1955. A three to seven year postoperative evaluation of 76 patients with severe hypertension treated by thoracolumbar sympathectomy. *Surg. Gynecol. Obstet.* 101:48–54.
5. Willner, C., and P. A. Low. 1997. Laboratory evaluation of complex regional pain syndrome. In *Clinical autonomic disorders,* ed. P. A. Low, 209–220. Philadelphia: Lippincott-Raven.
6. Lin, C. C., L. R. Mo, Y. W. Lin, and M. P. Yau. 1994. Bilateral thoracoscopic lower sympathetic-splanchnicectomy for upper abdominal cancer pain. *Eur. J. Surg. Suppl.* 572:59–62.
7. Strandness, D. E., Jr. 1966. Long-term value of lumbar sympathectomy. *Geriatrics* 21(10):144–155.
8. Matsumoto, Y., T. Ueyama, M. Endo, H. Sasaki, F. Kasashima, Y. Abe, and I. Kosugi. 2002. Endoscopic thoracic sympathectomy for Raynaud's phenomenon. *J. Vasc. Surg.* 36(1):57–61.
9. Noppen, M., P. Dendale, Y. Hagers, P. Herregodts, W. Vincken, and J. D'Haens. 1996. Changes in cardiocirculatory autonomic function after thoracoscopic upper dorsal sympathicolysis for essential hyperhidrosis. *J. Auton. Nerv. Syst.* 60(3):115–120.
10. Hederman, W. P. 1994. Present and future trends in thoracoscopic sympathectomy. *Eur. J. Surg. Suppl.* 572:17–19.

109

Physical Measures

Wouter Wieling
Department of Medicine
Amsterdam Medical Center
Amsterdam, The Netherlands

PHYSICAL COUNTER MANEUVERS

Specific treatment of the underlying disease in patients with autonomic failure usually is not possible; consequently, the goal in management is to obtain symptomatic improvement by other means. Physical maneuvers that are both easy to apply and effective in combatting orthostatic lightheadedness in daily life are, therefore, of obvious importance. Patients with autonomic failure have discovered several such maneuvers themselves. The beneficial effects of leg-crossing, squatting, abdominal compression, bending forward, and placing one foot on a chair have been described (Fig. 109.1). A great advantage of these maneuvers is that they can be applied immediately at the start of hypotensive symptoms. Physical counter maneuvers need to be related specifically to the individual patient. They may be difficult to perform in patients with multiple system atrophy, who may have motor disabilities and compromised balance.

LEG-CROSSING

Leg-crossing is the simplest maneuver to increase the standing time in a patient with autonomic failure. It has the advantage that it can be performed without much effort and without bringing much attention to the patient's problem. The maneuver is performed by crossing one leg in direct contact with the other while actively standing on both legs (see Fig. 109.1). The increase in mean arterial pressure and pulse pressure induced by leg-crossing can be attributed to compression of the muscles in the upper legs and abdomen with mechanical squeezing of venous vessels resulting in an increase in central blood volume, and thereby in cardiac filling pressures and cardiac output. Tensing of leg and abdominal muscles can increase this effect considerably (Fig. 109.2), most likely by the combination of a further increase in venous return and the mechanical effects of skeletal muscle tensing on the arterial circulation to the legs increasing systemic vascular resistance. Leg-crossing also can be used for the prevention of orthostatic lightheadedness in the sitting position (see Fig. 109.1).

Although the increase in upright blood pressure induced by leg-crossing alone is relatively small, with an average increase in mean arterial pressure of 10 to 15 mmHg (see Figs. 109.1 and 109.2), one should realize that medical treatment with fludrocortisone, erythropoietin, and midodrine results in similarly small blood pressure increases. Despite these small increases, the standing time improves markedly by all four methods, because they shift mean arterial pressure from just below to just above the critical level of perfusion of the brain. A driving pressure of about 40 mmHg is needed to maintain cerebral blood flow in young adult subjects in supine posture. Healthy subjects in the upright position need a mean arterial pressure of about 70 mmHg measured at heart level to compensate for the effects of gravity on the circulation. Patients with orthostatic hypotension tolerate a much lower standing mean pressure, occasionally as low as 50 mmHg, probably by adaption of autoregulatory mechanisms of the blood vessels in the brain.

Crossing one's legs often is applied unintentionally also by healthy humans when standing for prolonged periods (cocktail party posture). Studies show that instruction to apply physical counter maneuvers is helpful to otherwise healthy subjects with functional orthostatic disorders like the postural tachycardia syndrome (Fig. 109.3). The combination of leg-crossing and tensing of leg and abdominal muscles can abort an impending vasovagal reaction (Fig. 109.4).

SQUATTING

Squatting increases arterial mean pressure and pulse pressure (see Fig. 109.1) by two mechanisms. First, blood is squeezed from the veins of the legs and the splanchnic vascular bed, which increases cardiac filling pressures and cardiac output. Second, the mechanical impediment of the circulation to the legs increases systemic vascular resistance. Squatting is an effective emergency mechanism to prevent a loss of consciousness when presyncopal symptoms develop rapidly both in patients with autonomic failure and in patients with vasovagal episodes. Bending over as if to

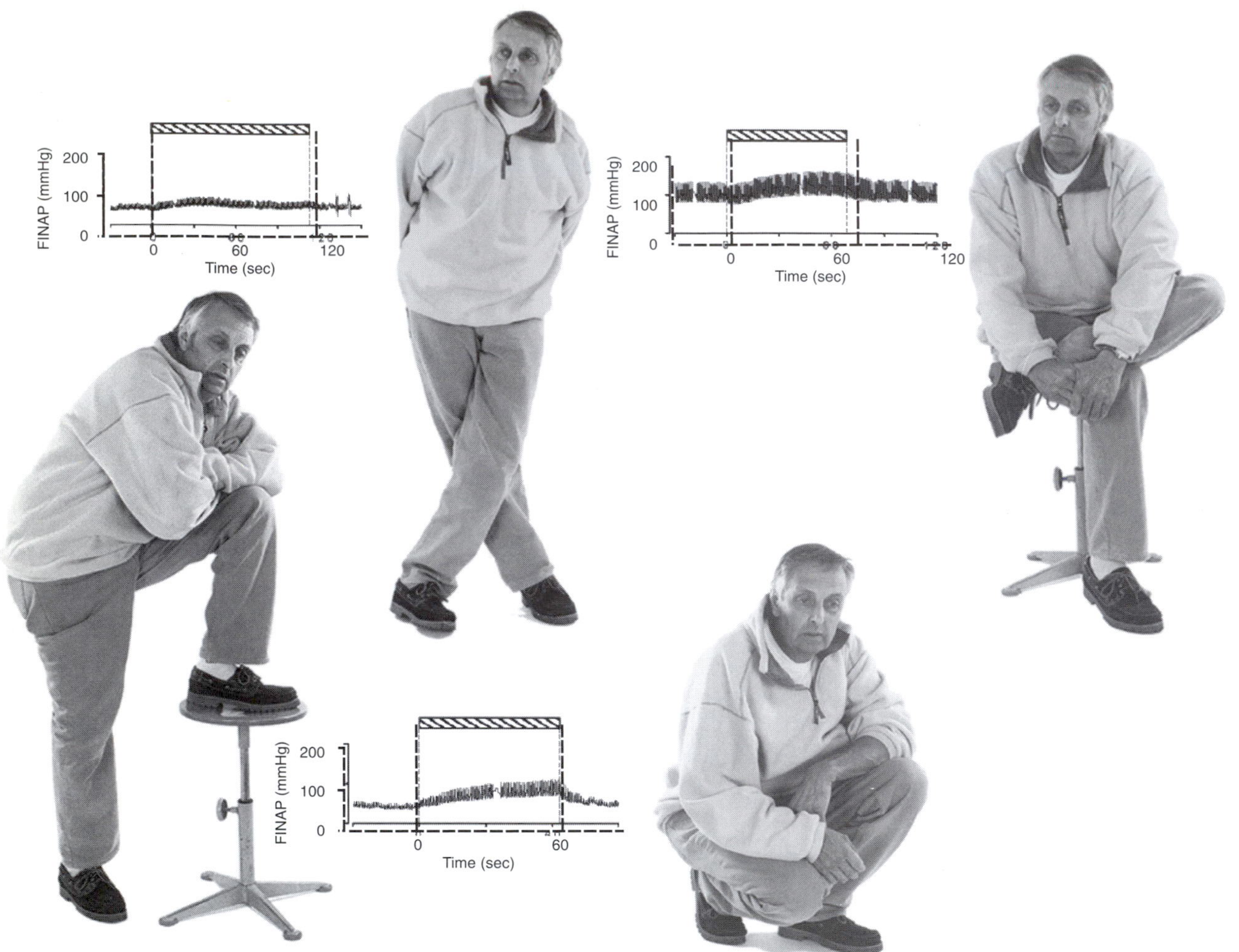

FIGURE 109.1 Physical counter maneuvers using isometric contractions of the lower limbs and abdominal compression. The effects of leg-crossing in standing and sitting position, placing a foot on a chair and squatting on finger arterial blood pressure (FINAP) in a 54-year-old male patient with pure autonomic failure and invalidating orthostatic hypotension. The patient was standing (sitting) quietly before the maneuvers. *Bars* indicate the duration of the maneuvers. Note the increase in blood pressure and pulse pressure during the maneuvers. (Courtesy M. P. M. Harms and W. Wieling, Amsterdam Medical Center, Amsterdam, The Netherlands.)

tie one's shoes has similar effects and is simpler to perform by elderly patients. The beneficial effects of sitting in knee-chest position or placing one foot on a chair while standing (see Fig. 109.1) are comparable to squatting. When rising again from the squatted position, immediate leg muscle tensing should be advised to prevent hypotension.

EXTERNAL SUPPORT

Applying external pressure to the lower half of the body substantially reduces venous pooling when upright; consequently, arterial pressure and cerebral perfusion are better maintained. External support can be applied by bandages firmly wrapped around the legs, or a snugly fitted abdominal binder, but it is best accomplished by a custom-fitted counterpressure support garment, made of elastic mesh, which forms a single unit extending from the metatarsals to the costal margin. External support garments are helpful in the treatment of a patient with incapacitating orthostatic hypotension, but have the disadvantage that the motivation of the patient must be strong, because they are uncomfortable to wear. In addition, counterpressure support garments prevent the formation of peripheral edema in the legs, which is considered to be an essential factor for effective therapy of orthostatic hypotension by acting as a perivascular water jacket that limits the vascular volume available for orthostatic pooling. We, therefore, only use an abdominal binder as a temporary external support expedient to achieve mobility in our most severely affected patients.

Small lightweight portable fishing chair or a derby chair, which is a cane when folded but a seat when unfolded, are

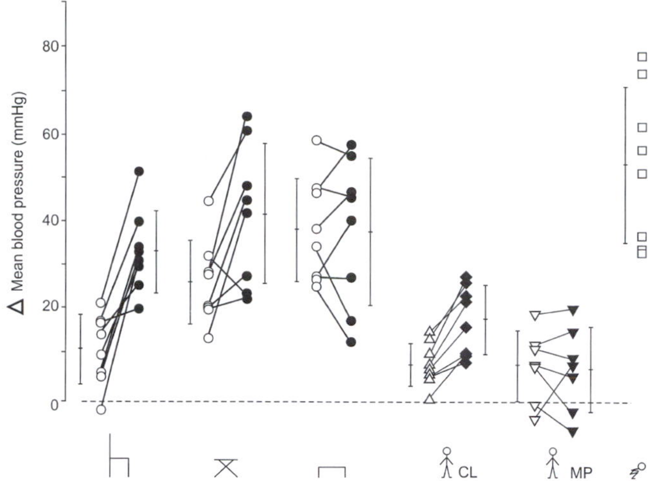

FIGURE 109.2 The efficacy of sitting, crossing legs, muscle pumping, and squatting to improve orthostatic hypotension in patients with autonomic failure. Mean finger arterial blood pressures are expressed as the blood pressure change during the intervention from the premaneuver standing blood pressure. **Left to right**, Sitting on a derby chair (height, 48 cm), a fishing stool (height, 38 cm), and a foot stool (height, 20 cm), without (O) and with crossed legs (●); standing in crossed-legs position (CL) without (▲) and with (◆) contraction of lower extremity musculature; standing while muscle pumping (MP), marching on the spot (▽), toe raising (▼), and squatting (□). The *vertical line* represents mean and SD. (From Smit, A. A. J., J. R. Halliwill, P. A. Low, and W. Wieling. 1999. Topical review. Pathophysiological basis of orthostatic hypotension in autonomic failure. *J. Physiol.* 519:1–10.)

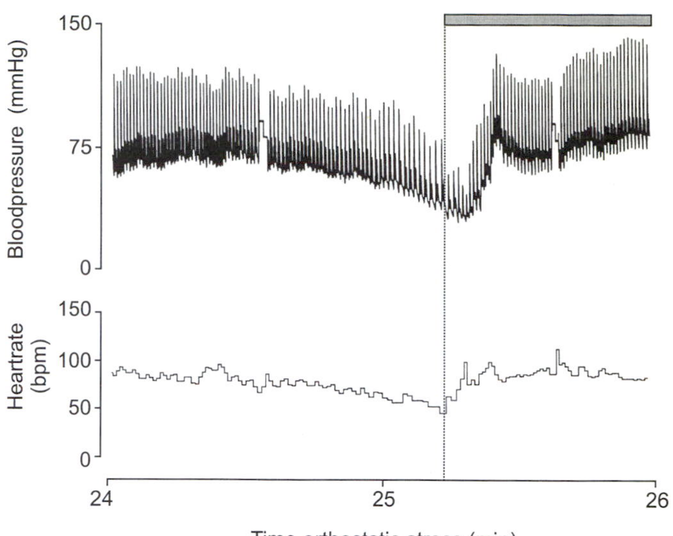

FIGURE 109.4 Aborting a vasovagal faint by the combination of leg-crossing and muscle tensing. Typical vasovagal syncope in a 24 year-old male subject with recurrent syncope during orthostatic stress testing on a tilt-table. Note progressive decrease in finger arterial pressure and heart rate. After crossing of the legs and tensing of leg and abdominal muscles, blood pressure and heart rate recover quickly. *Bar* indicates onset of leg-crossing and muscle tensing. (Courtesy C. T. P. Krediet and W. Wieling, Amsterdam Medical Center, Amsterdam, The Netherlands.)

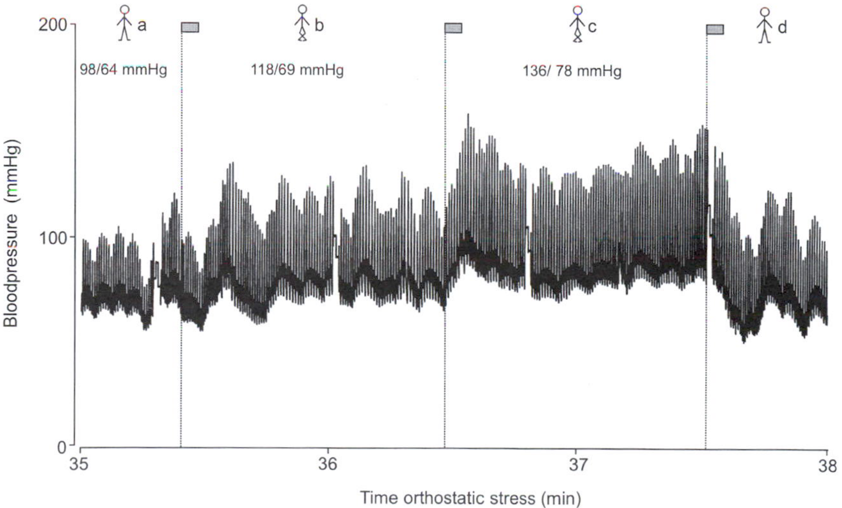

FIGURE 109.3 The effects of leg-crossing and tensing on orthostatic tolerance in a healthy subject. The effects of leg-crossing and leg-crossing combined with muscle tensing of the lower limbs in a 34-year-old woman reporting orthostatic intolerance. *a* and *d*, free standing; *b*, leg-crossing; *c*, leg-crossing combined with tensing of leg and abdominal muscles. Note the increase in blood pressure and pulse pressure during the maneuvers. Arterial pressure was monitored with a Finapres device. (Courtesy C. T. P. Krediet and W. Wieling, Amsterdam Medical Center, Amsterdam, The Netherlands.)

useful mechanical aids for severely affected patients. They enable the patients to sit for brief periods when presyncopal symptoms develop during standing. The lower the chair the more pronounced is the effect on blood pressure (see Fig. 109.2).

CONCLUSION

Mechanical maneuvers such as leg-crossing and squatting are simple to perform and can increase the standing time decisively of patients with orthostatic hypotension. Their beneficial effect is an increase in mean arterial pressure, small in magnitude but sufficient to guarantee adequate cerebral blood flow. The underlying mechanism is an augmentation of thoracic blood volume. Instruction in these maneuvers should be part of a treatment program for patients with orthostatic hypotension. It is our experience that after proper instruction and training, patients automatically apply leg-crossing in daily life.

References

1. Smit, A. A. J., J. R. Halliwill, P. A. Low, and W. Wieling. 1999. Topical review. Pathophysiological basis of orthostatic hypotension in autonomic failure. *J. Physiol.* 519:1–10.
2. Van Lieshout, J. J., A. D. J. Ten Harkel, and W. Wieling. 1992. Combating orthostatic dizziness in autonomic failure by physical maneuvers. *Lancet* 339:897–898.
3. Wieling, W., J. J. Van Lieshout, and A. M. Van Leeuwen. 1993. Physical maneuvers that reduce postural hypotension in autonomic failure. *Clin. Auton. Res.* 3:57–65.
4. Bouvette, C. M., B. R. McPHee, T. L. Opfer-Gehrking, and P. A. Low. 1996. Physical-countermanoeuvres: Efficacy and their augmentation by biofeedback training. *Mayo Clin. Proc.* 71:847–853.
5. Ten Harkel, A. D. J., J. J. Van Lieshout, and W. Wieling. 1994. Effects of leg muscle pumping and tensing on orthostatic arterial pressure: A study in normal subjects and in patients with autonomic failure. *Clin. Sci.* 87:533–558.
6. Krediet, C. T. P., N. Van Dijk, M. Linzer, J. J. Van Lieshout, and W. Wieling. 2002. Management of vasovagal syncope: Controlling or aborting faints by the combination of legcrossing and muscle tensing. *Circulation* 106:1684–1689.
7. Smit, A. A. J., M. A. Hardjowijono, and W. Wieling. 1997. Are portable folding chairs useful to combat orthostatic hypotension. *Ann. Neurol.* 42:975–978.
8. Denq, J. C., T. L. Opfer-Gehrking, M. Giuliani, J. Felten, V. A. Convertino, and P. A. Low. 1997. Efficacy of compression of different capacitance beds in the amelioration of orthostatic hypotension. *Clin. Auton. Res.* 7:321–326.
9. Tanaka, H., H. Yamaguchi, and H. Tamai. 1997. Treatment of orthostatic intolerance with an inflatable abdominal band [Letter]. *Lancet* 349:175.

110 Treatment of Orthostatic Hypotension: Nutritional Measures

Jens Jordan
Franz-Vohard-Klinik
Humboldt University
Berlin, Germany

Patients with autonomic failure are particularly sensitive to changes in vascular tone or volume status. Dietary components that do not cause a major change in healthy subjects may elicit profound cardiovascular responses. For example, drinking water and ingesting salt elicit a pressor response. Dietary components that increase blood pressure can be exploited in the treatment of orthostatic and postprandial hypotension. Ethanol ingestion and consumption of a meal decrease blood pressure and may exacerbate orthostatic hypotension.

Dietary components can affect blood pressure through different mechanisms. They may directly influence vascular tone. Ethanol and ingestion of a meal, for example, cause vasodilation. They may modulate sympathetic activity. Tyramine and water drinking increase norepinephrine release through different mechanisms. Dietary components may also influence sodium homeostasis. Obviously, sodium intake is important in the regulation of sodium balance, and thereby volume status. Similarly, potassium, calcium, and magnesium intake all play a role in blood pressure regulation. Less appreciated is that the diet may contain substances, such as components in licorice, chewing tobacco, and certain "health foods" that interfere with sodium regulation. Dietary stimuli that do not change blood pressure in healthy subjects may elicit profound blood pressure changes in patients with autonomic failure. In patients with severe orthostatic hypotension caused by autonomic failure, the efferent limb of the baroreflex is disrupted. Therefore, patients with autonomic failure are exquisitely sensitive to changes in vascular tone or changes in cardiac preload. Dietary components that elicit a pressor response may be useful to treat orthostatic hypotension. Components that decrease blood pressure and ingestion of larger meals may need to be avoided during the day. Yet, they may be useful to attenuate supine hypertension during the night. All dietary constituents that influence blood pressure may cause side effects and interfere with medications that are used for the treatment of orthostatic hypotension. The following sections provide an overview of dietary interventions that have been tested in patients with orthostatic hypotension. That the number of published interventions in this area is few suggests that the potential for nutritional measures in the treatment of orthostatic hypotension has not been fully explored.

WATER: A PRESSOR AGENT

Drinking water elicits a profound pressor response in a large subgroup of patients with autonomic failure [1–3]. Drinking 480 ml tap water increases seated systolic blood pressure 33 mmHg in patients with multiple system atrophy and 37 mmHg in patients with pure autonomic failure (Fig. 110.1) [2]. Older control subjects, who ingest 480 ml water, exhibited a moderate increase in systolic blood. In contrast, drinking water does not increase blood pressure in healthy young subjects. The pressor effect has a rapid onset within 5 minutes after drinking water. The maximal increase in blood pressure is reached after 30 to 40 minutes. The water pressor response is sustained for more than 1 hour. The sensitivity to water varies markedly between patients.

The water pressor response appears to be mediated by an increase in systemic vascular resistance rather than volume expansion. Several lines of evidence suggest that the water pressor response might be related to sympathetic activation. In healthy subjects, drinking water increases muscle sympathetic nerve traffic and venous plasma norepinephrine concentrations. The time course of both sympathetic nerve traffic and plasma norepinephrine responses corresponds to the time course of the pressor effect. The pressor response can be abolished with interruption of ganglionic transmission. The stimulus that triggers sympathetic activation with water is not known. The water pressor response is not related to water temperature. Gastric distension increases sympathetic activity in humans and may be contributory.

Drinking water improves standing blood pressure and orthostatic tolerance in a large subgroup of patients with autonomic failure [4]. Drinking water may also improve orthostatic tolerance in patients with orthostatic intolerance ("POTS") and in healthy subjects exposed to severe orthostatic stress [4, 5]. The maximal pressor effect is achieved well before commonly used pressor agents even begin to increase blood pressure. The use of oral water may be

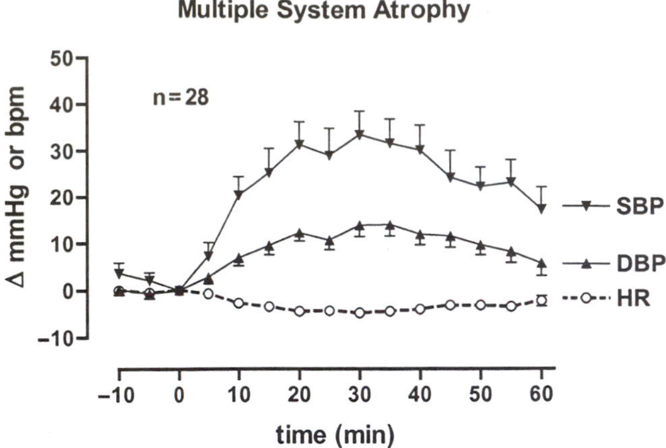

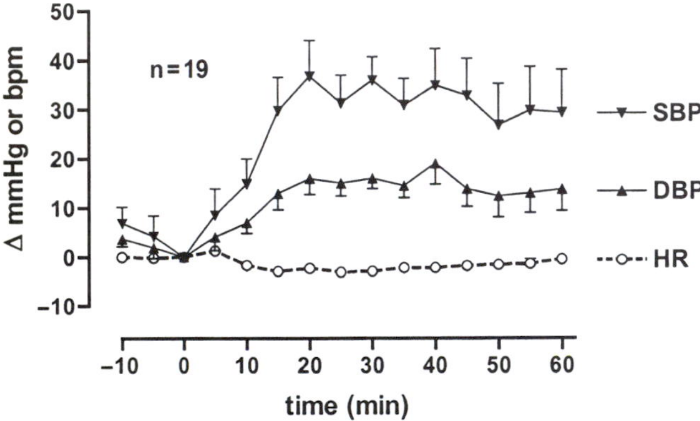

FIGURE 110.1 Changes in systolic blood pressure (SBP), diastolic blood pressure (DBP), and heart rate (HR) after patients with multiple system atrophy (**top**) and pure autonomic failure (**bottom**) drank 480 ml tap water. Patients started drinking at 0 minute. The blood pressure increase was evident within 5 minutes of drinking water, reached a maximum after approximately 20 to 30 minutes, and was sustained for more than 60 minutes. (From Jordan, J., J. R. Shannon, B. K. Black, Y. Ali, M. Farley, F. Costa, A. Diedrich, R. M. Robertson, I. Biaggioni, and D. Robertson. 2000. The pressor response to water drinking in humans: A sympathetic reflex? *Circulation* 101:504–509.)

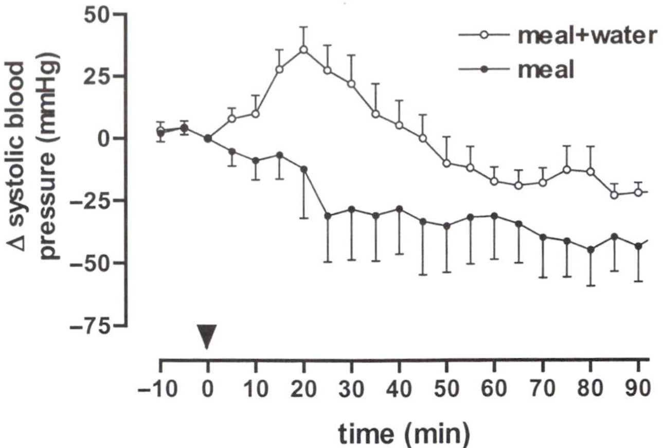

FIGURE 110.2 Change in systolic blood pressure in seven patients with primary autonomic failure (four multiple system atrophy, three pure autonomic failure) after ingestion of a standardized meal. The effect of 480 ml water taken just before ingestion of the meal is compared with the effect of the meal alone. Oral water substantially attenuated the hypotensive effect of food. (From Shannon, J. R., A. Diedrich, I. Biaggioni, J. Tank, R. M. Robertson, D. Robertson, and J. Jordan. 2002. Water drinking as a treatment for orthostatic syndromes. *Am. J. Med.* 355–360.)

particularly useful in conjunction with pressor drugs in the morning to provide a marked and rapid increase in blood pressure when orthostatic symptoms are more severe. Water taken just before a meal prevents postprandial hypotension (Fig. 110.2) [4]. We usually recommend that the daily fluid intake should be in the range of 2 to 3 liters. However, the timing of the water intake is of major importance. Patients should drink most of the water when their orthostatic symptoms tend to be worst. Drinking water should be avoided within the hour before bedtime in patients with supine hypertension.

CAFFEINE

The naturally occurring methylxanthine caffeine has been tested in patients with autonomic failure. The most important sources are coffee, tea, and caffeine-containing soft drinks. One cup of instant coffee or tea contains 5 to 70 mg caffeine, whereas filtered coffee contains approximately twice as much caffeine. Caffeine tablets also are available (typical dose, 250 mg). The pharmacologic effects of caffeine in humans are mainly related to nonselective adenosine receptor blockade. The receptor blockade attenuates adenosine-mediated vasodilatation and modulates sympathetic activity. Caffeine ingestion increases venous plasma norepinephrine and epinephrine concentrations, as well as plasma renin activity. Caffeine ingestion may also elicit a mild degree of phosphodiesterase inhibition. Phosphodiesterase inhibition decreases cyclic adenosine monophosphate (cAMP) breakdown and mimics the effect of those mediators that stimulate cAMP production.

Caffeine elicits an acute pressor response in healthy volunteers, patients with hypertension, and patients with severe autonomic failure [6, 7]. In patients with severe autonomic failure, seated systolic blood pressure increases 12 mm Hg within 1 hour after ingestion of 250 mg caffeine [7]. However, the response is heterogeneous [8]. Commonly used pressor agents, such as α-adrenoreceptor agonists or yohimbine, elicit a much greater pressor response than caffeine. However, compared with these agents, caffeine has a faster onset of the pressor effect. The fast effect of caffeine can be exploited in the treatment of postprandial hypotension. In one study in patients with severe autonomic failure, blood pressure decreased 28/18 mmHg after a standardized meal. When patients ingested 250 mg caffeine before the meal, blood pressure decreased only 11/10 mmHg.

Whether the beneficial pressor effect of caffeine in patients with autonomic failure is sustained in the long term is not known. Tachyphylaxis may occur. Methylxanthines have the potential to increase diuresis, which might negate the positive acute effect. Furthermore, patients may experience central nervous system side effects. We recommend that patients ingest caffeine with or before meals. Caffeine should be avoided before bedtime in patients with supine hypertension. Drinking water (see earlier) may be more efficacious in preventing orthostatic and postprandial hypotension than caffeine ingestion.

TYRAMINE

Tyramine-rich foods, such as aged cheddar cheese, in combination with monoamine inhibitors have been tested as a potential treatment of orthostatic hypotension [9, 10]. Tyramine is taken up in adrenergic neurons through the norepinephrine transporter and releases norepinephrine. Monoamine oxidase (MAO) inhibition profoundly augments the tyramine response by at least two mechanisms. MAO inhibition decreases the degradation of dietary tyramine in the gut wall and in the liver. The mechanism increases systemic bioavailability of tyramine. Moreover, MAO inhibition attenuates the metabolism of the norepinephrine released by tyramine. The combination of tyramine and MAO inhibitors can lead to unpredictable pressure surges and cannot be recommended as standard treatment of orthostatic hypotension. Furthermore, tyramine is not likely to be effective in patients who lost most of their sympathetic terminals (e.g., severe pure autonomic failure).

SODIUM

When healthy subjects are exposed to a low-sodium diet, renal sodium excretion decreases according to intake. Sodium homeostasis is restored within several days to the new level. The decrease in sodium excretion is explained by an increase in sodium reabsorption through activation of sympathetic efferents to the kidney and activation of the renin-angiotensin system. Activation of both the sympathetic and the renin-angiotensin system are impaired in patients with severe autonomic failure. When sodium intake is restricted in these patients, sodium excretion is not sufficiently suppressed. With insufficient sodium intake, patients experience a negative sodium balance, weight loss, and worsening of orthostatic hypotension [11–13]. The inability to conserve sodium provides a rationale for the therapeutic use of sodium. We recommend that patients ingest 150 to 200 mmol sodium per day. It may be necessary to supplement the diet with salt tablets. Clearly, patients with autonomic failure with severe orthostatic hypotension need to avoid low-sodium diets. Regular weighing is the most reliable method to assess chronic changes in sodium balance. Monitoring of 24-hour urinary sodium excretion can be useful to assess compliance with a high-sodium diet. Sufficient sodium ingestion is necessary in patients who are treated with fludrocortisone to attain an increase in blood pressure.

In addition to more long-term diet-related changes in sodium homeostasis, patients with autonomic failure experience substantial fluctuations in sodium balance with changes in posture. These fluctuations are probably related to fluctuations in blood pressure. In the upright position, as blood pressure is low, sodium is retained. Thus, orthostatic hypotension tends to improve during the day. In the supine position, as blood pressure is high, sodium excretion increases (i.e., pressure natriuresis). The excessive sodium loss worsens orthostatic hypotension in the morning. There are no data to suggest that changes in dietary sodium intake can attenuate the postural changes in sodium balance.

LICORICE

Licorice, and surprisingly many other "food" sources, contains glycyrrhizin, which inhibits 11β-hydroxysteroid dehydrogenase (11-HSD) activity. The enzyme is located in most mineralocorticoid target tissues. Normally, aldosterone is a much stronger mineralocorticoid than cortisol *in vivo* even though the mineralocorticoid receptors have identical *in vitro* affinities for these hormones. The specificity of the receptors *in vivo* is the result of activity of 11-HSD. The enzyme converts cortisol to cortisone. The latter is inactive at the mineralocorticoid receptor. Inhibition of 11-HSD with licorice prevents the inactivation of cortisol, which results in mineralocorticoid receptor activation. Licorice ingestion has been used as a treatment of orthostatic hypotension in patients with diabetic autonomic neuropathy [14]. However, the glycyrrhizin content in licorice is not standardized, which limits its therapeutic use. Furthermore, individual responses to licorice are highly variable.

NUTRITIONAL TREATMENT OF SUPINE HYPERTENSION

Approximately 50% of the patients with severe orthostatic hypotension feature supine hypertension. Supine hypertension is associated with excessive nocturnal sodium excretion, which worsens orthostatic hypotension the next morning. Whether supine hypertension is associated with increased cardiovascular morbidity or mortality is not known. Nutritional measures may be useful in the management of patients with supine hypertension. Substances that increase blood pressure, such as water and caffeine, should be avoided before bedtime. Licorice ingestion may cause more chronic increases in supine blood pressure. A small meal ingested before retiring may attenuate nocturnal hypertension. Ethanol consumption can exacerbate orthostatic hypotension. However, ingested before bedtime, ethanol may decrease supine hypertension. Patients who eat or drink alcohol before bedtime have to be made aware that they may experience more severe orthostatic hypotension during the night.

References

1. Jordan, J., J. R. Shannon, E. Grogan, I. Biaggioni, and D. Robertson. 1999. A potent pressor response elicited by drinking water. *Lancet* 353:723.
2. Jordan, J., J. R. Shannon, B. K. Black, Y. Ali, M. Farley, F. Costa, A. Diedrich, R. M. Robertson, I. Biaggioni, and D. Robertson. 2000. The pressor response to water drinking in humans: A sympathetic reflex? *Circulation* 101:504–509.
3. Cariga, P., and C. J. Mathias. 2001. Haemodynamics of the pressor effect of oral water in human sympathetic denervation due to autonomic failure. *Clin. Sci. (Lond).* 101:313–319.
4. Shannon, J. R., A. Diedrich, I. Biaggioni, J. Tank, R. M. Robertson, D. Robertson, and J. Jordan. 2002. Water drinking as a treatment for orthostatic syndromes. *Am. J. Med.* 355–360.
5. Schroeder, C., V. E. Bush, L. J. Norcliffe, F. C. Luft, J. Tank, J. Jordan, and R. Hainsworth. 2002. Water drinking acutely improves orthostatic tolerance in healthy subjects. *Circulation* 106:2806–2811.
6. Robertson, D., J. C. Frolich, R. K. Carr, J. T. Watson, J. W. Hollifield, D. G. Shand, and J. A. Oates. 1978. Effects of caffeine on plasma renin activity, catecholamines and blood pressure. *N. Engl. J. Med.* 298: 181–186.
7. Onrot, J., M. R. Goldberg, I. Biaggioni, A. S. Hollister, D. Kingaid, and D. Robertson. 1985. Hemodynamic and humoral effects of caffeine in autonomic failure. Therapeutic implications for postprandial hypotension. *N. Engl. J. Med.* 313:549–554.
8. Jordan, J., J. R. Shannon, I. Biaggioni, R. Norman, B. K. Black, and D. Robertson. 1998. Contrasting actions of pressor agents in severe autonomic failure. *Am. J. Med.* 105:116–124.
9. Lewis, R. K., C. G. Hazelrig, F. J. Fricke, and R. O. Russell, Jr. 1972. Therapy of idiopathic postural hypotension. *Arch. Intern. Med.* 129:943–949.
10. Diamond, M. A., R. H. Murray, and P. G. Schmid. 1970. Idiopathic postural hypotension: Physiologic observations and report of a new mode of therapy. *J. Clin. Invest.* 49:1341–1348.
11. Wilcox, C. S., M. J. Aminoff, and J. D. Slater. 1977. Sodium homeostasis in patients with autonomic failure. *Clin. Sci. Mol. Med.* 53:321–328.
12. Wilcox, C. S., R. Puritz, S. L. Lightman, R. Bannister, and M. J. Aminoff. 1984. Plasma volume regulation in patients with progressive autonomic failure during changes in salt intake or posture. *J. Lab. Clin. Med.* 104:331–339.
13. Wieling, W., J. J. Van Lieshout, and R. Hainsworth. 2002. Extracellular fluid volume expansion in patients with posturally related syncope. *Clin. Auton. Res.* 12:242–249.
14. Basso, A., P. L. Dalla, G. Erle, M. Boscaro, and D. Armanine. 1994. Licorice ameliorates postural hypotension caused by diabetic autonomic neuropathy. *Diabetes Care.* 17:1356.

111

Fludrocortisone

Rose Marie Robertson
Division of Cardiology
Vanderbilt University
Nashville, Tennessee

Fludrocortisone is a frequent component of the medication regimen in patients with autonomic failure and orthostatic hypotension. Studies by Frick and by Liddle in the 1960s demonstrated that the addition of a fluorine atom to the cortisol molecule fundamentally altered the pharmacodynamics of the parent compound, producing a drug with potent mineralocorticoid, but minimal glucocorticoid effect. The overall effect of this agent in patients with autonomic failure is an increase in blood pressure, both in the supine and the upright postures, and fludrocortisone has been used as a pressor agent in these disorders for 40 years. It also has been helpful in the management of those patients with vasovagal syncope in whom maintaining an adequate fluid balance is otherwise difficult, but it has been tested and found not to be helpful in patients with the chronic fatigue syndrome without autonomic deficits.

Careful studies of the cardiovascular responses to fludrocortisone determined that the increase in blood pressure in patients with orthostatic hypotension is related to an initial increase in plasma volume, because of sodium retention. This effect, dependent on mineralocorticoid receptors within the nucleus and altered gene transcription, takes several days to weeks to reach its peak. Although the plasma volume may return to baseline subsequently, in many patients a residual beneficial pressor effect continues. At least in some patients, this has been demonstrated to be caused by increased peripheral resistance, and the enhanced response to infused norepinephrine seen in several studies suggests a mechanism through cell surface receptors acting through second messengers. Such mechanisms would be expected to be activated more rapidly and to follow a different time course than those requiring alteration of cellular transcription.

Over the past decade studies have improved our understanding of the pharmacokinetic profile of fludrocortisone. An assay for fludrocortisone was developed and has been used to demonstrate that the drug is rapidly absorbed after oral administration and declines with a half-life of about 2 to 3 hours. Although this relatively short half-life was unexpected, it provides an explanation for the clinical observation that the drug seems to be more efficacious when given twice daily rather than once a day. However, some patients clearly receive benefit even with a once daily regimen.

On the basis of this information, there are several issues to consider to ensure that fludrocortisone is being used most effectively. First, because the full pressor action of fludrocortisone is not seen for 1 to 2 weeks, doses should not be altered more frequently than at weekly or biweekly intervals. The initial dose should be 0.05 to 0.1 mg (usually the latter) orally daily, and weekly or biweekly titration by 0.1-mg increments per week should aim for a weight gain of 5 to 8 lb and mild ankle swelling. The patient should be educated about the expected time course of the effect. It will be rare to find additional benefit beyond 0.2 mg orally twice daily, but doses as high as 2.0 mg/day have been reported. There is little, if any, glucocorticoid effect at doses in the range of 0.1 to 0.2 mg daily, but reduced cortisol levels caused by adrenocorticotrophic hormone suppression have been seen after a single dose of 2.0 mg. Weight is a good guide to the required dose, and the weight gain caused by fluid retention should be limited to less than 15 lb. Because much of the blood pressure effect is related to this fluid retention, the addition of a waist-high compression garment helps to keep this fluid distributed in the most beneficial manner.

Fludrocortisone should not be used in patients who cannot tolerate increased fluid retention, but this is rarely an issue, because such patients will rarely have significant orthostatic hypotension. In fact, patients with preexisting mild autonomic failure may actually find that their orthostatic hypotension improves when congestive heart failure develops. If symptoms of pulmonary congestion or even of pulmonary edema do develop in patient with autonomic failure after a fludrocortisone-induced increase in plasma volume, these symptoms will respond rapidly with assumption of the seated or upright posture.

There are potential side effects and complications that can develop with the use of fludrocortisone. Hypokalemia will develop in nearly 50% of patient, and it can appear within the first week of treatment. It will respond to oral supplementation with potassium, which usually must be given chronically in such patients. Concomitant hypomagnesemia will develop in a smaller group, perhaps 5%; although correction of the hypokalemia often will lead to secondary correction of the hypomagnesemia, if this is not complete, small doses of magnesium sulfate can be added.

Fludrocortisone therapy commonly produces the side effect of headache, especially initially, and particularly in younger, healthier patients. For example, although transient fludrocortisone therapy would seem to be an ideal approach for astronauts, who commonly experience orthostatic intolerance when they return from the exposure to microgravity associated with space travel, headache has been a limitation. Likewise, young patients using fludrocortisone to prevent vasovagal syncope may find headache a limiting factor. However, patients with severe autonomic failure, in whom it is most helpful, do not usually describe headache with fludrocortisone. An additional important issue is the development of an excessive increase in blood pressure, especially in the supine posture. Although supine hypertension can be decreased acutely by raising the head of the bed, by having the patient sit or stand, and/or by giving a carbohydrate snack, if it persists, a reduction in dosage or discontinuation may be necessary. As with all drugs, interactions with other medications must be considered. Although it is rare for patients with the potential for falling caused by orthostatic hypotension to be treated with warfarin, occasionally some patients will require the latter for valvular heart disease or another indication. In some of these patients, fludrocortisone will lead to an increased warfarin requirement to achieve the same international normalized ratio.

A theoretic concern with the long-term use of fludrocortisone has arisen in recent years with the description of novel effects of aldosterone. Classically, aldosterone has been known to act at the epithelial cell level to induce sodium reabsorption and potassium excretion, leading to intravascular volume expansion, and the antagonism of aldosterone by spironolactone has been used to good effect in the treatment of congestive heart failure. However, in the Randomized Aldactone Evaluation Study (RALES), the addition of spironolactone to existing therapy in patients with heart failure led to a significant reduction in morbidity and mortality as well. Data have demonstrated that aldosterone has additional, nonepithelial effects in the kidney and in vascular smooth muscle, involving activation of the sodium/hydrogen antiporter, and it is possible that this can produce cardiovascular damage independent of the level of blood pressure. Because this cardiovascular damage in experimental settings can be prevented by administering a selective mineralocorticoid receptor antagonist, one must have some concern about the chronic use of a mineralocorticoid receptor agonist. However, fludrocortisone has been used chronically in patients with Addison's disease with good results, and in patients with severe orthostatic hypotension, the benefit would seem to outweigh this theoretic risk. It is prudent in all patients to be certain that all appropriate measures of cardiovascular protection and prevention are being used.

References

1. Frick, M. H. 1966. 9-Alpha-fluorohydrocortisone in the treatment of postural hypotension. *Acta. Med. Scand.* 179:293–299.
2. Chobanian, A. V., L. Volicer, C. P. Tifft, H. Gavras, C. S. Lian, and D. Faxon. 1979. Mineralocorticoid-induced hypertension in patients with orthostatic hypotension. *N. Engl. J. Med.* 301:68–73.
3. Mitsky, V. P., R. J. Workman, E. Nicholson, J. Vernikos, R. M. Robertson, and D. Robertson. 1994. A sensitive radioimmunoassay for fludrocortisone in human plasma. *Steroids* 59:555–558.
4. Goldstein, D. S., D. Robertson, M. Esler, S. E. Straus, and G. Eisenhofer. 2002. Dysautonomias: Clinical disorders of the autonomic nervous system. *Ann. Intern. Med.* 137:753–763.
5. Frishman, W. H., V. Azer, and D. Sica. 2003. Drug treatment of orthostatic hypotension and vasovagal syncope. *Heart Dis.* 5(1):49–64.
6. Blockmans, D., P. Persoons, B. Van Houdenhove, M. Lejeune, and H. Bobbaers. 2003. Combination therapy with hydrocortisone and fludrocortisone does not improve symptoms in chronic fatigue syndrome: A randomized, placebo-controlled, double-blind, crossover study. *Am. J. Med.* 114:736–741.
7. Rocha, R., and G. H. Williams. 2002. Rationale for the use of aldosterone antagonists in congestive heart failure. *Drugs* 62:723–731.

112 Midodrine and Other Sympathomimetics

Janice L. Gilden
Division of Diabetes and Endocrinology
University of Health Sciences/The Chicago Medical School
North Chicago, Illinois

The sympathomimetics used for treatment of neurogenic orthostatic hypotension have either direct α_1 (e.g., midodrine) or mixed direct and indirect actions (e.g., ephedrine). Midodrine, a direct α_1 agonist, produces vasoconstriction of the arteriolar and venous vasculature and decreases venous pooling. Because it does not cross the blood–brain barrier, there are no central nervous system side effects. Midodrine does not cause cardiac stimulation. Midodrine is a prodrug that is hydrolyzed in the liver to its active form, desglymidodrine. The peak activity is 1 hour after administration and its duration of action is 4 to 6 hours. Studies have demonstrated efficacy for improving both standing blood pressure and symptoms. Side effects are generally mild, dose related, and include piloerection, urinary retention, and supine hypertension. Other sympathomimetics, such as ephedrine, pseudoephedrine, phenylpropanolamine, and methylphenidate have both direct and indirect actions and cross the blood–brain barrier. These pharmacologic agents have a short duration of action and are associated with marked central nervous system and cardiac toxic effects. Comparative studies with these mixed sympathomimetics show less efficacy in terms of blood pressure and symptomatic improvement.

MIDODRINE

Mechanism of Action

Midodrine [(1-2′,5′-dimethoxyphenyl 1)-2 glycinamidoethanol (1)-hydrochloride] is a selective α_1 agonist and results in α-adrenergic receptor activation of the arteriolar and venous vasculature. These actions produce vasoconstriction of the blood vessels and a decrease in venous pooling, thereby increasing blood pressure in the upright position. In addition, midodrine does not stimulate β-adrenergic receptors. This agent lacks central nervous system side effects, because it does not cross the blood–brain barrier. In contrast to the nonselective sympathomimetic agents, midodrine also does not cause cardiac stimulation [1]. This drug has no known effects on the pulmonary, renal, or blood coagulation function, or changes in blood glucose and lipids [1].

Pharmacology

Midodrine is well absorbed after oral administration. In the liver, midodrine hydrochloride is converted through hydrolytic cleavage to its active metabolite, desglymidodrine, which is 93% bioavailable. Desglymidodrine is excreted primarily in the urine, whereas fecal elimination of the prodrug and its metabolite is not significant.

The half-life of desglymidodrine and midodrine in healthy subjects is 2 to 3 hours and 0.49 hour, respectively. The duration of action is longer than that of the other sympathomimetic agonists. The dose-response curve for the effect of midodrine on the standing systolic blood pressure shows a log linear dose relation [2]. In healthy individuals without autonomic dysfunction, the maximal pharmacologic effect is found to be 1 hour after administration and duration of action is generally 4 to 6 hours. In patients with neurogenic orthostatic hypotension, these effects may be somewhat variable. This may reflect the differences in receptor and postreceptor impairments of the autonomic nervous system.

Efficacy

Midodrine is effective for treating orthostatic hypotension in patients with either preganglionic (multiple system atrophy [MSA] and Parkinson's disease) or postganglionic (pure autonomic failure [PAF] and diabetes mellitus) lesions. Earlier studies by Kaufmann and colleagues [3] evaluated seven patients after treatment with midodrine and found an increase in mean arterial pressure of 15 mmHg compared with baseline levels in the three responders (two MSA and one PAF) with decreased orthostatic symptoms. Other studies demonstrated maintenance of blood pressure improvements over 15 months [1]. In a later study of 97 patients with varying causes of neurogenic orthostatic hypotension, the 10 mg three times daily dosage significantly increased standing systolic blood pressure by 22 mmHg without affecting heart rate. There was significant improvement of symptoms (dizziness, lightheadedness, syncope, and depressed feelings), even at doses lower than that required to show significant improvement in systolic blood pressure. Global evaluation scores assessed by patients and investigators also improved [4, 5]. A second study by Gilden and Kaufmann [6] evaluated 53 patients with severe neurogenic orthostatic hypotension treated in a double-blind fashion with three daily doses of 10 mg midodrine versus placebo. There was not only an increase in standing systolic blood pressure compared with placebo, but also improvement of symptoms, and a 50% increase in motionless standing time. In a 6-week, double-blind study of 162 patients with severe neurogenic orthostatic hypotension (10 mg three times daily), systolic blood pressure significantly improved by 22 mmHg in all 4 weeks of treatment with symptomatic improvement, as rated by patients and investigators [7]. Other studies also have demonstrated the effectiveness of midodrine for treating patients with familial dysautonomia, neurocardiogenic syncope, and intradialytic orthostatic hypotension.

In comparative studies with etilefrine, dimetofrine, and ephedrine, midodrine treatment resulted in a greater improvement in standing blood pressure. When compared with norefenefrine, midodrine therapy resulted in a greater improvement in symptoms [1]. Fouad-Tarazi and colleagues [8] compared midodrine with ephedrine and confirmed greater improvement in upright blood pressure and symptoms with midodrine.

When midodrine was combined with the β-adrenoreceptor agonist, denodopamine, postprandial hypotension was prevented by increasing cardiac output and peripheral vascular resistance [1]. A subanalysis of the study by Low and colleagues [7] showed that the effect of midodrine was not altered by fludrocortisone or support garment use.

Adverse Effects and Disadvantages

The most common side effects are related to piloerection (paraesthesia, pruritus of the scalp, goose pumps, and chills) and urologic problems (urgency, hesitancy, frequency, and retention). Therefore, this drug needs to be used with caution in patients with urinary retention, as well as in diabetics also taking fludrocortisone, because the latter is known to increase intraocular pressure and glaucoma. There also is the risk for supine hypertension, especially in greater doses [2, 4, 7]. Percentages for supine hypertension have generally ranged from 4 to 7% [4, 7]. However, one study observed an 11% rate for blood pressures greater than 200 mmHg in response to a single dose of 10 mg [2]. It also should be noted that supine hypertension is a common feature of more severe autonomic failure, even before treatment, and hypertensive cerebrovascular accidents are not increased in autonomic neuropathy. Cerebral hypoperfusion with ischemic strokes caused by the decreases in blood pressure during the daytime may occur. Nevertheless, it is still recommended to administer the final dose 4 hours before bedtime. Side effects of midodrine are generally dose related and can be reversed by standing or α receptor antagonist phentolamine. Midodrine is contraindicated in patients with severe organic heart disease, pheochromocytoma, or thyrotoxicosis. Patients with renal failure may require smaller doses, because the active metabolite is excreted renally. Furthermore, patients with hepatic dysfunction also should be treated with caution because of the hepatic metabolism.

Dosing

The dose of midodrine is quite variable and should be individualized. Because there is generally a marked variation in symptoms and decreases in blood pressures (generally more profound in the early morning hours), this agent may be administered orally from 2.5 to 10 mg every 3 to 4 hours up to a maximum of 50 to 60 mg per day, depending on the clinical response. In addition, those patients with postprandial exacerbation may be given a dose before meals, so that the peak effect of the medication coincides with the maximal postprandial decrease in upright blood pressure. This medication also can be withheld during recumbency in patients with supine hypertension. Studies are currently in progress to determine the most effective and optimal dose with the least side effects for specific causes of neurogenic orthostatic hypotension.

EPHEDRINE/OTHER α AGONISTS

Mechanism of Action

The other sympathomimetics such as ephedrine and pseudoephedrine are nonselective α agonists, having both direct and indirect effects. A comparison of the various sympathomimetics is listed in Table 112.1. These agents stimulate both α and β receptors. The effectiveness of these agents depends on the increase in receptor number and affinity and the reduction in baroreflex modulation that accompanies autonomic failure. Ephedrine produces smooth muscle relaxation and cardiac stimulation. This results in blood pressure increases with increased cardiac output and, to a lesser effect, peripheral vasoconstriction [9, 10].

Adverse Events and Disadvantages

Because ephedrine crosses the blood–brain barrier, central nervous system stimulation is similar to that produced by amphetamines. Frequent side effects, such as nervousness, anxiety, headaches, weakness, dizziness, tremulousness, and supine hypertension result from this

TABLE 112.1 Sympathomimetic Agents for Treatment of Neurogenic Orthostatic Hypotension

Pharmacologic agent	Mechanism of action	Dose	ΩSide effects
Direct actions			
Midodrine HCL	α_1-Adrenergic agonist with activation of arteriolar and venous vasculature, and decreases venous pooling	2.5–10 mg every 3–4 hr, to maximal dose of 50–60 mg	Piloerection, urinary retention supine, hypertension
Mixed direct and indirect actions			
Ephedrine Pseudoephedrine	Stimulation α/β receptors action depends on receptors and baroreceptor defects	12.5–25 mg three times daily, 30–60 mg three times daily	Nervousness, tremors, anxiety, insomnia, agitation, arrhythmias, supine hypertension
Phenylpropanolamine Methylphenidate	Action depends on norepinephrine release from postganglionic neurons	12–25 mg three times daily, 5–10 mg three times daily dosage before 6 PM	Nervousness, tremors, anxiety, insomnia, agitation, arrhythmias, supine hypertension

class of pharmacologic agents. Furthermore, angina and potentially fatal arrhythmias may be provoked in patients with ischemic heart disease. Ephedrine may also constrict renal blood vessels and decrease urine production. Other disadvantages can occur including tachyphylaxis (tolerance), which often develops within weeks [9, 10].

Dosing

The doses required for effective treatment of neurogenic orthostatic hypotension with these α sympathomimetic agents are often greater than those contained in commonly used decongestants. Ephedrine doses of 12.5 to 25 mg three times daily are the most commonly used. Other over-the-counter sympathomimetics, such as pseudoephedrine (30 to 60 mg three times daily) and phenylpropanolamine (12.5 to 25 mg three times daily), are also included in this class. Phenylpropanolamine has been found to be associated with a small but significant risk for cerebrovascular accident and has been removed from the market by the Food and Drug Regulation Administration. Methylphenidate and dextromethorphan sulfate also have indirect and amphetamine-like actions [9, 10]. The vasoconstrictor effect results from norepinephrine release from postganglionic neurons, and it may be more effective in patients with partial or incomplete lesions. Doses required for methylphenidate are 5 to 10 mg three times daily with meals, with the last dose being given before 6 PM. Common side effects include agitation, tremor, insomnia, and hypertension. This pharmacologic agent also has central nervous system stimulation, which limits its use, and it is also a controlled substance.

References

1. McTavish, D., and K. L. Goa. 1989. Midodrine. A review of its pharmacological principles and therapeutic use in orthostatic hypotension and secondary hypotensive disorders. *Drugs* 38:757–777.
2. Wright, R. A., H. C. Kaufmann, R. Perera, T. L. Opfer-Gehrking, M. A. McElligott, K. N. Sheng, and P. A. Low. 1998. A double-blind, dose response study of midodrine in neurogenic orthostatic hypotension. *Neurology* 51:120–124.
3. Kaufmann, H., T. Brannan, L. Krakoff, M. D. Yahr, and J. Mandeli. 1988. Treatment of orthostatic hypotension due to autonomic failure with a peripheral alpha-adrenergic agonist (midodrine). *Neurology* 38:951–956.
4. Jankovic, J., J. L. Gilden, B. C. Hiner, H. Kaufmann, D. C. Brown, C. H. Coghlan, M. Rubin, and F. M. Fouad-Tarazi. 1998. Neurogenic orthostatic hypotension: A double-blind placebo controlled study with midodrine. *Am. J. Med.* 95:38–48.
5. Gilden, J. L. 1993. Midodrine in neurogenic orthostatic hypotension: A new treatment. *Int. Angiol.* 12:125–131.
6. Gilden, J. L., and H. Kaufmann. 1994. Midodrine therapy for neurogenic orthostatic hypotension. A double-blind placebo controlled study [Abstract]. *Clin. Auton. Res.* 4:203.
7. Low, P. A., J. L. Gilden, R. Freeman, K. Sheng, M. A. McElligott, for the Midodrine Study Group. 1997. Efficacy of midodrine vs placebo in neurogenic orthostatic hypotension: A randomized, double-blind multicenter study. *JAMA.* 277:1046–1051.
8. Fouad-Tarazi, F., M. Okabe, and H. Goren. 1995. Alpha sympathomimetic treatment of autonomic insufficiency with orthostatic hypotension. *Am. J. Med.* 99:604–610.
9. Grubb, B. P., and B. Karas. 1999. Clinical disorders of the autonomic nervous system associated with orthostatic intolerance: An overview of classification, clinical evaluation, and management. *Pacing Clin. Electrophysiol.* 22:798–810.
10. Robertson, D., and T. L. Davis. 1995. Recent advances in the treatment of orthostatic hypotension. *Neurology* 45(Suppl 5):S26–S32.
11. Grubb B. P., D. J. Kosinski, and Y. Kanjwal. 2003. Orthostatic hypotension: Causes, classification and treatment. *Pacing Clin Electrophysiol* 26:892–901.

113 Dihydroxyphenylserine

Roy Freeman
Center for Autonomic and Peripheral Nerve Disorders
Beth Israel Deaconess Medical Center
Boston, Massachusetts

Norepinephrine plays a major role in central and peripheral blood pressure control. It is the primary neurotransmitter at the peripheral autonomic neurovascular junction and an important neurotransmitter in those brainstem regions involved in the maintenance of blood pressure. Neurogenic orthostatic hypotension results from impaired noradrenergic neurotransmission; postganglionic sympathetic neurons do not release norepinephrine appropriately [1]. This defect in norepinephrine release can be caused by disorders of central and peripheral autonomic neurons and, rarely, by an enzymatic defect in catecholamine synthesis [2].

The successful therapy of Parkinson's disease, a disorder of dopaminergic neurotransmission, with the dopamine precursor, L-dihydroxyphenylalanine (L-Dopa), suggested that 3,4-dihydroxyphenylserine (DOPS), a synthetic precursor of norepinephrine, might improve noradrenergic neurotransmission and relieve orthostatic hypotension in patients with autonomic failure.

DOPS has two asymmetric carbons and four stereoisomers, but only one of the stereoisomers—L-threo-DOPS—is converted to biologically active L-norepinephrine by the enzyme L-aromatic amino acid decarboxylase (L-AADC). Because pure L-DOPS was unavailable in the United States, most studies have used the racemic mixture of DOPS (which contains 50% D- and 50% L-threo DOPS) [3]. It has been suggested, however, that the D isoform may inhibit the decarboxylation of the L isoform to L-norepinephrine, which may explain the lack of therapeutic efficacy of racemic DOPS in several clinical studies [4].

PRECURSOR THERAPY FOR ORTHOSTATIC HYPOTENSION

There is a large body of preclinical evidence showing that DOPS, both orally and parenterally, produces noradrenergic effects, thereby counteracting some effects of norepinephrine depletion [5]. Of special interest are the observations that DOPS had cardiovascular effects, particularly (1) the production of a chronotropic effect in isolated rat atria; (2) the production of a long-lasting pressor response in rats; (3) an increase in mean arterial blood pressure and regional cerebral blood flow; and (4) an improvement in postural hypotension in anesthetized rats.

Biaggioni and Robertson [2] and Man in't Veld and colleagues [6] first showed that administration of DOPS could be used to treat orthostatic hypotension. These investigators reported that L-DOPS improved orthostatic hypotension in autonomic failure caused by deficiency of the enzyme dopamine β-hydroxylase (the enzyme that catalyzes the conversion of dopamine to norepinephrine). L-DOPS replenished norepinephrine stores and treated orthostatic hypotension in these patients because its conversion to norepinephrine is catalyzed by the ubiquitous enzyme, L-AADC, and thus bypasses the deficient dopamine β-hydroxylase (Fig. 113.1).

The role of DOPS in the treatment of orthostatic hypotension caused by the more prevalent degenerative disorders of central and peripheral autonomic neurons is unresolved. Most studies have been small, open-label, single-blinded, and individual case studies. For example, a placebo-controlled study using racemic DL-threo-DOPS in six patients with autonomic failure (caused by diabetic autonomic neuropathy and pure autonomic failure) showed no improvement in orthostatic hypotension, and only 2% of the administered DOPS converted to norepinephrine [7].

Using a greater dosage of DL-DOPS, we showed a pressor effect in patients with autonomic failure and an increased plasma concentration of norepinephrine. This effect was present in patients with orthostatic hypotension [8, 10] and postprandial hypotension [11] caused by peripheral and central autonomic disorders. The pressor effect was associated with an increase in forearm vascular resistance. The pressor response had a gradual onset and a long duration. The maximum supine blood pressure occurred 300 minutes after ingestion of medication (Fig. 113.2) [8]. In addition, in studies using L-DOPS in a small number of patients, a significant improvement in orthostatic hypotension was demonstrated, particularly in patients with multiple system atrophy [12]. An open-label trial with a larger number of patients with autonomic failure showed that DOPS improved orthostatic hypotension [13].

The mechanism(s) whereby DOPS improves blood pressure control in autonomic failure also is unresolved.

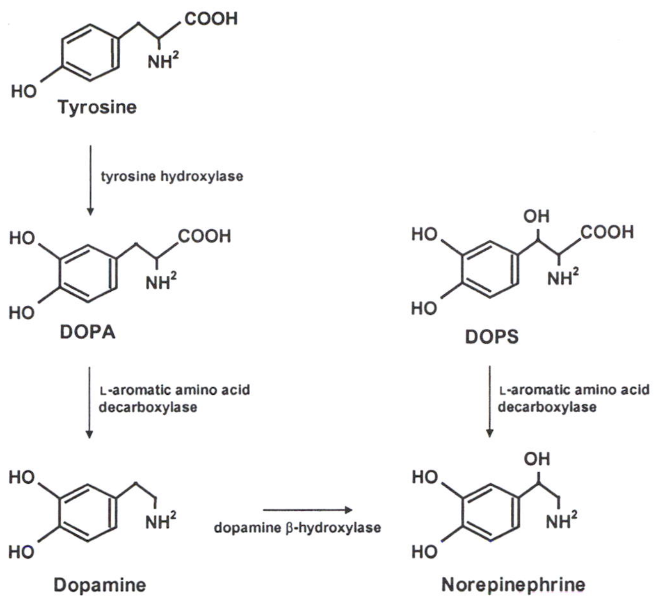

Tyrosine

tyrosine hydroxylase

DOPA

DOPS

L-aromatic amino acid decarboxylase

L-aromatic amino acid decarboxylase

Dopamine

dopamine β-hydroxylase

Norepinephrine

FIGURE 113.1 The formation of norepinephrine from dihydroxyphenylserine (DOPS). (Modified from Freeman, R., L. Landsberg, and J. Young. 1999. The treatment of neurogenic orthostatic hypotension with 3,4-DL-threo-dihydroxyphenylserine: A randomized, placebo-controlled, crossover trial. *Neurology* 53:2151–2157.)

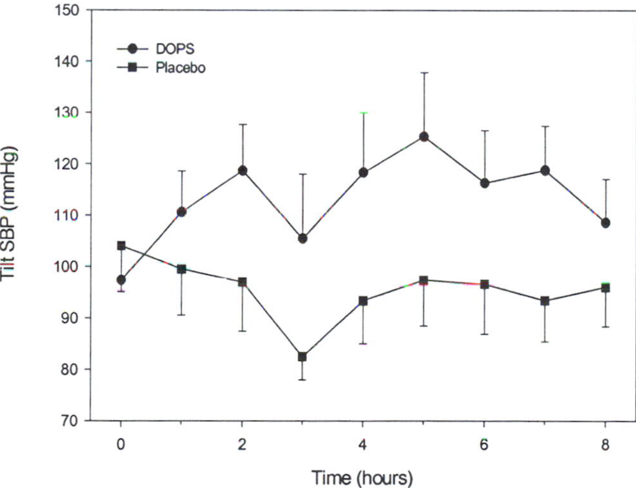

FIGURE 113.2 The systolic blood pressure (SBP) response to DL-dihydroxyphenylserine (DOPS) and placebo. Note the attenuation of the postprandial blood pressure decrease after the midday meal approximately 3 hours after ingestion of medication. (Modified from Freeman, R., L. Landsberg, and J. Young. 1999. The treatment of neurogenic orthostatic hypotension with 3,4-DL-threo-dihydroxyphenylserine: A randomized, placebo-controlled, crossover trial. *Neurology* 53:2151–2157.)

Investigators have proposed central and peripheral mechanisms. In patients with autonomic failure caused by dopamine β-hydroxylase deficiency, DOPS is most likely decarboxylated to norepinephrine in intact sympathetic neurons, and the generated norepinephrine acts as a neurotransmitter [2]. Investigators have suggested that DOPS exerts its effect after entry into the central nervous system, thereby stimulating sympathetic outflow [14]. However, it seems more likely that DOPS is converted to norepinephrine outside sympathetic neurons because the enzyme L-AADC is ubiquitously distributed in tissues, including kidney, gut, and liver. The generated norepinephrine then acts as a circulating vasoconstrictor hormone.

Although more recent data suggest that precursor therapy with DOPS increases plasma norepinephrine and effectively treats orthostatic hypotension [9], it is not yet known whether supplementation of the depleted neurotransmitter offers additional advantages over direct agonist therapy, with agents such as midodrine, a direct α-adrenergic agonist. Precursor therapy may be helpful for those patients who do not respond to standard therapies. The different mechanisms of action, pharmacokinetics, and duration of effect suggest that combination therapy with a precursor and direct α-adrenoreceptor agonist may be beneficial in some patients. Such an approach has been successfully implemented in the treatment of extrapyramidal dysfunction in patients with Parkinson's disease.

References

1. Goldstein, D. S., R. J. Polinsky, M. Garty, D. Robertson, R. T. Brown, I. Biaggioni, R. Stull, and I. J. Kopin. 1989. Patterns of plasma levels of catechols in neurogenic orthostatic hypotension. *Ann. Neurol.* 26:558–563.
2. Biaggioni, I., and D. Robertson. 1987. Endogenous restoration of noradrenaline by precursor therapy in dopamine-beta-hydroxylase deficiency. *Lancet* 2:1170–1172.
3. Bartholini, J., J. Constantinidis, M. Puig, R. Tissot, and A. Pletscher. 1975. The stereoisomers of 3,4-dihydroxyphenylserine as precursors of norepinephrine. *J. Pharmacol. Exp. Ther.* 193:523–532.
4. Inagaki, C., H. Fujiwara, and C. Tanaka. 1976. Inhibitory effect of (+)threo-3,4-dihydroxy-phenylserine (DOPS) on decarboxylation of (−)threo-dops. *Jpn. J. Pharmacol.* 26:380–382.
5. Satoh, S., A. Oyabe, M. Tanno, and M. Suzuki-Kusaba. 1989. Beneficial attenuating effect of L-threo-3,4-dihydroxyphenylserine on postural hypotension in anesthetized rats. *Arzneimittel-Forschung.* 39:1123–1129.
6. Man in't Veld, A. J., F. Boomsma, A. H. van den Meiracker, and M. A. Schalekamp. 1987. Effect of unnatural noradrenaline precursor on sympathetic control and orthostatic hypotension in dopamine-beta-hydroxylase deficiency. *Lancet* 2:1172–1175.
7. Hoeldtke, R. D., K. M. Cilmi, and K. Mattis-Graves. 1984. DL-Threo-3,4-dihydroxyphenylserine does not exert a pressor effect in orthostatic hypotension. *Clin. Pharmacol. Ther.* 36:302–306.
8. Freeman, R., L. Landsberg, and J. Young. 1999. The treatment of neurogenic orthostatic hypotension with 3,4-DL-threo-dihydroxyphenylserine: A randomized, placebo-controlled, crossover trial. *Neurology* 53:2151–2157.

9. Kaufman, H., D. Saadia, A. Voustianiouk, D. S. Goldstein, C. Holmes, M. D. Yahr, R. Nardin, and R. Freeman. 2003. Norepinephrine precursor therapy in neurogenic orthostatic hypotension. *Circulation* 108:724–738.
10. Freeman, R., and L. Landsberg. 1991. The treatment of orthostatic hypotension with dihydroxyphenylserine. *Clin. Neuropharmacol.* 14:296–304.
11. Freeman, R., J. B. Young, L. Landsberg, and L. A. Lipsitz. 1996. The treatment of postprandial hypotension in autonomic failure with 3,4-DL-threo-dihydroxyphenylserine. *Neurology* 47:1414–1420.
12. Kaufmann, H., E. Oribe, and M. D. Yahr. 1991. Differential effect of L-threo-3,4-dihydroxyphenylserine in pure autonomic failure and multiple system atrophy with autonomic failure. *J. Neural. Transm. Park Dis. Dement. Sect.* 3:143–148.
13. Mathias, C. J., J. M. Senard, S. Braune, L. Watson, A. Aragishi, J. E. Keeling, and M. D. Taylor. 2001. L-threo-dihydroxyphenylserine (L-threo-DOPS; droxidopa) in the management of neurogenic orthostatic hypotension: A multi-national, multi-center, dose-ranging study in multiple system atrophy and pure autonomic failure. *Clin. Auton. Res.* 11:235–242.
14. Kachi, T., S. Iwase, T. Mano, M. Saito, M. Kunimoto, and I. Sobue. 1988. Effect of L-threo-3,4-dihydroxyphenylserine on muscle sympathetic nerve activities in Shy-Drager syndrome. *Neurology* 38:1091–1094.

114 Adrenergic Agonists and Antagonists in Autonomic Failure

Roy Freeman
Center for Autonomic and Peripheral Nerve Disorders
Beth Israel Deaconess Medical Center
Boston, Massachusetts

Neurogenic orthostatic hypotension in autonomic failure is caused by impaired release of norepinephrine from postganglionic sympathetic neurons. The α_1-adrenoreceptor agonists are the primary therapeutic agents in the treatment of this disorder. The direct (those that act directly on the α-adrenoreceptor) and mixed (those that act directly on the α-adrenoreceptor and release norepinephrine from the postganglionic sympathetic neuron) are the most widely used agents. The indirect agonists and α_2-adrenoreceptor agonists and antagonists may have therapeutic benefits in selected patients.

Neurogenic orthostatic hypotension is in large part a consequence of the failure to release the adrenoreceptor agonist, norepinephrine, from sympathetic neurons, which results in impaired vasoconstriction in response to postural change. Thus, once intravascular volume is replete with varying combinations of fluid, sodium chloride, and fludrocortisone acetate, the adrenergic agonists and antagonists are used to treat this disorder. The pressor response of these agents is caused by the reduction in venous capacity and constriction of the resistance vessels.

SYMPATHOMIMETIC AGENTS

The effectiveness of the sympathomimetic agents is most likely dependent on the increase in receptor number and affinity and the reduction in baroreceptor modulation that accompanies autonomic failure. These drugs do not increase blood pressure significantly in patients who do not have autonomic failure.

The available α_1-adrenoreceptor agonists include those with direct and indirect effects (ephedrine, pseudoephedrine, and phenylpropanolamine), those with direct effects (midodrine and phenylephrine), and those with only indirect effects (methylphenidate and dextroamphetamine sulphate).

The peripheral, selective, direct, α_1-adrenoreceptor agonist, midodrine, is the only agent approved by the U. S. Food and Drug Administration (FDA) for the treatment of orthostatic hypotension [1]. The pressor effect of midodrine is caused by both arterial and venous constriction. The efficacy of this agent has been demonstrated in double-blind, placebo-controlled studies [1–3]. The prodrug midodrine is activated to desglymidodrine, the active α-adrenoreceptor agonist. Midodrine is rapidly absorbed from the gastrointestinal tract. There is 93% bioavailability after oral administration. The peak plasma concentration of midodrine occurs in 20 to 40 minutes. Midodrine has an elimination half-life of 0.5 hour and is undetectable in plasma 2 hours after an oral dose. There is minimal protein binding and the agent undergoes enzymatic hydrolysis (deglycination) in the systemic circulation to form the active agent, desglymidodrine. Desglymidodrine is 15 times more potent than midodrine and is primarily responsible for the therapeutic effect. The elimination half-life of desglymidodrine is 2 to 4 hours. Desglymidodrine is predominantly excreted by the kidneys.

Patient sensitivity to this agent varies and the dose should be titrated from 2.5 to 10 mg three times a day. The peak effect of this agent occurs 1 hour after ingestion [3]. Potential side effects of midodrine include pilomotor reactions, pruritus, supine hypertension, gastrointestinal complaints, and urinary retention. Central nervous system side effects occur infrequently.

The mixed α-adrenoreceptor agonists, which act directly on the α-adrenoreceptor and release norepinephrine from the postganglionic sympathetic neuron, include ephedrine, pseudoephedrine, and phenylpropanolamine. Ephedrine is an agonist of α, β_1, and β_2 receptors. The β_2 vasodilatory effects may attenuate the pressor effect of this drug. Pseudoephedrine, a stereoisomer of ephedrine, and phenylpropanolamine (D,L-norephedrine), an ephedrine metabolite, have similar pharmacologic and therapeutic properties. Phenylpropanolamine may have less β-adrenoreceptor agonists than ephedrine and less central sympathomimetic effects [4]. Typical doses of these indirect agonists are ephedrine (25–50 mg three times a day), pseudoephedrine (30–60 mg three times a day), and phenylpropanolamine (12.5–25 mg three times a day). Because the effectiveness of the indirect agonists is at least in part because of the release of norepinephrine from the postganglionic neuron, these medications are in theory most likely to benefit patients with partial or incomplete lesions [5–7].

The indirect agonists, methylphenidate and dextroamphetamine, that release norepinephrine from postganglionic neurons are infrequently used to treat orthostatic hypotension.

There are few head-to-head comparisons of the α-adrenoreceptor agonists. In a small clinical trial, midodrine (mean dosage 8.4 mg three times daily) improved standing blood pressure and orthostatic tolerance more than ephedrine (22.3 mg three times daily) [8]. Phenylpropanolamine (12.5 mg) and yohimbine (5.4 mg) produced equivalent increases in standing systolic blood pressure, whereas methylphenidate failed to increase standing systolic blood pressure significantly [4].

The use of the sympathomimetic agents (with the possible exception of midodrine) may be complicated by tachyphylaxis, although efficacy may be regained after a short drug holiday. The central sympathomimetic side effects such as anxiety, tremulousness, and tachycardia that invariably accompany the use of these agents are frequently intolerable to patients. Midodrine, which does not cross the blood–brain barrier, does not have these central sympathomimetic side effects. Although phenylpropanolamine may result in less central nervous system stimulation than the other agents, recent data suggest that phenylpropanolamine increases the risk for hemorrhagic stroke in women [9]. The FDA is examining the toxicity of this and other indirect and mixed α-adrenoreceptor antagonists and has suggested that phenylpropanolamine be removed from all drug products.

CLONIDINE

Clonidine is an α_2 antagonist that usually produces a central, sympatholytic effect and a consequent decrease in blood pressure. In patients with autonomic failure who have little central sympathetic efferent activity, the effect of this agent on postsynaptic α_2-adrenoreceptors may predominate. These receptors may be more numerous on veins than arterioles. The use of clonidine (0.1–0.6 mg/day) could, therefore, result in an increase in venous return without a significant increase in peripheral vascular resistance. The use of this agent, at least theoretically, is limited to patients with severe central autonomic dysfunction in whom there is no ostensible effect of further sympatholysis and the peripheral effect may dominate. The hypertensive effect is inconsistent, and, in some patients, residual sympathetic activity could be inhibited. The agent may cause profound hypotension in patients with autonomic failure. Other side effects include dry mouth and sedation [10, 11].

YOHIMBINE

Yohimbine is a centrally and peripherally active selective α_2-adrenoreceptor antagonist that increases sympathetic nervous system efferent output by antagonizing central or presynaptic α_2-adrenoreceptors, or both. Yohimbine (2.5–5.4 mg three times daily) enhances norepinephrine release from postganglionic sympathetic neurons and produces a modest pressor effect. This agent, theoretically, should be more effective in patients that have some residual sympathetic nervous system output, although this has not always been borne out in clinical studies. Side effects of yohimbine include anxiety, tremor, palpitations, diarrhea, and supine hypertension [4, 12].

References

1. Low, P. A., J. L. Gilden, R. Freeman, K. N. Sheng, and M. A. McElligott. 1997. Efficacy of midodrine vs placebo in neurogenic orthostatic hypotension. A randomized, doubleblind multicenter study. Midodrine Study Group. *JAMA*. 277:1046–1051.
2. Kaufmann, H., T. Brannan, L. Krakoff, M. D. Yahr, and J. Mandeli. 1988. Treatment of orthostatic hypotension due to autonomic failure with a peripheral alpha-adrenergic agonist (midodrine). *Neurology* 38:951–956.
3. Wright, R. A., H. C. Kaufmann, R. Perera, T. L. Opfer-Gehrking, M. A. McElligott, K. N. Sheng, and P. A. Low. 1998. A double-blind, dose-response study of midodrine in neurogenic orthostatic hypotension. *Neurology* 51:120–124.
4. Jordan, J., J. R. Shannon, I. Biaggioni, R. Norman, B. K. Black, and D. Robertson. 1998. Contrasting actions of pressor agents in severe autonomic failure. *Am. J. Med.* 105:116–124.
5. Ghrist, D. G., and G. E. Brown. 1928. Postural hypertension with syncope: Its successful treatment with ephedrine. *Am. J. Med. Sci.* 175:336–349.
6. Davies, B., R. Bannister, and P. Sever. 1978. Pressor amines and monoamine-oxidase inhibitors for treatment of postural hypotension in autonomic failure. Limitations and hazards. *Lancet* 1:172–175.
7. Biaggioni, I., J. Onrot, C. K. Stewart, and D. Robertson. 1987. The potent pressor effect of phenylpropanolamine in patients with autonomic impairment. *JAMA*. 258:236–239.
8. Fouad-Tarazi, F. M., M. Okabe, and H. Goren. 1995. Alpha sympathomimetic treatment of autonomic insufficiency with orthostatic hypotension. *Am. J. Med.* 99:604–610.
9. Kernan W. N., C. M. Viscoli, L. M. Brass, J. P. Broderick, T. Brott, E. Feldmann, L. B. Morgenstern, J. L. Wilterdink, and R. I. Horwitz. 2000. Phenylpropanolamine and the risk of hemorrhagic stroke. *N. Engl. J. Med.* 343:1826–1832.
10. Robertson, D., M. R. Goldberg, A. S. Hollister, D. Wade, and R. M. Robertson. 1983. Clonidine raises blood pressure in idiopathic orthostatic hypotension. *Am. J. Med.* 74:193–199.
11. Robertson, D., M. R. Goldberg, C. S. Tung, A. S. Hollister, and R. M. Robertson. 1986. Use of alpha 2 adrenoreceptor agonists and antagonists in the functional assessment of the sympathetic nervous system. *J. Clin. Invest.* 78:576–581.
12. Onrot, J., M. R. Goldberg, I. Biaggioni, R. G. Wiley, A. S. Hollister, and D. Robertson. 1987. Oral yohimbine in human autonomic failure. *Neurology* 37:215–220.

115 Erythropoietin in Autonomic Failure

Italo Biaggioni
Vanderbilt University
Nashville, Tennessee

Patients with severe autonomic failure have a high incidence of anemia, which may contribute to their symptoms. Sympathetic failure can contribute to this anemia by blunting of the expected compensatory erythropoietin response. Recombinant erythropoietin reverses anemia of autonomic failure, improves upright blood pressure, and may ameliorate symptoms of orthostatic hypotension. In the absence of controlled studies, a drug trial with erythropoietin in selected patients who do not respond to other treatment options may be warranted. The long-term safety of this treatment, however, is not known.

MODULATION OF ERYTHROPOIETIN PRODUCTION BY THE AUTONOMIC NERVOUS SYSTEM

Animal studies suggest that the sympathetic nervous system modulates erythropoiesis. The reticulocyte response to acute bloodletting was greatly diminished in rats when their kidneys were functionally denervated. Intravenous administration of the β-adrenergic agonist, salbutamol, increased plasma concentrations of erythropoietin-like factor in rabbits. Conversely, β-blockers blunted the erythropoietin response to hypoxia in rabbits and rats. Thus, β_2-adrenoreceptors could positively modulate erythropoiesis by stimulating erythropoietin production.

THE ANEMIA OF AUTONOMIC FAILURE

Studies in patients with autonomic failure reveal the physiologic significance of the animal experiments described above, and their relevance to humans. Patients with severe autonomic failure have an unusually high incidence of anemia; if World Heath Organization criteria are followed (hemoglobin <120 g/liter for women and <130 g/liter for men), up to 38% of patients are anemic [1] without obvious cause. The anemia of autonomic failure is mild to moderate and is not accompanied by a compensatory increase in reticulocytes, suggesting an inadequate erythropoietic response. Furthermore, an inappropriately low serum erythropoietin is evident in those patients with lower hemoglobin levels.

Lack of sympathetic stimulation may thus result in decreased erythropoietin production and the development of anemia in patients with autonomic failure. In support of this hypothesis, it has been found that the magnitude of sympathetic impairment correlates with the severity of the anemia, and that plasma norepinephrine levels are lowest in patients with the most severe anemia. These results support the hypothesis that sympathetic innervation is required for an adequate erythropoietin response. However, the acute renal denervation does not affect levels of mRNA encoding erythropoietin in animals. It is not certain, therefore, if the anemia of autonomic failure is solely caused by the lack of sympathetic input to erythropoietin-producing cells in the kidney.

That anemia can be associated with low erythropoietin levels in autonomic failure led to its treatment with recombinant erythropoietin (epoetin alfa). This therapy has successfully corrected anemia [1–3], even when used at modest doses (25–50 U/kg body weight, subcutaneously, three times a week). This response further confirms that inadequate erythropoietin production underlies anemia in these patients. Recombinant erythropoietin also increases supine and upright blood pressure in autonomic failure patients and may be effective in ameliorating orthostatic hypotension. This pressor response is expected, because it is a well documented side effect of erythropoietin treatment in chronic renal failure.

RECOMBINANT HUMAN ERYTHROPOIETIN IN THE TREATMENT OF ORTHOSTATIC HYPOTENSION

Treatment of orthostatic hypotension remains a challenge in patients with autonomic failure, and treatment with erythropoietin may provide a therapeutic alternative. These patients are sensitive to volume changes, which explains why administration of fludrocortisone often is the first step in their treatment. Fludrocortisone increases plasma volume only transiently and at the expense of expanding interstitial space. Its effectiveness may be explained by potentiation of pressor hormones rather than by volume changes. Treatment with erythropoietin, therefore, has the theoretic advantage of selectively increasing intravascular volume. This, however, may not be the only explanation for the increase in blood pressure produced by erythropoietin. Erythropoietin increases blood pressure in animals with experimental chronic renal failure, even if anemia is not corrected because of iron deficiency. Therefore, the mechanism by which erythropoietin increases blood pressure is not clear and is likely to be multifactorial. Several mechanisms have been explored, including increased sensitivity to the pressor effects of norepinephrine and angiotensin II, increased plasma endothelin levels, enhanced renal tubular sodium reabsorption, impaired nitric oxide production, and increased cytosolic free calcium in vascular smooth muscle [4]. Hemoglobin can bind nitric oxide, and it has been proposed that anemia can contribute to hypotension because of increased nitric oxide. Treatment of anemia with erythropoietin could increase blood pressure by limiting nitric oxide availability [5]. The relevance of these findings to its pressor effect in autonomic failure remains speculative.

Even though long-term, placebo-controlled studies are lacking, improvement of orthostatic hypotension by erythropoietin has been a consistent finding of published reports. In our anecdotal experience, erythropoietin has been extremely successful in many patients with autonomic failure, but others did not believe that the cost and inconvenience of the treatment justified the modest symptomatic improvement. Thus, a therapeutic trial aimed at normalizing hematocrit often is useful in patients that do not respond to other treatment options.

Potential limitations of this therapy should be considered. Up to 50% of patients with severe autonomic failure also experience significant supine hypertension, and erythropoietin therapy can worsen this problem. This side effect, however, is probably common to all currently available therapies. Other limitations include the inconvenience of injectable administration and the high cost of this medication. It is not known if erythropoietin will prove superior to currently available therapeutic alternatives. The long-term safety of treatment with erythropoietin is not known. Notably, patients with chronic renal failure, in whom hematocrit was "normalized" (to 42%) with erythropoietin, had a greater mortality rate than those in whom correction of anemia was less aggressive (hematocrit, 30%). Notably, however, both groups received similar doses of erythropoietin. These results may not be applicable to patients with autonomic failure, in whom anemia is moderate at worst, but they may be a reason to use this medication with caution.

References

1. Biaggioni, I., D. Robertson, S. Krantz, M. Jones, and V. Haile. 1994. The anemia of autonomic failure: Evidence for sympathetic modulation of erythropoiesis in humans and reversal with recombinant erythropoietin. *Ann. Intern. Med.* 121:181–186.
2. Hoeldtke, R. D., and D. H. P. Streeten. 1993. Treatment of orthostatic hypotension with erythropoietin. *N. Engl. J. Med.* 329:611–615.
3. Perera, R., L. Isola, and H. Kaufmann. 1995. Effect of recombinant erythropoietin on anemia and orthostatic hypotension in primary autonomic failure. *Clin. Auton. Res.* 5:211–213.
4. Vaziri, N. D. 2001. Cardiovascular effects of erythropoietin and anemia correction. *Curr. Opin. Nephrol. Hypertens.* 10:633–637.
5. Rao, S. V., and J. S. Stamler. 2002. Erythropoietin, anemia, and orthostatic hypotension: The evidence mounts. *Clin. Auton. Res.* 12:141–143.

116 Bionic Baroreflex

Takayuki Sato
Department of Cardiovascular Control
Kochi Medical School
Kochi, Japan

André Diedrich
Division of Clinical Pharmacology
Vanderbilt University
Nashville, Tennessee

Kenji Sunagawa
Department of Cardiovascular Dynamics
National Cardiovascular Center Research Institute
Osaka, Japan

A novel therapeutic strategy against central baroreflex failure is proposed on the basis of bionic technology. A recent innovation, bionic baroreflex system (BBS), was achieved to revitalize baroreflex function through a neural interface approach. In the BBS, arterial pressure is sensed through a micromanometer placed in the aortic arch and fed into a computer ambitious of functioning as an artificial vasomotor center. On the basis of measured changes in arterial pressure, the artificial vasomotor center commands an electrical stimulator to provide a stimulus of the appropriate frequency to the vasomotor sympathetic nerves. Although the BBS is not currently available for clinical practice, the future advance in its development is expected.

The arterial baroreflex is the most important negative feedback system to suppress the effects of rapid daily disturbances in arterial pressure [1]. Therefore, in patients with autonomic failure without baroreflex control of arterial pressure, the simple act of standing would cause a decrease in arterial pressure, reducing perfusion of the brain, and resulting potentially in loss of consciousness. The functional restoration of the arterial baroreflex is essential to patients with baroreflex failure caused by autonomic failure.

In patients with central baroreflex failure such as baroreceptor deafferentation, Shy–Drager syndrome, and spinal cord injuries, peripheral sympathetic nerves are still functional but not controlled by the brain. A novel therapeutic strategy has been proposed to use a BBS with a neural interface approach to control arterial pressure [2, 3]. A bionic system is an artificial device for functional replacement of a physiologic system able to mimic its static and dynamic characteristics. In the proposed BBS (Fig. 116.1), arterial pressure is sensed through a micromanometer placed in the aortic arch and fed into a computer ambitious of functioning as an artificial vasomotor center. On the basis of measured changes in arterial pressure, the artificial vasomotor center commands an electrical stimulator to provide a stimulus of the appropriate frequency to the vasomotor sympathetic nerves. This recent innovation, BBS, was achieved to revitalize baroreflex function in an animal model of central baroreflex failure.

BIONIC BAROREFLEX SYSTEM

Theoretic Background

It is of critical importance to identify the algorithm of the artificial vasomotor center—that is, how to determine the stimulation frequency (STM) of the vasomotor sympathetic nerves in response to changes in arterial pressure (AP). On the basis of expertise of bionics and systems physiology, the algorithm has been determined as transfer function by a white-noise system identification method [2]. First, the functional characteristics to be mimicked by the BBS—that is, the open-loop transfer function of native baroreflex (H_{native})—is identified in healthy subjects (Fig. 116.2). Second, the open-loop transfer function of the AP response to STM ($H_{STM \to AP}$) is determined in patients with central baroreflex failure. Finally, a simple process of division, $H_{Native}/H_{STM \to AP}$, could yield the transfer function required for the artificial vasomotor center of the BBS—that is, $H_{AP \to STM}$.

Implementation of Algorithm of Artificial Vasomotor Center in Bionic Baroreflex System

To operate in real time as the artificial vasomotor center, the computer was programmed to automatically calculate instantaneous STM in response to instantaneous AP changes according to a convolution algorithm [2, 3]:

$$\mathrm{STM}(t) = \int_0^\infty \mathrm{h}(\tau) \cdot \mathrm{AP}(t - \tau)\, d\tau$$

where $h(t)$ is an impulse response function computed by an inverse Fourier transform of $H_{AP \to STM}$.

Efficacy of Bionic Baroreflex System

In a prototype of the BBS for rats with central baroreflex failure, the celiac ganglion was selected as the sympathetic vasomotor interface [3]. The efficacy of the BBS against orthostatic hypotension during head-up tilting (HUT) is shown in Figure 116.3. Without the activation of the BBS, HUT produced a rapid progressive decrease in AP by

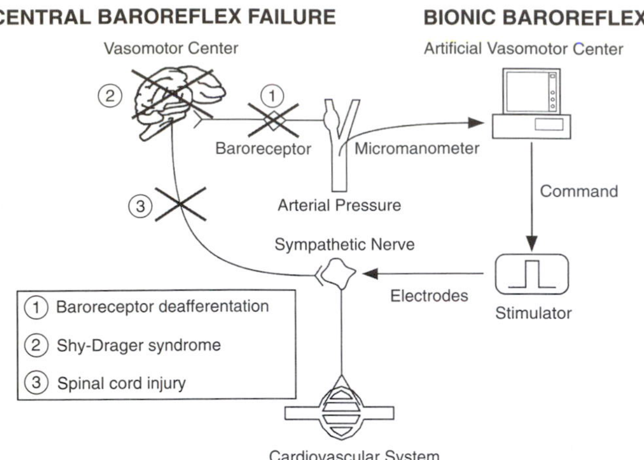

FIGURE 116.1 Central baroreflex failure and its functional replacement by a bionic baroreflex system.

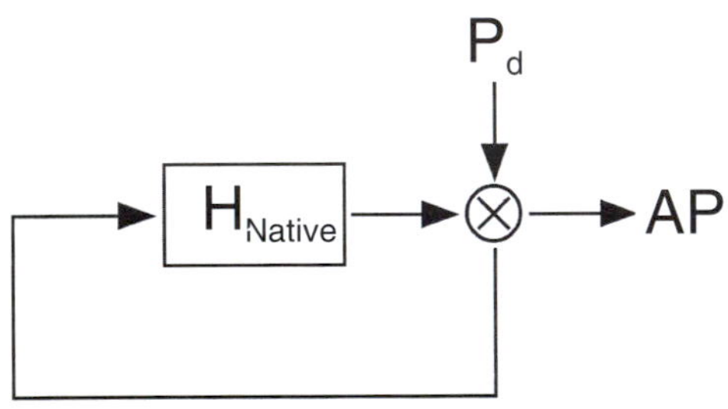

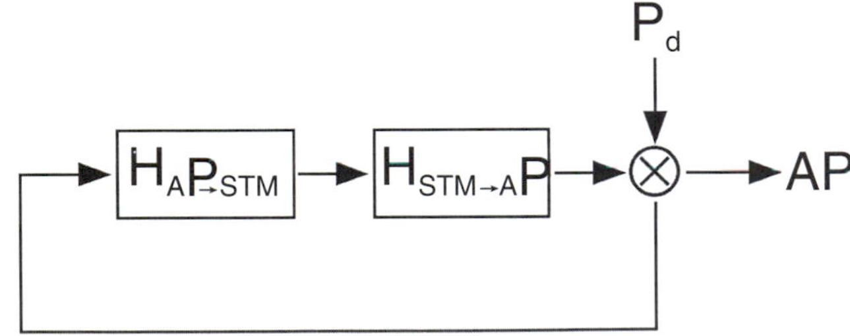

FIGURE 116.2 Block diagrams of native and bionic baroreflex systems. H_{Native} denotes the open-loop transfer function of the native baroreflex system. $H_{AP \rightarrow STM}$ and $H_{STM \rightarrow AP}$ are the open-loop transfer functions from arterial pressure (AP) to the frequency of electrical stimulation (STM) and from STM to AP, respectively. P_d is an external disturbance in pressure. (Modified from Sato, T., T. Kawada, M. Sugimachi, and K. Sunagawa. 2002. Bionic technology revitalizes native baroreflex function in rats with baroreflex failure. *Circulation* 106:730–734.)

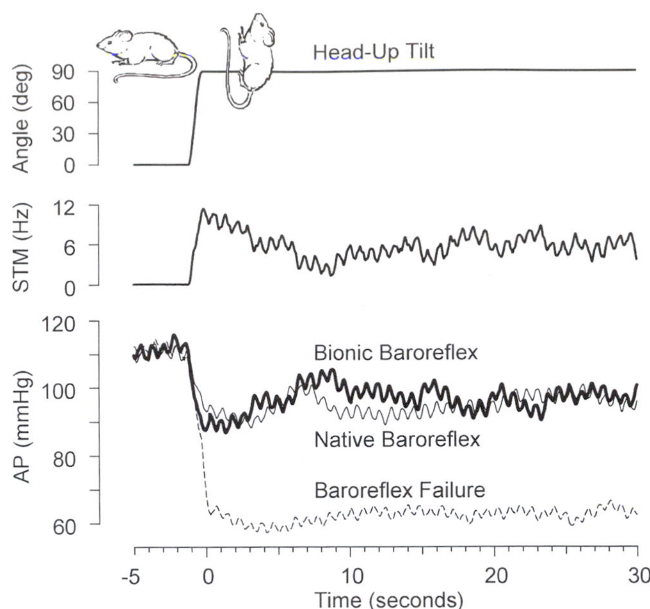

FIGURE 116.3 Real-time operation of the bionic baroreflex system during head-up tilting (HUT). In a model of central baroreflex failure (*broken line*), when the bionic baroreflex system was inactive, arterial pressure (AP) decreased rapidly and severely immediately after HUT. Conversely, whereas the bionic baroreflex system was activated (*thick line*), such an AP decrease was buffered as if the native baroreflex function (*thin line*) was restored. Although sensing changes in AP, the bionic baroreflex system automatically computed the frequency of electrical stimulation (STM) of the sympathetic nerves and drove a stimulator. (Modified from Sato, T., T. Kawada, M. Sugimachi, and K. Sunagawa. 2002. Bionic technology revitalizes native baroreflex function in rats with baroreflex failure. *Circulation* 106:730–734.)

40 mmHg only in 2 seconds. In contrast, whereas the BBS was activated, it automatically computed STM and appropriately stimulated the sympathetic nerves to quickly and effectively attenuate the AP decrease. Such an AP response to HUT during the real-time execution of the BBS was indistinguishable from that during functioning of the native baroreflex system. Therefore, the BBS was considered to revitalize the native baroreflex function.

EPIDURAL CATHETER APPROACH FOR HUMAN BIONIC BAROREFLEX SYSTEM

To apply BIONIC technology to patients, a neural interface with quick and effective controllability of AP in humans is needed. Here we proposed an epidural catheter approach for the human BBS [4]. We percutaneously placed an epidural catheter with a pair of electrodes at the level of Th9-11, and then we randomly altered the stimulation frequency between 0 and 20 Hz (Fig. 116.4A). The step response computed by the transfer function analysis showed that AP

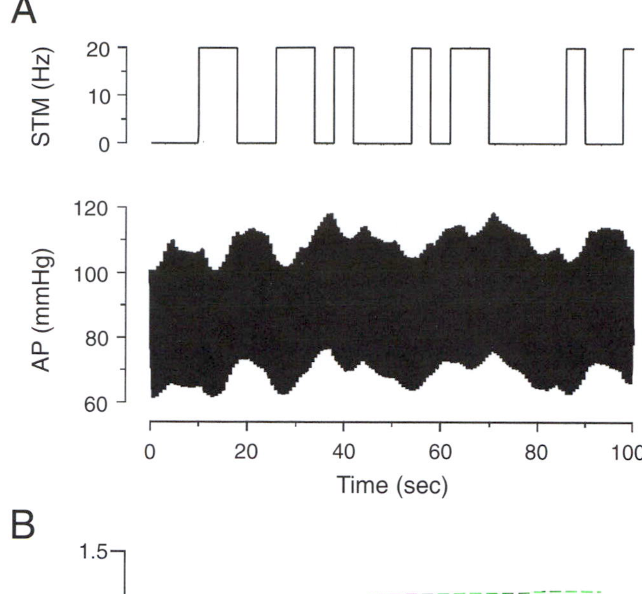

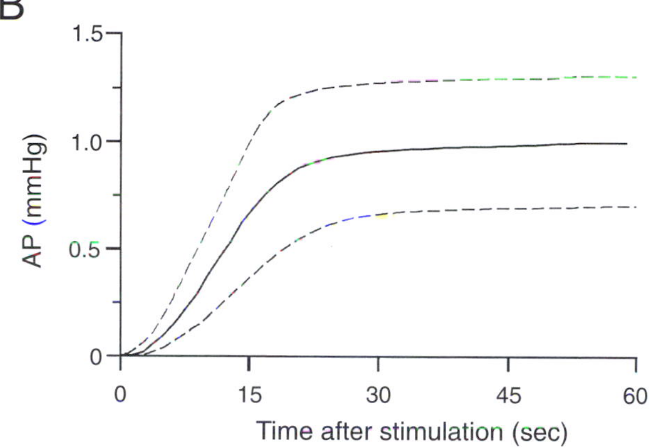

FIGURE 116.4 The response of arterial pressure (AP) to spinal cord stimulation at Th9-11 (**A**) and the step response estimated from the transfer function analysis (**B**).

quickly responded to the electrical stimulation and reached 90% of the steady-state response at 21 ± 5 seconds (see Fig. 116.4B). The gain was 1.0 ± 0.3 mm Hg/Hz. Therefore, the epidural approach would be a potential interface for the human BBS.

CLINICAL IMPLICATIONS

For practical use of the BBS for patients with central baroreflex failure, clinically applicable materials and devices should be developed—that is, a pressure sensor, an implantable stimulator, and stimulating electrodes. Fortunately, certain difficulties posed by these challenges have been already addressed in other areas of clinical practice to some degree, and may be readily adaptable for use with the BBS. For example, a tonometer has been developed as a noninvasive continuous monitor of AP [5]. Implantable pulse generators such as cardiac pacemakers can serve as permanent electrical stimulators. Also, implantable wire leads for nerve stimulation and epidural catheters for spinal stimulation have been approved for the long-term treatment of some neurologic disorders [6].

References

1. Sato, T., T. Kawada, M. Inagaki, T. Shishido, H. Takaki, M. Sugimachi, and K. Sunagawa. 1999. New analytic framework for understanding sympathetic baroreflex control of arterial pressure. *Am. J. Physiol. Heart Circ. Physiol.* 276:H2251–H2261.
2. Sato, T., T. Kawada, T. Shishido, M. Sugimachi, J. Alexander, Jr., and K. Sunagawa. 1999. Novel therapeutic strategy against central baroreflex failure: A bionic baroreflex system. *Circulation* 100:299–304.
3. Sato, T., T. Kawada, M. Sugimachi, and K. Sunagawa. 2002. Bionic technology revitalizes native baroreflex function in rats with baroreflex failure. *Circulation* 106:730–734.
4. Sato, T., M. Ando, and F. Yamasaki. 2002. New potential interface of bionic system for revitalization of baroreflex function: Epidural catheter approach in humans. *Circulation* 106(Suppl II):II–110.
5. Sato, T., M. Nishinaga, A. Kawamoto, T. Ozawa, and H. Takatsuji. 1993. Accuracy of a continuous blood pressure monitor based on arterial tonometry. *Hypertension* 21:866–874.
6. Shimoji, K., H. Kitamura, E. Ikezono, H. Shimizu, K. Okamoto, and Y. Iwakura. 1974. Spinal hypalgesia and analgesia by low-frequency electrical stimulation in the epidural space. *Anesthesiology* 41:91–94.

117

Acupuncture

John C. Longhurst
Department of Medicine
University of California, Irvine
Irvine, California

Acupuncture has been practiced for more than 3000 years in China [1], an important component of traditional Chinese medicine (TCM). TCM includes evaluation of the pulse, the tongue, and the general appearance of the patient and treatment using acupuncture, massage, and herbal therapy. Traditional physicians use acupuncture in a variety of disease conditions, which they describe as either having a deficiency or excess of Qi (pronounced "Chi"), a term for energy that flows through meridians and organ systems. The organs are named similarly, but they are not anatomically identical to the Western equivalent, including the heart, pericardium, lung, spleen, kidney, liver, gallbladder, stomach, small and large intestine, bladder and triple burner (no Western correlate). The use of acupuncture has spread to other countries, including Korea and Japan, and more recently to the United States and Europe. In practice, acupuncture is applied at one or more of the greater than 600 acupuncture points (also called acupoints) located along the meridians using thin (~32 ga) needles that are inserted and left in place or sometimes manipulated manually, or stimulated electrically during electroacupuncture (EA). The actual practice varies from country to country and from physician to physician, but generally one acupuncture point, or more commonly a combination of acupoints, is stimulated in an attempt to restore Qi that is circulating through the meridians and their associated organ systems. As alternatives to acupuncture, acupressure or heat (called moxibustion) can be applied to the acupoint. In addition to the classical 12 meridians, auricular acupuncture, originating recently from Europe, is frequently used in treatment.

WESTERN UNDERSTANDING OF ACUPUNCTURE

It is difficult to reconcile all aspects of acupuncture according to our knowledge of anatomy and physiology. However, many, if not all, of the meridians and their associated acupoints are located over major peripheral somatic neural pathways that can be stimulated by acupuncture needles, pressure, or heat. Stimulated action potentials then are transmitted by fine afferent nerve fibers to the central nervous system (CNS) where they lead to the release of neurotransmitters and neuromodulators that can have a profound effect on several regions concerned with pain and neural humoral regulation of the cardiovascular system. The type of neuromodulator released depends on the afferent stimulus. Low-frequency EA (2–6 Hz) leads to the release of endogenous opioids, including endorphins and enkephalins, because the effects can be substantially reduced by naloxone (Fig. 117.1) [2]. Other neurotransmitters that may play a role in low-frequency EA include γ-aminobutyric acid and serotonin [3]. Preliminary data suggest that nociceptin also may play a role in low-frequency EA [4]. High-frequency EA (>100 Hz) also leads to the release of opioids, particularly dynorphin [5]. Low-frequency EA has been used most extensively in treatment of pain and cardiovascular conditions, although there also may be a role for high-frequency EA, both in treatment of pain and in clinical conditions associated with hypotension. The increase in blood pressure evoked by high-frequency EA in hypotensive conditions may be associated with release of the neurotransmitter acetylcholine [3]. Low-frequency EA does not alter resting blood pressure of normotensive subjects, but it can reduce blood pressure during sympathoexcitatory reflex responses.

NEUROLOGIC SUBSTRATE

Direct multiunit and single-unit recordings show that stimulation of group III and probably group IV somatic afferents constitute the predominate sensory input to the CNS during acupuncture [6]. During percutaneous acupuncture or transcutaneous epidermal nerve stimulation, to simulate EA, most patients report a sensation of heaviness, tingling, numbness, or mild pain that is called DeQi by physicians of TCM. These sensations, including the absence of sharp pain, suggest that group III afferents form the predominate afferent pathway stimulated by low-frequency, low-intensity EA. Histologic mapping studies, using c-Fos, have shown that the hypothalamic supramammillary bodies, arcuate nucleus, midbrain ventrolateral periaqueductal gray (PAG), and caudal raphe, as well as the raphe obscurus and

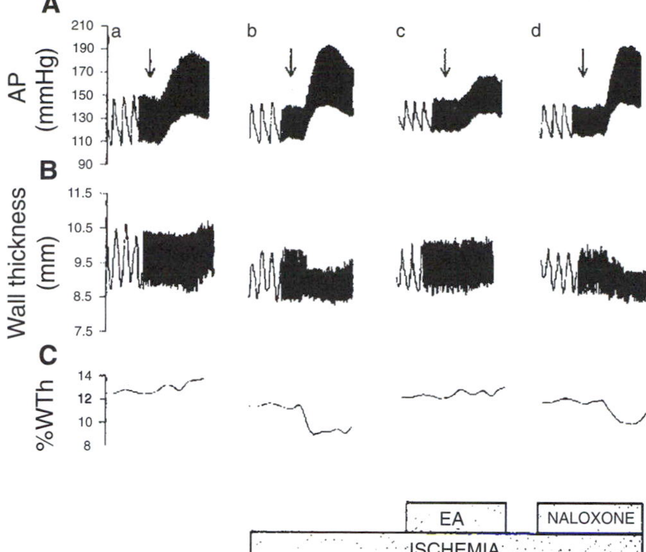

FIGURE 117.1 Reflex increases in arterial blood pressure and regional myocardial function after application of bradykinin 10 μg/ml) to the gallbladder (*arrows*). Regional function was measured with a single crystal sonomicrometer system that assessed wall thickening (WTh), which was measured online with a computer and expressed as percentage WTh. From left to right are shown responses to blood pressure and cardiac function after treatment with bradykinin under control normal coronary artery flow conditions (**A**), after occlusion of a diagonal branch of the left anterior descending coronary artery to create ischemia during gallbladder stimulation (**B**), superimposition of 30 minutes of electroacupuncture (EA) (**C**) at the *Neiguan* acupoints bilaterally, which are situated over the median nerve and following intravenous administration of naloxone (0.4 mg/kg) (**D**). Naloxone was administered 5 to 10 minutes after termination of EA, at a time when EA has been shown to significantly inhibit the ischemic responses to the increased oxygen demand produced by the reflex increases in arterial blood pressure after coronary artery occlusion. Because naloxone reversed the effect of EA, these results suggest that EA modulates the reflexly induced myocardial ischemic response through an opioid mechanism. (From Chao, D. M., L. L. Shen, S. Tjen-A-Looi, K. F. Pitsillides, P. Li, and S. C. Longhurst. 1999. Naloxone reverses inhibitory effect of electroacupuncture on sympathetic cardiovascular reflex responses. *Am. J. Physiol.* 276:H2127–H2134, with permission.)

rostral ventral lateral medulla (rVLM), among other regions, are activated during EA (Fig. 117.2) [3, 5, 7]. The arcuate nucleus represents an important source of opioid peptides that are either transported through direct neural connections through the cerebrospinal fluid or via the circulatory system to other regions such as the PAG and rVLM. Pharmacologic studies have shown that μ- and δ-, but not κ-opioid receptors, in the rVLM are responsible for much of the inhibitory effect of EA on sympathoexcitatory reflexes (Fig. 117.3) [8]. This information suggests that β-endorphin, endomorphin, and met-enkephalin, but not dynorphin, serve as important control neurotransmitters in low-frequency EA brainstem modulation of sympathetic outflow to the cardiovascular system. Likewise, preliminary studies indicate that nociceptin in the rVLM also may play a role in this response [4]. Much work remains to be done to fully define the complex central neural interconnections and neurotransmitter systems involved in EA regulation of sympathetic outflow to the cardiovascular system.

CLINICAL ROLE OF ACUPUNCTURE

Strong randomized blinded controlled studies are available suggesting that acupuncture can be used clinically to treat many, but not all, forms of pain [1, 5, 9–11]. For example, a number of studies indicate that this therapy reduces dental pain. There is a rich history in China of the use of acupuncture as anesthesia. Currently, acupuncture is used mainly as an adjunctive measure to decrease the doses of injectable and inhalational anesthetics. There also is good evidence suggesting that acupuncture reduces nausea and vomiting [11]. A number of isolated studies indicate that acupuncture also may be helpful in treatment of several cardiovascular disorders including hypertension, possibly hypotensive disorders, myocardial ischemia (see Fig. 117.1), and certain arrhythmias [3]. It appears that acupuncture, especially EA, is useful in the treatment of these cardiovascular disorders through its ability to alter premotor sympathoexcitatory outflow from medullary regions like the rVLM. The capability of acupuncture in reducing blood pressure in hypertensive states and during excitatory reflexes or to increase blood pressure in hypotensive conditions has been documented both experimentally and clinically, but deserves further study. Currently, prospective, randomized, controlled, clinical studies are ongoing to more rigorously define the role of acupuncture in treating hypertension and other cardiovascular disorders.

OUTSTANDING ISSUES IN ACUPUNCTURE RESEARCH

Studies of acupuncture present a number of challenges. Although we understand a great deal about this treatment modality, much remains to be learned about the mechanism by which acupuncture influences autonomic outflow and, hence, the cardiovascular function. It is clear that the system is complex, involving a number of neurotransmitters/neuromodulators and regions of the brain and spinal cord, with many interactions likely and with different regions (e.g., pain vs. cardiovascular autonomic influences) playing a role depending on the underlying condition and the specific acupuncture input. Most acupuncturists perform an individualized form of therapy involving a combination of acupoints that can vary from practitioner to practitioner [1, 5]. Point specificity, or the ability of a specific acupoint or a combination of acupoints to cause a specific response, needs further study. Another area is the substantial concern by

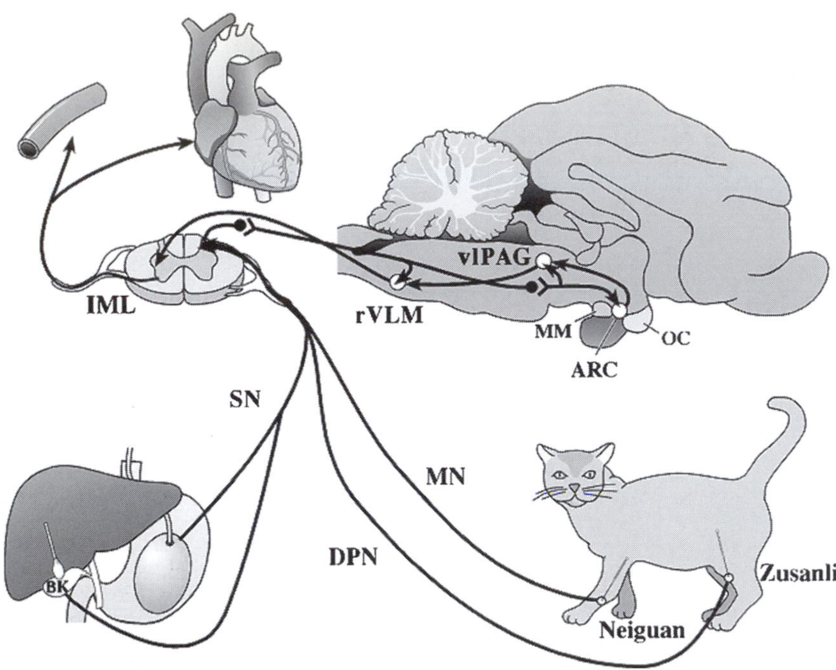

FIGURE 117.2 Diagram of neural pathways and regions in central nervous system through which electroacupuncture (EA) modifies sympathetic outflow and cardiovascular function. Because EA has the potential to attenuate sympathoexcitatory cardiovascular reflexes, this model illustrates such reflex input through the splanchnic nerve (SN) from gallbladder and stomach, which are stimulated by application of noxious chemicals like bradykinin (BK) or mechanical stimulation with a balloon. Superimposed on this reflex is 30 minutes of EA at acupoints *Neiguan* and *Zusanli* (pericardial or PE 6 and stomach or ST 36, located over the median [MN] and deep peroneal somatic nerves [DPN], respectively). Somatic and visceral afferents enter spinal cord through dorsal horn and ascend through polysynaptic connections to the brainstem and hypothalamus. Both somatic (EA) and visceral (reflex) input ascend to the midbrain ventral lateral periaqueductal gray (vlPAG) and rostral ventral lateral medulla (rVLM) as shown by *solid lines*. In addition, EA provides input to the arcuate nucleus (ARC) in the hypothalamus, an important site of production of opioid peptides. Opioid peptides, including both endorphins and enkephalins, acting through μ- and δ-opioid receptors in the rVLM, modify activity of premotor sympathoexcitatory neurons that project to the intermediolateral columns (IML) of the spinal cord, which contain sympathetic motor fibers that innervate the heart and blood vessels. Thus, EA acting through an opioid mechanism modulates sympathetic outflow during excitatory reflex stimulation. Such modulation has the potential capacity to limit demand-induced myocardial ischemia (as shown in Figure 117.1), arterial hypertension, and cardiac arrhythmias.

many scientists and practitioners that the acupuncture response may simply represent a placebo effect that is not much more than can be seen with sham intervention [11]. In fact, placebo responses occur in many as 30 to 40% of treated subjects and acupuncture leads to beneficial response in only 70 to 80% of cases, suggesting a narrow difference in response rate between the two treatments. Furthermore, the mechanism of placebo, like acupuncture, involves the endogenous opioid system [12]. A final issue that has to be addressed with acupuncture is the difficulty of blinding the subject and the acupuncturist [5, 11]. Experimental studies are not complicated by this latter problem because anesthesia is used. However, future clinical trials will need to consider each of these issues.

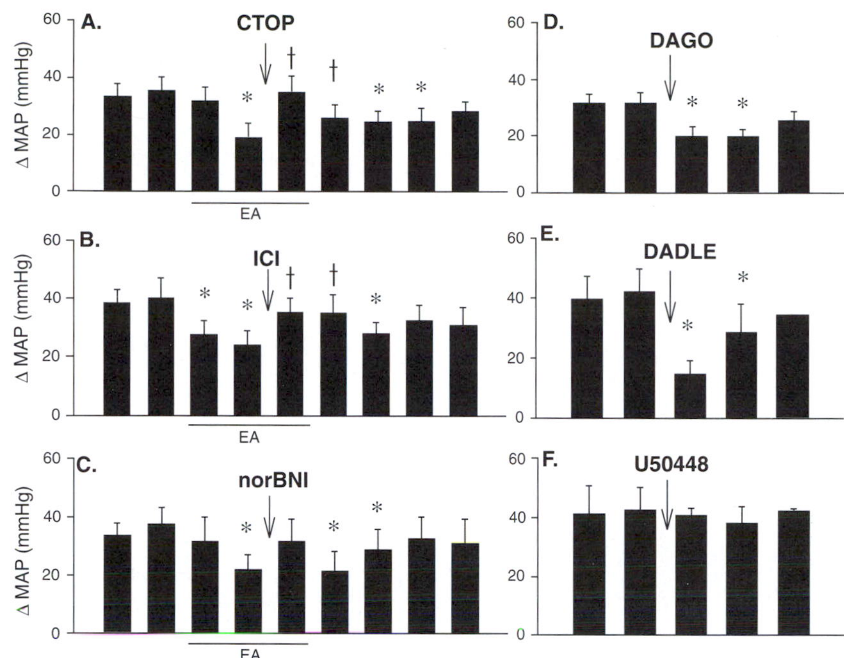

FIGURE 117.3 Reflex changes in mean arterial pressure (ΔMAP) during repeated stimulation of the gallbladder with bradykinin and modulation of the reflex by electroacupuncture (EA) at the *Neiguan* acupoint. Immediately after termination of 30 minutes of EA, either antagonists (**left**) or, as a surrogate to EA, agonists (**right**) of one of three opioid receptors were microinjected unilaterally into the rostral ventral lateral medulla (rVLM). There was reversal of EA-related inhibition of reflex responses by the μ- and δ-opioid receptor antagonists, CTOP (**B**) and ICI-174-864 (**A**), and transient reversal by the κ-opioid receptor antagonist, nor-BNI (**C**). Similarly, the μ- (**D**) and δ-opioid (**E**), but not the κ-opioid (**F**) receptor agonists (as a surrogate for EA), modulated the reflex response to gallbladder stimulation. Thus, endorphins (possibly endomorphin) and enkephalins, the ligands for the μ- and δ-opioid receptors, but not dynorphin, the ligand for κ-opioid receptors, are responsible in the rVLM for modulation of cardiovascular excitatory reflexes by EA. (Modified from Li, P., S. Tjen-A-Looi, and J. C. Longhurst. 2001. Rostral ventrolateral medullary opioid receptor subtypes in the inhibitory effect of electroacupuncture on reflex autonomic response in cats. *Auton. Neurosci.* 89:38–47, with permission.)

References

1. Longhurst, J. C. 1998. Acupuncture's beneficial effects on the cardiovascular system. *Prev. Cardiol.* 1:21–33.
2. Chao, D. M., L. L. Shen, S. Tjen-A-Looi, K. F. Pitsillides, P. Li, and J. C. Longhurst. 1999. Naloxone reverses inhibitory effect of electroacupuncture on sympathetic cardiovascular reflex responses. *Am. J. Physiol.* 276:H2127–H2134.
3. Cheung, L., P. Li, and C. Wong. 2001. *The mechanism of acupuncture therapy and clinical case studies*. London: Taylor & Francis.
4. Crisostomo, M., S. Tjen-A-Looi, and J. Longhurst. 2001. Nociceptin and classical opioids in the rostral ventral lateral medulla (rVLM) reduce electroacupuncture (EA) inhibition on gastric distention-induced pressor reflex in rats. 31st Annual Meeting of Neuroscience, 260.
5. Ernst, E., and A. White. 1999. *Acupuncture: A scientific appraisal.* Oxford, UK: Butterworth Heinemann.
6. Li, P., K. F. Pitsillides, S. V. Rendig, H.-L. Pan, and J. C. Longhurst. 1998. Reversal of reflex-induced myocardial ischemia by median nerve stimulation: A feline model of electroacupuncture. *Circulation* 97:1186–1194.
7. Dai, J. L., Y. H. Zhu, X. Y. Li, D. K. Huang, and S. F. Xu. 1992. C-fos expression during electroacupuncture analgesia in rats-an immunohistochemical study. *Acupunct. Electrother. Res.* 17:165–176.
8. Li, P., S. Tjen-A-Looi, and J. C. Longhurst. 2001. Rostral ventrolateral medullary opioid receptor subtypes in the inhibitory effect of electroacupuncture on reflex autonomic response in cats. *Auton. Neurosci.* 89:38–47.
9. Longhurst, J. 2001. The ancient art of acupuncture meets modern cardiology. *Cerebrum: The Dana Forum on Brain Science* 3:48–59.
10. Longhurst, J. C., M. P. Kaufman, G. A. Ordway, and T. I. Musch. 1984. Effects of bradykinin and capsaicin on endings of afferent fibers from abdominal visceral organs. *Am. J. Physiol.* 247:R552–R559.
11. Mayer, D. J. 2000. Acupuncture: An evidence-based review of the clinical literature. *Ann. Rev. Med.* 51:49–63.
12. Riet, G., A. Craen, A. Boer, and A. Kessels. 1998. Is placebo analgesia mediated by endogenous opioids? A systemic review. *Pain* 76: 273–275.
13. Tjen-A-Looi, S., P. Li, and J. C. Longhurst. 2003. Prolonged inhibition of rostral ventral lateral medullary premotor sympathetic neurons by electroacupuncture in cats. *Auton. Neurosci.* 106(2):119–131.

P A R T XIV

EXPERIMENTAL AUTONOMIC NEUROSCIENCE

118 Autonomic Disorders in Animals

Matthew J. Picklo, Sr.
Department of Pharmacology, Physiology and Therapeutics
University of North Dakota School of Medicine and Health Sciences
Grand Forks, North Dakota

Autonomic failure in animals is studied as a means to determine the role of the autonomic nervous system in physiologic regulation, the compensation as a result of denervation, and the therapeutic modalities for autonomic failure. Experimentally, lesioning of the sympathetic nervous system (sympathectomy) by numerous methods is well characterized. These methods are reviewed in this chapter. Less documented, but equally as important, are selective methods to create experimental sympathetic and parasympathetic autonomic failure in adult animals. Pathologic cases of autonomic failure in animals are noted in the veterinary literature and also are described in this chapter.

SYMPATHECTOMY

The term *sympathectomy* used in this discussion refers mainly to the lesioning of postganglionic noradrenergic (NA) neurons and fibers except where noted. Although norepinephrine depletion commonly is the desired effect, other costored neurotransmitters (e.g., ATP, NPY, and enkephalins) are depleted by sympathetic denervation. The multitude of research studying the effects of sympathetic loss is made possible by the morphologically defined anatomy of the postganglionic sympathetic chains, the sensitivity of postganglionic NA neurons to nerve growth factor (NGF) deprivation, and the phenotypic specialty of these neurons that allows for the selective uptake of neurotoxins. A number of relatively facile methods of inducing irreversible and reversible sympathectomy in a number of species ranging from nonhuman primates to mice have been described. However, all possess advantages and disadvantages related to the completeness of the lesion and age of susceptibility to the toxin. In addition, methods that selectively target the NA neurons would spare the non-NA sympathetic neurons such as those that innervate the sweat glands.

SURGICAL SYMPATHECTOMY

Historically, surgical removal of the sympathetic chains from cats by Arthur Cannon and co-workers was the first method described to affect sympathetic nervous system loss. This method, however, is tedious and impractical for small laboratory animals. Although immunologic and chemical methods to kill NA neurons have been developed, surgical ablation of non-NA sympathetic neurons and the adrenal medulla are the only methods to remove these sympathetic influences.

ANTI–NERVE GROWTH FACTOR IMMUNOSYMPATHECTOMY

Treatment of neonates using anti-NGF antisera induces sympathectomy in a number of species by deprivation of the necessary NGF signaling, resulting in apoptosis of the NA neuron. This treatment causes a 50% decrease in vascular NA innervation with sparing of the adrenal chromaffin cells. Immunosympathectomy can be performed antenatally by injection of the antiserum to the pregnant female. In this case, sensory and sympathetic neuron loss occurs. Similar results are observed in NGF knockout mice. The effects of anti-NGF on adult mice is not well characterized but is less severe than in neonates.

IMMUNE-MEDIATED SYMPATHECTOMY

Immune-mediated forms of sympathetic lesioning include treatment with anti-dopamine β-hydroxylase (anti-DBH) antibodies and with anti-acetylcholinesterase (AChE) antibodies. The anti-DBH treatment causes reversible, complement-mediated damage of the NA neuronal terminal in guinea pigs. Conversely, administration of anti-AChE to rats leads to reversible, immune-mediated damage to the preganglionic sympathetic terminals. This results in an alteration in plasma catecholamine levels and decreases in adrenal medullary catecholamines without damage to sensory neurons.

CHEMICAL SYMPATHECTOMY

6-Hydroxydopamine (6-OHDA), guanethidine, and *N*-(2-chloroethyl)-*N*-ethhyl-2-bromobenzylamine (DSP4) administration are three popular means of destroying NA neurons and fibers on the basis of the selective uptake of these chemicals by the presynaptic norepinephrine transporter. 6-OHDA, after uptake into the NA fiber, undergoes redox cycling leading to the formation of cytotoxic reactive oxygen species. 6-OHDA lesioning in neonates of multiple species causes irreversible loss of NA neurons, whereas in adult animals it causes reversible damage to the synaptic terminal. Adrenal catecholamines are not decreased by 6-OHDA.

Chronic guanethidine treatment, in contrast, causes irreversible, immune system–dependent destruction of NA neurons in adults and neonates. However, in adult animals, the treatment period entails daily injection of guanethidine for approximately 6 weeks to affect a complete lesion. Although guanethidine is transported into adrenal chromaffin cells, adrenal catecholamine levels are not altered. Interestingly, although guanethidine is used clinically without neuronal damage, a related congener, guanacline was sympathotoxic to humans causing irreversible orthostatic hypotension, reduced urinary catecholamine levels, and parotid gland innervation.

The mechanism of action of DSP4 is unclear. It is able to cross the blood–brain barrier and causes both peripheral and central toxicity after intraperitoneal administration. Recovery of peripheral catecholamine levels and histofluorescence suggest a reversibility of the lesion. DSP4 lesions serotonergic neurons through uptake by the serotonin reuptake transporter.

IMMUNOTOXIN SYMPATHECTOMY

A highly selective method of ablating peripheral NA neurons was formed by chemically linking a monoclonal antibody against DBH to the ribosome-inactivating protein, saporin. The selectivity of this immunotoxin, anti-DBH –saporin, is based on the binding and internalization of the anti-DBH antibody to the membrane-bound form of DBH, allowing entry of saporin, a potent cytotoxin, into the neuron. Administration of anti-DBH-saporin causes irreversible loss of NA neurons in adults and neonates within 3 days of a single injection without damage to the nodose or dorsal root ganglia. Although the immunotoxin accumulates in the outer layer of adrenal chromaffin cells, plasma epinephrine levels are not decreased.

Another immunotoxin, 192-saporin, was formed using saporin linked to a monoclonal antibody against the low affinity, p75 NGF receptor. This immunotoxin destroys peripheral, p75-expressing NA neurons and sensory neurons of the nodose and dorsal root ganglia. The physiologic consequences after peripheral administration of 192-saporin are not well characterized.

PATHOLOGIC AUTONOMIC FAILURE IN ANIMALS

Autonomic failure consisting of parasympathetic and sympathetic degeneration is documented in horses, dogs, and cats. In horses, *equine grass sickness* consists of symptoms and pathology demonstrating peripheral autonomic failure. A similar if not identical disease, the *Key–Gaskell syndrome*, is observed in dogs and cats. Histologic analyses of sympathetic and parasympathetic ganglia from affected dogs show a marked loss or chromatolysis of neurons with satellite cell infiltrate. The cause of this form of peripheral autonomic failure is unknown. An incidence of 1/10,000 dogs has been noted in the rural midwestern United States. These syndromes have high morbidity and current treatments are for symptomatic relief only.

References

1. Picklo, M. J. 1997. Methods of sympathetic degeneration and alteration. *J. Auton. Nerv. Syst.* 62:111–125.
2. Thoenen, H. 1972. Surgical, immunological and chemical sympathectomy. In *Catecholamines*, ed. H. Blaschko, and E. Muscholl, 814–844. Berlin: Springer-Verlag.
3. O'Brien, D. P., and G. C. Johnson. 2002. Dysautonomia and autonomic neuropathies. *Vet. Clin. North Am. Small Anim. Pract.* 32:251–265.

119 Transgenic Strategies in Autonomic Research

Kazuto Kobayashi
Department of Molecular Genetics
Institute of Biomedical Sciences
Fukushima Medical University
Fukushima, Japan

Toshiharu Nagatsu
Institute of Comprehensive Medical Science
Fujita Health University
Toyoake, Japan

TRANSGENIC ANIMAL MODEL

Activity of the autonomic nervous system including sympathetic and parasympathetic pathways is controlled under the brain and spinal cord functions. Development of several autonomic disorders is closely linked to degeneration of specific cell types in the central and peripheral nervous systems [1]. In particular, pure autonomic failure or idiopathic orthostatic hypotension is mainly characterized by lesion of the sympathetic nervous system [2]. For a clearer understanding of the etiology and pathogenesis of autonomic disorders, it is necessary to have animal models in which degeneration of the causative neuronal types can be induced. Immunotoxin-mediated cell targeting (IMCT) is a technique for conditional genetic ablation of specific cell types in transgenic mice [3, 4]. IMCT provides a useful approach for generating animal models for human neurodegenerative disorders. It also has been used to eliminate selective neuronal types from the complex neuronal network in the brain [5, 6]. In this chapter, we describe the strategy of IMCT and its use to generate a transgenic mouse model for autonomic neuropathy derived from disruption of the peripheral catecholaminergic cell types [7].

EXPERIMENTAL STRATEGY OF IMMUNOTOXIN-MEDIATED CELL TARGETING TECHNIQUE

IMCT is designed on the basis of the species-specific action of anti-Tac–based recombinant immunotoxin (IT), which selectively kills the cell type bearing human interleukin-2 receptor α-subunit (IL-2Rα) [8, 9]. The recombinant IT is composed of the variable heavy and light chains of the anti-Tac antibody, a monoclonal antibody against human IL-2Rα fused a truncated form of *Pseudomonas* exotoxin. It selectively recognizes human IL-2R, but does not cross-react with murine IL-2R. In the strategy of IMCT (Fig. 119.1), transgenic mice are generated that express human IL-2Rα under the control of a cell type-specific gene promoter. Subsequently, these animals are treated with an appropriate dose of IT, which is internalized by the cells bearing human IL-2Rα, resulting in elimination of these cells through inhibition of protein synthesis. Because human IL-2R does not respond to murine IL-2, the expression of transgene products causes no biological effects on the transgenic animals. In addition, the IT treatment is nontoxic to healthy animals because of the specificity of IT. Therefore, some phenotypic influences can be induced as a consequence of the selective cell loss in the transgenic mice treated with IT.

MODEL FOR AUTONOMIC NEUROPATHY

IMCT was used to generate an animal model that exhibits autonomic failure caused by ablation of the peripheral catecholaminergic cell types [7]. To express human IL-2Rα in these cell types, the dopamine β-hydroxylase gene promoter was used (Fig. 119.2A). In the transgenic mice, IL-2Rα was expressed in the adrenal medulla chromaffin cells and the sympathetic ganglion principal neurons (see Fig. 119.2B). Systemic treatment of adult mice with IT (1.5 μg/mouse intravenously) induced degeneration of the peripheral catecholaminergic cell types in the transgenic mice, and, in particular, the sympathetic nerve fibers terminating the peripheral tissues were markedly decreased (Fig. 119.3). The histopathologic examination indicated no apparent damages in many other cell types in the treated transgenic mice. However, blood congestion in vessels in various tissues and pulmonary edema were seen in the transgenic mice showing signs of cardiovascular deficits. The degeneration was accompanied by a reduction in noradrenaline and adrenaline levels in the peripheral tissues. The treated transgenic mice displayed progressive phenotypic abnormalities including cardiac dysfunction and hypothermia (Fig. 119.4). The cardiac dysfunction was mainly characterized by a marked reduction in heart rate and prolongation of the P-Q interval in electrocardiography. These abnormalities reflected deficits in autonomic regulation of heart function

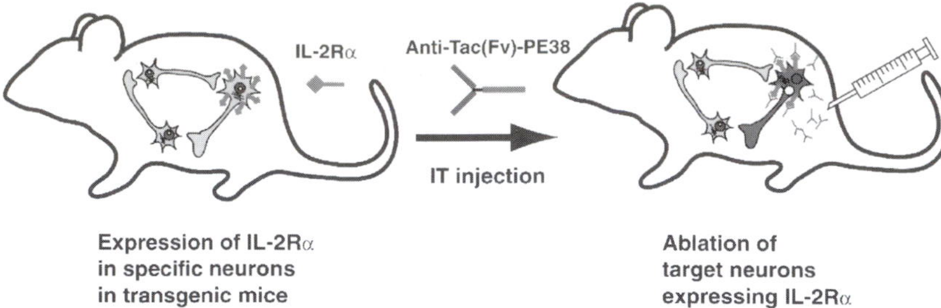

FIGURE 119.1 Strategy for immunotoxin-mediated cell targeting. Human interleukin-2 receptor α-subunit (IL-2Rα) is expressed in specific cell types in transgenic mice under the control of an appropriate tissue-specific gene promoter. Adult transgenic mice are treated with anti-Tac-based immunotoxin (IT), and the cells bearing the receptor are disrupted by the cytotoxic activity of the IT. (See Color Insert)

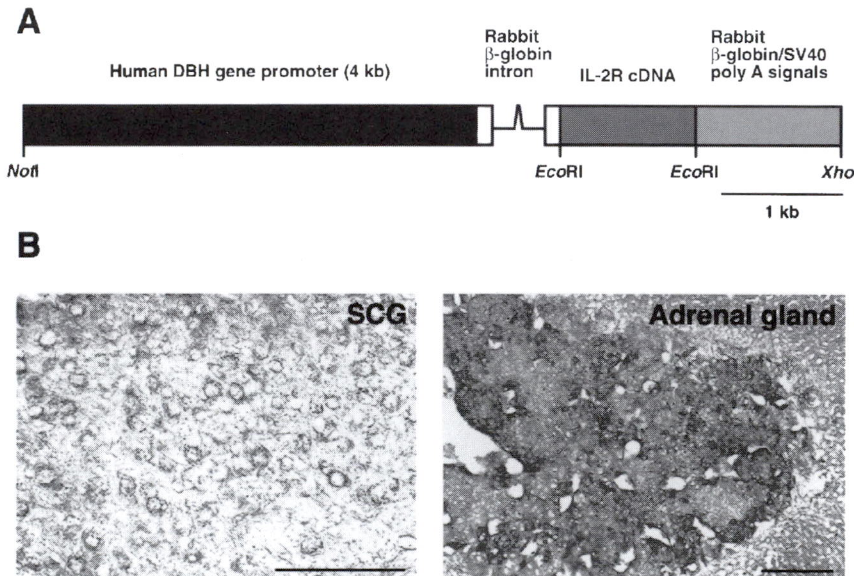

FIGURE 119.2 Generation of transgenic mice expressing interleukin-2 receptor α-subunit (IL-2Rα) in specific cell types. (**A**) Transgene containing the 4-kb promoter of the human dopamine β-hydroxylase (DBH) gene connected to the human IL-2Rα gene cassette. (**B**) Expression of human IL-2Rα in the superior cervical ganglion (SCG) and adrenal gland in the transgenic mice revealed by immunohistochemistry with anti-Tac antibody. Scale bar = 100 μm.

and cardiovascular system because of ablation of the peripheral catecholaminergic cell types.

FUTURE ASPECTS

IMCT provides a technique for conditionally ablating specific neuronal types involved in autonomic functions. It is possible to differentially target the central and peripheral nervous systems depending on the impermeability of IT across blood–brain barrier. The intracerebroventricular injection is applicable for targeting the cells in the central nervous system [3], whereas the intravenous injection is applicable for targeting the cells in the peripheral nervous system [7]. To optimize the human IL-2Rα expression in the transgenic mice, the knockin strategy with gene targeting is feasible that introduces the transgene cassette into the target gene locus of the interest. Furthermore, the knockin of the cassette located downstream of an internal ribosome entry site into the 3′-untranslated region of the target gene enables IL-2Rα expression in the restricted cell types, while preserving the intact target gene expression [10]. IMCT will be useful for elucidating the role of different neuronal types and their interactions in the development and in the symptoms of autonomic disorders.

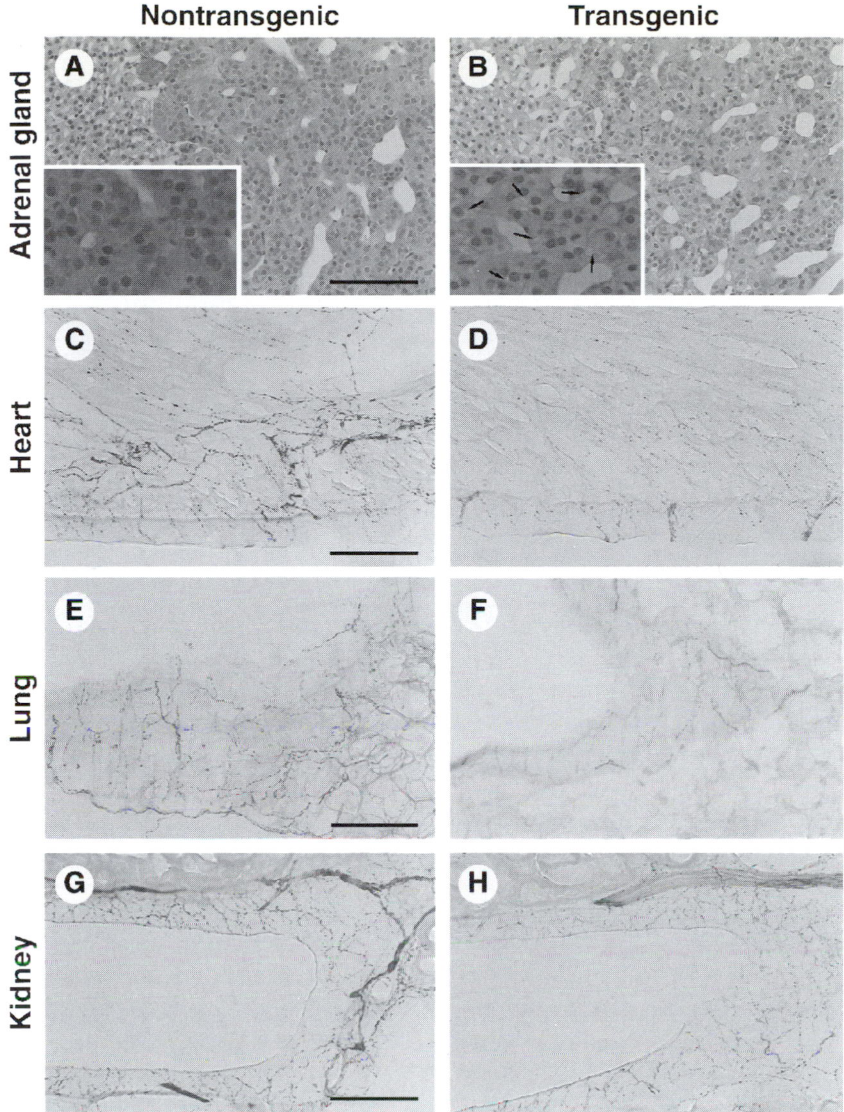

FIGURE 119.3 Ablation of the target cell types by immunotoxin (IT) injection. Histology of tissue sections prepared from the IT-injected mice 3 days after the injection. (**A** and **B**) Hematoxylin and eosin staining. The *insets* show four-fold magnifications. In the transgenic section, a decrease in staining intensity and vacuolation in the cytosol in the medullary cells are evident, indicating cell degeneration as a consequence of IT action. (**C–H**) Immunostaining with anti–tyrosine hydroxylase antibody. In the transgenic mice, degeneration and loss of the sympathetic nerve fibers innervating the heart, lung, and kidney are remarkable. Scale bar = 100 μm.

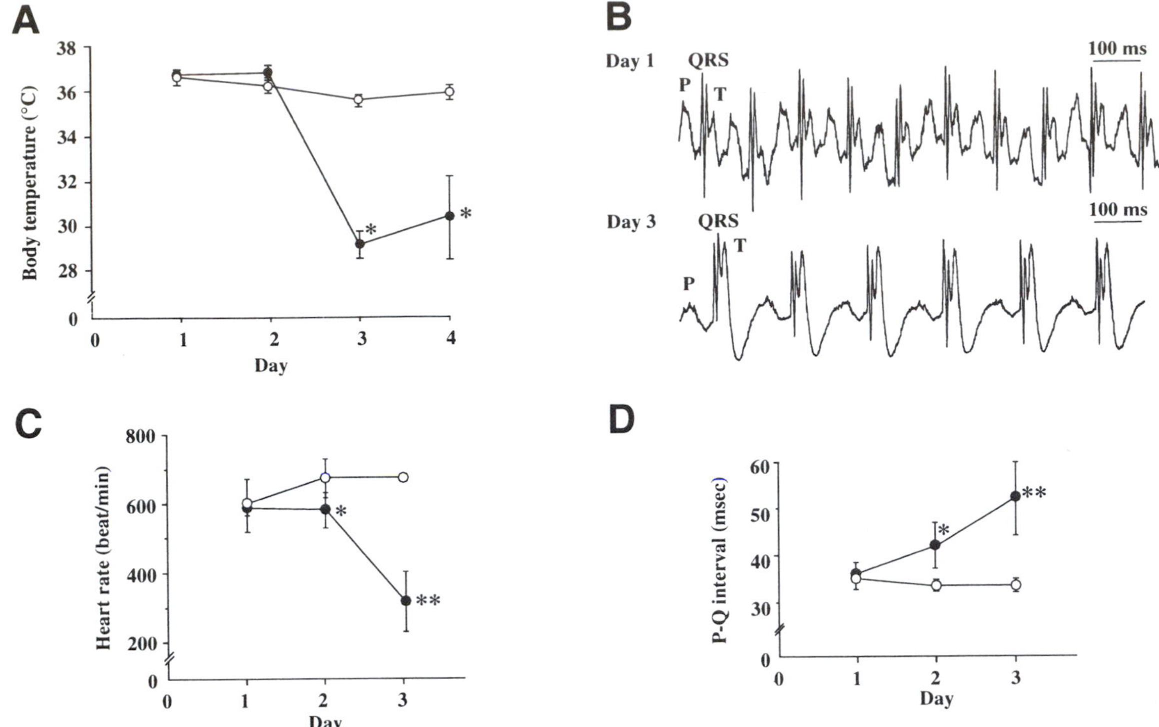

FIGURE 119.4 Autonomic phenotypes caused by ablation of the target cell types. Several physiologic parameters were monitored daily after immunotoxin injection. **A**, Body temperature. **B**, Typical electrocardiography patterns of the injected transgenic mice. **C**, Heart rate. **D**, P-Q interval. *Open circle*, nontransgenic mice (n = 4); *closed circle*, transgenic mice (n = 4). $^*P < 0.05$, $^{**}P < 0.01$, significantly different from nontransgenic mice according to Student's *t*-test.

References

1. Robertson, D., and I. Biaggioni. 1995. *Disorders of the autonomic nervous systems*. Luxembourg: Harvard Academic Publishers.
2. Robertson, D., C. Beck, T. Gary, and M. Picklo. 1993. Classification of autonomic disorders. *Int. Angiol.* 12:93–102.
3. Kobayashi, K., S. Morita, H. Sawada, T. Mizuguchi, K. Yamada, I. Nagatsu, K. Fujita, R. J. Kreitman, I. Pastan, and T. Nagatsu. 1995. Immunotoxin-mediated conditional disruption of specific neurons in transgenic mice. *Proc. Natl. Acad. Sci. USA* 92:1132–1136.
4. Kobayashi, K., I. Pastan, and T. Nagatsu. 1997. Controlled genetic ablation by immunotoxin-mediated cell targeting. In *Transgenic animals: Generation and use*, ed. L. M. Houdebine, 331–336. Amsterdam: Harwood Academic Publishers.
5. Watanabe, D., H. Inokawa, K. Hashimoto, N. Suzuki, M. Kano, R. Shigemoto, T. Hirano, K. Toyama, S. Kaneko, M. Yokoi, K. Moriyoshi, M. Suzuki, K. Kobayashi, T. Nagatsu, I. Pastan, and S. Nakanishi. 1998. Ablation of cerebellar Golgi cells disrupts synaptic integration involving GABA inhibition and NMDA receptor activation in motor coordination. *Cell* 95:17–27.
6. Kaneko, S., T. Hikida, D. Watanabe, H. Ichinose, T. Nagatsu, R. J. Kreitman, I. Pastan, and S. Nakanishi. 2000. Synaptic integration mediated by striatal cholinergic interneurons in basal ganglia function. *Science* 289:633–637.
7. Sawada, H., K. Nishii, T. Suzuki, K. Hasegawa, T. Hata, I. Nagatsu, R. J. Kreitman, I. Pastan, T. Nagatsu, and K. Kobayashi. 1998. Autonomic neuropathy in transgenic mice caused by immunotoxin targeting of the peripheral nervous system. *J. Neurosci. Res.* 51:162–173.
8. Chaudhary, V. K., C. Queen, R. P. Junghans, T. A. Waldmann, D. J. FitzGerald, and I. Pastan. 1989. A recombinant immunotoxin consisting of two antibody variable domains fused to *Pseudomonas* exotoxin. *Nature* 339:394–397.
9. Kreitman, R. J., P. Bailon, V. K. Chaudhary, D. J. P. FitzGerald, and I. Pastan. 1994. Recombinant immunotoxins containing anti-Tac(Fv) and derivatives of *Pseudomonas* exotoxin produce complete regression in mice of an interleukin-2 receptor-expressing human carcinoma. *Blood* 83:426–434.
10. Kobayashi, T., Y. Kida, T. Kaneko, I. Pastan, and K. Kobayashi. 2001. Efficient ablation by immunotoxin-mediated cell targeting of the cell types that express human interleukin-2 receptor depending on the internal ribosome entry site. *J. Gene Med.* 3:505–510.

120

Mouse Homologous Recombination Models

Nancy R. Keller
Autonomic Dysfunction Center
Vanderbilt University
Nashville, Tennessee

Disruption or overexpression of targeted mouse genes has been a boon to understanding the effect of individual genes in mammalian physiology. There has been an avalanche of reports describing historically well recognized genes, as well as a number of seemingly unrelated genes, that have a significant impact on autonomic nervous system (ANS) function. This review focuses primarily on knockout and transgenic mice with an autonomic phenotype characterized by altered blood pressure, cardiac function, sympathetic nerve activity, or catecholamine levels. Certain ancillary mouse models also have been included for their notable autonomic phenotypes, such as those with an exaggerated pressor response, hyperactivity, altered metabolism, or end organ dysfunction. Because of the sheer number of transgenic animals currently being studied, some will undoubtedly be underrepresented or left out. In particular, animals reported to have a behavioral phenotype, learning or memory deficit, altered nociception, motor difficulties, or an atypical pharmacologic response may, in fact, also reflect altered autonomic function. Without specific testing, however, prediction of a correlative autonomic phenotype is mere speculation; therefore, refer to the many excellent reviews for descriptions of these animal models [1–6].

A large number of publications are available that describe knockout and transgenic mouse models with autonomic phenotypes characterized by altered blood pressure, heart rate, or nerve activity measurements. Table 120.1 lists representative data compiled from reports of baseline heart rate and blood pressure measurements, weight, fertility, catecholamine levels and sympathetic tone, and phenotypic descriptions relevant to autonomic regulation of the heart and vasculature. Among those of particular interest are mouse models that may broaden our understanding of the pathophysiology of human autonomic disorders with discernible hemodynamic aberrations, such as multiple system atrophy (α_{1B}-adrenergic receptor (AR) overexpression) [7], pure autonomic failure (α_{1B} [$Ca_V2.2$] N-type voltage-dependent Ca^{2+} channel (VDCC) knockout) [8], dopamine β-hydroxylase (DBH) deficiency [9], the circadian variation of heart rate ($G_{s\alpha}$) [10], dopamine and norepinephrine uptake kinetics (monoamine oxidase type A [MAO-A] knockout) and dissection of central versus peripheral regulation of heart rate and blood pressure (MAO-A/B double knockout) [11], the role of nicotinic acetylcholine receptor (nAChR) subunits in neurotransmitter release and orthostatic tachycardia (α_3 and α_7 nAChR knockouts) [12], ANS-independent regulation of blood pressure (endothelial [eNOS] and neuronal nitric oxide synthase [nNOS] knockouts) [13, 14], the role of norepinephrine and dopamine in cardiovascular development (tyrosine hydroxylase [TH] knockout) [15], and sudden death (vesicular monoamine transporter 2 heterozygote) [16].

Regrettably, the number of transgenic mouse models tabulated in this report has been limited to conserve space. Among the excluded are genetic manipulations resulting in embryonic or neonatal death. However, despite the obvious limitations in assessment of an adult phenotype, many are nonetheless worthy of brief mention. For example, there is an estimated 70% and 90% embryonic mortality rate in mice homozygous for the deletion of the β_1-adrenoreceptor on a mixed strain background versus a fixed 129/Sv background, respectively [53]. Intuitively, one may assume that baseline heart rate would be decreased because β_1-AR signaling mediates cardiac sympathetic activity, yet adult survivors exhibit normal baseline heart rate and blood pressure, although they lack chronotropic and inotropic responses to β-AR agonists. Similar embryonic lethality occurs with deletion of the G protein–coupled receptor kinase, βARK1 [54], which encodes the cytosolic enzyme responsible for phosphorylation of β_1-AR and receptor desensitization. Phenotypic analysis has revealed that embryonic knockouts are smaller in size with an enlarged right atrium, myocardial thinning, and overall myocardial hypoplasia. Decreased cardiac ejection was visualized with intravital microscopy *in utero*, suggesting heart failure as a probable cause of death with underlying ventricular chamber dysfunction and an associated thin myocardium syndrome. Similar cardiac developmental defects are seen with genetic deletion of the transcription factors RXRα [55], N-*myc* [56], TEF-1 [57],

Text continued on p. 444

TABLE 120.1 Autonomic/Cardiovascular Phenotypes of Knockout (–) and Transgenic (OE) Mice

Gene or Gene Product	Exp	Fert	Wt	BP	HR	CAT Source	NE	Epi	DA	DOPAC	HVA	5HT	5HIAA	Phenotype	Model of Human Disease	References
α_{1A}-AR	–	↔	↔	↓										↓cardiac contractility; ↓pressor response to PE	cardiac development; contractile diversity of vascular beds	[17]
α_{1B}-AR	OE (+/–)	↓ (+/+)	↓	↓	↓									age-related neurodegeneration; ↓TH in substantia nigra; grand mal seizure; hindlimb dysfunction; cardiac hypertrophy; ↓total plasma catecholamines (NE + Epi)	multiple system atrophy (MSA); epilepsy; contractile dysfunction; cardiac hypertrophy	[17, 18]
α_{1D}-AR	–	↔	↔	↓	↔	CATs ↔								↓agonist-induced pressor response & contractility in aorta & mesenteric arterial bed; <↑BP after subtotal nephrectomy & salt diet	efficacy of α_{1D}-AR antagonists in salt-sensitive hypertension; contractile diversity of vascular beds; comparative role of α_{1A}-AR	[19]
α_{2A}-AR	–	↔	↔	↑	↑	P T/H	↑ ↓	↔						↑sympathetic tone; shortened onset of salt-sensitive hypertension	α_2-AR sympathoinhibition; hypertension	[20–22]
α_{2B}-AR	–	↔	↔	↔	↔	P	↔							↓Mendelian ratios (12% at weaning); ↓body fat	immediate hypertensive response to α2-AR agonists; hypertension; metabolism	[23, 24]
α_{1B} (Ca_v2.2) N-type VDCC	–	↔	↔	↑	↑	P	↔							↓sympathetic tone; <<↓BP with bilateral carotid artery occlusion; ↑aortic contractility with PE or thromboxane A_2; diabetes	PAF; N-type VDCC regulation of sympathetic neurotransmitter release; baroreflex; hypertension; diabetes	[8, 25]
α_{1D} (Cacna 1d) L-type VDCC	–	↔	↔		↓	P	↔							bradycardia; arrhythmias; myocardial ischemia; deafness; ↓Mendelian ratios (15%)	congenital deafness; SA node pacemaker activity; CHF	[26]
β_1-AR	OE[d]				↔									↓sympathetic tone; ↔BRS; ↓HRV; ↑exercise capacity	exercise tolerance	[27, 28]
β_2-AR	OE[f]			±[g]	↑									cardiac hypertrophy	pheochromocytoma	[29]
αCGRP	–		↔	↑	↑	U	↑[a]	↑[a]	↑[a]		↑			↑sympathetic tone; ↓vagal tone; ↓HRV	baroreflex-mediated tachycardia	[30]
COMT	–	↔	↔	↔		T/B U	↔ ↑		 ↑[a]	 ↔		↔	↔	↓HVA : DOPAC in brain; ↑DA in ♂ frontal cortex; baroreflex-mediated tachycardia; ↓natriuresis; ↑anxiety (♀); ↑♂ aggression (+/–)	Na^+ excretion; salt-sensitive hypertension; sex differences in catecholamine metabolism; anxiety syndromes & OCD; gene dosage effect	[31, 32]
D_2DAR	–	↔		↑	↑	U	↔	↑	↔					↑sympathetic tone; ↑weight (+/–)	endothelin B-mediated hypertension; Na^+ excretion	[33]

D_5DAR	–	↔	↔	↑[i]		T/A	↔	↔						↑sympathetic tone; ↑E/NE ratio; ↓BP > post α-AR blockade or adrenalectomy; ↓BP with oxytocin antagonist; cardiac hypertrophy	hypertension; role of oxytocin dependent sensitization of vasopressin & non-NMDA glutamatergic receptors in modulation of sympathetic outflow	[34]
DβH	–	↓[j] ♂	↔			T	ND	ND	↑	ND				↑embryonic death, fetal rescue with maternal DOPS; ↑NE in kidney & pancreas with DOPS; ptosis; hyperphagia; ↑metabolic rate; ↓UCP1 in brown fat	DβH deficiency; role of NE in development, metabolism & thermoregulation; peripheral amine precursor uptake & decarboxylation	[9]
ER-β	–	↔	↔	↑[i]	↔									↑aortic NO release (♀); ↑vasoconstriction; ↑anxiety (♀); progressive neuronal hypocellularity, including LC & NTS, ♂ > ♀; ↑astroglia	age-dependent hypertension; role of ER in NO release, CNS neuronal maintenance & lifespan; sex differences in neurodegeneration & anxiety	[35–38]
$G_{s\alpha}$	OE[f]			↑	↑									↓circadian HR variation; ↑respiratory rate; ↓LF, ↓HF, ↓LF:HF, ↓TP, ↓SDRR	role of Gs protein in β-AR signaling; circadian variation of HR; cardiomyopathy	[10]
KKA^y	OE		↑	↑	↔	U	↑	↑						↑sympathetic tone; hyperphagia; ↑insulin; ↑leptin; ↑urine output	role of leptin in mature-onset obsesity-related hypertension, diabetes, & melanocortin antagonism	[39]
Leptin	OE		↓	↑	↔	U	↑	↑						↑sympathetic tone; hypophagia; loss of AT; ↓insulin; ↑leptinemia; insulin hypersensitivity	role of leptin in sustained hypertension with caloric restriction; hypothalamic melanocortin system	[39]
MAO-A	–	↔[n]	↓	↓	↓	T/B	↑		↑	↓		↑	↓	↔MAO-B, ↔COMT; ↑BRS; atypical 5-HT uptake by DAT & NET in fetal & neonatal hypothalamus & brainstem (LC); altered thermoregulation; ↓motor function; behavioral changes	BRS; role of 5-HT & NE in development/maturation of somatosensory & locomotor neuronal networks; DAT & NET uptake kinetics; 5-HT metabolism via MAO-B; thermoregulation; behavior	[11, 40]
MAO-B	–	↔	↔	↓	↓	T/B	↔		↔	↔	↔	↔	↔	↑phenylethylamine (PEA); ↔MAO-A; ↔COMT; ↔behavior; absence of MPTP-induced neurodegeneration	PEA modulation of central sympathetic activity & peripheral VSM contraction; PEA inhibition of DA, NE, 5-HT uptake	[11]

(*continues*)

TABLE 120.1 *(continued)*

Gene or Gene Product	Exp	Fert	Wt	BP	HR	CAT Source	NE	Epi	DA	DOPAC	HVA	5HT	5HIAA	Phenotype	Model of Human Disease	References
MAO-A/B	M[o] /–	↔	↓	↓	↓[a]	T/B U	↑		↑			↑	ND ND	♂ test group; ↑PEA; ↑BRS; ↑vagal tone; ↔HRV; ↑VLF, ↑LF, ↑↑HF; hyperreactivity to handling	role of NE, 5-HT & PEA in central vs. peripheral HR/BP regulation; ANS function in Norrie's disease & pheochromocytoma	[11, 41, 42]
$M_{2,3}$ mAChR	—	↔	↓	↔										↓sympathetic tone; ↓BRS; ↔GI morphology; ↓salivation; ↑urinary retention (♂); ↑mydriasis	BRS; cholinergic regulation of GI motility & sex differences in urination; role of M_2 in pupil dilation	[43]
α_3 nAChR	–		↓											↑neonatal/postnatal death; ↑pupil dilation, ↓response to light; mydriasis/ptosis; bladder distention, ↓contractility	megacystis-microcolon-intestinal hypoperistalsis syndrome; idiopathic autonomic neuropathy, orthostatic tachycardia	[12, 44]
α7 nAChR	–		↔	↔	↔	T/H	↔							↓NE release; ↓baroreflex-mediated tachycardia; β-AR supersensitivity	baroreflex; syncope; hypertension; CHF; role of nACHRs in neurotransmitter release	[12, 45]
β2,4 nAChR	—		↓											↑neonatal death (>90%); ↑pupil dilation, ↓response to light; mydriasis/ptosis; bladder distention, ↓↓contractility; hypoperistalsis	multiorgan autonomic dysfunction; megacystis-microcolon-intestinal hypoperistalsis syndrome	[46]
NKCCI	–	↓ ♂	↓	↓	↔									↑weanling mortality; GI bleeding; ↓salivation; deaf; ↓astrocyte EAA release; ↓venous contractility	hypotension; efficacy of furosemide in venous return; impaired K^+ & Cl^- secretion	[47, 48]
eNOS (NOS3)	–	↔	↓	↑	↓									↑BP variability; ↔BRS; ↑LF; cardiac hypertrophy; ↑contractility; ↓kidney renin	ANS-independent regulation of BP; eNOS modulation of βAR signaling & L-type VDCC activation	[14, 49, 50]
nNOS (NOS1)	–	↔	↔	↔	↑									↓vagal tone; ↓HRV; cardiac hypertrophy; ↔BRS; ↓ΔHR & ↓HRV pressor response with G protein inactivation; ↓ACh release in small intestine	HRV; NO central vs. peripheral regulation of parasympathetic activity; nNOS modulation of βAR- & G protein–independent cardioinhibition	[13, 14, 51]

ob	–		↑	↔	↓	U	↔	↓[a]						leptin deficient; obese; >↑BP with leptin despite weight loss	role of leptin in sympathetic tone, hypertension & metabolism	[39]
TH	–	N/A	↓											↑embryonic death (≥97%), postnatal death by 4 wk; embryonic bradycardia	role of NE & DA in cardiovascular development	[15]
VMAT2	–		↓	↑	↔	T/B	↓		↓	↔	↑	↓	↑	neonatal death; hypoactive; hypothermia; ↓suckling;	impaired monoamine storage and release	[52]
VMAT2	+/–	↔	↔						↓	↑		↓	↓	↑QT interval; sudden death; psychostimulant sensitization	impaired monoamine storage and release; gene dose effect; sudden death	[16, 52]

↑ increased; ↓ decreased; ↔ no changes; 5-HT, 5-hydroxytryptamine (serotonin); 5-HIAA, 5-hydroxyindole acetic acid; A, adrenal; ANS, autonomic nervous system; B, brain; blank, not reported; BP, blood pressure; BRS, baroreflex sensitivity; CGRP, calcitonin gene–related peptide; CHF, congestive heart failure; CNS, central nervous system; COMT, catechol-*O*–methyl transferase; DA, dopamine; DBH, dopamine β-hydroxylase; DOPS, dihydroxyphenylserine; eNOS, endothelial nitric oxide synthase; Epi, epinephrine; GI, gastrointestinal; H, heart; HF, high frequency; HR, heart rate; HVA, homovanillic acid; K, kidney; KO, knockout; LF, low frequency; M, mutation; mAChR, muscarinic acetylcholine receptor; MAO-A, monoamine oxidase type A; MAO-B, monoamine oxidase type B; MSA, multiple system atrophy; N/A, not applicable; nAChR, nicotinic acetylcholine receptor; ND, below limit of detection; NE, norepinephrine; NET, norepinephrine transporter; NMDA, *N*-methyl-D-aspartate; nNOS, neuronal nitric oxide synthase; NO, nitric oxide; NTS, nucleus tractus solitarii; OE, overexpression/transgenic; P, plasma; PAF, pure autonomic failure; PEA, phenylethylamine; SA, sinoatrial; T, tissue; TH, tyrosine hydroxylase; U, urine; UE, underexpression; VMAT, vesicular monoamine transporter.

[a] Notable trend, not statistically significant.
[b] Outbred.
[c] Response to graded treadmill exercise.
[d] 8× atrial OE.
[e] Response to exercise or epinephrine.
[f] Cardiac expression.
[g] Gene dose-dependent BP increase or decrease.
[h] Peptide inhibitor of βARK1 × calsequestrin.
[i] Age dependent.
[j] Improved 55% with DOPS.
[k] Guanosine triphosphate cyclohydrolase I (e.g., TH) deficiency in *hph-l* mouse mutant.
[l] Liver-inducible, inactivated at 4 weeks.
[m] Greater in female individuals (♀).
[n] Altered reproductive behaviors.
[o] X-linked mutation of MAO-A in MAO-B (–/–) males.
[p] TH knockout with DβH targeted expression in noradrenergic neurons.

and WT-1 [58], suggesting a convergence in the developmental expression of these transcription factors and G protein–coupled receptor signaling during cardiogenesis [54].

Abnormal cardiac development also occurs in α_{1AB}-AR double knockout mice with a reduced adult heart size [17], whereas cardiac hypertrophy is a common finding in mice overexpressing α_{1B}-AR, and animals deficient in α_{2AC}-AR, β_2-AR, endothelial- or neuronal-derived NOS (eNOS, nNOS, and the e/nNOS double knockout), as well as the gene encoding the natriuretic peptide receptor A, *Npr1* [14, 24, 59, 60]. These and other seemingly tangential mouse models may also provide insight into autonomic compensatory mechanisms that develop in an attempt to maintain hemodynamic balance. Future interest in the characterization of autonomic phenotype is predicted for mice deficient in β_1-AR or $\beta_{1,2}$-AR (exercise tolerance) [61], the estrogen receptor α (ER-α; cardiac L-type Ca^{2+} channels and arrhythmia) [62], the G protein–activated inwardly rectifying potassium channel, GIRK4 (HRV postmyocardial infarction) [63], and the G protein–coupled receptor kinase, GRK3 (role of M_2 muscarinic AChR in cardioinhibition) [64]. Of similar appeal are genetic deletions that at first glance would not arouse expectations for a significant impact on the cardiovasculature, but may nevertheless reveal autonomic abnormalities, such as the adenosine A_{2a} receptor (hyperaggression, hypoalgesia) [65], the α_{2C}-AR (thermoregulation) [66], the β_3- and $\beta_{1,2,3}$-ARs (obesity, cold intolerance) [67, 68], the dopamine (hyperactivity, psychosis) and serotonin transporters (thermogenesis) [69, 70], the guanosine triphosphate cyclohydrolase I, GTP-CHI (TH deficiency, progressive dystonia) [71], and the M_2 and M_3 muscarinic AChRs (pupil dilation, sex differences in micturition) [72].

Other homologous recombinants are noteworthy for profound developmental abnormalities in the ANS. Mice lacking various constituents of the glial cell line–derived neurotrophic factor (GDNF) family of ligands were studied by Enomoto and colleagues [73], including the receptor tyrosine kinase RET, GDNF, GDNF/neurturin (NRTN), and the GDNF family receptor α2 (GFRα). These molecules are essential for the development of cranial parasympathetic ganglia; RET, in particular, is required for development of sphenopalatine, otic, and submandibular ganglia, whereas GDNF is crucial in RET/GFRα_1 signaling that stimulates proliferation and migration of ganglionic neuronal precursors. A maturational switch in neurotrophic signaling is presumed because before ganglionic formation, parasympathetic neuronal precursors are dependent on GDNF [74]. Later, however, NRTN assumes the role of neuronal trophic support in the neonate, and receptor expression shifts accordingly to reflect signaling through GFRα_2. Targeted disruption of upstream transcription factors that induce RET expression further highlights the complex interdependence of regulatory pathways affecting neural development before RET/GFRα_1 signaling. For example, expression of MASH1 precedes that of Phox2a, which, in turn, stimulates expression of RET. As might be expected, neuronal development is severely blunted in both MASH1- and Phox2a-deficient mice, and knockout animals die shortly after birth [75]. The central effects of this elaborate genetic cascade are revealed by the total absence of the locus ceruleus in both MASH1- and Phox2a-deficient mice. Precursor neurons of the peripheral ANS, in contrast, undergo incomplete differentiation in MASH1 knockout embryos and most sympathetic neurons, certain enteric neurons, and paracardiac parasympathetic ganglia undergo midgestational degeneration. The remaining parasympathetic ganglia, however, are apparently normal. This is in contrast to the phenotype of Phox2a-deficient mice in which parasympathetic ganglia are completely missing. Ganglion formation, therefore, is believed to require Phox2a activity in the presence of MASH1, yet these results raise the possibility that parasympathetic ganglion development in the absence of MASH1 does not require Phox2a. Differentiation of sympathetic ganglia, however, apparently requires MASH1-induced expression of Phox2a or an alternate factor (e.g., Phox2b), because the neuronal primordia of Phox2a knockouts express midgestational DβH, whereas the DβH gene remains silent in MASH1-deficient mice [75]. Together, these data suggest that alternative transcription factors may compensate for the absence of MASH1 or Phox2a, thereby allowing parasympathetic ganglion formation, whereas both factors are required for normal development of the noradrenergic phenotype.

In good conscience, a cautionary statement must be offered with regard to interpretation of results from this, or any, report of genetic manipulation or hemodynamic assessment in a mouse model. Although deletion or overexpression of an individual gene may truly reflect the effect of that single gene on a particular outcome, it is also quite possible that the underlying mechanisms of the observed phenotype are, in fact, multifactorial. Phenotypic evaluation of animal models designed to mimic human behavior and psychiatric disorders has demonstrated that genetic makeup alone does not dictate complex functional changes, and developmental adaptation, background strain, and environmental variables also must be considered when assigning phenotype [22, 76]. For example, adaptation may manifest itself as increased or decreased expression of related genes in compensation for the missing element, thus masking the true physiologic uniqueness of the targeted gene. Moreover, multiple genes are known to regulate blood pressure and cardiac function [77], and phenotypic evaluation can be dramatically distorted by factors such as age, sex, detection method, anesthesia, postoperative recovery period, restraint, isolation, environmental novelty or stress, background strain(s) used to generate the homologous recombinant, and the appropriate matching of control subjects [78–81]. Baseline catecholamine levels are equally dependent on many of the same variables, the most important being anesthesia, handling, restraint, and stress or fear [82]. In this review, therefore, hemodynamic values are preferentially reported from conscious, unrestrained animals with telemetric data preferred over intraarterial catheterization, which, in turn, is preferable to the tail-cuff method.

The true impact of targeted manipulation of the mouse genome and its usefulness as a portal into the mechanistic world of disease is yet to be fully realized, although results gathered thus far have undeniably expanded medical and scientific knowledge exponentially, with the future promising even greater returns. And, although objectionable to some, such murine sacrifice will not be in vain so long as we humans do not allow ourselves to forget that we are but mere mammalian counterparts; on a loftier perch perhaps, but atop branches of the same evolutionary tree. It is, therefore, more than a philosophic obligation as not-so-distant relatives to be thorough in extracting all possible information from a given animal model; this is a goal best achieved with an interdisciplinary approach and a commitment to continue search beyond the most obvious outcome. This strategy is particularly applicable to the unobtrusive and often overlooked ANS. The information provided here, therefore, is offered in anticipation that more presumably disparate genetic models of human disease will be recognized for their underlying autonomic phenotype.

References

1. Morimoto, S., and C. D. Sigmund. 2002. Angiotensin mutant mice: A focus on the brain renin-angiotensin system. *Neuropeptides* 36(2–3):194–200.
2. Kingery, W. S., G. S. Agashe, T. Z. Guo, S. Sawamura, M. F. Davies, J. D. Clark, B. K. Kobilka, and M. Maze. 2002. Isoflurane and nociception. *Anesthesiology* 96(2):367–374.
3. Gainetdinov, R. R., T. D. Sotnikova, and M. G. Caron. 2002. Monoamine transporter pharmacology and mutant mice. *Trends Pharm. Sci.* 23(8):367–373.
4. Kobayashi, K. 2001. Role of catecholamine signaling in brain and nervous system functions: New insights from mouse molecular genetic study. *J. Investig. Dermatol. Symp. Proc* 6:115–121.
5. Takahashi, N, and O. Smithies. 1999. Gene targeting approaches to analyzing hypertension. *J. Am. Soc. Nephrol.* 10:1598–1605.
6. Thompson, M. W., D. C. Merrill, G. Yang, J. E. Robillard, and C. D. Sigmund. 1995. Transgenic animals in the study of blood pressure regulation and hypertension. *Am. J. Physiol.* 269(5 Pt 1):E793–E803.
7. Zuscik, M. J., S. Sands, S. A. Ross, D. J. J. Waugh, R. J. Gaivin, D. Morilak, and D. M. Perez. 2000. Overexpression of the α_{1B}-adrenergic receptor causes apoptotic neurodegeneration: Multiple system atrophy. *Nat. Med.* 6:1388–1394.
8. Mori, Y., M. Nishida, S. Shimizu, M. Ishii, T. Yoshinaga, M. Ino, K. Sawada, and T. Niidome. 2002. Ca^{2+} channel α_{1B} subunit (Ca_V 2.2) knockout mouse reveals a predominant role of N-type channels in the sympathetic regulation of the circulatory system. *Trends Cardiovasc. Med.* 12(6):270–275.
9. Thomas, S. A., B. T. Marck, R. D. Palmiter, and A. M. Matsumoto. 1998. Restoration of norepinephrine and reversal of phenotypes in mice lacking dopamine β-hydroxylase. *J. Neurochem.* 70:2468–2476.
10. Uechi, M., K. Asai, M. Osaka, A. Smith, N. Sato, T. E. Wagner, Y. Ishikawa, H. Hayakawa, D. E. Vatner, R. P. Shannon, C. J. Homcy, and S. F. Vatner. 1998. Depressed heart rate variability and arterial baroreflex in conscious transgenic mice with overexpression of cardiac $G_{s\alpha}$. *Circ. Res.* 82:416–423.
11. Holschneider, D. P., K. Chen, I. Seif, and J. C. Shih. 2001. Biochemical, behavioral, physiologic, and neurodevelopmental changes in mice deficient in monoamine oxidase A or B. *Brain Res. Bull.* 56(6): 453–462.
12. Wang, N., A. Orr-Urtreger, and A. D. Korczyn. 2002. The role of neuronal nicotinic acetylcholine receptor subunits in autonomic ganglia: Lessons from knockout mice. *Prog. Neurobiol.* 68:341–360.
13. Jumrussirikul, P., J. Dinerman, T. M. Dawson, V. L. Dawson, U. Ekelund, D. Georgakopoulos, L. P. Schramm, H. Calkins, S. H. Snyder, J. M. Hare, and R. D. Berger. 1998. Interaction between neuronal nitric oxide synthase and inhibitory G protein activity in heart rate regulation in conscious mice. *J. Clin. Invest.* 102:1279–1285.
14. Barouch, L. A., R. W. Harrison, M. W. Skaf, G. O. Rosas, T. P. Cappola, Z. A. Kobeissi, I. A. Hobai, C. A. Lemmon, A. L. Burnett, B. O'Rourke, E. R. Rodriguez, P. L. Huang, J. A. C. Lima, D. E. Berkowitz, and J. M. Hare. 2002. Nitric oxide regulates the heart by spatial confinement of nitric oxide synthase isoforms. *Nature* 2002. 416: 337–339.
15. Zhou, Q., C. J. Qualife, and R. D. Palmiter. 1995. Targeted disruption of the tyrosine hydroxylase gene reveals that catecholamines are required for mouse fetal development. *Nature* 374:640–643.
16. Uhl, G. R., L. Su, N. Takahashi, K. Itokawa, Z. Lin, M. Hazama, and I. Sora. 2000. The VMAT2 gene in mice and humans: Amphetamine responses, locomotion, cardiac arrhythmias, aging, and vulnerability to dopaminergic toxins. *FASEB J.* 14:2459–2465.
17. Tanoue, A., T. Koshimizu, and G. Tsujimoto. 2002. Transgenic studies of α_1-adrenergic receptor subtype function. *Life Sci.* 71:2207–2215.
18. Zuscik, M. J., D. Chalothorn, D. Hellard, C. Deighan, A. McGee, C. J. Daly, D. J. J. Waugh, S. A. Ross, R. J. Gaivin, A. J. Morehead, J. D. Thomas, E. F. Plow, J. C. McGrath, M. T. Piascik, and D. M. Perez. 2001. Hypotension, autonomic failure, and cardiac hypertrophy in transgenic mice overexpressing the α_{1B}-adrenergic receptor. *J. Biol. Chem.* 276:13738–13743.
19. Tanoue, A., Y. Nasa, T. Koshimizu, H. Shinoura, S. Oshikawa, T. Kawai, S. Sunada, S. Takeo, and G. Tsujimoto. 2002. The α_{1D}-adrenergic receptor directly regulates arterial blood pressure via vasoconstriction. *J. Clin. Invest.* 109:765–775.
20. Altman, J. D., A. U. Trendelenburg, L. MacMillan, D. Bernstein, L. Limbird, K. Starke, B. K. Kobilka, and L. Hein. 1999. Abnormal regulation of the sympathetic nervous system in α_{2A}-adrenergic receptor knockout mice. *Mol. Pharmacol.* 56:154–161.
21. Makaritsis, K. P., C. Johns, I. Gavras, J. D. Altman, D. E. Handy, M. R. Bresnahan, and H. Gavras. 1999. Sympathoinhibitory function of the α_{2A}-adrenergic receptor subtype. *Hypertension* 34:403–407.
22. Kable, J. W., L. C. Murrin, and D. B. Bylund. 2000. *In vivo* gene modification elucidates subtype-specific functions of α_2-adrenergic receptors. *J. Pharm. Exp. Ther.* 293(1):1–7.
23. Link, R. E., K. Desai, L. Hein, M. E. Stevens, A. Chruscinski, D. Bernstein, G. S. Barsch, and B. K. Kobilka. 1996. Cardiovascular regulation in mice lacking α_2-adrenergic receptor subtypes b and c. *Science* 273:803–805.
24. Hein, L., J. D. Altman, and B. K. Kobilka. 1999. Two functionally distinct α_2-adrenergic receptors regulate sympathetic neurotransmission. *Nature* 402:181–184.
25. Ino, M., T. Yoshinaga, M. Wakamori, N. Miyamoto, J. Sonoda, T. Kagaya, T. Oki, T. Nagasu, Y. Nishizawa, I. Tanaka, K. Imoto, S. Aizawa, S. Koch, A. Schwartz, T. Niidome, K. Sawada, and Y. Mori. 2001. Functional disorders of the sympathetic nervous system in mice

lacking the α_{1B} subunit (CaV 2.2) of N-type calcium channels. *Proc. Natl. Acad. Sci. USA* 98(9):5323–5328.

26. Platzer, J., J. Engel, A. Schrott-Fischer, K. Stephan, S. Bova, H. Chen, H. Zheng, and J. Striessnig. 2000. Congenital deafness and sinoatrial node dysfunction in mice lacking Class D L-type Ca^{2+} channels. *Cell* 102:89–97.
27. Mansier, P., C. Medigue, N. Charlotte, C. Vermeiren, E. Coraboeuf, E. Deroubal, F. Carre, T. Dahkli, B. Bertin, P. Briand, D. Strosberg, and B. Swynghedauw. 1996. Decreased heart rate variability in transgenic mice overexpressing atrial β_1-adrenoceptors. *Am. J. Physiol.* 271(4 Pt 2):H1465–H1472.
28. Rohrer, D. K., E. H. Schauble, K. H. Desai, B. K. Kobilka, and D. Bernstein. 1998. Alterations in dynamic heart rate control in the β_1-adrenergic receptor knockout mouse. *Am. J. Physiol.* 274(4 Pt 2): H1184–H1193.
29. Liggett, S. B., N. M. Tepe, J. N. Lorenz, A. M. Canning, T. D. Jantz, S. Mitarai, A. Yatani, and G. W. Dorn. 2000. Early and delayed consequences of β_2-adrenergic receptor overexpression in mouse hearts. *Circulation* 101:1707–1714.
30. Oh-hashi, Y., T. Shindo, Y. Kurihara, T. Imai, Y.-M. Wang, H. Morita, Y. Imai, Y. Kayaba, H. Nishimatsu, Y. Suematsu, Y. Hirata, Y. Yazaki, R. Nagai, T. Kuwaki, and H. Kurihara. 2001. Elevated sympathetic nervous activity in mice deficient in αCGRP. *Circ. Res.* 89: 983–990.
31. Gogos, J. A., M. Morgan, V. Luines, M. Santha, S. Ogawa, D. W. Pfaff, and M. Karayiorgou. 1998. Catechol-*O*-methyltransferase-deficient mice exhibit sexually dimorphic changes in catecholamine levels and behavior. *Proc. Natl. Acad. Sci. USA* 95:9991–9996.
32. Odlind, C., I. I. Reenila, P. T. Mannisto, R. Juvonen, S. Uhlen, J. A. Gogos, M. Karayiorgou, and P. Hansell. 2002. Reduced natriuretic response to acute sodium loading in COMT gene deleted mice. *BMC Physiol.* 2(1):14.
33. Li, X. X., M. Bek, L. D. Asico, Z. Yang, D. K. Grandy, D. S. Goldstein, M. Rubinstein, G. M. Eisner, and P. A. Jose. 2001. Adrenergic and endothelin B receptor-dependent hypertension in dopamine receptor type-2 knockout mice. *Hypertension* 38:303–308.
34. Hollon, T. R., M. J. Bek, J. E. Lachowicz, M. A. Ariano, E. Mezey, R. Ramachandran, S. R. Wersinger, P. Soares-da-Silva, Z. F. Liu, A. Grinberg, J. Drago, W. S. I. Young, H. Westphal, P. E. Jose, and D. R. Sibley. 2002. Mice lacking D_5 dopamine receptors have increased sympathetic tone and are hypertensive. *J. Neurosci.* 22(24):10801–10810.
35. Krezel, W., S. Dupont, A. Krust, P. Chambon, and P. F. Chapman. 2001. Increased anxiety and synaptic plasticity in estrogen receptor β-deficient mice. *Proc. Natl. Acad. Sci. USA* 98:12278–12282.
36. Wang, L., S. Andersson, M. Warner, and J. A. Gustafsson. 2001. Morphological abnormalities in the brains of estrogen receptor-β knockout mice. *Proc. Natl. Acad. Sci. USA* 98(5):2792–2796.
37. Darblade, B., C. Pendaries, A. Krust, S. Dupont, M. J. Fouque, J. Rami, P. Chambon, F. Bayard, and J. F. Arnal. 2002. Estradiol alters nitric oxide production in the mouse aorta through the α-, but not β-, estrogen receptor. *Circ. Res.* 90:413–419.
38. Zhu, Y., B. Zhao, P. Lu, R. H. Karas, L. Bao, D. Cox, J. Hodgin, P. W. Shaul, P. Thoren, O. Smithies, J. A. Gustafsson, and M. E. Mendelsohn. 2002. Abnormal vascular function and hypertension in mice deficient in estrogen receptor β. *Science* 295(5554):505–508.
39. Aizawa-Abe, M., Y. Ogawa, H. Masuzaki, K. Ebihara, N. Satoh, H. Iwai, N. Matsuoka, T. Hayashi, K. Hosoda, G. Inoue, Y. Yoshimasa, and K. Nakao. 2000. Pathophysiological role of leptin in obesity-related hypertension. *J. Clin. Invest.* 105(9):1243–1252.
40. Cases, O., C. Lebrand, B. Giros, T. Vitalis, E. De Maeyer, M. G. Caron, D. J. Price, P. Gaspar, and I. Seif. 1998. Plasma membrane transporters of serotonin, dopamine, and norepinephrine mediate serotonin accumulation in atypical locations in the developing brain of monoamine oxidase A knock-outs. *J. Neurosci.* 18:6914–6927.
41. Holschneider, D. P., O. U. Scremin, D. R. Chialvo, K. Chen, and J. C. Shih. 2002. Heart rate dynamics in monoamine oxidase-A and -B deficient mice. *Am. J. Physiol. Heart Circ. Physiol.* 282(5):H1751–H1759.
42. Holschneider, D. P., O. U. Scremin, K. P. Roos, D. R. Chialvo, K. Chen, and J. C. Shih. 2002. Increased baroreceptor response in mice deficient in monoamine oxidase A and B. *Am. J. Physiol. Heart Circ. Physiol.* 28223(3):H964–H972.
43. Matsui, M., D. Motomura, T. Fujikawa, J. Jiang, S. Takahashi, T. Manabe, and M. M. Taketo. 2002. Mice lacking M_2 and M_3 muscarinic acetylcholine receptors are devoid of cholinergic smooth muscle contractions but still viable. *J. Neurosci.* 22:10627–10632.
44. Xu, W., S. Gelber, A. Orr-Urtreger, D. Armstrong, R. A. Lewis, C. N. Ou, J. W. Patrick, L. W. Role, M. DeBiasi, and A. L. Beaudet. 1999. Megacystis, mydriasis, and ion channel defect in mice lacking the α3 neuronal nicotinic acetylcholine receptor. *Proc. Natl. Acad. Sci. USA* 96:5746–5751.
45. Franceschini, D., A. Orr-Urtreger, W. Yu, L. Y. Mackey, R. A. Bond, D. Armstrong, J. W. Patrick, A. L. Beaudet, and M. De Biasi. 2000. Altered baroreflex responses in α7 deficient mice. *Behav. Brain Res.* 113:3–10.
46. Xu, W., A. Orr-Urtreger, F. Nigro, S. Gelber, C. B. Sutcliffe, D. Armstrong, J. W. Patrick, L. W. Role, A. L. Beaudet, and M. DeBiasi. 1999. Multiorgan autonomic dysfunction in mice lacking the β2 and the β4 subunits of neuronal nicotinic acetylcholine receptors. *J. Neurosci.* 19:9298–9305.
47. Meyer, J. W., M. Flagella, R. L. Sutliff, J. N. Lorenz, M. L. Nieman, C. S. Weber, R. J. Paul, and G. E. Shull. 2002. Decreased blood pressure and vascular smooth muscle tone in mice lacking basolateral Na^+-K^+-2Cl cotransporter. *Am. J. Physiol. Heart Circ. Physiol.* 283: H1846–H1855.
48. Su, G., D. B. Kintner, M. Flagella, G. E. Shull, and D. Sun. 2002. Astrocytes from Na^+-K^+-2Cl cotransporter-null mice exhibit an absence of swelling and decrease in EAA release. *Am. J. Physiol. Heart Circ. Physiol.* 282:C1147–C1160.
49. Shesely, E. G., N. Maeda, H. S. Kim, K. M. Desai, J. H. Krege, V. E. Laubach, P. A. Sherman, W. C. Sessa, and O. Smithies. 1996. Elevated blood pressures in mice lacking endothelial nitric oxide synthase. *Proc. Natl. Acad. Sci. USA* 93:13176–13181.
50. Stauss, H. M., B. Nafz, and P. B. Persson. 2000. Blood pressure control in eNOS knockout-mice: Comparison with other species under NO blockade. *Acta. Physiol. Scand.* 168:155–160.
51. Mang, C. F., S. Truempler, D. Erbelding, and H. Kilbinger. 2002. Modulation by NO of acetylcholine release in the ilium of wild-type and NOS gene knockout mice. *Am. J. Physiol. Gastrointest. Liver Physiol.* 283:G1132–G1138.
52. Wang, Y.-M., R. R. Gainetdinov, F. Fumagalli, F. Xu, S. R. Jones, C. B. Bock, G. W. Miller, R. M. Wightman, and M. G. Caron. 1997. Knockout of the vesicular monoamine transporter 2 gene results in neonatal death and supersensitivity to cocaine and amphetamine. *Neuron* 19:1285–1296.
53. Rohrer, D. K., K. H. Desai, J. R. Jasper, M. E. Stevens, D. P. Regula Jr., G. S. Barsh, D. Bernstein, and B. K. Kobilka. 1996. Targeted disruption of the mouse β1-adrenergic receptor gene: Developmental and cardiovascular effects. *Proc. Natl. Acad. Sci. USA* 93:7375–7380.
54. Jaber, M., W. J. Koch, H. A. Rockman, B. Smith, R. A. Bond, K. K. Sulik, J. J. Ross, R. J. Lefkowitz, M. G. Caron, and B. Giros. 1996. Essential role of β-adrenergic receptor kinase 1 in cardiac development and function. *Proc. Natl. Acad. Sci. USA* 93:12974–12979.
55. Kastner, P., J. M. Grondona, M. Mark, A. Gansmuller, M. LeMeur, D. Decimo, J.-L. Vonesch, P. Dolle, and P. Chambon. 1994. Genetic analysis of RXRα developmental function: Convergence of RXR and RAR signaling pathways in heart and eye morphogenesis. *Cell* 78:987–1003.
56. Charron, J., B. A. Malynn, P. Fisher, V. Stewart, L. Jeanotte, S. P. Goff, E. J. Robertson, and F. W. Alt. 1992. Embryonic lethality in mice

homozygous for a targeted disruption of the N-myc gene. *Genes Dev.* 6:2248–2257.

57. Moens, C. B., B. R. Stanton, L. F. Parada, and J. Rossant. 1993. Defects in heart and lung development in compound heterozygotes for two different targeted mutations at the N-myc locus. *Development* 119:485–499.
58. Kreidberg, J. A., H. Sariola, J. M. Loring, M. Maeda, J. Pelletier, D. Housman, and R. Jaenisch. 1993. WT-1 is required for early kidney development. *Cell* 74:679–691.
59. Chruscinski, A. J., D. K. Rohrer, E. H. Schauble, K. H. Desai, D. Bernstein, and B. K. Kobilka. 1999. Targeted disruption of the β2 adrenergic receptor gene. *J. Biol. Chem.* 274:16695–16700.
60. Oliver, P. M., J. E. Fox, R. Kim, H. A. Rockman, H. S. Kim, R. L. Reddick, K. N. Pandey, S. L. Milgram, O. Smithies, and N. Maeda. 1997. Hypertension, cardiac hypertrophy, and sudden death in mice lacking natriuretic peptide receptor A. *Proc. Natl. Acad. Sci. USA* 94:14730–14735.
61. Rohrer, D. K., A. Chruscinski, E. H. Schauble, D. Bernstein, and B. K. Kobilka. 1999. Cardiovascular and metabolic alterations in mice lacking both β1- and β2-adrenergic receptors. *J. Biol. Chem.* 274: 16701–16708.
62. Johnson, B. D., W. Zheng, K. S. Korach, T. Scheuer, W. A. Catterall, and G. M. Rubanyi. 1997. Increased expression of the cardiac L-type calcium channel in estrogen receptor-deficient mice. *J. Gen. Physiol.* 110:135–140.
63. Wickman, K., J. Nemec, S. Gendler, and D. E. Clapham. 1998. Abnormal heart rate regulation of GIRK4 knockout mice. *Neuron* 20(1):103–114.
64. Walker, J. K. L., K. Peppel, R. J. Lefkowitz, M. G. Caron, and J. T. Fisher. 1999. Altered airway and cardiac responses in mice lacking G protein-coupled receptor kinase 3. *Am. J. Physiol. Regulatory Integrative Comp. Physiol.* 45:R1214–R1221.
65. Ledent, C., J. M. Vaugeois, S. N. Schiffmann, T. Pedrazzini, M. El Yacoubi, J. J. Vanderhaeghen, J. Costentin, J. K. Heath, G. Vassart, and M. Parmentier. 1997. Aggressiveness, hypoalgesia and high blood pressure in mice lacking the adenosine A_{2a} receptor. *Nature* 388:674–678.
66. Sallinen, J., R. E. Link, A. Haapalinna, T. Viitamaa, M. Kulatunga, B. Sjoholm, E. MacDonald, M. Pelto-Huikko, T. Leino, G. S. Barsh, B. K. Kobilka, and M. Scheinin. 1997. Genetic alteration of α_{2C}-adrenoceptor expression in mice: Influence on locomotor, hypothermic, and neurochemical effects of dexmedetomidine, a subtype-nonselective α_2-adrenoceptor agonist. *Mol. Pharm.* 51:36–46.
67. Susulic, W. S., R. C. Frederich, J. Lawitts, E. Tozzo, B. B. Kahn, M.-E. Harper, J. Himms-Hagen, J. S. Flier, and B. B. Lowell. 1995. Targeted disruption of the β_3-adrenergic receptor gene. *J. Biol. Chem.* 270:29483–29492.
68. Bachman, E. S., H. Dhillon, C. Y. Zhang, S. Cinti, A. C. Bianco, B. K. Kobilka, and B. B. Lowell. 2002. βAR signaling required for diet-induced thermogenesis and obesity resistance. *Science* 297:843–845.
69. Bosse, R., F. Fumagalli, M. Jaber, B. Giros, R. R. Gainetdinov, W. C. Wetsel, C. Missale, and M. G. Caron. 1997. Anterior pituitary hypoplasia and dwarfism in mice lacking the dopamine transporter. *Neuron* 19:127–138.
70. Sora, I., F. S. Hall, A. M. Andrews, M. Itokawa, X. F. Li, H. B. Wei, C. Wichems, K. P. Lesch, D. L. Murphy, and G. R. Uhl. 2001. Molecular mechanisms of cocaine reward: Combined dopamine and serotonin transporter knockouts eliminate cocaine place preference. *Proc. Natl. Acad. Sci. USA* 98:5300–5305.
71. Maeda, T., S. Haeno, K. Oda, M. Daisuke, H. Ichinose, N. Toshiharu, and T. Suzuki. 2000. Studies on the genotype-phenotype relation in the hph-1 mouse mutant deficient in guanosine triphosphate (GTP) cyclohydrolase I activity. *Brain Dev.* 22:S50–S53.
72. Matsui, M., D. Motomura, H. Karasawa, T. Fujikawa, J. Jiang, Y. Komiya, S. Takahashi, and M. M. Taketo. 2000. Multiple functional defects in peripheral autonomic organs in mice lacking muscarinic acetylcholine receptor gene for the M_3 subtype. *Proc. Natl. Acad. Sci. USA* 97:9579–9584.
73. Enomoto, H., R. O. Heuckeroth, J. P. Golden, E. M. Johnson, Jr., and J. Milbrandt. 2000. Development of cranial parasympathetic ganglia requires sequential actions of GDNF and neurturin. *Development* 127:4877–4889.
74. Rossi, J., K. Luukko, D. Poteryaev, A. Laurikainen, Y. F. Sun, T. Laakso, S. Eerikainen, R. Tuominen, M. Lakso, H. Rauvala, U. Arumae, M. Pasternack, M. Saarma, and M. S. Airaksinen. 1999. Retarded growth and deficits in the enteric and parasympathetic nervous system in mice lacking GFRα2, a functional neurturin receptor. *Neuron* 22:243–252.
75. Hirsch, M.-R., M. C. Tiveron, F. Guillemot, J. F. Brunet, and C. Goridis. 1998. Control of noradrenergic differentiation and Phox2a expression by MASH1 in the central and peripheral nervous system. *Development* 125:599–608.
76. Murphy, D. L., C. Wichems, Q. Li, and A. Heils. 1999. Molecular manipulations as tools for enhancing our understanding of 5-HT neurotransmission. *Trends Pharmacol. Sci.* 20:246–252.
77. Smithies, O. 1997. A mouse view of hypertension. *Hypertension* 30:1318–1324.
78. Doevendans, P. A., M. J. Daemen, E. D. de Muinck, and J. F. Smits. 1998. Cardiovascular phenotyping in mice. *Cardiol. Res.* 39:34–49.
79. Homanics, G. E., J. J. Quinlan, and L. L. Firestone. 1999. Pharmacologic and behavioral responses of inbred C57BL/6J and strain 129/SvJ mouse lines. *Pharmacol. Biochem. Behav.* 63(1):21–26.
80. Kass, D. A., J. M. Hare, and D. Georgakopoulos. 1998. Murine cardiac function: A cautionary tail. *Circ. Res.* 82:519–522.
81. Mattson, D. L. 2001. Comparison of arterial blood pressure in different strains of mice. *Am. J. Hypertens.* 14:405–408.
82. Harikai, N., T. Fujii, S. Onodera, and S. Tashiro. 2002. Increases in plasma dihydroxyphenylacetic acid levels in decapitated mice after exposure to various stresses. *Biol. Pharm. Bull.* 25:823–826.

Index

A

B

O

P

Q

R

T

U

V

W

Y